Manual of Sports Medicine

Manual of Sports Medicine

Edited by

Marc R. Safran, M.D.
Co-Director, Sports Medicine
Department of Orthopedic Surgery
Kaiser Permanente, Orange County
Anaheim Hills, California
Assistant Clinical Professor, Orthopedic Surgery
University of California, Irvine and
University of California, San Diego
Assistant Team Physician
University of California, Irvine
Irvine, California

Douglas B. McKeag, M.D., M.S.
Past President, American Medical Society for Sports Medicine
Arthur J. Rooney Sr. Professor and Vice Chairman
Departments of Family Medicine/Clinical Epidemiology and Orthopaedic Surgery
University of Pittsburgh School of Medicine
Pittsburgh, Pennsylvania

Steven P. Van Camp, M.D.
Past President, American College of Sports Medicine
Assistant Clinical Professor
Department of Pathology
University of California-San Diego School of Medicine
Alvarado Medical Group
San Diego, California

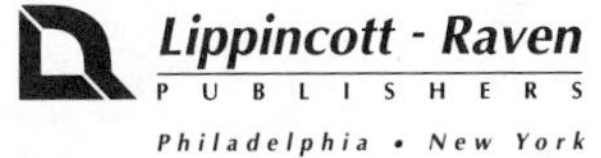

Acquisitions Editor: Danette Knopp
Developmental Editor: Juleann Dob
Manufacturing Manager: Kevin Watt
Production Manager: Robert Pancotti
Production Editor: Jeff Somers
Indexer: Robert Elwood
Compositor: Circle Graphics
Printer: RR Donnelley

Printed in the United States of America

9 8 7 6 5 4 3 2 1

Library of Congress Cataloging-in-Publication Data

Manual of sports medicine / edited by Marc R. Safran, Douglas B. McKeag, Steven P. Van Camp
p. cm.
Includes bibliographical references and index.
ISBN 0-7817-1222-X (alk. paper).
1. Sports medicine—Handbooks, manuals, etc. I. Safran, Marc R. II. McKeag, Douglas, 1945– . III. Van Camp, Steven P.
[DNLM: 1. Athletic Injuries. 2. Sports Medicine. QT 261 S759 1998]
RC1211.S65 1998
617.1′027—DC21
DNLM/DLC
for Library of Congress

Care has been taken to confirm the accuracy of the information presented and to describe generally accepted practices. However, the editors, authors and publisher are not responsible for errors or omissions or for any consequences from application of the information in this book and make no warranty, express or implied, with respect to the contents of the publication.

The editors, authors and publisher have exerted every effort to ensure that drug selection and dosage set forth in this text are in accordance with current recommendations and practice at the time of publication. However, in view of ongoing research, changes in government regulations, and the constant flow of information relating to drug therapy and drug reactions, the reader is urged to check the package insert for each drug for any change in indications and dosage and for added warnings and precautions. This is particularly important when the recommended agent is a new or infrequently employed drug.

Some drugs and medical devices presented in this publication have Food and Drug Administration (FDA) clearance for limited use in restricted research settings. It is the responsibility of the health care provider to ascertain the FDA status of each drug or device planned for use in their clinical practice.

To my wife, Lee, and daughter, Janna, who gave me the encouragement, love, and understanding to allow this dream to come to fruition. To my father, the voracious reader, who passed on before he could read this book. To my mother, sister, and my friends for their support and encouragement, and to all my teachers for their guidance.

—MRS

To my family—my wife, Diane, and my children, Heather, Kelly and Ian—for the love and support you provided me in good times and bad.

And to my sports medicine fellows, without whom academic sports medicine would be inconsequential.

—DBM

To sports medicine physicians, trainers, and students; continuously striving to improve medical care for athletes of stadium and sand lot.

—SPVC

Contents

Contributing Authors xv

Preface xxv

Acknowledgments xxvii

I. Medical Supervision of the Athlete

1. Team Physician, Athletic Trainer and Training Room 3
Douglas B. McKeag and Jeffrey S. Monroe

2. The Preparticipation Physical Examination 10
Jeffrey R. Kovan

3. Limiting Conditions for Sports Participation 21
James L. Moeller and David A. Stone

4. Evaluating the Injured Athlete 33
Robert J. Johnson

5. Emergencies on the Field

A. Preparation for Emergencies in Sport 37
Gordon O. Matheson, Paul Ford, Peter Brukner, Robert M. Brock, and Robert L. Norris

B. Management of On-the-Field Emergencies 43
Aaron L. Rubin and Robert E. Sallis

6. Event Coverage 54
William O. Roberts

II. Conditioning

7. Building Aerobic Power 69
Carl Foster and Curtis Brackenbury

8. Building Strength 77
William J. Kraemer and Fred S. Harman

9. Flexibility 84
Karl Anthony Salesi

III. Environmental Concerns

10. Thermoregulation 91
Peter B. Raven

11. Exercise in the Heat and Heat Injuries 95
James Moriarity

12. Exercise in the Cold and Cold Injuries 106
Wayne K. Gersoff

13. High Altitude 110
Robert B. Schoene

14. Diving-Related Illnesses 114
Alfred A. Bove and Tom S. Neuman

IV. Protective Equipment

15. Protective Equipment 121
Arthur L. Boland and Shawn D. Sieler

V. Nutrition

16. Nutrition 129
Ann C. Grandjean, Kristin J. Reimers, and Jaime S. Ruud

VI. Pharmacology

17. Performance Enhancers 141
John A. Lombardo

18. Recreational Drugs 148
Gary I. Wadler

19. Drug Testing 156
Christopher A. McGrew

VII. Special Groups

20. Young Athletes 163
Lyle J. Micheli and Craig M. Mintzer

21. Special Concerns of the Female Athlete 171
Aurelia Nattiv and Mary Lloyd Ireland

22. Activity for Older Persons and Mature Athletes 184
Henry C. Barry

23. The Athlete with a Disability 190
Brian C. Halpern and Dennis A. Cardone

VIII. Medical Problems

24. Infections in Athletes 201
Thomas L. Sevier and Matthew B. Roush

25. Endocrinology 216
David O. Hough and Michael J. Woods

26. Cardiology 226
Steven P. Van Camp

27. Pulmonary 244
Bryan W. Smith and John M. MacKnight

28. Hematology 255
E. Randy Eichner

29. Dermatology 260
Wilma F. Bergfeld and Thomas N. Helm

30. Gastrointestinal Disorders 267
Peter Bruno

IX. Neurological Problems

31. Head Injuries 275
Robert C. Cantu

32. Injuries of the Cervical Spine 280
Joseph S. Torg and James J. Guerra

33. Peripheral Nerve Injuries of the Shoulder Girdle 287
Robert D. Leffert

34. Exercise-Related Headaches 293
John M. Henderson

35. The Athlete with Epilepsy 299
Gregory L. Landry and David T. Bernhardt

X. Musculoskeletal Injuries

36. Imaging 305
Leanne L. Seeger and Lawrence Yao

37. Fractures 316
Peter J. Fowler and Bruce C. Twaddle

38. Soft Tissue and Overuse Injuries 322
Wayne B. Leadbetter

39. The Shoulder—Musculotendinous Injuries 342
Russell F. Warren

40. The Shoulder—Instability and Miscellaneous 351
Jon J.P. Warner and Ronald A. Navarro

41. The Clavicle 361
William N. Levine, Evan L. Flatow, and Louis U. Bigliani

42. The Elbow 368
Champ L. Baker, Jr. and Charles A. Gottlob

43. The Wrist and Hand—Bone and Ligament Injuries 381
Arthur C. Rettig and Dipak V. Patel

44. The Wrist and Hand—Soft Tissues 388
Frank C. McCue III and Andrew M. Schuett

45. The Hand and Fingers 393
Charles P. Melone, Jr. and Sharon L. Hame

46. The Spine and Low Back 402
Robert G. Watkins

47. Injuries to the Pelvis, Groin, and Buttock 412
Per A. F. H. Renström

48. Hip Injuries 418
Cato T. Laurencin and Michael T. Rowland

49. The Groin and Thigh 424
Barry P. Boden and William E. Garrett

50. Knee-Ligaments 431
John A. Bergfeld and Marc R. Safran

51. Knee-Cartilage 440
Christopher D. Harner and Ronald A. Navarro

52. Uncommon Causes of Knee Pain in the Athlete 448
Freddie H. Fu and Marc R. Safran

53. Knee-Patellofemoral 454
John P. Fulkerson

54. The Leg 460
Robert A. Pedowitz and Anthony J. Saglimbeni

55. The Ankle 467
William G. Hamilton

56. The Foot 476
G. James Sammarco and Frank G. Russo-Alesi

XI. Face/ENT/Dental

57. Maxillofacial Injuries 489
John Downs

58. The Ear, Nose, and Throat 491
Jeffrey W. Bailet

59. The Eye 497
John B. Jeffers

60. Dental 500
John F. Wisniewski

XII. Other Injury

61. The Thorax 509
Harry L. Galanty and Douglas E. White

62. The Abdomen 518
Jeffrey L. Tanji

63. Genitourinary Injuries 523
Brent S.E. Rich

XIII. Rehabilitation

64. General Principles of Rehabilitation 529
W. Benjamin Kibler and Stanley A. Herring

XIV. Specific Sports

65. Baseball and Softball 541
Jan Fronek

66. Basketball 544
David N.M. Caborn and Michael J. Coen

67. Boxing 546
Barry D. Jordan

68. Cricket 549
Answorth A. Allen

69. Cycling: Road, Velodrome, and Mountain Biking 551
Robert E. Hunter

70. Dance 553
Marie D. Schafle

71. Diving: Platform and Springboard 556
Benjamin D. Rubin

72. Endurance Events: Marathon, Ultramarathon, Triathlon 558
Warren A. Scott

73. Equestrian Activities 562
Anastasios V. Korompilias and Anthony V. Seaber

74. Fencing 564
Rebecca Jaffe and Julie Moyer Knowles

75. Field Hockey 566
Cato T. Laurencin and W. Jay Gorum II

76. Football 568
James P. Bradley and Michael J. Rytel

77. Golf 571
William J. Mallon

78. Gymnastics 573
Bert R. Mandelbaum and Aurelia Nattiv

79. Ice Hockey 575
Arthur R. Bartolozzi III, Michael Palmeri, and Peter F. DeLuca

80. Lacrosse 578
Stephen J. O'Brien, Eva M. Anisko, and Answorth A. Allen

81. Martial Arts 580
Answorth A. Allen

82. Mountaineering and Climbing 583
Allan Bach

83. Power Lifting, Weight Lifting, and Body Building 586
William F. Luetzow and David Hackley

84. Rodeo 589
Jack Harvey

85. Rafting/Rowing/Kayaking/Canoeing 592
David M. Jenkinson

86. Rugby 595
Peter Brukner

87. Speed Skating, In-Line Skating, Figure Skating 597
Wade Smith

88. Alpine Skiing 600
J. Richard Steadman and Mark T. Dean

89. Soccer: Futsal and Indoor 602
Jonathan B. Ticker

90. Soccer: Outdoor 604
Darren L. Johnson and Ray L. Neef

91. Surfing 606
Marvin Bergsneider and Ronald A. Navarro

92. Swimming 609
Allen B. Richardson

93. Tennis and Other Racket Sports 611
Marc R. Safran and David A. Stone

94. Track and Field 613
R. Douglas Shaw

95. Volleyball 615
H. Paul Hirshman

96. Water Polo 616
John A. Gansel

97. Waterskiing: Standard and Wakeboarding 618
George L. Caldwell, Jr.

98. Wrestling 620
Edward M. Wojtys and John E. Kuhn

Appendices

1. Injections 625
Marc R. Safran

2. Athletic Taping and Bandaging 635
Gary B. Johnson

3. Banned Drugs 651
Marc R. Safran

4. Contents of the Medical Bag 655
Marc R. Safran and George C. Fareed

5. Rehabilitation Programs 659
W. Benjamin Kibler and Robert G. Watkins

6. Physical Examination—Special Tests 669
Marc R. Safran

Subject Index 693

Contributing Authors

Answorth A. Allen, M.D.
Instructor, Department of Orthopedics, Cornell University Medical College, 1300 York Avenue, New York, New York 10021, Associate Team Physician, New York Mets, Assistant Team Physician, St. John's University, Orthopedic Consultant, West Indies Cricket Team, Associate Team Physician, Long Island Rough Riders, Assistant Team Physician, New York Saints Lacrosse, The Hospital for Special Surgery, New York, New York, Northshore University Hospital at Glen Cove, Glen Cove, New York, North General Hospital, New York, New York.

Eva M. Anisko, M.D.
Hospital for Special Surgery, 535 East 70th Street, New York, New York 10021

Allan Bach, M.D.
Clinical Professor, Department of Orthopedics, University of Washington, Seattle, Washington, 98159, Seattle Hand Surgery Group, 600 Broadway #440, Seattle, Washington 98122

Jeffrey W. Bailet, MSPH, M.D.
Clinical Assistant Professor, Department of Otolaryngology—Head and Neck Surgery, University of Washington School of Medicine, Box 356515, Seattle, Washington 98195-6515, Department of Otolaryngology—Head and Neck Surgery and Chief of Surgery, Pacific Medical Center, 1101 Madison Medical Tower, Suite 301, Seattle, Washington 98104

Champ L. Baker Jr, M.D.
Clinical Assistant Professor, Department of Orthopedics, Tulane University School of Medicine, Team Physician, Columbus State University, Columbus, Georgia, President and Staff Physician, The Hughston Clinic, P.C., 6262 Veterans Parkway, Columbus, Georgia 31909

Henry C. Barry, M.D., M.S.
Associate Professor, Senior Associate Chair, Department of Family Practice, Michigan State University, B-100 Clinical Center, East Lansing, Michigan 48824-1315

Arthur R. Bartolozzi, III, M.D.
Vice Chairman, Department of Orthopedic Surgery, Surgeon and Chief, Department of Sports Medicine, Allegheny University Hospitals–Graduate, Philadelphia, Pennsylvania, 3B Orthopedics, 1800 Lombard Street, 1st Floor, Philadelphia, Pennsylvania 19146

John A. Bergfeld, M.D.
Head, Section of Sports Medicine, Department of Orthopedic Surgery, Cleveland Clinic Foundation, 9500 Euclid Avenue, Desk A41, Cleveland, Ohio 44195-5027, Team Physician, Baltimore Ravens, National Football League, Cleveland Cavaliers, National Basketball Association, Cleveland Ballet

Wilma F. Bergfeld, M.D.
Professor of Dermatology and Pathology, Department of Dermatology and Pathology, The Cleveland Clinic, 9500 Euclid Avenue, Cleveland, Ohio 44195, Consultant, Cleveland Browns, National Football League, Consultant, Cleveland Cavaliers, National Basketball Association, Consultant Cleveland Indians, Major League Baseball

Marvin Bergsneider, M.D.
Assistant Professor of Surgery, Division of Neurosurgery, UCLA Medical Center, Harbor/UCLA Medical Center, 10833 Le Conte Avenue, Box 956901, Los Angeles, California 90095-6901

David T. Bernhardt, M.D.
Assistant Professor, Department of Pediatrics, University of Wisconsin Medical School, 600 Highland Avenue, Madison, Wisconsin 53792, Team Physician, University of Wisconsin Athletic Teams

Louis U. Bigliani, M.D.
Chief, The Shoulder Service, Professor of Orthopedic Surgery, Professor, Columbia-Presbyterian Medical Center, 161 Fort Washington Avenue, New York, New York 10032

Barry P. Boden, M.D.
Clinical Instructor, Uniformed Services University Health Sciences, 2101 Medical Park Drive, Silver Spring, Maryland 20902

Arthur L. Boland, M.D.
Assistant Clinical Professor of Orthopedic Surgery, Department of Orthopedic Surgery, Harvard Medical School, Massachusetts General Hospital, 10 Hawthorne Place, Suite 114, Boston, Massachusetts 02114

Alfred A. Bove, M.D., Ph.D.
Chief of Cardiology, Bernheimer Professor of Medicine, Department of Medicine, Temple University Medical School, 3400 N. Broad Street, Philadelphia, Pennsylvania 19148

Curtis Brackenbury
Director of Hockey Operations/Head Coach, Mohawk Valley Prowlers Hockey Club, 400 Oriskany Street West, Utica, New York 13502

James P. Bradley, M.D.
Clinical Assistant Professor, Department of Orthopedic Surgery, University of Pittsburgh Medical Center, 200 Lothrop Street, Pittsburgh, Pennsylvania 15213

Robert M. Brock, M.D. FRCS (C), DABOS, FAAOS
Lecturer, Department of Family Medicine, University of Toronto, 1333 Sheppard Avenue E, Toronto, Ontario M2J 1V1, Canada

Peter Brukner, M.B.B.S., FACSP
Clinic Director, Olympic Park Sports Medicine Centre, Swan Street, Melbourne, Vic 3144, Australia

Peter Bruno, M.D.
Associate Professor of Medicine, Department of Medicine, New York University School of Medicine, 110 East 59th Street, Suite 9A, New York, New York 10022

David N.M. Caborn, B.S., MB Ch.B.
Associate Professor, Department of Orthopedics, Section of Sports Medicine, University of Kentucky, 740 South Limestone, K401 Kentucky Clinic, Lexington, Kentucky 40536-0284

George L. Caldwell, Jr., M.D.
Associate Clinical Professor, Department of Orthopedics, University of Miami School of Medicine, 6000 North Federal Highway, Fort Lauderdale, Florida 33308, Assistant Team Physician, Miami Dolphins, National Football League, Consulting Team Physician, Florida Marlins, Major League Baseball

Robert C. Cantu, M.D., M.A.
Chief, Neurosurgery Service, Director, Sports Medicine Service, Department of Neurosurgery, Emerson Hospital, 131 Ornac, Concord, Massachusetts 01742

Dennis A. Cardone, D.O.
Assistant Professor, Director, Sports Medicine Center, Department of Family Medicine, UMDNJ/Robert Wood Johnson Medical School, One Robert Wood Johnson Place, New Brunswick, New Jersey 08903

Michael J. Coen, M.D., M.S.
Holmes County Orthopedics and Sports Medicine, 212 N. Washington Street, Millersburg, Ohio 44654

Mark T. Dean, M.D.
Hilton Head Orthopedics and Sports Medicine, 95 Matthews Drive, Hilton Head Island, South Carolina 29926

Peter F. DeLuca, M.D.
Attending Physician, The Orthopaedic Hospital at Allegheny University Hospitals–Graduate, Assistant Professor, Department of Orthopaedic Surgery, MCP◇Hahnemann School of Medicine AUHS, Philadelphia, Pennsylvania 19146

John Downs, D.D.S., M.S., D.O.
Professor of Surgery, Department of Surgical Specialists, Michigan State University, B405 W. Fee Hall, East Lansing, Michigan 48824

E. Randy Eichner, M.D.
Professor of Medicine, Department of Medicine, University Hospital, University of Oklahoma Health Sciences Center, PO Box 26901, Oklahoma City, OK 73190

George C. Fareed
U.S. Davis Cup Team Physician, P.O. Box 1397, Brawley, California 92227

Evan L. Flatow, M.D.
Professor of Orthopedic Surgery, The Shoulder Service, Columbia-Presbyterian Medical Center, 161 Fort Washington, New York, New York 10032

Paul Ford, M.D.
Assistant Professor of Medicine, Department of Medicine, Stamford Medical Group, 900 Blake Wilbur Drive, W2080, Stamford, California 94305-5320

Carl Foster, Ph.D.
Professor of Medicine, University of Wisconsin Medical School, Milwaukee Heart Institute, 960 North Twelfth Street, Milwaukee, Wisconsin 53201-0342, Chair, Sports Medicine Committee, United States Speed Skating

Peter J. Fowler, M.D., F.R.C.S. (C)
Professor of Orthopedic Surgery, Department of Surgery, University of Western Ontario, London, Canada N6A 3K7, Fowler-Kennedy Sports Medicine Clinic, 3M Centre, University of Western Ontario, London, Canada N6A 3K7

Jan Fronek, M.D.
Clinical Assistant Professor, Department of Orthopedic Surgery: Knee and Shoulder, University of California, San Diego, Scripps Clinic and Research Foundation, 10666 North Torrey Pines Road, San Diego, California 92037

Freddie H. Fu, M.D.
Head Team Physician, Athletic Department, Center for Sports Medicine, University of Pittsburgh, 4601 Baum Boulevard, 2nd Floor, Pittsburgh, Pennsylvania 15213

John P. Fulkerson, M.D.
Clinical Professor of Orthopedic Surgery, Department of Orthopedic Surgery, University of Connecticut School of Medicine, Suite 364, The Exchange, 270 Farmington Avenue, Farmington, Connecticut 06032, Head Team Physician, Hartford Whalers, National Hockey League

Harry L. Galanty, M.D.
Assistant Professor, Department of Orthopedics, Texas Tech University, 3601 4th Street, Room 4A149, Lubbock, Texas 79430

John A. Gansel, M.D.
Department of Orthopedic Surgery, Kaiser Santa Rosa Medical Center, 401 Bicentennial Way, Santa Rosa, California 95403

William E. Garrett, M.D., Ph.D.
Professor of Orthopedic Surgery, Department of Orthopedic Surgery, Duke University Medical Center, Box 3435, Durham, North Carolina 27710

Wayne K. Gersoff, M.D.
4500 East Ninth Avenue, #540-S, Denver, Colorado 80220, Team Physician, Colorado Rockies, Major League Baseball, Team Physician, Colorado Rapids Soccer

W. Jay Gorum II, M.D.
Department of Orthopaedic Surgery, Allegheny University of Health Sciences, Allegheny University Hospitals, Hahnemann/MCP Divisions, 3300 Henry Avenue, Philadelphia, Pennsylvania 19129

Charles A. Gottlob, M.D.
Assistant Clinical Professor, Orthopedic Surgery, University of Illinois, 680 North Lake Shore Drive, Suite 1206 A, Chicago, Illinois 60611

Ann C. Grandjean, ED.D.
Director, International Center for Sports Nutrition, 502 S. 44th Street, Suite 3007, Omaha, Nebraska 68105

James J. Guerra, M.D.
Head, Section of Sports Medicine, Department of Orthopedic Surgery, Cleveland Clinic Florida, 3000 West Cypress Creek Road, Fort Lauderdale, Florida 33309-1743

David Hackley, M.D.
San Dieguito Orthopedic Medical Group, Inc., 9850 Gennessee, La Jolla, California 92037

Brian C. Halpern, M.D.
Clinical Assistant Professor, Department of Family Medicine, UMDNJ, Sports Medicine New Jersey, 475 Country Road 520, Marlboro, New Jersey 07746

Sharon L. Hame, M.D.
Clinical Instructor, Department of Orthopedic Surgery, University of California Los Angeles, 33 Le Conte Avenue, Los Angeles, California 90095

William G. Hamilton, M.D.
Clinical Professor of Orthopedic Surgery, Columbia University College of Physicians and Surgeons, St. Lukes-Roosevelt Hospital, 1000 10th Avenue, New York, New York 10019, Orthopedist for New York City Ballet, American Ballet Theatre, and the School of American Ballet, Foot and Ankle Consultant, New York Knicks, National Basketball Association

Fred S. Harman, M.S.
Doctoral Research Fellow, Department of Kinesiology/Laboratory for Sports Medicine, The Pennsylvania State University, 21 Rec Building, University Park, Pennsylvania 16802

Christopher D. Harner, M.D.
Professor of Orthopedic Surgery, Director, Sports Medicine Fellowship, Center for Sports Medicine, Department of Orthopedic Surgery, University of Pittsburgh, 4601 Baum Boulevard, 2nd Floor, Pittsburgh, Pennsylvania 15213, Head Team Physician, University of Pittsburgh, Head Team Physician, Robert Morris College, Head Team Physician, Woodland Hills High School

Jack Harvey, M.D.
Chief, Sports Medicine, Orthopedic Center of the Rockies, 2923 Ginnala Drive, Loveland, Colorado 80538, Director, Orthopedic Center of the Rockies/HealthSouth National Rodeo Sports Medicine Program, Chief Physician, USA Wrestling

Thomas N. Helm, M.D.
Assistant Clinical Professor of Dermatology, State University of New York at Buffalo, 6255 Sheridan Drive, Building B, Suite 208, Williamsville, New York 14221

John M. Henderson, D.O.
Director, Primary Care Sports Medicine, Department of Family Practice, The Hughston Sports Medicine Center, 2300 Manchester Expressway, Building G, Columbus, Georgia 31904

Stanley A. Herring, M.D.
Puget Sound Sports and Spine Physicians, P.S., 1600 E. Jefferson, Suite 401, Seattle, Washington 98122, Clinical Associate Professor, Departments of Rehabilitation and Orthopedics, University of Washington, Seattle, Washington 98195, Team Physician, Seattle Seahawks, National Football League

H. Paul Hirshman, M.D.
Department of Orthopedics, Scripps Clinic, 10666 North Torrey Pines Road, La Jolla, California 92037

David O. Hough, M.D. (Deceased)

Robert E. Hunter, M.D.
Clinical Associate Professor of Orthopedics, Orthopedic Associates of Aspen and Glenwood, University of Colorado, 100 East Main Street #101, Aspen, Colorado 81611

Mary Lloyd Ireland, M.D.
Orthopedic Surgeon, Operating Surgeon, Shriner's Hospital, Lexington, Kentucky, Director, Kentucky Sports Medicine Clinic, 601 Perimeter Drive, #200, Lexington, Kentucky 40517, Team Physician, Eastern Kentucky University, Richmond, Kentucky

Rebecca Jaffe, M.D.
Medical Center of Delaware, 3105 Limestone Road, Suite 200, Wilmington, Delaware 19808

John B. Jeffers, D.V.M., M.D.
Assistant Clinical Professor, Department of Opthamology, Thomas Jefferson University/Wills Eye Hospital, 900 Walnut Street, Philadelphia, Pennsylvania 19107

David M. Jenkinson, D.O.
Assistant Professor, Department of Family Medicine and Orthopedic Surgery, University of Pittsburgh, 1010 Kaufmann Building, 3471 Fifth Avenue, Pittsburgh, Pennsylvania 15213

Darren L. Johnson, M.D.
Chief, Section of Sports Medicine, Assistant Professor of Orthopedic Surgery, Department of Orthopedic Surgery, University of Kentucky, Kentucky Clinic, Kentucky 431, Lexington, Kentucky 40536-0284, Team Physician, University of Kentucky, Head Team Physician, Kentucky Thoroughblades

Gary B. Johnson, B.S., M.S.
Head Athletic Trainer, Department of Athletics, San Diego State University, 5500 Campanile Drive, San Diego, California 92182-4304

Robert J. Johnson, M.D.
Director, Primary Care Sports Medicine, Department of Family Practice, Hennepin County Medical Center, Five West Lake Street, Minneapolis, Minnesota 55408

Barry D. Jordan, M.D., M.P.H.
Instructor, Department of Neurology, University of California, Los Angeles, School of Medicine, 710 Westwood Plaza, Los Angeles, California 90095

W. Benjamin Kibler, M.D.
Medical Director, The Lexington Clinic Sports Medicine Center, 1221 South Broadway, Lexington, Kentucky 40504

Julie Moyer Knowles, Ph.D.
3105 Limestone Road, #101, Wilmington, Delaware 19808

Anastasios V. Korompilias, M.D., Ph.D.
Fellow in Orthopedics, Department of Surgery, Division of Orthopedic Surgery, Duke University Medical Center, MSRB Research Drive, Durham, North Carolina 27710

Jeffrey R. Kovan, D.O.
Director of Sports Medicine, Department of Family Practice, Michigan State University, Sports Medicine Clinic, 2900 Hannah Boulevard, Suite 104, East Lansing, Michigan 48823

William J. Kraemer, Ph.D.
Professor of Applied Physiology, Department of Kinesiology/Laboratory for Sports Medicine, The Pennsylvania State University, 21 Rec Building, University Park, Pennsylvania 16802

John E. Kuhn, M.D.
Assistant Professor, Division of Sports Medicine, Section of Orthopedic Surgery, University of Michigan Medical School, 24 Frank Lloyd Wright Drive, Ann Arbor, Michigan 48106-0363

Gregory L. Landry, M.D.
Professor of Pediatrics, Department of Pediatrics, University of Wisconsin Hospital, 600 Highland Avenue, Madison, Wisconsin, 53792-4116, Team Physician, University of Wisconsin Athletic Teams

Cato T. Laurencin, M.D., Ph.D.
Associate Professor of Orthopedic Surgery, Department of Orthopedic Surgery, Allegheny University of the Health Sciences, University Hospitals MCP Division, 3300 Henry Avenue, Philadelphia, Pennsylvania 19129

Wayne B. Leadbetter, M.D., B.S.
Senior Partner, The Orthopedic Center, P.A., 9711 Medical Center Drive, Suite 201, Rockville, M.D. 20850, Clinical Assistant Professor of Orthopedic Surgery, Georgetown University Hospital, 3800 Reservoir Road NW, Washington, D.C. 20007

Robert D. Leffert, M.D.
Professor of Orthopedic Surgery, Harvard Medical School, Massachusetts General Hospital, 55 Fruit Street, Boston, Massachusetts 02114

William N. Levine, M.D.
Clinical Instructor, Division of Orthopedic Surgery, University Sports Medicine, University of Maryland Medical System, Baltimore, Maryland 21207

John A. Lombardo, M.D.
Ohio State University, Sports Medicine Center, 2050 Kenny Road, Columbus, Ohio 43221

William F. Luetzow, M.D.
8231 Camino del Oro, #5, La Jolla, California 92037, Kaiser Permanente Medical Center, San Diego, California, San Diego Knee and Sports Medicine Fellowship, Clinical Instructor, University of California, San Diego School of Medicine, Department of Orthopedic Surgery

John M. MacKnight, M.D.
Assistant Professor of Clinical Internal Medicine and Sports Medicine, Division of General Internal Medicine, University of Virginia Health Sciences Center, Box 494, Charlottesville, Virginia 22908

William J. Mallon, M.D.
Clinical Assistant Professor, Department of Orthopedics, Duke University Medical Center and University of North Carolina School of Medicine, 2609 North Duke Street, Suite 900, Durham, North Carolina 27704-9464

Bert R. Mandelbaum, M.D.
Fellowship Director, Santa Monica Orthopedic and Sports Medicine Group, 1301 Twentieth Street, Suite 150, Santa Monica, California 90404

Gordon O. Matheson, M.D., Ph.D.
Associate Professor and Chief, Division of Sports Medicine, School of Medicine, Head Team Physician, Department of Athletics, Director of Sports Medicine, Stanford University, Burnham Pavilion, Stanford, California 94305-6175

Frank C. McCue, III, M.D.
Alfred R. Shands Professor of Orthopedic Surgery, and Plastic Surgery of the Hand, Director, Division of Sports Medicine and Hand Surgery, Department of Surgery, Team Physician, Department of Athletics, University of Virginia School of Medicine, Box 243, Charlottesville, Virginia 22908

Christopher A. McGrew, M.D.
Associate Professor of Family Practice and Orthopedics, Department of Family and Community Medicine and Department of Orthopedics and Rehabilitation, University of New Mexico Health Sciences Center, 2211 Lomas NE, Albuquerque, New Mexico 87106

Douglas B. McKeag, M.D., M.S.
Past President, American Medical Society for Sports Medicine, Arthur J. Rooney Sr. Professor and Vice Chairman, Departments of Family Medicine/Clinical Epidemiology and Orthopaedic Surgery, University of Pittsburgh School of Medicine, Pittsburgh, Pennsylvania 15213

Charles P. Melone Jr, M.D.
Chief of Orthopedic Hand Surgery, Beth Israel Medical Center, Professor, Department of Orthopedic Surgery, New York University Medical Center, 317 East 34th Street, New York, New York 10016

Lyle J. Micheli, M.D.
Associate Clinical Professor of Orthopedic Surgery, Harvard Medical School, Children's Hospital, 300 Longwood Avenue, Boston, Massachusetts 02115, Attending Physician, Boston Ballet

Craig M. Mintzer, M.D.
Staff Orthopedist, Jewett Orthopedic Clinic, 1285 Orange Avenue, Winter Park, Florida 32789

James L. Moeller, M.D.
Assistant Residency Director, Director, Primary Care Sports Medicine, Department of Family Practice, William Beaumont Hospital, 44199 Dequindre, Troy, Michigan 48098

Jeffrey S. Monroe, B.S., M.S.
Specialist/Head Athletic Trainer, Departments of Kinesiology and Athletics, Michigan State University, Duffy Daugherty Building, East Lansing, Michigan 48824-1214

James Moriarity, M.D.
Head Team Physician, University Health Center, University of Notre Dame, Notre Dame, Indiana 46556

Aurelia Nattiv, M.D.
Assistant Professor, Department of Family Medicine and Department of Orthopedic Surgery, Team Physician, UCLA Department of Intercollegiate Athletics, University of California, Los Angeles, 50-071 Center for Health Sciences, 10833 LeConte Avenue, Los Angeles, California 90095-1683

Ronald A. Navarro, M.D.
Assistant Clinical Professor, Department of Orthopedic Surgery, Harbor-UCLA Medical Center, Kaiser Permanente Southern California Permanente Medical Group, 25825 S. Vermont Avenue, Harbor City, California 90710

Ray L. Neef, M.D. (Deceased)

Tom S. Neuman, M.D.
Professor of Medicine and Surgery, Department of Emergency Medicine, University of California San Diego Medical Center, 200 W. Arbor, San Diego, California 92103-8676

Robert L. Norris, M.D., FACEP
Assistant Professor of Surgery, Departments of Surgery, Division of Emergency Medicine, Stanford University, 300 Pasteur Drive-H1249, Stanford, California 94305

Stephen J. O'Brien, M.D.
Associate Attending Orthopedic Surgeon, Sports Medicine and Shoulder Service, Hospital for Special Surgery, 535 East 70th Street, New York, New York 10021, Associate Professor of Surgery, Department of Orthopedics, Cornell University Medical College, Assistant Team Physician, New York Giants, National Football League

Michael Palmeri, M.D.
Rothman Institute, 800 Spruce Street, Philadelphia, Pennsylvania 19107

Dipak V. Patel, M.D., M.S., MSc Orth, FCPS Orth
Sports Medicine Fellow, Cornell University Medical Center and Hospital for Special Surgery, 535 East 70th Street, New York, New York 10021

Robert A. Pedowitz, M.D., Ph.D.
Assistant Professor In-Residence, Department of Orthopedics, University of California San Diego, 200 W. Arbor Drive, San Diego, California 92103

Peter B. Raven, M.D.
Professor and Chair, Department of Integrative Physiology, University of North Texas Health Science Center, 3500 Camp Bowie Boulevard, Fort Worth, Texas 76107

Kristin J. Reimers, M.S., R.D.
Associate Director, International Center for Sports Nutrition, 502 S. 44th Street, Suite 3007, Omaha, Nebraska 68105-1065

Per A.F.H. Renström, M.D., Ph.D.
Department of Orthopedics, Professor of Sports Medicine and Orthoroscopy, Karolinska Hospital, S-171.76, Stockholm, Sweden

Arthur C. Rettig, M.D.
Associate Clinical Professor, Department of Orthopedic Surgery, Indiana University School of Medicine, 201 Pennsylvania Parkway, Suite 200, Indianapolis, Indiana 46280

Brent S.E. Rich, M.D., ATC
Team Physician, Arizona State University, Team Physician, Arizona Diamondbacks, Major League Baseball, Team Physician, Mountain Pointe High School, University Sports Medicine, 777 South Pointe Parkway, Phoenix, Arizona 85044

Allen B. Richardson, M.D.
Chairman, Division of Orthopedic Surgery, John A. Burns School of Medicine, University of Hawaii, 1380 Lusitana Street, #608, Honolulu, Hawaii 96813

William O. Roberts, M.D., M.S.
Associate Clinical Professor, Department of Family Practice, University of Minnesota Medical School, MinnHealth Sports Care Consultants, 4786 Banning Avenue, White Bear Lake, Minnesota 55110

Matthew B. Roush, M.D.
Co-Director, Sports Medicine Fellowship, Department of Family Practice, Ball Memorial Hospital, 100 North Tillotson Avenue, Muncie, Indiana 47304

Michael T. Rowland, M.D.
Resident in Orthopedic Surgery, Allegheny University of the Health Sciences, MCP Division, 3300 Henry Avenue, Philadelphia, Pennsylvania 19129

Aaron L. Rubin, M.D., FACSM
Director, Kaiser-Permanente S.P.O.R.T. Fellowship Program, Fontana, California. Team Physician, University of California, Riverside.

Benjamin D. Rubin, M.D.
Assistant Clinical Professor, Department of Orthopedic Surgery, University of California Irvine, 302 W. LaVetta Avenue, Suite 202, Orange, California 92866

Frank G. Russo-Alesi, M.D.
Attending, Department of Orthopedic Surgery, Harbin Clinic, 1825 Martha Berry Boulevard, Rome, Georgia 30165

Jaime S. Ruud, M.S., R.D.
Nutrition Consultant, International Center for Sports Nutrition, 502 S. 44th Street, Suite 3007, Omaha, Nebraska 68105-1065

Michael J. Rytel, M.D.
Oakland Orthopedic Associates, 5820 Centre Avenue, Pittsburgh, Pennsylvania 15206

Marc R. Safran, M.D.
Co-Director, Sports Medicine, Department of Orthopedic Surgery, Kaiser Permanente, Orange County, Anaheim Hills, California, Assistant Clinical Professor of Orthopedic Surgery, University of California, Irvine and University of California, San Diego, Assistant Team Physician, University of California, Irvine, Medical Director, Toshiba Women's Professional Tennis Tournament, La Costa, California

Anthony J. Saglimbeni, M.D.
Clinical Instructor, Department of Family and Preventive Medicine, University of California, San Diego, 9500 Gilman Drive, La Jolla, California 92093

Karl Anthony Salesi, A.T.C., LPT
Head Athletic Trainer, University of Pittsburgh, Men's Soccer, Men's Basketball, Women's Tennis. Clinical Instructor, HPRED, University of Pittsburgh School of Education, 140 Trees Hall, Pittsburgh, Pennsylvania 15261

Robert E. Sallis, M.D., FAAFP, FACSM
Director of Residents, Kaiser Permanente Medical Center, Administration Faculty, Family Medical Resident and Sports Medicine Fellowship Program, Assistant Clinical Professor of Family Medicine, University of California, Riverside.

G. James Sammarco, M.D.
Past President, American Orthopedic Foot and Ankle Society, Volunteer Professor of Orthopedics, Department of Orthopedic Surgery, University of Cincinnati, 2624 Clifton Avenue, Cincinnati, Ohio 45220

Marie D. Schafle, M.D.
511 Kelmore, Moss Beach, California 94038

Robert B. Schoene, M.D.
Professor of Medicine, Adjunct Professor of Orthopedics and Sports Medicine, Division of Pulmonary and Critical Care Medicine, University of Washington, Harborview Medical Center, 325 9th Street, Seattle, Washington 98104

Andrew M. Schuett, M.D.
Orthopedic Surgeon, 490 Cherry Avenue, Bluefield, West Virginia 24701

Warren A. Scott, M.D.
Clinical Instructor in Surgery, Division of Emergency Medicine, Stanford University, Stanford, California, Department of Sports Medicine, Kaiser Permanente Medical Center, 900 Kiely Boulevard, Santa Clara, California 95051

Anthony V. Seaber
Laboratory Director Orthopedic Surgery, Department of Orthopedic Surgery, Duke University Medical Center, 375 MSRB Research Drive, Durham, North Carolina 27710

Leanne L. Seeger, M.D.
Associate Professor, Chief, Musculoskeletal Imaging, Department of Radiological Sciences, University of California Los Angeles School of Medicine, 200 Medical Plaza, Suite 165-59, Los Angeles, California 90095-6952

Thomas L. Sevier, M.D.
Director, Sports Medicine Fellowship, Department of Internal Medicine, Ball Memorial Hospital, 100 North Tillotson Avenue, Muncie, Indiana 47304

R. Douglas Shaw, M.D.
Santa Barbara Medical Foundation Clinic 2776 Puesta Del Sol, Santa Barbara, California 93105

Shawn D. Sieler, M.D.
Attending Physician, Department of Orthopedic Surgery, Robert Wood Johnson University Hospital, 21 Kilmer Drive, Building 2, Suite A, Morganville, New Jersey 07751

Bryan W. Smith, M.D., Ph.D.
UNC Student Health Services, CB 7470, Clinical Assistant Professor of Pediatrics and Orthopedics, University of North Carolina School of Medicine, Sports Medicine Physician, University of North Carolina Student Health Service, Head Team Physician, University of North Carolina at Chapel Hill, Chapel Hill, North Carolina 27599-7470

Wade Smith, M.D.
SVSM, P.O. Box 2064, Ketchum, Idaho 83340

J. Richard Steadman, M.D.
Steadman/Hawkins Clinic, 181 West Meadow Drive, #400, Vail, Colorado 81657

David A. Stone, M.D.
Assistant Professor of Orthopedics, Department of Sports Medicine, University of Pittsburgh, 4601 Baum Boulevard, Pittsburgh, Pennsylvania 15213-1217

Jeffrey L. Tanji, M.D.
UCDMC, Department of Family Practice, 2221 Stockton Boulevard, Sacramento, California 95817

Jonathan B. Ticker, M.D.
Island Orthopedic & Sports Medicine, PC, 660 Broadway, Massapequa, New York 11758, Chairman, Sports Medicine Committee, United States Fustal Federation, National Teams Physician, United States Soccer Federation

Joseph S. Torg, M.D.
Professor of Orthopedic Surgery, Orthopedic Institute, Allegheny University Hospitals, Hahnemann, 219 North Broad Street, Third Floor, Philadelphia, Pennsylvania 19107

Bruce C. Twaddle, MbChB, FRACS
Department of Orthopedics, Auckland Hospital, Park Road, Private Bag 92024, Auckland 1, New Zealand

Steven P. Van Camp, M.D.
Past President, American College of Sports Medicine, Assistant Clinical Professor, Department of Pathology, University of California–San Diego School of Medicine, Alvarado Medical Group, San Diego, California 92120

Gary I. Wadler, M.D., F.A.C.P., FACSM
Associate Professor of Clinical Medicine, Department of Medicine, New York University School of Medicine, 1380 Northern Boulevard, Manhasset, New York 11030

Jon J.P. Warner, M.D.
Chief, Harvard Shoulder Service, Associate Professor, Harvard Combined Orthopedic Surgery Program, Boston, Massachusetts 02114

Russell F. Warren, M.D.
Chief, Department of Orthopedic Surgery, Professor of Orthopedic Surgery, Hospital for Special Surgery/Cornell Medical College, 535 East 70th Street, New York, New York 10021, Team Physician, New York Giants, National Football League

Robert G. Watkins, M.D.
Professor of Orthopedic Surgery, Director, The Center for Spinal Surgery at University of Southern California, University of Southern California University Hospital, 1500 San Pablo, Los Angeles, California 90033

Douglas E. White, M.D.
Departments of Family Medicine and Primary Care Sports Medicine, Intermountain Health Care, 955 East 11400 South, Sandy, Utah 84094

John F. Wisniewski, M.D.
Associate Professor of Dentistry, Department of General and Hospital Dentistry, University of Medicine and Dentistry of New Jersey, New Jersey Dental School, 110 Bergen Street, Newark, New Jersey 07103-2400, Dental Consultant, Atlanta Braves, Major League Baseball, Dental Educational Consultant, Florida Marlins, Houston Astros, and Kansas City Royals, Major League Baseball

Edward M. Wojtys, M.D.
Professor of Surgery, Department of Orthopedics, University of Michigan, MedSport, 24 Frank Lloyd Wright Drive, Ann Arbor, Michigan 48106

Michael J. Woods, D.O.
Team Physician, Harrisburg Heat, Professional Soccer, Team Physician, Dickinson College, Carlisle, Pennsylvania, Arlington Rehab and Sports Medicine, 805 Sir Thomas Court, Harrisburg, Pennsylvania 17109

Lawrence Yao, M.D.
Associate Professor, Department of Radiology, Georgetown University Medical Center, 3800 Reservoir Road NW, Washington, D.C. 20007

Preface

Welcome to the *Manual of Sports Medicine*. We feel that this contribution to sports medicine literature should rank high among those texts that emphasize practicality and comprehensive coverage of this special interest area. In these times, one rarely gets the opportunity to sit down and read about a subject for any significant period of time. Thus, the editors of this book—specializing in orthopaedic surgery, family medicine, and cardiology—hope that this reference manual is easy to use, contains practical and up-to-date information, and is presented in an informal, understandable style.

It is our intent to continue the excellent tradition of the spiral manual series by presenting a volume meant for the practicing sports medicine physician. Each of our contributors represents a recognized and respected leader in sports medicine. It is also the goal of the editors and contributors to have compiled and produced a quick and easy-to-use, practical guide that can be carried in your pocket or your doctors' or trainers' bag when assisting in the care of the athlete.

As sports medicine continues to evolve, we felt that this would be an ideal time to compile a thorough, complete, and practical pocket guide for the practitioner who cares for the athlete. Sports Medicine has become more organized, academically rigorous, and important in its impact on medicine in general. Sports Medicine has also evolved to include multiple disciplines and specialties, with its basic premise not founded in glitz and glamour but in profoundly improving medical care for the athlete. We would submit to you that the benefactor of these changes (and indeed, the teachings of this book) is not simply the elite or competitive athlete, but a much larger population loosely defined as anyone who uses exercise for prevention, therapy, recreation, avocation, or vocation.

In multi-authored texts, some overlap of material is inevitable. Recognizing this we have chosen not to attempt to eliminate it entirely, thus allowing the reader to be exposed to different presentations and, at times, approaches. It also avoids excessive internal cross-referencing, thereby improving readability. We hope this approach is beneficial for the reader.

We, along with the contributors, hope you find this textbook a worthy addition to your medical library. May its cover and pages become "dog-eared" from overuse.

Marc R. Safran, M.D.
Douglas B. McKeag, M.D., M.S.
Steven P. Van Camp, M.D.

Acknowledgments

We extend much thanks and appreciation to each of our respected contributors for their willingness, effort, and time in addressing their areas of expertise. We also thank our editors, Danette Knopp and Juleann Dob, for their support, assistance, and patience, which allowed us to complete this book in keeping with our standards and goals.

I. MEDICAL SUPERVISION OF THE ATHLETE

1. TEAM PHYSICIAN, ATHLETIC TRAINER, AND TRAINING ROOM

Douglas B. McKeag and Jeffrey S. Monroe

I. Changes in Sports and Medicine

The justification for considering the special interest area of sports medicine separately from the rest of medicine resides in reviewing the changes that have taken place in both sports and medicine. The trends indicate favorable consideration of this subject for most practitioners of medicine and especially for primary care physicians as they minister to the needs of their patients. Sports medicine is unique in a variety of ways:

A. The injuries of athletes are not always treated like those of injured non-athletes. Return-to-play considerations are affected by significantly different forces than return-to-function considerations.
B. Sources of information in sports medicine remain relatively inconsistent and confusing.
C. Sophistication regarding the personal health of today's athletes has increased considerably. Because biomechanics and biopharmacology aid in training, more athletes than ever before have studied applied human physiology and the ability to change that physiology.
D. The number of sports- and exercise-related injuries has increased exponentially. Some of the reasons for this include but are not limited to:
   1. Increased participation.
   2. Growing number of sports offered.
   3. Disappearance of "natural selection"; borrowing from Darwinian theory, this terminology refers to persons who may have, for a variety of reasons, elected not to participate and who suddenly find themselves instead participating in a particular sport.
   4. Increased opportunities to play; this is especially true from the standpoints of socioeconomics and gender.
   5. Increased sophistication of sports, which has required many young athletes to pay a much higher price (in time and effort) to be successful in a sport
   6. Training intensity, duration, and frequency, which appear to have increased across the general population of athletes.
   7. Apparent lack of a concurrent advancement of coaching technique or knowledge that keeps up with the above-described changes
E. Current trends in medicine are more community oriented, especially with regard to health-care issues. For most of the sports activities in this country, the community is the organizing point.
F. Sports medicine remains an excellent marketing tool. Athletes and active individuals represent an excellent health-risk population. Generally, such persons are well motivated, with above-average resources available to them.
G. The area of sports medicine lacks quality assurance. Because of the multidisciplinary nature of sports medicine, defining the type of expertise needed to take care of active individuals becomes extremely difficult. One movement in that direction, however, has been the establishment of a certificate of added qualification (CAQ) in sports medicine offered to board-certified physicians in the specialties of family medicine, emergency medicine, internal medicine and pediatrics.
H. There is a relative lack of formal sports medicine education. This is especially true in the medical school setting. Because of its multidisciplinary nature, formal sports medicine education or even musculoskeletal education is not taught comprehensively or well at the graduate medical level.
I. The field of sports medicine continues to involve many disciplines and, to a certain degree, remains outside the mainstream of medical politics. Resources to support its academic underpinnings are certainly insufficient.

J. The concepts that have evolved from the special needs of athletes have now been expanded and used for the treatment of non–exercise-related problems. Dogma, which once burdened physicians, concerning the treatment of certain musculoskeletal injuries has been eliminated with the experience of years of new techniques and protocols practiced on highly motivated and elite athletes.
K. Exercise remains one of the most powerful, positive preventive tools available to physicians today. It is relatively low-cost and carries with it the ability to modulate a significant number of risk factors in humans.
L. Exercise has been shown to be highly effective adjunct therapy in a variety of chronic disorders such as epilepsy, diabetes mellitus, asthma, and manic depression.

II. Sports Medicine Team

A. The team physician should be
   1. A physician treating clinical problems (not a researcher or paramedic).
   2. The extension of the athlete's personal physician.
   3. Capable of offering quality, continuous primary care to the athlete or group in question (this does not include interacting only on an episodic or sporadic basis).
   4. Head "gatekeeper" of a support network surrounding the athlete that includes other allied health personnel and consultants.
   5. Medically answerable to no one but peers.
   6. Competent in the special interest area of sports medicine. The team physician must possess an adequate knowledge base to take care of all needs of an athlete in all situations that might arise.

B. The athletic trainer should
   1. Provide the athletic program and medical community with a connection to health care services including but not limited to emergency procedures, preventive measures, and rehabilitation services.
   2. Coordinate, guide, and triage all care given to athletes.

C. The athletic training room should be
   1. Administered by athletic trainers with direction from the athletic director and the team physician.
   2. Limited to treatment of minor medical procedures under the protocols set by the team physician.
   3. The repository of all athletic medical files.
   4. A "safe haven" for student athletes from members of the press and fans.

D. Consultants
   1. Consultants represent a vital part of the sports medicine team. A list of consultants who are willing to work with the special needs of athletes and who understand the demands that exercise places on the athlete is important. It is recommended that the clinicians in following specialty areas become members of the sports medicine team:
      a. Cardiology
      b. Nutrition
      c. Orthopaedic surgery
      d. Gynecology
      e. Physical medicine and rehabilitation
      f. Otorhinolaryngology
      g. Psychology
      h. Psychiatry
      i. Neurosurgery/neurology
      j. Ophthalmology/optometry
      k. Radiology
      l. General surgery
      m. Plastic surgery/hand surgery
      n. Podiatry
      o. Biomechanics

2. The "perfect" sports medicine consultant
   a. is able to see the patient in a timely manner.
   b. understands the need of team physician to participate in providing care.
   c. provides proper feedback to team physician and network.
   d. promises confidentiality.
   e. understands the "sense of urgency" in providing medical care.
   f. agrees with the network "philosophy of care" concerning injuries and/or illnesses.

III. The Sports Medicine Network

A. Philosophy
1. Precompetition: major responsibility is the *prevention* of injury
   a. Preseason
      (1) Assessment of community/system epidemiology
         (a) Community needs/allotment of resources
         (b) Injury patterns of sport
         (c) Severity of injury
         (d) Existing network of medical care
         (e) Successful disposition of injured athlete
      (2) Establishment of sports medicine network
         (a) Coverage of events
         (b) Chain of command/decision making
         (c) Legal issues and their delineation
         (d) Transportation of injured athletes
         (e) Consultation principals and protocols
         (f) Continuing education in sports medicine for network members
      (3) Preseason conditioning/preparticipation evaluation and screening
         (a) Preexisting conditions
         (b) Physical conditioning
         (c) Provide forum for presentation of biopsychosocial concerns (sexual activity, drug use, and so on)
         (d) Assessment of appropriate maturation and matching
      (4) Season-long competitive environment
         (a) Playing conditions/environmental factors
         (b) Adequacy of facilities/field of play
         (c) Up-to-date training techniques/coaching
         (d) Health care maintenance of current injuries
         (e) Athlete education/monitoring of high-risk behavior
         (f) Equipment safety
      (5) Postseason
         (a) Review of network functioning
         (b) Complete follow-up of all injuries/illnesses (exit physical examinations)
         (c) Evaluation of health care rendered
         (d) Future network needs
2. Competition: *Triage* is the priority during competition.
   a. Physician coverage data
   b. Recognition of early signs of sports-induced injuries
   c. "Sideline" philosophy, chain of command for evaluation
   d. Return-to-play criteria and appropriate triage
   e. On-the-field initial examination
      (1) "Golden" postinjury period, defined as the time immediately following injury when the athlete may remain stunned, (the first five minutes after injury). Swelling may be minimal and guarding of the injured area nonexistent. It is during this period that the most accurate postinjury clinical examination is usually obtained.

(2) Take your time on the field, rule out serious injury, then transport athlete to acceptable site.
(3) Take a history, with appropriate emphasis on the biomechanics of the injury.
(4) Perform a focused physical examination.
(5) Assessment of the problem on the sidelines should include
  (a) diagnosis.
  (b) assessment of the severity and extent of the injury.
  (c) need for diagnostic services.
  (d) determination of the mode of transportation if necessary.
(6) More complete physical after removal from competition should include:
  (a) the concept of serial examination.
  (b) return-to-play guidelines as well as planning rehabilitation and treatment.
  (c) consideration and examination of peripheral body areas that may be involved.
  (d) confirmatory re-examination of injured area.

3. Postcompetition: The major responsibility of the postcompetition period is to develop an efficient, effective, and fast *rehabilitation* program.
   a. Close follow-up and assessment should be included.
   b. Rehabilitation oriented toward the active individual, stressing the following points:
      (1) early initiation of rehabilitation.
      (2) maintenance of conditioning.
      (3) early mobilization when possible.
      (4) return to play as soon as possible.
   c. Appropriate use of therapeutic modalities and medications
   d. Return-to-play guidelines evaluated and updated to include:
      (1) restoration of full function, strength, and range of motion (ROM).
      (2) restoration of strength, sensation, including proprioception and balance.
      (3) psychologically readiness of athlete to return to play
   e. Concept of relative rest: Most injured athletes do not need absolute rest but can be "shunted" to other activities or to a milder form of the normal sporting activity.
   f. Light-intensity training (LIT): In this concept, athletes are considered participants in their own rehabilitation. When athletes are worked back into a sports activity from which they have been disqualified, they should be told to begin functional rehabilitation, with cessation of all symptoms on activities of daily living. Activities should begin with minimal distance and with very low intensity level. Athletes then have three choices in evaluation of whether to progress in rehabilitation.
      (1) If pain or swelling develops *during* activity, the athlete should immediately *stop* and *back down* one step in the process.
      (2) If pain or swelling develops *after* activity, the athlete should continue that activity but *not increase* it until no pain is present after activity.
      (3) If *asymptomatic* during and after activity, the athlete should *increase* activity in predetermined gradients, with physician consultation.

IV. Roles and Responsibility Clarification

A. The team physician is *not*
   1. a policeman.
   2. a punisher
   3. an extension of the coach or trainer or of administrative policies.
   4. a fan.

5. Medically answerable to anyone except peer review or law.
6. Provider of 100% of health care.

B. The team physician *is*
1. coordinator of all health care.
2. provider of continued care.
3. overseer of the sports medicine network.
4. knowledgeable and current regarding on sports medicine practices.
5. contributor to feel
6. a resource to community and colleagues.
7. aware of rules.

V. Legal Issues

As sports medicine becomes a more recognized special-interest area it is only natural that its practitioners will be held to higher medical standards commensurate with increased duties and responsibilities that they have assumed and that the community expects of them.

A. Avoiding lawsuits. Risk of litigation over medical treatment of athletes can be reduced if sports physicians
1. follow established guidelines (these may even be ones that they have helped formulate).
2. generate a written contract with the school or group with which you are working.
3. if at all possible, work with athletic trainers. The physician may be able to help bring athletic trainers into a particular system.
4. generate a thorough preparticipation sports physical exam (see chapter 2).
5. use sound judgment concerning the athlete's return to competition. Recent and future guidelines are being established in a variety of areas.
6. institute early and proper care.
7. seek informed consent for treatment before athletic activity begins.
8. be careful and conservative with release of information.
9. make decisions based on medical knowledge, not competition concerns.
10. know when to refer.

VI. Ethics in Medical Decision Making

Sports medicine, like any other special-interest area involving physicians with conflicting priorities (e.g., prison, occupational, military medicine) is subject to medical decision-making issues that require ethical analysis for a rational solution. These are often termed *conflict of interest* or *divided loyalty* dilemmas. Such dilemmas result from being situated between two or more parties, each evoking a strong sense of commitment and/or duty from the care provider. These conflicts may differ, depending on the level of sport covered (professional, college, high school or youth programs) but remain a continuing problem and major factor in medical decision-making in sports.

A. Conflicts of interest
1. Role of team physician versus role of fan: Most sports physicians are involved in sports because they enjoy them and are fans. At times, this can create a conflict of interest in the treatment of an injury and judgment concerning return to play. Obviously, the role of the fan/booster must be subservient to the role of the team physician.
2. Welfare of the athlete versus welfare of the team: The conflict between the welfare of the individual athlete and the welfare of the team is probably the most common dilemma occurring at all levels of competition. It becomes more of a conflict as the pressure to win takes priority over medical values in a program. Established return-to-play criteria for a program can help tremendously in guiding a physician or physicians.
3. Welfare of the athlete versus wishes of the athlete: The principle that should prevail when one confronts the problem of an athlete's wishes versus welfare is "Physician do no harm." The team physician must think about long-term consequences versus short-term benefit. In addi-

tion, the physician should ask whether the athlete is making the decision due to coercion, either overt or covert. The athlete may not be old enough to consider the ramifications of his or her actions fully.

4. Welfare of the athlete versus wishes of the family: Occasionally, though not often, the wishes of the athlete's family unit may conflict with the long-term welfare of the athlete.

B. Minimizing dilemmas: Ambiguity and misunderstandings should be avoided at all times and certain principles should be followed:
   1. Clarify the *nature of the relationship* between you and the other parties involved (e.g., coaches, parents, athletes, school administrators, team owners) at the onset.
   2. Insist on *professional autonomy* over all medical decisions.
   3. Anticipate, identify, then *insulate* yourself formally from all possible coercive pressures to insure such autonomy. Give clear directions to the athletic trainer.
   4. Communicate the principles and guidelines under which you intend to deliver care and make decisions before becoming the care provider.
   5. Eliminate or at least recognize and minimize any *personal biases* you may have that might adversely effect your function as team physician.

C. The handling of a potential medical problem: With the onset of injury
   1. Remove the athlete from the field/court of play to a quieter less open environment.
   2. Carry out an unhurried, thorough examination.
   3. Decide whether return to play is possible (triage), always considering potential risk of further injury. If you decide that an athlete cannot return to play, inform the athlete first of your decision and then inform the appropriate coach. If you decide the athlete can be continue to play proceed as follows:
      a. Discuss return to play with the athlete only, exclusive of others.
      b. In the case of a young athlete, insist on discussion to clarify the athlete's wishes and then confer with appropriate family members.
      c. Any doubts expressed by the athlete about return to play should strongly bias the physician to eliminate the athlete from further play in that contest regardless of what the physician thinks.
      d. Act as an athlete advocate when dealing with the coach concerning a decision not to play.
      e. Be very clear on the limits of your responsibility as team physician. If a physician concludes that an athlete can return to play, but at a diminished level of performance, it becomes the coach's decision as to whether the injured athlete is more valuable to the team than a healthy backup.

VII. Helpful Hints

Consider the following list before becoming or agreeing to become a team physician. These are recommendations only but they may help you put your participation as team physician in perspective.

A. Do you have current training in cardiopulmonary resuscitation (CPR, BCLS)?
B. Do you know how to manage an acutely traumatized athlete with an injury to the head, neck or back?
C. Will your malpractice insurance extend to sports medicine coverage?
D. Does the team or program sponsoring the activity you are covering have liability insurance to cover a team physician?
E. Are the athletes to be covered provided with a consent form for treatment of non-emergency injuries?
F. Are you comfortable with your knowledge base concerning re-entry into a sporting event following an injury (return to play guidelines)?
G. Can you recognize your own limitations and call in other specialists when necessary?
H. Are you willing to put in the time and to be on call for athletic team needs?

VIII. Issues to Consider as Team Physician

A. Medical/legal
   1. Catastrophic injury, emergency care, notification of family, administration, media relations
   2. Disqualification
      Medically
      Psychological
      Return from disqualification
   3. Malpractice: assumed responsibility
   4. Confidentiality/record keeping

B. Substance abuse: policy
   1. Detection
   2. Education
   3. Treatment/records

C. Performance improvement
   1. Consultants
   2. Medical education
   3. Research

D. Prevention
   1. Coaching techniques
   2. Risk-taking behavior by athletes
   3. Equipment
   4. Preparticipation screening
   5. Injury rehabilitation

E. Nutrition
   1. Behavior modification
   2. Eating disorders
   3. Supplements

2. THE PREPARTICIPATION PHYSICAL EXAMINATION

Jeffrey R. Kovan

The preparticipation physical examination (PPPE) of children, adolescents, and young adults is one of the most common reasons for a visit to a physician. As the frequency of office visits among adolescents decreases with increasing age, the PPPE offers one of the few opportunities for direct contact between the physician and the child/adolescent. The purpose of the PPPE is to assist young athletes by reviewing previous medical concerns, preventing injury or illness, and ultimately weighing the benefit of exercise and sports participation against the risk of exacerbating any preexisting medical condition.

The primary goal of the PPPE is to help maintain the health and safety of athletes in training and competition. In allowing an athlete to participate, a major objective of the physician is to limit exclusion of healthy athletes from participation and to promote a safe environment in which to compete. Approximately 1% of athletes are denied clearance during their PPPE and 3% to 15% require further evaluation. The PPPE is not intended to substitute for an athlete's regular health maintenance examination. Nevertheless, due to the lack of compliance of patients in visiting a physician, the PPPE has often provided the only direct contact between the athlete and the medical community. According to the forthcoming PPPE monograph, the primary objectives of the preparticipation physical are (1) detect any condition that may predispose an athlete to an injury or illness during competition; (2) detect any medical or health condition that may limit an athlete's safe participation, and (3) address any legal or insurance requirements.

PPPEs are used as a screening tool to assess athletes who may be at risk for injury, illness, or abusive behaviors. Assessment of athletes' fitness level and risk in participation are common goals that should be shared by all.

Implementation

Provider

The PPPE should ultimately be performed by physicians competent in preventive screening of athletes. Individual states certify which practitioners are qualified to perform such examinations, and many states allow health care professionals other than physicians to perform them. In general, the PPPE should be completed by a physician (M.D./D.O.) and by assisting medical personal (i.e., physician assistants, medical students, and residents). The primary provider should review all records and cosign all completed portions of that examination as the director of the medical team.

Timing

The PPPE should be performed approximately 6 weeks before the beginning of preseason practice. This allows further evaluation for any necessary referrals as well as adequate time for any rehabilitation from previous injuries. If a longer time is allocated before the examination, other injuries that may subsequently occur may not be evaluated before the athlete participates in sports.

Frequency

Optimum timing intervals for the PPPE have not been fully established. Often based on school or state requirements, level of risk of the student athlete, out-of-pocket costs, as well as availability of qualified personnel, the frequency of performance of the PPPE varies markedly at different age levels. It is generally recommended that entry-level screening evaluation should be performed before an athlete enters a new school level, i.e., middle school, high school, or college, and be followed by an interim yearly evaluation to assess any problems incurred during the previous year and follow up on previous pertinent medical conditions or injuries.

Method/Setting

Office-based Physical Examination

Although not time efficient or cost effective, the office-based PPPE offers the most comprehensive examination and provides the best avenue for continuity of care. If the physician has treated an athlete throughout his or her childhood and has an adequate record of that athlete's previous history, any pertinent medical problems are less likely to be missed on the examination. Unfortunately, not all physicians have equal interest in sports participation among adolescents and are often unaware of an athlete's particular sport and its demands. This may lead to performance of an incomplete examination and ultimately to a feeling of uneasiness about the care provider with regard to determining clearance for an athlete with a particular medical or physical condition.

Station

The Garrick "station" method of examination uses several examiners, each focusing on a particular region of the body during the PPPE. Often the most cost-effective and efficient method with regard to the examination, the station-based evaluation has become quite useful when several providers are available and can focus on a particular body part during their examination. Unfortunately, the station-based examination limits continuity of care among examining physicians, and any need to delve into pertinent private issues of the athlete is often hindered. Physicians often are rushed through the examination because of time constraints and are unable to provide an overall general screening of the athlete's entire body, leading to a disjointed approach (Table 2-1).

Locker Room

The locker room examination necessitates an approach similar to the station-based examination, with the focus on a one-on-one encounter. Each physician performs a complete PPPE on an individual athlete, providing continuity of care not achieved with the station-based examination. Concerns similar to those arising in the station-based examination arise regarding confidentiality, privacy issues, and a quiet environment for the evaluation. Despite these concerns, time efficiency, cost effectiveness, and a more detailed level of continuity of care have caused the locker room examination to be the most widely used method today.

Content

History

The medical history alone provides a 92% sensitivity in detecting significant musculoskeletal injuries and a 63% to 74% identification rate with history alone.

Table 2-1. Organization of examination stations

Station	Task	Personnel
1	Registration; fill out history	Teacher, administrator
2	Vital signs taken	Teacher, coach, trainer
3	Blood pressure and pulse	Nurse, coach, trainer
4	Urine sample taken	Nurse, coach, trainer
5	Assessment of visual acuity: Snellen chart	Nurse, coach, trainer
6	Assessment of hearing acuity	Nurse, coach, trainer
7	General medical examination and Tanner staging	Physician
8	Student athlete exits the examination area; gathering of materials for completeness	Teacher, administrator

Unfortunately, significant variation occurs between completion of the historical information by the athlete alone versus completion by the athlete and parent together. Statewide PPPEs of athletes who are minors require the signature of parents or guardian before review. Joint completion of the medical history by parents and athletes would dramatically improve the history evaluation and is recommended. The

Preparticipation Physical Evaluation

HISTORY

DATE OF EXAM ______________

Name ______________ **Sex** ______ **Age** ______ **Date of birth** ______

Grade ______ **School** ______________ **Sport(s)** ______________

Address ______________ **Phone** ______________

Personal physician ______________

In case of emergency, contact

Name ______________ **Relationship** ______ **Phone (H)** ______ **(W)** ______

Explain "Yes" answers below.
Circle questions you don't know the answers to.

	Yes	No
1. Have you had a medical illness or injury since your last check up or sports physical?	☐	☐
Do you have a chronic illness?	☐	☐
2. Have you ever been hospitalized overnight?	☐	☐
Have you ever had surgery?	☐	☐
3. Are you currently taking any prescription or nonprescription (over-the-counter) medications or pills or using an inhaler?	☐	☐
Have you ever taken any supplements or vitamins to help gain or lose weight or improve your performance?	☐	☐
4. Do you have any allergies (for example, to pollen, medicine, food, or stinging insects)?	☐	☐
Have you ever had a rash or hives develop during or after exercise?	☐	☐
5. Have you ever passed out during or after exercise?	☐	☐
Have you ever been dizzy during or after exercise?	☐	☐
Have you ever had chest pain during or after exercise?	☐	☐
Do you get tired more quickly than your friends during exercise?	☐	☐
Have you ever had racing of your heart or skipped heartbeats?	☐	☐
Have you had high blood pressure or high cholestrol?	☐	☐
Have you ever been told you have a heart murmur?	☐	☐
Has any family member or relative died of heart problems or of sudden death before age 50?	☐	☐
Have you had a severe viral infection (for example, myocarditis or mononucleosis) within the last month?	☐	☐
Has a physician ever denied or restricted your participation in sports for any heart problems?	☐	☐
6. Do you have any current skin problems (for example, itching, rashes, acne, warts, fungus, or blisters)?	☐	☐
7. Have you ever had a head injury or concussion?	☐	☐
Have you ever been knocked out, become unconscious, or lost your memory?	☐	☐
Have you ever had a seizure?	☐	☐
Do you have frequent or severe headaches?	☐	☐
Have you ever had numbness or tingling in your arms, hands, legs, or feet?	☐	☐
Have you ever had a stinger, burner, or pinched nerve?	☐	☐
8. Have you ever become ill from exercising in the heat?	☐	☐
9. Do you cough, wheeze, or have trouble breathing during or after activity?	☐	☐
Do you have asthma?	☐	☐
10. Do you use any special protective or corrective equipment or devices that aren't usually used for your sport or position (for example, knee brace, special neck roll, foot orthotics, retainer for your teeth, hearing aid?	☐	☐
11. Have you had any problems with your eyes or vision?	☐	☐
Do you wear glasses, contacts, or protective eyewear?	☐	☐
12. Have you ever had a sprain, strain, or swelling after injury?	☐	☐
Have you broken or fractured any bones or dislocated any joints?	☐	☐
Have you had any other problems with pain or swelling in muscles, tendons, bones, or joints?	☐	☐

If yes, check appropriate box and explain below.

☐ Head	☐ Neck	☐ Back
☐ Chest	☐ Shoulder	☐ Upper arm
☐ Elbow	☐ Forearm	☐ Wrist
☐ Hand	☐ Finger	☐ Hip
☐ Thigh	☐ Knee	☐ Shin/calf
☐ Ankle	☐ Foot	

	Yes	No
13. Do you want to weigh more or less than you do now?	☐	☐
Do you lose weight regularly to meet requirements for your sport?	☐	☐
14. Do you feel stressed out?	☐	☐

15. Record the dates of your most recent immunizations (shots) for:

Tetanus ______ Measles ______

Hepatitis B ______ Chicken Pox ______

FEMALES ONLY

16. When was your first menstrual period? ______

When was your most recent menstrual period? ______

How much time do you usually have from the start of one to the start of another? ______

How many periods have you had in the last year? ______

What was the longest time between periods in the last year? ______

Explain "Yes" answers here: ______________

I hearby state that, to the best of my knowledge, my answers to the above questions are complete and correct.

Signature of athlete ______________ Signature of parent/guardian ______________ Date ______

Fig. 2-1. Preparticipation physical evaluation form with recommended baseline history.

recommended baseline medical history is shown in Fig. 2-1. Specific highlights concerning the medical history include evidence of exercise-induced syncope; family history of myocardial infarction or sudden death at age less than 50 years; current medications, including over-the-counter products; and allergies to medications and other outside irritants. Any significant past medical history of seizure disorders, sin-

Preparticipation Physical Evaluation continued

PHYSICAL EXAMINATION

Name ______ Date of birth ______

Height ______ Weight ______ % Body fat (optional) ______ Pulse ______ BP ___/___, ___/___, ___/___

Vision R 20/___ L 20/___ Corrected: Y N Pupils: Equal ______ Unequal ______

	NORMAL	ABNORMAL FINDINGS	INITIALS*
Appearance			
Eyes/Ears/Nose/Throat			
Heart			
Pulses			
Lungs			
Abdomen			
Genitalia (males only)			
Skin			
Other			
MUSCULOSKELETAL			
Neck			
Back			
Shoulder/arm			
Elbow/forearm			
Wrist/hand			
Hip/thigh			
Knee			
Leg/ankle			
Foot			

* Station-based examination only

CLEARANCE

☐ Cleared

☐ Cleared after completing evaluation/rehabilitation for: ______

☐ Not cleared for: ______ Due to: ______

Recommendations: ______

Name of physician (print/type) ______ Date ______

Address ______ Phone ______

Signature of physician ______, MD or DO

Fig. 2-1. *Continued.*

gle organs, previous head injuries with loss of consciousness (LOC) or previous concussions, and significant musculoskeletal injuries should be included. A general review of systems is warranted only to focus on specific positive findings. Tetanus vaccination may be indicated and should be emphasized. Use of any other previous medical appliances, such as mouth guards, hearing aids, and so on, is significant. Finally, review of potential eating disorder behaviors or illicit drug use in all athletes, as well as of menstrual history in female athletes, should be included.

Physical Examination

Adequate exposure of the athlete is imperative for the physical examination. Shorts and light shirts and/or tank tops are recommended for both men and women. Please see Fig. 2-1 for the PPPE to be completed by the physician.

Height and Weight

Height and weight should be measured with each examination and be recorded. Follow-up from previous examinations is necessary to assess any concerns of eating disorders, steroid use, or other potentially harmful practices.

Head, Ears, Eyes, Nose, and Throat

Visual acuity, measured with the standard Snellen Chart, should be established on baseline evaluations and evaluated annually unless proof of completion by the school system since the previous physical has been documented. Athletes who wear glasses and/or contact lenses should be informed of the risks of participating in sports with them, and proper protective eyewear should be recommended. Specific focus of the eye examination is based on pupil size (anisocoria) and should be reported to coaches and/or trainers if there is any asymmetry. The remainder of the examination of head, ears, eyes, nose, and throat should focus on conditions that may be harmful to the athlete, including oral ulcerations, leukoplakia, gingival atrophy, and decreased enamel such as results from eating disorders and chewing tobacco use.

Cardiovascular System

Yearly blood pressure (BP) measurements with a cuff of appropriate size are recommended. If an athlete's BP is initially elevated recheck it after 10 to 15 minutes. If further concerns arise, referring the athlete back to the primary care provider is recommended. Heart murmurs require further evaluation if a new-onset murmur is detected. Particular attention should be paid to the presence and character of any murmurs, the timing of the murmur in relation to S1 and S2, extra heart sounds, or clicks. Any systolic murmur greater than 2/6 in severity, any diastolic murmur, or any murmur that becomes louder when a Valsalva maneuver is executed should be further evaluated before the athlete is cleared for participation. Concerns over arrhythmias require a follow-up evaluation by the athlete's primary provider. The 26th Bethesda Conference guidelines are an excellent resource for the primary care physician on the cardiovascular evaluation and specific clearance guidelines.

Pulmonary

Any obvious signs of wheezing or abnormal breath sounds should be reviewed and may require a more thorough examination. In general, a normal resting examination does not exclude exercise-induced asthma and, if the physician is concerned an appropriate history should be obtained to further rule out this and other pulmonary conditions.

Abdomen

The abdominal examination should be performed with the athlete supine. Palpation of any hepato- or splenomegaly must exclude the athlete's from participation in contact sports. Any evidence of masses, tenderness, rigidity, or enlargement requires further evaluation before the athlete receives clearance to return to play. Previous history of increased alcohol intake, hepatitis, or mononucleosis warrants a through abdominal examination.

Genitalia

Males: The genitourinary examination, although somewhat stressful to the athlete, is imperative in ruling out athletes with one testicle, as well as in screening for any testicular cancers. Although testicular cancer is an uncommon cause of cancer deaths in men, it does occur most commonly in males aged 18 to 35 years. Performing the examination allows the physician an opportunity to counsel the athlete on performing self-examinations at home. Athletes with undescended testicles or absence of a testicle should be counseled with regard to protective gear. Potential Restrictions from contact sports are listed in the recommendations for participation in competitive sports of the American Academy of Pediatrics (Table 2-2).

Females: Examination of the female genitalia is not a routine part of the general PPPE. If warranted, based on the athletes' medical history, such examination should be performed later in a more private setting.

Tanner staging for both males and females is recommended, although sometimes difficult to achieve in a locker room or station-based examination. A general screening is indicated to help set baseline levels for competition.

Skin

A general evaluation of the integument is recommended to assess for any rashes, infections, and infestations. Specifically, herpetic lesions, scabies, and other transmissible infections are necessary for evaluation so that treatment can be instituted before the athlete participates in sports.

Musculoskeletal System

The musculoskeletal examination has received much scrutiny lately because of its lack of depth on evaluation. Previously, a 13-point screening examination that offered the care provider an opportunity to perform a baseline evaluation of musculoskeletal weakness and asymmetries was instituted by Lombardo, et al. Many researchers have advocated joint-specific testing as a means for screening. Time constraints, physician comfort levels, and access to an adequate examination environment limit this method. In accordance with the two approaches described, I advocate a 13-point musculoskeletal screening, with addition of some general rotator cuff tests, knee ligament testing and ankle stability testing.

First, the athlete stands facing the examiner, allowing the examiner to evaluate symmetry of the trunk, the upper and lower extremities, and alignment of the lower extremities. The athlete then actively moves their neck through a full range of motion (flexion-extension, right and left lateral bending and rotation). Next, the athlete abducts their shoulders 90 degrees then flex and extend their elbows through the full range of motion looking for loss of motion. The athlete then, with the shoulders in 90 degrees of abduction and the elbows in 90 degrees of flexion, rotate their shoulders into full active internal and external rotation assessing symmetry (throwing athletes will often have non-pathologic increased external rotation of their throwing shoulder as compared with their non-throwing shoulder). The examiner then can assess shoulder abduction deltoid strength as the patient attempts to resist a downward force, applied by the examiner, to the athlete's abducted arm. Additionally, rotator cuff strength can be assessed with the supraspinatus (empty-the-can) test (see appendix 6). Trapezius strength is next tested by having the athlete stand with their arms at their sides and the examiner push down on the athlete's shoulder. The athlete then attempts to shrug their shoulders. With the athlete's arms at their sides and their elbows flexed 90 degrees, the examiner can assess hand and finger range of motion. This is done by first by assessing the athlete's ability to open and close their hands as a fist looking for symmetry. Next, with the patient's fingers extended, the athlete is

(text continues on page 18)

Table 2-2. Recommendations for participation in competitive sports

Physical condition	Contact/ collision	Limited contact/ impact	Noncontact—strenuous	Noncontact—moderately strenuous	Noncontact—nonstrenuous
Atlantoaxial instability	No	No	Yes; in swimming, no butterfly, breast stroke, or diving starts	Yes	Yes
Acute illness	Requires individual assessment (e.g., contagiousness, exacerbation of illness)				
Cardiovascular carditis	No	No	No	No	No
Hypertension					
Mild	Yes	Yes	Yes	Yes	Yes
Moderate	Requires individual assessment				
Severe	Requires individual assessment				
Congenital heart disease	Patients with mild forms can be allowed a full range of physical activities; patients with moderate or severe forms or those who are postoperative should be evaluated by a cardiologist before athletic participation				
Absence or loss of function in one eye	Eye guards may allow the athlete to participate in most sports, but this must be judged on an individual basis				
Detached retina	Consult an ophthalmologist				
Inguinal hernia	Yes	Yes	Yes	Yes	Yes
Absence of one kidney	No	Yes	Yes	Yes	Yes
Enlarged liver	No	No	Yes	Yes	Yes

Musculoskeletal disorders	Requires individual assessment				
History of serious head or spine trauma, repeated concussions or craniotomy	Requires individual assessment		Yes	Yes	Yes
Convulsion disorder					
Poorly controlled	Yes	Yes	Yes	Yes	Yes
Well controlled	No	No	Yes; no swimming or weight lifting	Yes	Yes; no archery or riflery
Absence of one ovary	Yes	Yes	Yes	Yes	Yes
Pulmonary insufficiency	May be allowed to compete if oxygenation remains satisfactory during a graded stress test				Yes
Asthma	Yes	Yes	Yes	Yes	Yes
Sickle cell trait	Yes	Yes	Yes	Yes	Yes
Skin: Boils, herpes, impetigo, scabies	While contagious, no contact sports or gymnastics using mats		Yes	Yes	Yes
Enlarged spleen	No	No	No	Yes	Yes
Absent or undescended testicle	Yes; certain sports may require a protective cup		Yes	Yes	Yes

Adapted with permission from American Academy of Pediatrics Committee on Sports Medicine. Recommendations for participating in competitive sports. Pediatrics 1988;81:737–9.

asked to move their fingers in an abduction/adduction maneuver (spreading the fingers and bringing them next to each other again). The last upper extremity test is to look for elbow pronation supination range of motion and symmetry. This is performed while the athlete's arms are still at their sides, elbows flexed 90 degrees and they are asked to rotate the forearm so that the palms are first up, then down. The athlete then stands on both heels facing the examiner, again looking for equal stance, balance and symmetry of the lower extremity. The athlete next attempts to touch their toes while their knees are straight. The athlete then is asked to squat and perform a "duck walk" looking for full squatting and symmetry.

The athlete is next asked to turn and faces away from the examiner. Symmetry of the trunk, upper and lower extremities is then evaluated. Then, the athlete is asked to touch their toes while standing with their knees straight assessing for scoliosis, deformity or other asymmetry. Next, the patient hyperextends their back to allow a search for evidence of pain or gross "step-off" deformities to rule out spondylolysis or spondylolisthesis. The patient is then asked to stand on their toes. Evaluation is to look for symmetry of the lower extremities and ability to stand on both feet equally.

With the patient supine, the knee is tested with the Lachman maneuver and posterior sag and posterior drawer tests (see appendix 6).

With the patient seated, ankle stability testing with anterior drawer and talar tilt can be performed (see appendix 6).

When a history of injury or surgery suggests, further detailed testing is performed. Many of these specific examinations are shown in appendix 6.

Neurological

In general, most neurological function will be screened through the musculoskeletal examination. Additional neurological examination occasionally may be warranted if an athlete has recurrent stingers and burners or if any evidence of parethesias or motor weakness is elicited. History of previous concussions demands a neurological screening to assess the athlete for cognitive and motor/sensory changes.

Additional Screening Tests

At present, no specific laboratory screening tests are recommended for the PPPE. Determinations of height, weight, BP, pulse, and visual acuity are recommended yearly, with visual acuity being assessed again only as needed on the interim evaluation. If state and other governing bodies have other specific requirements for PPPEs, they should be followed.

Clearance

After completion of the PPPE, the physician must determine the ability of the athlete to participate in sports. Whether restrictions or full participation is recommended, documentation on the medical record to provide coaches, trainers, and athletic directors with a baseline for the athlete's participation is indicated. Almost all athletes are cleared for full participation. Occasionally, a few athletes require further evaluation of previous injuries before participation is allowed. On very rare occasions, an athlete will not be cleared for sports and, in that setting, further evaluation by either the athlete's primary care provider or other specialists may be warranted. The American Academy of Pediatrics Committee in Sports Medicine from 1988 (Table 2-2) provides recommendations for participation in competitive sports. A list of contact versus non-contact sports from the American Academy of Pediatrics is shown in Table 2-3.

Others

Several other concerns affecting adolescent and young adult athletes are frequently missed or bypassed during the PPPE. These issues (although personal and generally requiring a more developed rapport) warrant further discussion based on the athletes' social and physical habits. Included are alcohol and drug use, recent acute ill-

Table 2-3. Classification of sports by contact

Contact/collision	Limited contact	Noncontact
Basketball	Baseball	Archery
Boxing[a]	Bicycling	Badminton
Diving	Cheerleading	Body building
Field hockey	Canoeing/kayaking (white water)	Canoeing/kayaking (flat water)
Football Flag Tackle	Fencing	Crew/rowing
Ice hockey	Field High jump Pole vault	Curling
Lacrosse	Floor hockey	Dancing
Martial arts	Gymnastics	Field Discus Javelin Shot put
Rodeo	Handball	Golf
Rugby	Horseback riding	Orienteering
Ski jumping	Racquetball	Power lifting
Soccer	Skating Ice In-line Roller	Race walking
Team handball	Skiing Cross-country Downhill Water	Riflery
Water polo	Softball	Rope jumping
Wrestling	Squash	Running
	Ultimate Frisbee	Sailing
	Volleyball	Scuba diving
	Windsurfing/ surfing	Strength training
		Swimming
		Table tennis
		Tennis
		Track
		Weight lifting

[a] Participation not recommended by the American Academy of Pediatrics (AAP); the American Academy of Family Practice (AAFP), American Medical Society for Sports Medicine (AMSSM), American Osteopathic Academy of Sports Medicine (AOASM), and American Orthopedic Society for Sports Medicine (AOSSM) have no stand against boxing.

Reprinted with permission [pending] from American Academy of Pediatrics Committee on Sports Medicine and Fitness: Medical conditions affecting sports participation. *Pediatrics* 1994; 94:757–60.

nesses, exposure to blood-borne pathogens, disordered eating, pregnancy in a female athlete, and previous history of heat illnesses.

Medical and Legal Considerations

A few important medical/legal issues associated with the PPPE have been described. Physicians are often asked to provide athletes clearance for participation when prior injury or illness may predispose the athlete to complications. If an athlete should obtain clearance for participation from an outside source, regardless of the designated team physician's recommendation, the school administration must then assume responsibility for the decision whether or not to allow the athlete to compete. In the event the athlete is allowed to participate, the designated team physician should obtain an exculpatory waiver or risk release to protect their interests and beliefs regarding the athlete's participation.

With regard to potential sexual harassment claims, physician must use common sense when evaluating an athlete. The physician should inform the athlete of the thoroughness of the examination and provide an appropriate setting. A chaperone may be necessary during breast and genital assessment in the PPPE. The physician should be discreet in comment and action during the examination. Additional portions of the examinations may require a chaperone depending on involvement of the examination and comfort level of the athlete.

Finally, with regard to the Good Samaritan statute, it is imperative that physicians know the state statutes regarding group participation and, whether they wish to be protected according to this title. If their interest in the Good Samaritan statute is to be protected, physicians should not accept any form of remuneration for their services.

Conclusions

The PPPE provides a basic framework for screening a generally healthy group before they participate in sports. A thoroughly completed medical history with significant parental input appears to offer the examiner a reasonable baseline to conduct the examination. Among adolescents, athletic participation must continue a pleasant to be an enjoyable experience. As providers of health care, physicians must continue to promote such expererience in a safe and risk-free environment.

Suggested Reading

Bracker MD. Environmental and thermal injury. *Clin Sports Med* 1992; 2:419.

Gersoff WK, Motz, HA, Environmental factors in athletic performance. In: *Sports injuries, mechanisms, prevention, treatment.* Baltimore: Williams & Wilkins, 1994.

Hamlet MD. An overview of medically related problems in the cold environment. *Milit Med* 1987; 152:393–6,

Hamlet, MD. Cold injuries, Raynaud's disease, and hypothermia. In: Casey MJ, Foster C, Hixson EG, (eds.) *Winter sports medicine.* F.A. Davis: Philadelphia, 1990; Chap. 18.

Hixson EG, Cold injury. In: *Orthopaedic sports medicine, principles and practice, vol. 1,* W.B. Saunders, Philadelphia: Ch. 12, section B.

McKeag DB. Preparticipation screening of the potential Athletes. *Clin Sports Med* July 1989; 8:373–97.

Tanji JL. The Preparticipation Physical Examination for Sports, *AFP* 1990;00: 397–403.

Wilkerson JA Avoiding hypothermia. In: Wilkerson JA, Bangs CC, Hayward JS, eds., *Hypothermia, frostbite, and other cold injuries.* Seattle: The Mountaineers, 1986; Ch. 2.

3. LIMITING CONDITIONS FOR SPORTS PARTICIPATION

James L. Moeller and David A. Stone

I. Cardiovascular System

Athletes with an underlying cardiovascular abnormality may place themselves at increased medical risk during competitive sports due to an increase in workload on the heart or stress on the cardiovascular system. Risk of sudden death, life-threatening cardiovascular alterations, or disease progression may all be increased. Recommendations for participation of an athlete with a cardiovascular disorder are based on the type of cardiac abnormality, severity of disease, and the static or dynamic demands of the sport. The classification of sports in Table 3-1 was developed by The 26th Bethesda Conference participants based on the dynamic and static demands of competitive sports.

A. Hypertrophic Cardiomyopathy (HCM)

1. HCM is the leading cause of sudden cardiac death in athletes aged less than 30 years.
   a. The prevalence of HCM is approximately 0.1% to 0.2% in the general population.
   b. Sudden death due to HCM usually occurs in the absence of previous symptoms.
2. History of exertional syncope, dizziness or chest pain with activity should alert the physician or athletic trainer to the possibility of HCM.
3. Physical examination may disclose a systolic murmur that increases with Valsalva maneuver. Often, no murmur is present on physical examination.
4. If history and physical examination findings raise the suspicion of HCM, diagnostic tests should be undertaken, including electrocardiogram (ECG) 24-hour Holter monitor, and echocardiogram.
   a. Echocardiogram will disclose a thickened ventricular septum (>15 mm) as compared with the ventricular free wall in most patients with HCM. Left ventricular cavity size is generally unchanged but left ventricular filling and compliance is impaired.
      (1) Some patients affected with HCM will have a wall thickness less than 15 mm.
      (2) A subgroup of highly trained male athletes without cardiovascular disease may show wall thickness of 12 to 16 mm (physiologic "athlete's heart").
      (3) Screening echocardiography is not recommended as part of the preparticipation physical examination (PPPE).
5. A familial form of HCM has been identified and has been attributed to genetic defects involving contractile proteins and mutations of the beta-myosin heavy-chain gene. DNA diagnosis by genetic testing may be possible.
   a. Screening echocardiography in patients with a family history of HCM may be warranted.
6. Recommendations for athletic participation
   a. Symptomatic athletes should not be allowed to participate in competitive sports.
   b. Asymptomatic athletes should be allowed to participate only in low-intensity (class IA) sports.

B. Hypertension (HTN)

Blood pressure (BP) readings which indicate HTN differ for different age groups (Table 3-2). HTN is diagnosed by three elevated BP readings obtained on separate occasions.

1. Patients with mild to moderate HTN without end organ damage or concomitant heart disease should not be restricted from competitive sports.

Table 3-1. Classification of sports (based on dynamic and static components during competition)

	A. Low Dynamic	B. Moderate Dynamic	C. High Dynamic
I. Low static	Billiards Bowling Cricket Curling Golf Riflery	Baseball Softball Table tennis Tennis (doubles) Volleyball	Badminton Cross-country skiing Field Hockey[a] Orienteering Race walking Racquetball Running (long distance) Soccer[a] Squash Tennis (singles)
II. Moderate static	Archery Auto Racing[a,b] Diving[a,b] Equestrian[a,b] Motorcycling[a,b]	Fencing Field events (jumping) Figure skating[a] Football (American)[a] Rodeoing[a,b] Rugby[a] Running (sprint) Surfing[a,b] Synchronized swimming[a]	Basketball[a] Ice hockey[a] Cross-country skiing (skating technique) Football (Australian)[a] Lacrosse[a] Running (middle distance) Swimming Team handball
III. High static	Bobsledding[a,b] Field events (throwing) Gymnastics[a,b] Karate/judo[a] Luge[a,b] Sailing Rock climbing[a,b] Waterskiing[a,b] Weight lifting[a,b] Windsurfing[a,b]	Body building[a,b] Downhill skiing[a,b] Wrestling[a]	Boxing[a] Canoeing/kayaking Cycling[a,b] Decathlon Rowing Speed skating

[a] Danger of bodily collision.
[b] Increased risk if syncope occurs.

   a. Moderate dynamic/static exercise should be encouraged to help decrease BP.
2. Patients with severe and very severe HTN should be restricted from high static sports until HTN is controlled.
   a. Control may entail the use of medications and lifestyle modification.

C. Infective Carditis

Infective carditis (myocarditis) is usually caused by Coxsackie B virus, but may be difficult to detect clinically.

1. History will usually include a respiratory illness complicated by other symptoms such as fatigue, dyspnea, syncope, palpitations, arrhythmias, or acute congestive heart failure (CHF).

Table 3-2. Classification of hypertension by age in children and adolescents

	MAGNITUDE OF HYPERTENSION[a]			
Age group	Mild (stage 1) (mm Hg)	Moderate (stage 2) (mm Hg)	Severe (stage 3) (mm Hg)	Very severe (stage 4) (mm Hg)
Children				
6–9 yr				
Systolic BP	120–124	125–129	130–139	≥140
Diastolic BP	75–79	80–84	85–89	≥90
10–12 yr				
Systolic BP	125–129	130–134	135–144	≥145
Diastolic BP	80–84	85–89	90–94	≥95
Adolescents				
13–15 yr				
Systolic BP	135–139	140–149	150–159	≥160
Diastolic BP	85–89	90–94	95–99	≥100
16–18 yr				
Systolic BP	140–149	150–159	160–179	≥180
Diastolic BP	90–94	95–99	100–109	≥110
Adults				
>18 yr				
Systolic BP	140–159	160–179	180–209	≥210
Diastolic BP	90–99	100–109	110–119	≥120

BP, blood pressure.

[a] Applies to patients who are not receiving antihypertensive drugs and who are not acutely ill. When the systolic and diastolic BP measurements fall into different categories, the higher category should be selected to classify that patient's BP status. In adults, isolated systolic hypertension is defined as a systolic BP ≥140 mm Hg and a diastolic BP <90 mm Hg and staged appropriately. Blood pressure values are based on the average of three or more readings taken at each of two or more visits after the initial screening. Classifications taken from the 26th Bethesda Conference on Recommendations for Determining Eligibility for Competition in Athletes with Cardiovascular Abnormalities.

2. Physical examination may disclose a new or increasing murmur, an enlarged heart, or signs of heart failure.
3. Diagnostic tests include ECG, chest radiograph, and echocardiogram to detect arrhythmias, signs of heart failure, and cardiac enlargement, ventricular size, and cardiac function.
4. Endomyocardial biopsy may be helpful in confirming the diagnosis.
5. Because infective carditis may cause dangerous arrhythmias, patients with the disease should be withdrawn from sports for 6 months from the onset of symptoms. Patients may return to competition when ventricular function is normal, cardiac dimensions are normal, and no clinically relevant arrhythmias are present on Holter monitoring.

D. Mitral Valve Prolapse (MVP)

MVP is a relatively common condition with a prevalence of approximately 5% in the general population. Many athletes with this condition participate in competitive sports at a very high level.

1. MVP is characterized by systolic protrusion of the mitral valve leaflets into the left atrium, as demonstrated by echocardiography or angiography.
2. History may be negative or may include palpitations, dizziness, or exertional syncope.
3. Physical examination may disclose the hallmark auscultatory finding of a midsystolic click with or without a late systolic murmur.

a. This murmur differs from the murmur of HCM in that Valsalva maneuver should not increase the intensity of the murmur, but may increase its length.

4. If history and physical examination findings raise the suspicion of MVP, further diagnostic tests including ECG and echocardiography may be warranted. These tests are not considered necessary if the patient is asymptomatic and the heart murmur found on physical examination is clinically "innocent."
5. Recommendations for athletic participation
   a. All patients with MVP should be allowed to participate competitive sports in so long as the following conditions do not exist.
      (1) History of syncope documented to be arrhythmogenic
      (2) Family history of sudden death associated with MVP
      (3) Repetitive forms of sustained venticular tachycardia (SVT) or complex ventricular arrhythmias
      (4) Moderate to marked mitral regurgitation
      (5) Occurrence of a prior embolic event
   b. If any of the above criteria are met, the patient may participate in low-intensity competitive sports only.

E. Congenital Coronary Artery Anomalies

Congenital coronary artery abnormality are an important cause of SCD in young athletes. Most commonly, the left main coronary artery originates from the anterior right sinus of Valsalva and courses between the pulmonary trunk and the anterior of the aorta. However, other anomalies have been described, including anomalous right coronary arteries and origin of the left coronary artery from the pulmonary trunk. If detected and associated with exercise-induced ischemia, this condition represents an absolute contraindication to participation, in sports.

F. Idiopathic Concentric Left Ventricular Hypertrophy has been described as a cause of SCD. In comparison with conditions in HCM, there is symmetrical left ventricular hypertrophy and left ventricular thickness. Echocardiography is the diagnostic procedure of choice. As with HCM, only low levels of athletic activity are permitted.

G. Marfan's Syndrome

Marfan's syndrome is an autosomal dominant disorder of the gene for the structural protein fibrillin. It affects a number of different organs, including the eyes (dislocated lens), joints (hypermobility and scoliosis), and the heart and cardiovascular system (cystic medial necrosis of the aorta, MVP, and mitral or aortic regurgitation). About 25% to 35% of cases occur sporadically, and the overall incidence is 1 in 20,000. A significant screening finding is dolichostenomelia (inappropriately long limbs relative to the trunk). Athletes should not participate in contact or collision sports, but can participate in low static and dynamic competitive sports if they do not have aortic route dilation, mitroregurgitation, or a family history of premature sudden death. Aortic root dimensions should be assessed at 6-month intervals.

H. Coronary Artery Disease

Coronary artery disease (CAD) is the most frequent cause of SCD in adults but has not been shown in all studies to be a consistent cause of death in young athletes. Patients should be screened for risk factors (hypertension, elevated chlolesterol level, diabetes mellitus, smoking, family history), and risk factors should be managed aggressively. See Chapter 26 and Bethesda Conference 26 guidelines for specific recommendations for persons with coronary artery disease.

I. Aortic Valve Stenosis

Aortic Valve Stenosis is not a common cause of SCD in athletes but is a common cause of sudden death. The rarity of aortic stenosis among athletic death victims is believed to due to repeated PPPE which allow the diagnosis to be made before progression of the condition. Athletes with aortic stenosis should undergo Doppler echocardiography, ECG, and exercise testing for arrhythmias. Athletes with mild stenosis can participate in all competitive sports. See Chapter 26 and Bethesda Conference 26 guidelines for specific recommendations for persons with aortic valve stenosis.

J. Wolff-Parkinson-White (WPW) Syndrome

The WPW syndrome generally carries a low risk-for sudden death. The risk can be increased with use of calcium channel blockers or digoxin or in patients who exhibit atrial fibrillation with a rapid ventricular response. Ablation is recommended by some authorities before participation in sports but optional management remains debatable. Athletes without structured heart disease, a history of palpitations, or tachycardia (particularly those age > 20 years) may be appropriate for clearance for full competition.

K. Congenital Long QT Interval Syndrome

Patients with congenital long QT interval syndrome are at risk of sudden death and should be restricted from participation in all sports. Two inherited forms exist; the more common form is autosomal dominant. An autosomal-recessive form is associated with deafness. The diagnosis has been based on a corrected QT interval (QT_c) of 440-450ms, although the QT interval is variable and at times even normal.

II. Neurological System

A. Seisure disorder. Participation in all sports is allowed for athletes whose seizures are well controlled with medication.

1. Special consideration should be made for certain sports including swimming, weight lifting, archery and riflery.
2. Patients with poorly controlled disease should be precluded from contact/collision sports (Table 3-3) and limited contact/impact sports.
   a. Swimming, weight lifting, archery and riflery should not be allowed.

B. Concussion. There are many different classification systems for concussion and gray areas exist in each classification system. Gray areas also exist with regard to return-to-play criteria.

1. An athlete who sustains a closed head injury should be disqualified from the current activity if the sensorium does not clear quickly or if other symptoms and signs are present, such as loss of consciousness (LOC) posttraumatic amnesia, confusion, dizziness, or headache.
2. Depending on severity of symptoms, a computed tomography (CT) scan may be required to seek intracranial bleeding.
3. An athlete who continues to have symptoms from a prior concussion should not be allowed to participate in contact sports until those symptoms clear. The time during which the patient must be asymptomatic before returning to play is a controversial issue.
   a. Athletes who exhibit symptoms are excluded from competition to avoid second-impact syndrome, which occurs when a second head injury is sustained before the symptoms of the first head injury have cleared.
      (1) Rapid cerebral swelling leads to rapid neurologic deterioration and death.
      (2) The second impact may be minor and may not even be direct to the head (e.g., Valsalva maneuver, strong blow to the chest, and so on).

C. Burner syndrome, also known as the "stinger," is generally the result of traction on the brachial plexus; caused by depression of the shoulder when a player makes contact with another player or the ground. An alternative mechanism is a compression injury to the fixed brachial plexus between the shoulder pad and the superior medial scapula at Erb's point. Most of these injuries are mild, and players are able to return to play within 3 weeks ; however, allowing an athlete to return to play before achieving complete re-

Table 3-3. Classification of sports

CONTACT		NONCONTACT		
Contact/ collision	Limited contact/ impact	Strenuous	Moderately strenuous	Nonstrenuous
Boxing	Baseball	Aerobic dancing	Badminton	Archery
Field hockey	Basketball	Crew	Curling	Golf
Football	Bicycling	Fencing	Table tennis	Riflery
Ice Hockey	Diving	Discus		
Lacrosse	Field	Javelin		
Martial arts	High Jump	Shot put		
Rodeo	Pole Vault	Running		
Soccer	Gymnastics	Swimming		
Wrestling	Horseback riding	Tennis		
	Skating	Track		
	Ice	Weight lifting		
	Roller			
	Skiing			
	Cross-country			
	Downhill			
	Water			
	Softball			
	Squash, handball			
	Volleyball			

covery is contraindicated. Use of an orthosis to protect Erb's point may be of value.

III. Respiratory

A. **Exercise-induced bronchospasm (EIB)** is a reversible transient increase in airway responsiveness involving large and small airways after 5 to 8 minutes of strenuous exercise. It generally presents as wheezing, cough, or excessive dyspnea, but can present as poor exercise performance or chest tightness and chest pain. The intensity of the exercise required to elicit symptoms is generally in the range of 75% to 85% of V_{O2max}. For the diagnosis to be made, a decrease in forced expiratory volume (FEV1) of 10% from pre-exercise level must be demonstrated. Sixty percent to 90% of asthmatic children and 40% of atopic children will demonstrate EIB symptoms. EIB is generally considered a relative contraindication to sports participation. Symptoms are generally worse during running than during cycling or swimming, and cold dry air is generally worse than warm moist air, although any sport played in an environment with poor air circulation may exacerbate symptoms. Sports such as baseball requiring short, intense exercise periods, may be best tolerated. Treatment before play in less than ideal circumstances may need to be modified. Athletes with upper respiratory infections, exacerbations of allergies, and poor conditioning may at times need to be removed from competition.

B. **Exercise-induced anaphylaxis** is a life-threatening emergency characterized by symptoms of upper respiratory obstruction, urticaria, cutaneous erythema, and vascular collapse. The exact mechanism is unknown, but is believed to involve exposure to allergens before or at the start of exercise. Various foods, alcoholic beverages, medications, and inhaled allergens have been implicated. Attacks are unpredictable and the condition is thought of as a continuum with EIB by some authors. Patients may be allowed to exercise but should use the buddy system and take special precautions not to expose themselves to known triggering agents before exercising.

IV. Dermatology

A. Herpes simplex

1. Patients with active skin lesions should be precluded from participating in sports in which intimate skin-to-skin contact may be made. These patients should also be disqualified from activities in which a mat is used, such as wrestling, gymnastics, karate, or judo.
2. Athletes may return to play when lesions are healed or a physician confirms that they are no longer contagious.

B. Impetigo

1. Patients with active skin lesions should be precluded from participation in sports in which intimate skin-to skin contact may be made. Like patients with herpes simplex, such patients should also be disqualified from activities in which a mat is used.
2. Athletes may resume participation when lesions are healed or when the lesions are no longer considered contagious.

C. Tinea corpora

1. Athletes with tinea corpora should be disqualified from sports involving intimate contact with mats or skin-to-skin when active lesions are present.
2. Athlete may resume participation when the lesions are healed or are no longer considered contagious.

D. Scabies

1. The recommendations for patients with active scabies are the same as those for herpes simplex, impetigo, and tinea corpora. Return to play should be withheld until treatment has been completed and the athlete is no longer considered contagious.

E. Molluscum contagiosum is a viral infection caused by a pox virus. It presents as a pearly white or flesh-colored papule which may be single or in clusters and is filled with keratogenous debris and virions. Common locations include the trunk, axilla, face, perineum, and thighs. The diagnosis is usually made clinically, and spontaneous remission is often noted. However, the lesion is considered infectious, and close-contact sports such as wrestling are contraindicated until healing occurs. The period of transmissibility of the lesion is unknown. For this reason, athletes are often treated with curettage which allows faster return to sports.

F. Furunculosis is a staphylococcal bacterial infection which presents as tender, red inflammatory nodules that may evolve into fluctuant abscesses. Diagnosis is made clinically and is confirmed by culturing the lesions. These athletes are often ill, presenting with low-grade fever. Athletes with furunculosis are disqualified from contact sports and swimming. Treatment consists of warm compresses, and benzoyl peroxide 5% to 10% solution two to three times daily, in addition to systemic antibiotics, usually dicloxacillin or cephalexin for 10 to 14 days. Incision and drainage is occasionally necessary, especially when lesions are not treated early. As with impetigo, clearance for return to play is given at 24 to 48 hours with appropriate treatment.

G. Pseudofolliculitis is an inflammatory papule caused by a foreign body reaction to ingrown hairs. Acute lesions often appear pustular and suggest an infection. The condition is common in African-American males and men with coarse curly beards. The condition is not a contraindication to participation, although secondary infection may occur, requiring Gram stain and culture to distinguish it from foreign body reaction.

H. Contact dermatitis secondary to irritants such as poison ivy, oak, or sumac may be a contraindication to play depending on the location and degree of skin involvement.

V. Viral Diseases

Viral illness is common in all age groups; the average adult is affected between 1 and 6 times per year and the average child 10 to 12 times a year. The effect of a single agent may vary considerably from person to person. While upper respiratory infection has been associated with sudden death there is no consistent association, and viral infection remains a relative contraindication to participation.

Bloodborne pathogens, in particular human immunodeficiency virus (HIV) and hepatitis B and C, pose complex problems for the sports medicine practitioner. The increase in medical information for both HIV and hepatitis C infection in particular may change guidelines dramatically in the future. Present guidelines to limit play are therefore based on information available. In general, contact sports pose the greatest risk for the transmission of these agents, but very little evidence of spread of any of these conditions in athletic participation has been documented.

A. HIV transmission through sports contact is alleged in only one case report. Because of the prevalence of HIV infection and the lack of its documented transmission through sports participation, it is believed that transmission on the playing field is unlikely, but not impossible. HIV infection is not considered an absolute contraindication to sports participation, but decisions regarding continued participation should be based on the athlete's medical status, the required intensity of training, potential stress, risk of transmission (see Chapter 24), and nature of the sport.

B. Hepatitis B virus transmission has been documented in sumo wrestlers but in no other sports to date. Infection is not an absolute contraindication to participation. Clinical status, in particular hepatosplenomegaly, is a consideration in limiting participation, however, acute infection should be considered similar to any other viral infection.

C. Hepatitis C virus infection is viewed as is hepatitis B and is not a contraindication to participation in sports.

D. Epstein-Barr virus (EBV) infection remains a conflicting problem for sports participation. Initial guidelines on return to play were not based on resolution of splenic abnormalities and reflected a belief that splenic rupture could occur after clinical and serologic resolution of the infection. These guidelines emphasized a conservative approach to return to play, limiting participation for a minimum of 2 to 3 months and, if possible, to 6 months. Subsequent information has demonstrated an enlarged spleen by ultrasound in 100% of patients scanned, but with complete resolution by 28 days. No outcome data are available on athlete return to play at early time periods, but the guidelines in Section VI and in Chapter 24 are recommended.

VI. Abdomen

A. Splenomegaly. Under normal circumstances, the spleen is protected by the rib cage. Enlargement of the spleen increases its risk for injury because portions of the spleen may no longer be protected by the rib cage.

1. Athletes with splenomegaly should be precluded from contact/collision, limited contact/impact, and strenuous noncontact sports.
2. The athlete may return to sports when the spleen has returned to normal size or is at least non palpable on physical examination.
   a. Return-to-play decisions should be individualized according not only to the size of the spleen but to the type of activity in which the athlete participates (e.g., return to a strenuous noncontact sport may be advisable whereas return to a contact/collision sport may not).

b. The usefulness of serial measurements of the spleen by ultrasound is controversial as the spleen may be significantly enlarged but completely protected by the rib cage.

3. **Infectious mononucleosis** is a very common cause of splenomegaly in adolescents and young adults.
   a. Splenic rupture, though rare, is the most common cause of death in infectious mononucleosis and most commonly occurs in the initial 3 weeks of the illness.
   b. It is recommended that patients with infectious mononucleosis be disqualified from strenuous noncontact as well as all contact sports for the first 3 weeks of illness.
   c. Return-to-play criteria depends on physical examination findings and type of activity in which the athlete participates.
      (1) After 3 weeks, if the patient is feeling up to activity and the spleen in nonpalpable, a return to strenuous noncontact sports is permitted.
      (2) Disqualification for contact sports should be continued for an additional week (one full month) after the onset of the illness. When the athlete resumes contact sports, the spleen should be non palpable.

B. Hepatomegaly. The liver is normally protected by the rib cage. The liver is at increased risk of injury when it is enlarged due to loss of bony protection.
1. Athletes with an enlarged liver should be disqualified from contact/collision and limited contact/impact sports.
2. Return to play may be allowed when the liver returns to normal size.

C. Active hepatitis. Active hepatitis may cause hepatomegaly which would put the patient at increased risk for liver injury, as described in the hepatomegaly section above. Patients with active hepatitis also pose a risk to teammates and competitors because the different forms of hepatitis are transmissible through blood products as well as through the fecal/oral route. Therefore, patients with active hepatitis should be precluded from competitive sports in which the risk of transmission is high.

D. Inguinal hernia
1. Athletes with small inguinal hernias may participate in all levels of athletics.
2. Surgical repair should be considered for patients with large or symptomatic inguinal hernias because the risk of incarceration and strangulation is increased.

VII. Musculoskeletal System

The following are general return-to-play recommendations for athletes who have sustained an acute musculoskeletal injury. Specific injuries, their diagnosis, treatment, and return-to-play recommendations are discussed afterwards and elsewhere in this book.

A. Range of motion. The athlete should attain normal, pain-free range of motion (ROM) before return to play is considered.
1. Range of motion exercises are incorporated early into the rehabilitative process. ROM may be facilitated by performance of exercises in an ice slush and later facilitated by use of local heat.

B. Muscular strength. Strength of the injured side should be within 90% of that of the uninjured side.
1. This is usually assessed during physical examination; however, certain instruments are available for assessing muscular strength and may be utilized in certain situations (e.g., Cybex testing in a patient with a knee injury).
2. Antagonist muscle group should be adequately strong to prevent further injury (e.g., patients with underdeveloped hamstring musculature as opposed to quadriceps musculature may be at increased risk for anterior cruciate ligament injuries).

C. Pain-free activity at functional levels. Sports-specific activities should be included in the rehabilitation program. Athletes who are unable to complete sport-specific activities successfully in a pain-free manner should be precluded from return to their sport until they can do so.

D. Fractures. In general, an athlete with a fracture should not be allowed to participate in competitive athletics, especially if the fracture is unstable or displaced. In many situations, an athlete may participate with an acute fracture.
   1. Patients with nondisplaced scaphoid fractures may compete in a short arm thumb spica cast (if the sport allows players to compete in casts).
   2. Patients with stable metacarpal or phalangeal fractures may also participate with the appropriate cast if the sport allows casts to be worn during competition.

E. Spine injuries represent the most significant of all musculoskeletal limiting conditions.
   1. Spinal cord injury documented by magnetic resonance imaging (MRI) is generally accepted as an absolute contraindication to further participation. Injuries with symptoms referable to the spinal cord but without documented MRI lesions such as spinal cord neurapraxia may be considered a relative contraindication.
   2. Spinal column instability as defined by the criteria of White et al. is an absolute contraindication to return to sports. These criteria include (1) more than 3.5 mm horizontal displacement of adjacent vertebrae evident on lateral or flexion-extension views, (2) more than 11 degrees of rotation difference to either adjacent vertebrae evident on lateral view or flexion-extension view of the cervical spine.
   3. Acute spine fractures of either the body of the vertebrae or the posterior elements are an absolute contraindication to participation. In general, however, when these fractures heal, return to play is acceptable. Notable exceptions include (1) vertebral body fracture with a sagittal component; (2) comminuted fractures of the vertebral body with displacement into the spinal canal; (3) healed fractures associated with pain, neurologic findings, or limitations in ROM; (4) healed displaced fractures involving the lateral masses with resulting facet incongruity; and (5) fracture of the vertebral body with or without displacement, with associated posterior arch fractures and/or ligamentous laxity.

F. Congenital anomalies of the cervical spine in some cases also represent an absolute contraindication to participation in contact sports.
   1. Os odontoideum, odontoid hypoplasia, and odontoid agenesis are absolute contraindications to contact sports.
   2. Congenital fusion of one or two segments of the upper cervical spine (Kipple-Feil anomaly) and atlantooccipital fusion are also absolute contraindications to participation in contact sports (21).
   3. Mass fusion or fusion of one or two segments of cervical spine with limitation of motion, instability, disc disease, or degenerative changes also represent a contraindication to return to contact sports.
   4. Congenital stenosis of the cervical spinal canal is a relative contraindication to participation in contact sports. However, congenital spinal stenosis associated with intervertebral disc disease, ligamentous instability, neurologic symptoms lasting more than 36 hours, degenerative changes, or MRI evidence of cord defects or swelling are absolute contraindications to participation.
   5. Chiari I malformation has also been associated with spinal cord injury in one case report and may also be considered a contraindication to contact sports.

G. Acute cervical disc herniations are a contraindication to participation. Disc–osteophyte complexes associated with cord neurapraxia are also a contraindication to participation. Disc herniations associated with limitations in ROM are also a contraindication. However a conservatively treated disc herniation with no neurologic deficits and normal ROM is not a contraindication to play.

H. Cervical spine fusion is not a contraindication to contact sports if the patient is asymptomatic and neurologically intact with normal ROM. Two- or three-level fusion is a relative contraindication to participation. Fusion of more than two levels is an absolute contraindication to return to sports.

I. Joint instability represents a relative contraindication to sports participation. In certain cases, unstable joints can be braced to reduce symptoms and allow participation. These cases are often determined by the level of play of the athlete, his or her size, and the sports in which they are participating. Rugby, for example, has strict criteria about bracing, and standard derotational braces are illegal. In some cases, the athlete will not feel comfortable or stable enough in a brace to play or the brace may simply not control joint laxity.

VIII. Single-Organ Athletes

There has been a great deal of controversy surrounding disqualification criteria for single-organ athletes. In the past, the loss of a paired organ resulted in disqualification from contact sports and many healthcare professionals still believe that this is a wise course of action. Due to advances in protective equipment, single-organ athletes may now safely participate in many athletic endeavors.

A. The singled eye athlete

1. American Medical Association (AMA) guidelines suggest that single-eye athletes should not participate in contact sports.
    a. Many experts now believe that, with proper eye protection, most athletes with only on eye should be allowed to participate in sports.
        1. Regular streetwear glasses are not adequate protection. Protective eyewear should be made of coated polycarbonate plastic.
        2. Protective eyewear should meet either Canadian Standards Association or American Society for Testing and Materials guidelines.
    b. It is important that the single-eye athlete wear eye protection not only during competitive sports but also during recreational activities.
    c. The proper use of face masks and shields will also help decrease the likelihood of injury to the athlete's remaining eye.
2. One-eyed athletes should not participate in some sports. Among these are boxing and wrestling since protective eye devices are not available for these sports and the risk of eye injury is high.

B. The single-kidney athlete

1. Even though there is very little risk of losing a kidney due to contact sports, guidelines preclude collision sports for athletes with a normal solitary kidney.
2. Protective equipment such as flak jackets may make limited contact/impact sports very safe.
3. Patients whose solitary kidney is abnormal (including pelvic kidney, iliac kidney, multicystic kidney or kidney with an anatomic variance) should be precluded from contact sports.

C. The single-testicle athlete. With use of a protective cup, athletes with a single testicle may participate in all types of sports. Specifically, a cup is required for all contact and collision as well as most limited contact/impact sports. The current widespread use of protective cups makes this issue less controversial than it was in the past, but many athletes are precluded from participation in certain sports due to lack of one testicle.

IX. Miscellaneous Conditions

A. Diabetes is not a contraindication to sports participation unless control is poor and the risk of ketosis and dehydration is significant. Athletes with proliferative retinopathy may be at increased risk of developing retinal and vitreous hemorrhage during exercise. Retinal detachment may also occur. Athletes with diabetes with peripheral neuropathy may be at more risk for foot and ankle injuries, and high-impact exercise and sports may be relatively contraindicated for them. Strategies to prevent hypoglycemia in such athletes during intense exercise should first be devised to minimize risks of symptomatic hypoglycemia during training.

B. Sickle cell trait is not considered a contraindication to sports participation but has been associated with exertional rhabdomyolysis. (See Chapter 28)

X. Conclusion

Medical conditions requiring participation restrictions should be reviewed with the athlete, coaches, parents, and other significant persons. In some cases, the athlete may be redirected to different sports or to treatment options that will allow return to play. The physician should actively assist the athlete in making a decision if treatment options exist and should explain restrictions in terms that all participants in the process of disqualification can understand.

Suggested Reading

American Academy of Pediatrics Committee on Sports Medicine. Recommendations for Participation in Competitive Sports. *Pediatrics* 1988;81(5):737–739.

Dorsen, PJ. Should athletes with one eye, kidney or testicle play contact sports? *Physician Sports Med* 1986;14:130–8.

Nelson WE, Jane JA, Gieck JH. Minor head injury in sports. A new system of classification and management. *Physician Sports Med* 1984;12: 103–7.

The 26th Bethesda Conference. Recommendations for Determining Eligibility for Competition in Athletes with Cardiovascular Abnormalities. January 6–7, 1994. *J Am Coll Cardiol* 1994;24:845–899.

4. EVALUATING THE INJURED ATHLETE

Robert J. Johnson

I. Assessment of the Athlete

A. Assessing the injured athlete on the field, on the sideline, or in the training room is a truly unique medical experience. Physicians must rely only on their history-taking and physical examination skills. Laboratory tests and radiographs are not readily available. In addition, many decisions must be made under the pressure of allowing an athlete to return to practice or competition. These decisions may have a direct effect on the success of the athlete and team. A dictum by which the sideline and team physician must operate is: "When in doubt, the athlete is out."

B. Ethical responsibilities on the field and sideline.
   1. To the athlete
      a. Allow the athlete to participate safely.
      b. Protect the athlete from injury, reinjury, permanent disability, and inadvertent self-inflicted injury.
      c. Provide optimal health care.
      d. Preserve confidentiality regarding dissemination of the athlete's injury or health information.
   2. To the team
      a. Facilitate team success.
   3. To the coach
      a. Facilitate team success.
      b. Educate the coach in matters of importance to the health and well-being of athletes during practice and competition.
      c. Protect from future liability regarding medical issues.
   4. To the institution
      a. Facilitate success.

C. Be certain that the physician's and trainer's roles are well-defined.
   1. Establish protocols and standing orders to be followed in the physician's absence.
   2. These protocols and orders must apply to specific situations:
      a. Emergency care [cardiopulmonary resuscitation (CPR) C-spine stabilization, fractures, dislocations].
      b. Communication.
      c. Emergency transport.
      d. Methods used on the field and in the training room.
      e. Dispensing medications.

II. On the Field

A. Physician responsibilities
   1. Ensure availability of general medical equipment and supplies
   2. Ensure availability of emergency equipment and transport.
   3. Ensure appropriate hospital referral based on specific resources required for the injury or illness.
   4. Ensure proper consultations for the athletes.
   5. Develop proper communications network to
      a. Athlete.
      b. Coach.
      c. Parents.
   6. Provide appropriate supervision of athletic trainers.
      a. Procedures and protocols
      b. Triage
      c. Education

B. The physician must be able to perform a triage function to make one of three decisions.
   1. Transfer the athlete to an emergency department for further evaluation and treatment.
   2. Remove the athlete from the field, with no return to play, and with appropriate and timely follow-up.
   3. Remove the athlete from the field; follow this with observation of the athlete for possible return to play in the same game or practice.
C. In determining if an athlete can return to practice or competition, the physician must keep two questions in mind.
   1. If the athlete returns to play, will the athlete risk furthering the injury?
   2. If the athlete returns to play, is the athlete at increased risk of a second injury at another site?
D. If the physician is working with an athletic trainer, the trainer will make the first assessment on the field. He or she may ask for physician evaluation.
E. If no certified athletic trainer is present, the sideline physician must assume this role and its responsibilities. Use proper bloodborne pathogen precautions.
   1. Be a good observer, watching for injury situations and mechanisms of injuries.
   2. When an athlete is "down," enter the field of play after the official halts play and the game officials permit your entry.
   3. If the situation is emergent, be prepared to use advanced trauma life support (ATLS) techniques.
      a. Airway and C-spine. May have to remove a facemask. May have to use a "log-roll" to gain airway access.
      b. Breathing/ventilation. If stridor with respiration or hoarseness with speech is present, consider laryngeal fracture.
      c. Circulation. Check the carotid pulse for quality, rate, regularity of pulse.
      d. Disability. Conduct a brief survey, which may include a neurologic examination.
      e. Exposure. Inspect the extremities for possible fractures/deformities.
   4. For nonemergent situations, calm and reassure the athlete.
   5. Obtain a brief history about the site and characteristics of the injury.
   6. Perform a brief examination.
      a. Inspect for deformity or swelling.
      b. Palpate for localizing pain or crepitus.
      c. Ask the athlete to perform active ROM and observe the extent of motion or degree of pain associated with attempted motion.
      d. For dislocations and suspected fractures, check CMS (color, motion, sensation).
   7. Determine how to remove the athlete from the field, e.g., with or without assistance, weightbearing.
F. For unconscious or minimally responsive athletes, assume C-spine injury along with closed head injury. Stabilize the cervical spine and transport the athlete to an emergency department for further evaluation and treatment. (See Chapter 5B.)
G. The athlete with brief loss of consciousness or confusion. (See Chapter 5B.)
H. Medicolegal expectations of the physician on the sideline.
   1. The team physician is expected to carry a medical bag with appropriate equipment and to ensure the availability of proper equipment on the sideline (see Chapter 5A and Appendix 4).
   2. The team physician has a duty to provide emergency resuscitative equipment.
   3. The team physician has a duty to provide advanced cardiac life support (ACLS) or have someone immediately available who can provide this service.

III. On the Sideline

The key to the sideline assessment of an athlete is to establish a definite diagnosis or, at least, a critical nondiagnosis.

A. Take a more thorough history, including more detailed information about the mechanism of injury, site of injury, and pain characteristics.

B. Conduct a more thorough focused examination at the site of injury. Remove any protective equipment to simplify visualization and examination of the injured site.
   1. Inspect the injured site.
   2. Palpate the injured site and adjacent areas.
   3. Have athlete perform active, passive, and resisted ROM for comparison of findings for better determination of soft tissue injury as distinct from osseous injury and of stability of injured site.
   4. Perform special tests to establish tentative diagnosis. This may also include appropriate neurologic testing.

C. Determine athlete's status.
   1. If you determine that the athlete's injury requires further and immediate investigation, make the appropriate referral.
   2. If you determine that the athlete cannot return to play but does not need urgent evaluation, ice injuries as appropriate and appropriately protect or immobilize the athlete
   3. If return to play is uncertain, rest and ice the injury as appropriate briefly (10 to 15 minutes), then reevaluate. If symptoms appear improved on reassessment, consider the possibility of the athlete's return to play. The examination should show nearly symmetric ROM and nearly symmetric strength in comparison of injured and uninjured extremities.
   4. If return to play is likely, perform functional testing. Observe for symmetry of function, comparing injured with uninjured sides.

D. Functional tests to perform on the sideline
   1. Upper extremity
      a. Nearly complete ROM
      b. Nearly symmetric strength
      c. Ability to perform upper-extremity skills specific to the sport (throwing, reaching, blocking) effectively and almost pain-free
   2. Lower extremity
      a. Nearly complete ROM
      b. Nearly symmetric strength
      c. Hopping on injured extremity symmetric with uninjured extremity
      d. Performing skills specific to sport (starting, sprinting, cutting, backward running, cross-over step) without significant limp and in a coordinated manner
   3. Head injury. See Chapter 5B and Chapter 31 for return-to-play suggestions.
   4. For other nonmusculoskeletal injuries, return to play is based on physician's clinical judgment and experience.

E. Finally, if the decision is made to permit the athlete to return to play, you must ask the athlete; "Do you feel you are ready to play?" An athlete who answers "no," should not be permitted to return regardless of a physician's clinical decision. Do not force an athlete to return to play if he or she does not feel prepared to participate.

F. When the athlete is prepared to return to play, notify the coach.

G. On the athlete's return to play, observe a series of plays/exchanges to ensure that the athlete performs without favoring the injury. If the athlete favors the injury during the conduct of play, it is prudent to remove the athlete from play.

IV. In the Training Room

In the training room, athletes may present with overuse injuries as well as acute injuries.

A. Acute injuries. Acute injuries may be handled in same way as injuries incurred on the sideline, but there are no audience pressures or urgencies to increase the difficulty of decision making.

B. Overuse injuries.

1. History. The history is likely to differ significantly since most overuse injuries have an insidious onset. The improvement of symptoms with use often seduce an athlete into unwittingly furthering the injury by failing to alter the training routine or to intervene by taking other appropriate measures.

a. It is important for the physician to determine when the athlete's pain occurs during competition or training. Does it hurt only at the start of the workout? Does it feel worse later in the workout or after the workout is completed? Does it hurt throughout the workout? This determination enables the physician to classify the injury by severity based on the training and competition restrictions forced by the injury.

b. Obtain other historical information, including changes in equipment, training, surface, or sport.

2. Examination. The examination for overuse injuries is essentially the same as any diagnostic musculoskeletal examination. It is important to develop a specific diagnosis to enable the sports medicine team to establish a directed treatment program. Examining running shoes or other equipment may assist the physician in making a diagnosis and correcting contributory factors.

V. Risk Management on the Field and in the Training Room

The four Cs of risk management are commonly cited to reduce liability risk.

A. Compassion and concern for the athlete.

B. Communication. It is important to discuss diagnoses, options for treatment, likely outcomes, and the risks of each option fully (i.e., informed consent).

C. Competence. Stay current in all areas of sports medicine.

D. Charting. A complete, legible medical record is a key ally for the physician and athletic trainer.

VI. Summary

Caring for athletes on the field and in the training room is a clinically challenging experience, yet professionally and personally rewarding. By following these guidelines, the physician can provide a safe environment for athletic competition.

Suggested Reading

Baker CP, ed. *The Hughston Clinic sports medicine field manual.* Baltimore: Williams & Wilkins, 1996.

Gallup EM. *Law and the team physician.* Champaign, IL: Human Kinetics Publishers, 1995.

Herbert DL. *Legal aspects of sports medicine.* Canton, OH: Professional Reports Corporation, 1990.

Mellion MB, Walsh WM, Shelton GL, eds. *The team physician's handbook.* Philadelphia: Hanley and Belfus, 1990.

5. EMERGENCIES ON THE FIELD

A. Preparation for Emergencies in Sport

Gordon O. Matheson, Paul Ford, Peter Brukner,
Robert M. Brock, and Robert L. Norris

Most injuries or illnesses that occur during organized sporting events are not immediately life-threatening but occasionally the practitioner is presented with a full-blown life and death situation that requires immediate diagnosis, intervention, and transportation. The most important factors in the successful treatment of serious emergencies are anticipation and preparedness. Because life-threatening emergencies are relatively rare in organized sports, there is a tendency to minimize or even ignore preparedness. In addition, because sports are vastly different in their potential for serious trauma and illness and because wide variation exists in the physical and environmental conditions of sporting venues, it is not possible to develop a single plan for emergency coverage that applies to all events. However, a few general principles exist which, if followed, will provide the practitioner with some measure of assurance in the handling of emergencies if they occur.

The treatment of specific injuries and illnesses is discussed in the second part of this chapter and the reader is referred to the suggested readings at each section's end for literature that covers treatment of specific emergencies. We discuss the two issues of preparedness: factors related to emergency events occurring at venues and factors related to preparedness of the individual medical practitioner.

Venue Preparedness

Many different types of life-threatening emergencies confront the practitioner planning medical coverage, depending on the sport and the event. For example, collision sports such as ice hockey, football, and rugby or high-velocity sports such as luge or alpine skiing carry the small but ever present risk of severe neurologic or musculoskeletal trauma. It is fortunate that organized sporting events usually include provision for the possibility of transport of emergency cases and most often are held at sites from which immediate transfer to a tertiary care facility is available. Nevertheless, it is incumbent on the physician accepting responsibility for emergency coverage to be sure that the following six factors have been addressed prior to the sporting event. Planning meetings should be held well in advance of the event to provide ample time for implementation and should include not only medical staff but also members of the sporting event organizing staff.

Equipment

Equipment checklists are unique to the event and venue, but almost always include spinal immobilization boards and defibrillators or full crash carts. Most often, equipment for full cardiopulmonary resuscitation and transport is supplied by paramedical personnel providing ambulance backup. Because the extent of the inventory of resuscitation and transport equipment and supplies varies with the ambulance company and the training of the ambulance attendants, it is important to review this inventory prior to the sporting event. In addition to a spinal immobilization board, standard equipment should include traction splints, limb splints, oxygen, blankets, and heart rate (HR) and rhythm monitoring equipment.

Other necessary equipment may include tents to protect from heat or inclement weather during treatment of patients, tables or cots for physical examination and treatment, and splints for musculoskeletal injury. The inventory of equipment requires some thought and consultation with other event organizers.

Personnel

Medical personnel at sporting events should, at minimum, have basic cardiac life support (BCLS) certification and physicians should ideally have both advanced cardiac life support (ACLS) and advanced trauma life support (ATLS) certifications. All medical personnel providing coverage should have clearly defined responsibilities in the event of an emergency, including their roles in communication and their areas of geographic coverage. Skill and experience are vital in the event of an emergency. For this reason, wherever possible, availability of a fully outfitted ambulance with trained paramedic personnel is desirable.

Protocols

In life-threatening emergencies, protocols that have been practiced prior to the event can make all the difference with respect to orderly resuscitation of patients and successful outcomes. Good protocols are brief and to the point, but must define such issues as specific job responsibility, lines of communication, lines of authority with respect to decision making, clothing that identifies medical personnel, and transportation routes. Many trivial issues assume great importance during an emergency, including, for example, who should accompany the victim in the ambulance and who cover the post vacated by staff attending the emergency if the event continues.

Protocols can be assessed by staging a mock-up or "walk-through" exercise during the planning phase. This step will help identify deficiencies in planning.

Communication

For medical coverage of sporting events over long distances, cellular phone or radio communication is essential. Medical personnel placed strategically at sites throughout the venue, or roving on any form of transportation from bicycles to skis to automobiles, are the initial contact people when an emergency occurs. Radios permit the implementation of protocols once an emergency occurs and allow a simultaneous sequence of events to be orchestrated, including arranging transportation and alerting the tertiary care center.

Transportation

Transportation must be arranged in advance. Routes to the nearest tertiary-care facility must be mapped out and must be familiar to ambulance personnel.

Tertiary care

Preparedness includes obtaining the cooperation of medical personnel at a tertiary care facility. Specific names and phone numbers of medical staff at the facility should be available for event coverage staff and ambulance attendants.

Individual Preparedness

Each of the medical personnel providing coverage at an event should be trained in BCLS, and, ideally, physicians should have both ACLS and advanced trauma life support (ATLS) certification. Other specific skills necessary for competence in emergency treatment and resuscitation are the subject of clinical training programs and are not covered herein. Physicians providing coverage at events in which there is a risk of serious injury or illness should be skilled in emergency care.

Each physician should have a portable emergency kit that contains the supplies and medications necessary for both minor and major emergencies. Medical kits have been the subject of several publications and different philosophical approaches have been advocated. We believe that a standardized kit should be developed and that it must be self-contained except for supplies normally earned by athletic therapists and trainers. Because emergencies are not common, many kits lack the equipment and supplies necessary for resuscitation. We believe that physicians should be responsible for their own emergency kit, including the equipment necessary for initial airway care and basic cardiopulmonary resuscitation (CPR). The kit then must be set up for life-threatening emergencies and also must contain the supplies and medications commonly needed for minor emergencies. Such a kit has been developed by the Canadian Academy of Sports Medicine. We have modified this kit to include the inventory shown in Table 5-1. The kit is portable and is equipped with back straps that permit travel by foot over longer distances (Fig. 5-1). It contains a number of

Table 5-1. Emergency kit checklist

Airway kit
- Bag valve mask (1)
- McGill forcep (1)
- Laryngoscope (1)
- Straight laryngoscope blade (1)
- Curved laryngoscope blade (1)
- Extra laryngoscope batteries (2)
- Extra laryngoscope bulbs (2)
- Endotracheal tubes, sizes 6–9 (1 each)
- Oral airways, sizes 5.5–12 (1 each)
- 60-cc syringe with catheter tip (1)
- 12-cc syringe (1)
- #11 scalpel blade on metal handle (1)
- cricothyrotomy kit (1)
- #14 intercatheter (1)

Intravenous kit
- Penrose tubing (1)
- Alcohol prep pads (5)
- 3-cc syringes (3)
- 12-cc syringes (3)
- #16 × 1.5″-gauge needles (6)
- #18 × 1.5″-gauge needles (6)
- #22 × 1.5″-gauge needles (6)
- #25 × 5/8″-gauge needles (6)
- Angiocatheters, sizes 14, 16, 18, 20 (6 each)
- Butterfly catheters, sizes 19, 21, 23 (6 each)
- 3x3 sterile gauze (10)
- Betadine swabs (5)
- 1″ Leukofix tape (1)
- $D_{50}W$ (1)
- Ringer's lactate 1,000 ml (2)
- Normal saline 1,000 ml (2)
- I.V. administration sets (4)
- Betadine swabs (4)
- Tube gauze

Eye kit
- Metal eye shield (1)
- Oval eye pads (5)
- Cotton-tipped applicators (5)
- Artificial tears (1)
- Eye irrigant solution (1)
- 1″ Leukofix tape (1)
- Fluorescein eye drops (5)
- Tobramycin drops (1)
- Proparacaine drops (1)
- Contact lens case (1)
- Cobalt blue light (1)
- Mirror (1)
- Pen light (1)

Injectable medication
- 0.25% bupivicaine (1)
- 0.50% bupivicaine (1)
- 1% lidocaine (1)
- 1% lidocaine with epinephrine (1)
- Diphenhydramine (2)
- Dimenhydrinate (2)
- Diazepam (2)
- Tetanus toxoid (2)
- Ketorolac (2)
- Morphine (2)
- Epi Pen (1)
- Prochlorperazine (2)

Injection kit
- 12-cc syringes (3)
- 3-cc syringes (3)
- #16 × 1.5″-gauge needles (3)
- #18 × 1.5″-gauge needles (3)
- #22 × 1.5″-gauge needles (3)
- #25 × 1.5″-gauge needles (3)
- Alcohol swabs (10)

Suture kit
- Alcohol prep pads (10)
- 4-wing Band-aids (5)
- Knuckle Band-aids (5)
- Extra-large Band-aids (5)
- 1″-strip Band-aids (5)
- 3×3 sterile gauze (10)
- 4×4 sterile gauze (5)
- #10, #11, and #15 disposable scalpels (2 each)
- 6-0 nylon (5)
- 5-0 nylon (PRE2 needle) (5)
- 5-0 nylon (FS2 needle) (5)
- 4-0 nylon (5)
- 4-0 Dexon (5)
- 3-0 Dexon (5)
- 12-cc syringes (3)
- 6-cc syringes (3)
- 3-cc syringes (3)
- #25 × 1.5″-gauge needles (5)
- #22 × 1.5″-gauge needles (5)
- #18 × 1.5″-gauge needles (5)
- #16 × 1.5″-gauge needles (5)
- Betadine swabs (5)
- 1/4″ Steri-strips (5)
- Betadine scrub brush (2)
- Purell antiseptic hand wash (1)
- Hibiclens solution (1)
- Triple-antibiotic ointment packs (10)

Save-A-Tooth kit

Antibiotic medications
- Amoxicillin (2)
- Erythromycin (2)
- Penicillin VK (2)
- Bactrim (2)
- Cephalexin (2)
- Doxycyline (2)
- Prochlorperazine (2)
- Cortisporin otic solution (1)

Table 5-1. *(continued)*

Other medications
- Ibuprofen 800 mg (4)
- Naproxen sodium (4)
- Diclofenac (4)
- Diphenhydramine (2)
- Docusate (2)
- Diphenoxylate (2)
- Acetaminophen with codeine (5)
- Albuterol inhaler (2)
- Lotrisone cream (2)

Dressing kit
- 3×3 sterile gauze (10)
- 4×4 sterile gauze (5)
- 4-wing Band-aids (5)
- Knuckle Band-aids (5)
- Extra-large Band-aids (5)
- 1″-strip Band-aids (5)
- Adhesive Telfa pads (5)
- Nonadhesive Telfa Pads (10)
- 2″ Kling rolled gauze (1)
- 3″ Kling rolled gauze (1)
- Duoderm (3)
- 1/4″ Steri-strips (3)
- Bioclusives (5)
- Adaptics (5)
- Benzoin swabs (5)
- Triple-antibiotic ointment packs (10)

Physician diagnostic kit
- Tongue depressors (10)
- Cotton-tipped applicators (10)
- Latex examination gloves (10 pair)
- Pen light (1)
- Sharpie pen (1)
- Black ink pen (1)
- Red ink pen (1)
- Oto/ophthalmoscope (1)
- Stethoscope (1)
- Sphygmomanometer (1)
- Reflex hammer (1)
- Tape measure (1)
- Goniometer (1)
- Alcohol prep pads (10)
- Urine dip sticks
- Oral and rectal thermometers

Large side pocket
- Sterile suture kits (2)
- Sterile gloves (5 pair)
- Nonsterile latex gloves
- Emergency cricothyrotomy set (1)
- Soft cervical collar (1)
- Hard cervical collar (1)
- Foil blanket (1)

Medium side pocket
- Athlete insurance information
- Injury assessment forms
- Prescription pads
- List of banned substances
- Sharps container

Small side pocket
- Biohazard bags

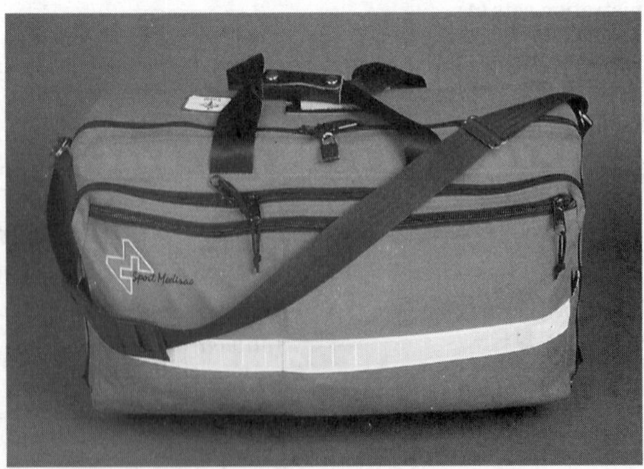

Fig. 5-1. Medical kit available from the Canadian Academy of Sport Medicine, Suite 507, 1600 James Naismith Drive, Gloucester, Ontario, K1B 5N4, Canada. The kit is equipped with shoulder straps that allow easier transport.

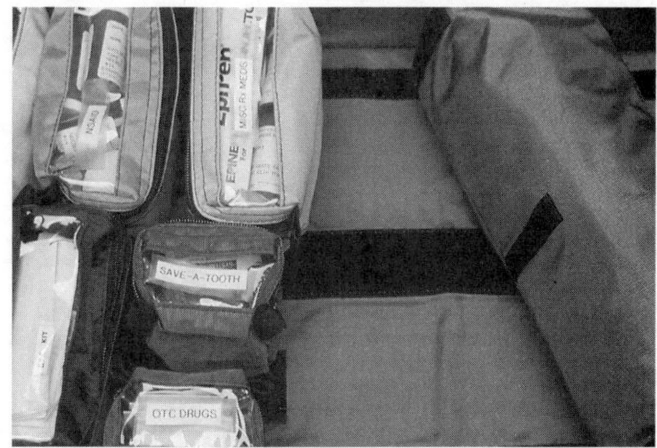

Fig. 5-2. Several smaller bags of differing sizes are held in place by velcro and are labeled for easy identification. The contents of each of these smaller kits is detailed in Table 5-1.

color-coded smaller kits held in place by velcro as shown in Fig. 5-2 (the specific contents of each of these kits is detailed in Table 5-1). When opened, the kits are clearly displayed, together with the examining instruments, intravenous bags, and injectable medications (Fig. 5-3). The emergency resuscitation kit is self-contained, lacking only an oxygen bottle (Fig. 5-4). The physician examining kit is also self-contained (Fig. 5-5).

Most of the kit is self-explanatory, but there are several points worthy of emphasis. Maintaining a patent airway is the most important part of treatment in life-threatening circumstances. The equipment described in Table 5-1 includes not only a mask

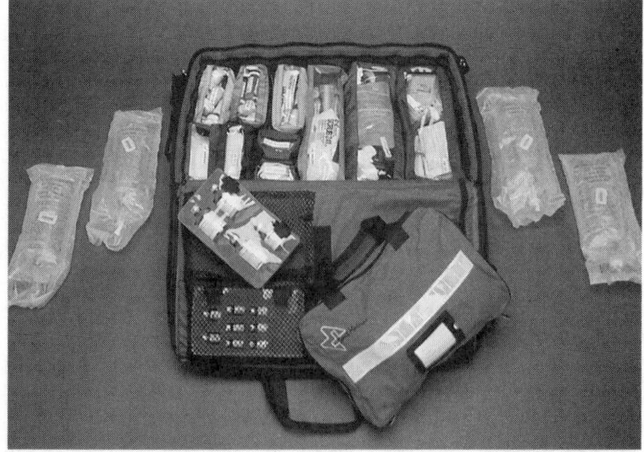

Fig. 5-3. When the bag is opened, immediate access is obtained to intravenous bags, injectable medications, and the physician diagnostic kit. After these are removed, each of the smaller kits is easily identifiable by color and by label and can be accessed and removed easily from the larger kit.

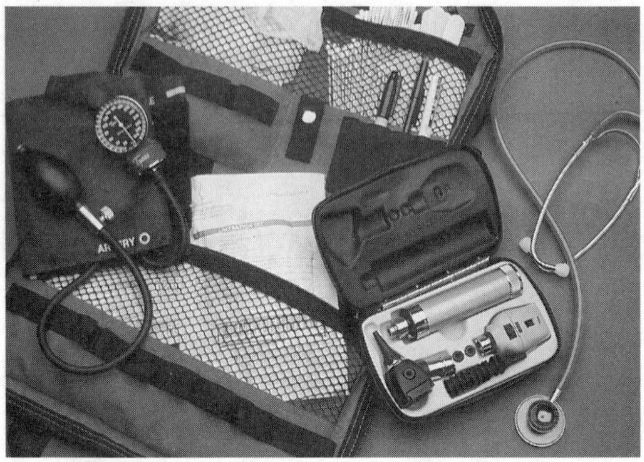

Fig. 5-4. The contents of the physician diagnostic kit (see also Table 5-1).

and airways for ventilating a patient, but also the equipment necessary for more invasive measures that may be required to maintain the airway. Different sizes of straight and curved laryngoscope blades are required to accommodate differences in oropharyngeal anatomy and varying patient size. Extra batteries and bulbs for the laryngoscope are essential. The 12-cc syringe is used to fill the cuff on the endotracheal tube, and the 60-cc syringe can be used as a means of portable suction for clearing the airway. A McGill forcep is essential for clearing the back of the throat in cases of foreign body aspiration. In cases of airway obstruction in which a surgical airway is required, we prefer the cricothyrotomy technique.

A good selection of intravenous catheters is important, depending on the athlete's size and the conditions at the sporting venue. Penrose tubing can be used for a tourniquet, and various needle sizes are included for direct intravenous or intramuscular injections of medications.

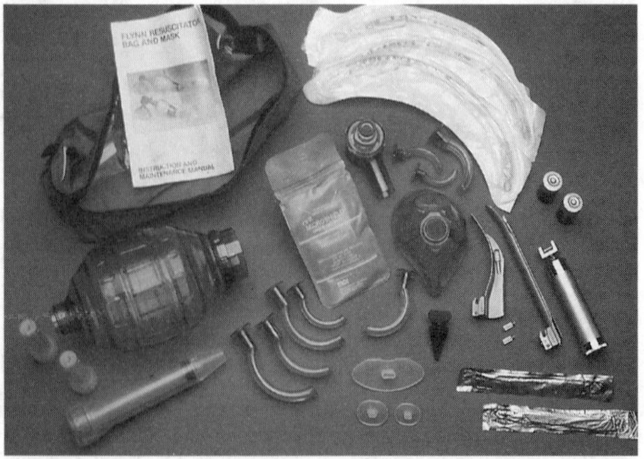

Fig. 5-5. The contents of the airway kit (see also Table 5-1).

The physician diagnostic kit is a separate bag attached by velcro to the top flap of the emergency kit, adjacent to the parenteral medications. This kit can be removed and transported to the field for diagnostic evaluation. Additional equipment is maintained in the side pockets of the bag (Table 5-1).

Summary

The most important aspects of emergency care are preparedness and selection of personnel trained in assessment and treatment of emergency conditions. Preparedness involves six factors: (1) equipment, (2) personnel, (3) protocols, (4) communication, (5) transportation, and (6) tertiary care. Each physician should have a single self-contained medical kit that holds all necessary supplies, equipment, and medication for treatment of minor and major emergencies. These kits are now commercially available, and only minor modifications are required to tailor the kit to the specific needs of the physician.

Suggested Readings

Bock HC, Cordell WH, Hawk AC, Bowdish GE. Demographics of emergency medical care at the Indianapolis 500 mile race (1983–1990). *Ann Emerg Med* 1992;21:1204–7.

Brock RM. The fallen athlete: emergencies of the musculoskeletal system in sport. In: Harries M, Williams C, Stanish WD, Micheli LJ eds. *Oxford textbook of sports medicine.* Oxford University Press, Oxford. 655–65. 1996

Halpern BL. Down man on the field. *Primary Care* 1993;18:883–50.

Haycock CF. How I manage abdominal injuries. *Physician Sports Med* 1986;14:86–99.

Howe WB. The team physician. *Primary Care* 1991;18:763–6.

Kujala UM, Heinonen LM, Lehto M., et al. Equipment, drugs and problems of the competition and team physician. *Sports Med* 1988;6:197–209.

Martinez R. Catastrophes at sporting events. A team physician's pivotal role. *Physician Sports Med* 1991;19:40–4.

Matheson GO. Emergency treatment of life threatening conditions. In: Jackson R, ed. *Sport medicine manual.* Calgary: International Olympic Committee Medical Commission, 1990:159–77.

Ray RL, ed. Emergency treatment of the injured athlete. *Clin Sports Med* (8)1, 1989;1:1–151.

Ray RL, Feld FX. The team physician's medical bag. *Clin Sports Med* 1989;8:139–46.

Rund DA. Management of emergencies. In: Strauss RH, ed. *Sports medicine,* 2nd ed. Philadelphia: W.B. Saunders, 1991.

Tom PA, Garmel GM, Auerbach PS. Environment-dependent sports emergencies. *Med Clin North Am* 1994;78:305–25.

B. Management of On-the-Field Emergencies

Aaron L. Rubin and Robert E. Sallis

I. Introduction: Though a relatively rare event, emergencies do arise during sports competitions. Sideline physicians must be prepared to handle emergency situations in their role as a team physician. The key to effectively providing necessary care to the seriously injured or sick athlete is prior planning and preparation. The sideline physician must take steps to insure they have proper equipment and training to handle the most common emergencies seen during athletic competition. This chapter will review some basic concepts of sideline management, and discuss the evaluation and management of some common emergencies.

II. Field Protocol/Medical Organization:

A. Sideline physicians must have a knowledge of field conditions and possible hazards prior to the onset of the competition. They should arrive at least 15–30 minutes prior to the beginning of the game to inspect the playing surface and introduce themselves to coaches and trainers. They should be updated on any potential injuries or problems existing prior to the game.

B. Sideline physicians should also meet with emergency medical personnel and determine exactly what resources are available should they be needed. They should also take care to locate the nearest phone and be prepared to call for emergency back up if it is not readily availalble.

C. It is also helpful for the sideline physician to introduce himself to the opposing teams coaches and trainers, as well as the referees so these individuals are aware of their presence.

D. During the game, the sideline physician should choose a vantage point that allows him close observation of the competition. Many times the ability to see an injury occur can be of great benefit in making a diagnosis and determining further treatment.

III. Sideline Medical Equipment:

A. Appropriate equipment is needed to manage many athletic injuries and is a reflection of the planning and organization above.

B. See Chapter 5A and appendix 4.

IV. The Decision Process:

A. Probably the most essential role of the sideline physician is determining whether or not an athlete can return to competition. In making this determination, the physician should consider the injured athlete's history, physical exam findings, past problems, and the wishes of the athlete.

1. In evaluating any injured athlete, the first consideration is whether or not emergency treatment is indicated. Usually this is quite evident, based on a brief history and exam.
2. The next consideration is if the athlete continues to compete, is there a potential for worsening of the injury? Injuries such as fractures, ligamentous tears, or severe head or neck injuries have the potential to worsen if an athlete continues in competition.
3. A third consideration is if the athlete continues to compete, will this injury predispose them to another injury? An athlete who is crippled by a leg injury may not have the speed and agility needed to effectively compete, and therefore put themselves at risk for another injury.
4. If the physician feels that the athlete's continued competition will predispose to a worsening of the injury or to another injury, then obviously these athletes need to be held from returning to play.
5. If it has been decided that the athlete may continue to compete, physicians should help suggest protective measures which may allow continued competition. Examples of such measures include taping for an ankle sprain, steri-stripping small lacerations, and padding contused extremities.
6. Underlying this entire decision making process is the necessity for the athlete, coach and parents (of minors) to understand any potential risks of the athlete's continued participation.

B. It is important that physicians take an impartial view in determining return to play issues. They must realize the importance of athletic competition to the athlete, coach and team and do their best to help athletes return quickly and safely to competition. However they must avoid letting coaching decisions affect their judgment. Whether the injured player is the star or a benchwarmer, should not influence the physician's decision making process. Similarly, there is often pressure during a close game to return a key player who is injured. Sideline physicians must not allow their personal allegiance to the team as a fan to cloud their decision process.

V. Disaster Plan:

A. It is critical that physicians who work on the field at athletic competitions have a well organized plan for potential emergencies. Such a plan would include whom to call, which hospitals to use, and who would be in charge in the event of a catastrophic injury.

B. The components of a basic disaster plan should include placing an individual in charge of making medical decisions. Generally this would be the physician, but in his absence a trainer or student trainer, or even a coach, may be called on to temporarily take charge. This individual would be in charge of all medical decisions pertaining to the injured athlete until more experienced personnel are present.

1. The disaster protocol would begin with an immediate on field evaluation to determine the extent of the injury. If a catastrophic injury is suspected, the person taking charge would direct the immediate care of the athlete.
2. Early activation of emergency medical services is critical. Plans should be made for who will carry out this task and how it will be done (i.e., via cell phone, pay phone, radio, walkie-talkie, etc.).
   a. Plans should be thought out as to how emergency transport services would enter the field to assist the downed athlete.
   b. A coach, assistant trainer, administrator, or security person would need to be in charge of opening gates and directing EMS personnel to the downed athlete.
3. Initiation of basic life support should begin with proper assessment of the injured athlete's airway, breathing, and circulation.
4. Other individuals would be in charge for caring for other team members, pulling the injured athlete's medical files, and notifying parents and school officials where needed.

VI. Principles of Injury Evaluation:

A. Potential on field emergencies can be grouped into three basic levels of priority.

1. The **first priority** are those injuries which pose an immediate threat to life. These injuries require immediate treatment followed by transport to a hospital. Such injuries include respiratory arrest, airway obstruction, acute respiratory failure, acute pulmonary edema, or pneumothorax. In addition, problems such as cardiac arrest, anaphylactic shock, seizures, and uncontrolled hemorrhage or hypovolemia, are also potential sideline emergencies of the first priority.
2. The **second priority** injuries are those that are urgent and potentially a threat to life. These injuries require urgent evaluation and treatment when indicated. Such injuries include severe head injuries, severe neck and back injuries, visceral injuries, facial injuries, myocardial infarctions, seizures, burns, severe musculoskeletal trauma, heat stroke, hypothermia, and near drowning.
3. The **third priority** of injuries are those which are not life threatening and are the most common. These include joint or other musculoskeletal injuries, lacerations, skin blisters or bullae, and puncture wounds.

VII. Specific Injuries: Always start with ABCDE: Airway, Breathing, Circulation, Disability, Exposure/Examination.

A. Airway Obstruction/Laryngeal Injuries

1. Airway management must include cervical spine control in the unconscious athlete.
2. The medical team should practice the "log-roll" to move the face down athlete to a position where the airway can be accessed. Facemask must be removed to gain access to the airway. Specialized tools have been developed to remove facemask attachments for football, hockey and other athletic masks. These procedures should be practiced by medical personnel under controlled circumstances on a regular basis.
3. **Airway obstruction** is most often secondary to the tongue falling back in the throat and can be easily treated by proper positioning of the head and neck. The head-tilt method should not be performed on anyone with potential cervical spine injury. The chin-lift or jaw-thrust methods may be used with someone maintaining neck stabilization.
4. The airway may also be obstructed by teeth, mouthguard, or vomitus, which must be cleared.

5. Airway may need to be maintained by use of an oral or nasal airway. If properly trained personnel and equipment are present, endotracheal intubation may be performed to secure the airway.
6. If the airway has been compromised by a neck injury such as a **laryngeal fracture** or **laryngeal edema,** a needle ***cricothytoidotomy*** should be performed.
   a. Find the cricothyroid membrane at the between the thyroid cartilage and cricoid cartilage.
   b. Prepare the area with skin antiseptic if time is available.
   c. Insert a 14 gauge or larger needle thought the membrane entering the trachea.
   d. Ventilate as described below.

B. Breathing

1. Opening the airway is often all that is needed for the athlete to begin breathing again.
2. If breathing does not start spontaneously, mouth-to-mouth, mouth-to-mask, bag-valve-mask resuscitation should be started. High concentration (100%) oxygen should be administered.
3. Asthma and anaphylaxis can also compromise breathing.
   a. Athletes with asthma should be identified during the pre-participation physical with attention to those with severe asthma and respiratory compromise. They should be instructed in prevention and keep an inhaler at the athletic venue.
   b. Treatment of **acute asthma** includes use of albuterol inhaler 2 puffs via a "spacer," 0.3–0.5 ml of 1:1000 epinephrine subcutaneously, 100% oxygen, and transport to medical facility for definitive therapy.
   c. **Anaphylaxis** is an acute allergic reaction that leads to respiratory difficulties. This can occur due to food, medications, or exposures such as a bee sting. Athletes with a history of anaphylaxis should have ***epinephrine injection*** in ready to use syringes that is available commercially. Treatment is the same as asthma with addition of IV fluids and closely monitoring patient for recurrent symptoms.
4. **Pneumothorax** can be caused by trauma as occurs with a penetrating injury to the chest or rib fracture puncturing the lung and allowing air into the pleural space compressing the lung and compromising respiration. Pneumothorax can also occur spontaneously. When this compresses the remaining lung tissue, a **tension pneumothorax** has occurred. Keys to diagnosis include tracheal deviation, hypotension, unilateral absence of breath sounds, distended neck veins, and difficulty breathing. This problem is treated by relieving the tension by placing a ***large bore needle*** into the ***second intercostal space*** along the midclavicular line. Air should return and ventilation should improve. Definitive treatment is provided at the emergency department.

C. Circulation and Cardiac Arrest

1. If the victim is pulseless after establishing airway and breathing, chest compression should be started.
2. Activation of the **Emergency Medical System** should be performed.
3. ***Early defibrillation*** has been shown to be important in survival of cardiac arrest and should not be delayed. If ***Advanced Cardiac Life Support*** and defibrillation is not readily available, the team physician should consider obtaining an ***Automated External Defibrillator*** (AED). These devices internally evaluate cardiac rhythms and deliver a shock when indicated.
4. Appropriate training in ***Basic Life Support*** should be the goal for all individuals working with athletes. All team physicians should have training in Advanced Cardiac Life Support.

D. Disability—Head Injuries

1. Along with neck injuries, head injuries are the most common cause of catastrophic sports injuries. A critical point in evaluating the uncon-

scious athlete is to assume that a cervical spine fracture is present until proven otherwise. It is important that the evaluation of the unconscious athlete begin with in-line traction of the athlete's neck until the cervical spine can be determined to not be injured.

2. **Cerebral concussion** is by far the most common head injury seen by the sideline physician. Milder forms can often times be evaluated and sent back to competition. However, athletes with persistent symptoms, especially memory loss or any loss of consciousness should not be allowed to return to competition.
   a. Evaluation of an athlete's mental status and neurologic status are imperative prior to making decisions on return to play.
   b. Various grading systems, such as those developed by the Colorado Medical Society and the American Academy of Neurology, can be quite useful in helping to make decisions on returning athletes to competition after a cerebral concussion (see Table 31-3).
3. **Cerebral contusions** represent a more severe sports related head injury. This injury is essentially a bruising of the brain. It can best be seen with an MRI, and cannot be diagnosed clinically.
   a. Symptoms include a persistent headache or neurologic defect, and in severe cases may include seizures.
   b. The treatment of cerebral contusion is entirely symptomatic and generally the symptoms resolve over time.
4. **Intracerebral hematomas** are a much more severe effect of sports related head injury. This occurs when there is bleeding into the brain substance itself. This also can be demonstrated on MRI as well as CT scanning.
   a. The symptoms of an Intracerebral Hematoma are similar to contusions but are often more severe and they may rapidly progress to death.
   b. These injuries should be promptly transported to a neurosurgical medical center, as surgical evacuation may be needed to reduce intracranial pressure. If available on the field, the athlete should be intubated and hyperventilated. Also, the administration of intravenous mannitol can help to reduce intracranial pressure as well.
5. **Epidural hematomas** occur from arterial bleeding between the skull and the dura of the brain. This is frequently associated with a temporal skull fracture and involves tearing of the middle meningeal artery. These injuries can also be quite readily seen with CT or MRI scanning.
   a. Classic symptoms of Epidural Hematoma include an initial short loss of consciousness followed by a lucid interval. This lucid period is associated with increasing headache, and a progressive deterioration in the level of consciousness usually within one to two hours.
   b. Treatment of an Epidural Hematoma is prompt surgical evacuation. This injury can be quite treatable if caught early, to prevent permanent neurologic injury. Therefore, quick transport from the field to a neurosurgical center is imperative.
6. **Subdural hematomas** can also occur in association with athletic competition. These are caused by a venous bleed between the brain surface and the dura. These injuries are often associated with damage to the underlying brain tissue. This injury is easily seen on CT scanning or MRI.
   a. Symptoms of a Subdural Hematoma typically depend on the acuity.
      (1) **Acute subdural hematomas** typically present with an unconscious athlete showing focal neurologic signs. This is often associated with significant underlying brain injury and generally has a poor outcome.
      (2) **Subacute or chronic subdural hematomas** can also be seen. These often present with relatively mild symptoms of headache along with mild mental, motor or sensory signs. Symptoms fre-

quently develop over 24 hours to two weeks or more. These are more often seen in older patients due to tearing of the bridging veins between the brain and the dura.

b. Treatment for Acute Subdural Hematoma is surgical evacuation which can lead to full recovery. Thus, stabilization (A, B, C), early recognition of the diagnosis and rapid transportation to a neurosurgical center with administration of high concentration oxygen is imperative.

E. Spine Injuries

1. Cervical spine injury should always be assumed in the unconscious or poorly responsive athlete.
2. Any athlete with neck pain, weakness, numbness, neck spasm or tenderness should be assumed to have a cervical spine injury until cleared by appropriate exam and radiological evaluation.
3. If suspected injury, the athlete should be moved only when adequately trained personnel and equipment are available. The contest should be stopped and the athlete moved directly to the ambulance after proper cervical spine immobilization and the athlete placed on a backboard. If a helmet is worn, it should be left on the athlete with any face guard removed to allow access to the airway. Equipment has been developed for removal of facemasks. The helmet is better removed in the emergency department after appropriate radiographs of the cervical spine have confirmed no fracture is present. Taping the helmet to the backboard and supporting the helmet with sandbags can provide excellent cervical spine immobilization. Shoulder pads should also be left in place, as it is difficult to properly immobilize the athlete if they are removed with the helmet in place.
4. If the athlete is in danger for other reasons, such as in diving accidents or if in respiratory arrest, they may have to be carefully moved so further treatment can take place. Careful immobilization of the spine during rolling the patient in the water or on the field must be accomplished.
5. Lower spine injury requires similar immobilization until complete evaluation in the emergency department has been performed.

F. Abdominal and Pelvis Injuries

1. Injury can rapidly lead to hypovolemic shock secondary to blood loss.
2. Most commonly injured organs are the spleen and liver. This is followed by injuries to the pancreas, bowel, kidney, bladder, and blood vessels.
3. Most athletic injuries involve blunt trauma as opposed to penetrating trauma.
4. Symptoms of significant injury include abdominal pain, nausea, vomiting, and symptoms of shock. Signs include abdominal tenderness, rigidity, and rebound, rigid abdomen, hematuria, and hypotension.
5. Treatment includes intravenous access and fluids, not allowing oral intake, transport to emergency department for definitive diagnosis and treatment.

G. Eye Injuries:

1. Severe eye injuries are occasionally encountered in association with sports participation. Basketball and baseball are two of the most likely sports in which a physician would encounter an ocular emergency.
2. Physicians should be prepared to undertake an appropriate ocular examination and initiate correct early diagnosis and treatment in cases of on-field ocular trauma. Even though most severe injuries will need treatment by an ophthalmologist, it is imperative that the sideline physician do a thorough initial evaluation of the athlete with an injured eye. In general, more mistakes are made because of not looking than not knowing about ocular injury.
3. Examination should begin with a baseline visual acuity test. Athletes who have decreased visual acuity in the injured eye must be assumed to have more serious injury until proven otherwise.

   a. Gross inspection of the eye is often revealing and can demonstrate contusions or lacerations. It is particularly important to observe the eyelids and orbit for symmetry and to look for ptosis of the eyelids or proptosis of the globe on the injured side.
   b. The cornea and the sclerae should be examined closely for signs of perforation or rupture, which is generally indicated by darkly pigmented uveal tissue herniating through a laceration.
   c. The anterior chamber should also be looked at closely for signs of bleeding or hyphema.
   d. Extraocular muscles should be tested in all directions. The pupils should also be checked for size, shape and reaction to light. Lastly, a fundoscopic examination should be undertaken to assess the ocular media as well as the status of the retina.
3. Probably the most common injuries seen by the sideline physician include corneal abrasions, foreign bodies and lacerations in and around the eyelids.
4. More severe injuries may require emergency treatment.
   a. **Lacerations to the globe** generally present with pain and decreased visual acuity. On exam there is often distortion and displacement of the pupil. When this injury is suspected, manipulation should be minimized, the eye shielded and the patient should be referred immediately to an ophthalmologist.
   b. **Orbital blow out fractures** can occur due to direct trauma to the eye, such as occurs with a baseball. These fractures most commonly involve the floor and the medial wall of the orbit, and present with diplopia, obscured maxillary sinus cavity on x-ray, and hypesthesia of the face. CT scanning can be quite helpful when such an injury is suspected. The eye should be covered with a patch and immediate referral for ophthalmologic evaluation as well as ENT evaluation is critical in treating this injury.
   c. **Retinal hemorrhage** and edema can occur as a result of direct trauma to the eye, or by transmission of force to the retinal surface from a contusion injury to the globe. These often present with decreased visual acuity or distortion of vision. These generally are treated symptomatically. The eye should be patched for comfort and the athlete transferred for appropriate evaluation from an ophthalmologist.
   d. **Retinal detachment** can also occur as a result of repeated trauma in and around the eye. These frequently present with complaints of lightening flashes or sparks in the visual field. These can be seen with an ophthalmoscope but often are difficult to visualize. Frequently, in order to see peripheral lens detachment, it is necessary that the pupil be dilated. When this injury is suspected, these need prompt ophthalmologic evaluation and treatment.
   e. **Hyphema** refers to the presence of blood in the anterior chamber of the eye. This usually occurs after a contusion to the globe. When present, this indicates more serious intraocular injury and a risk for delayed re-bleeding. The athlete should be kept quiet and calm and transported for prompt, urgent ophthalmologic evaluation.

H. Dental Injury:

1. The sideline physician may also encounter serious dental injuries as a result of sports related trauma. Generally the severity of the injury can be appreciated by direct inspection and physical examination. Most severe injuries need prompt treatment from ENT physicians and dentists.
2. **Tooth avulsions** are among the more common dental injuries treated on the sidelines. The tooth that is completely displaced from its socket can be replanted with varying degrees of success depending for the most part on the length of time it is out. In general, if it can be reinserted

within a few minutes after avulsion and if the periodontal ligament fibers attached to the roots have not been damaged by rough handling, the avulsed tooth may recover full function.

a. The vitality of the root surface elements can be maintained by replanting the tooth as soon as possible after avulsion. The tooth should be rinsed in tap water to remove loose debris, but the root surface should not be brushed or handled.
b. The tooth can be reinserted into the socket, after which the patient should bite on a piece of gauze or a tea bag to apply gentle pressure to completely seat the tooth. Follow-up evaluation by a dentist for definitive treatment is necessary as soon as possible.
c. If it is not possible to replant the tooth at the time of the accident, the patient should take the avulsed tooth to the dentist as quickly as possible. During transport the tooth should be kept moist. Keeping the tooth in the athlete's mouth inside the buccal vestibule is an excellent place for transport. However, this may not be feasible, especially in athletes who may have altered levels of consciousness. An excellent and often readily available transport medium is milk. Alternatives include commercially available media as well as saline, and a last resort is tap water.

I. Orthopedic Injuries: (see individual chapters for more detailed information)

1. Emergencies include open fractures, hip or knee dislocations, other dislocations and fractures with neurovascular compromise.
2. **Open fractures** should be covered with sterile dressing, splinted in position found and transported to the emergency department. Consider possible fracture with loss of skin integrity in vicinity of injury to be an open fracture until proven otherwise.
3. *Trained individuals* can reduce **knee dislocation** by providing linear traction and straightening the leg. Evaluate and document neurovascular status before and after treatment. The diagnosis of a hip or knee dislocation must be transported to the treating physician in the emergency department so studies can be performed to rule out vascular injury and fracture and to allow for definitive treatment.
4. Other injuries with neurovascular compromise should be splinted and transported to the emergency department. Reduction should be attempted if there will be a significant delay in treatment.
5. Reduction of **hip dislocations** should probably be performed in the hospital under general anesthesia and not on the field. These patients can generally be transported on a spine board for adequate immobilization.
6. Reduction of some dislocations, such as shoulder, finger or elbow, can be attempted to decrease pain unless fracture is suspected. Some dislocations are easier to reduce if done early, before muscle spasm and pain become a factor. All reductions should have follow-up radiological examination to rule out associated fractures. Reductions can generally await transport to the emergency department, and are done on the field for the comfort of the athlete. One should never attempt reduction without proper training and should not consider it inappropriate to refer to the emergency department if in doubt. Neurovascular status must always be checked and documented as part of the examination before and after reduction.
   a. **Shoulder dislocations** can often be reduced more easily soon after it occurs. There are multiple methods for reduction of an anterior-inferior dislocation of the gleno-humeral joint (the most common shoulder dislocation). Neuro-sensory testing must be performed and documented *before and after* reduction. If reduction does not easily occur, the athlete should be splinted in position and transferred to the emergency department. Several simple and effective techniques of on-the-field ***reduction*** of the anterior shoulder dislocation follow:
      (1) One easy method is to have the athlete clasp his hands together and, seated on the ground, wrap these over the knee. He then

leans back applying anterior traction to their shoulder. This usually results in relocation.

(2) If the dislocation is seen rapidly before pain and muscle spasm set in, the humeral head may be reduced by gentle in-line traction.

(3) With the athlete seated or lying down and as relaxed as possible, gradually bring the arm into an overhead position (Statue-of-Liberty) with the shoulder usually reducing when reaching overhead. Then bring arm down across the chest and placed in a sling.

(4) The athlete lies prone on a training table with the affected arm hanging off of the table. Traction is applied or weights applied (starting with 10 kg). Reduction should occur as the athlete relaxes. To aid in this reduction, the outer, lower edge of the scapula may be manipulated toward the midline to bring the glenoid over the humerus.

b. **Finger Dislocation**

(1) **Dislocation of the metacarpophalangeal joint** can be attempted by flexing the wrist and interphalangeal joint (finger), pulling gentle in-line traction and pushing the metacarpal head into position then flexing the MCP joint. The MCP joint is then splinted in mild (30 degrees) flexion and the athlete sent for appropriate radiography. Repeated attempts at reduction should not be attempted. These are often irreducible by closed means.

(2) **Dislocation of the interphalangeal joint** can be accomplished in a similar manner, pulling in-line traction, hyperextending the phalanx, sliding the base of the phalanx distally opposite the head of the proximal phalanx, and flexing the interphalangeal joint. This is the more common case of dorsal dislocation when the distal bone rides dorsally on the proximal bone. Splinting in 20–30 degrees of flexion and appropriate radiography should follow.

c. **Elbow Dislocation**

(1) Most common dislocation is posterior with the radius and ulna displaced posterior to the distal humerus.

(2) ***Reduction*** with an assistant providing counter-traction, the wrist is grasped and steady traction is applied. Sometimes this can be aided by the assistant gently pushing the olecranon while the wrist is being pulled.

(3) While traction is maintained, gently flex the forearm.

(4) Splint is applied and patient sent for radiographs.

(5) If the dislocation is not directly posterior, reduction in this manner may not be successful. Further, a fracture fragment may block reduction. Thus, if reduction is not easily performed on-the-field or in the training room, referral to an appropriate facility for radiographs and reduction is necessary. Splinting prior to transport will make the athlete more comfortable.

J. Heat Injuries: (see chapter 11 for more detailed information)

1. Heat injuries are commonly seen in athletes participating in sports during the summer months in which temperature and humidity are high. Severe heat injuries have been seen with decreasing frequency in football players, as coaches have come to realize that these injuries are preventable if their athletes consume adequate amounts of water.
2. The most important point is prevention of heat injuries that can be easily accomplished by adequate consumption of water. Athletes must be informed about the importance of drinking water before, during and after exercise.
3. There are spectrum of heat injuries in which the sideline physician will encounter.

a. **Effort-induced muscle cramps** are probably the most common, and early sign of heat related injury. These are thought to be generally due to sodium depletion, along with dehydration. Typically these cramps occur in the calf muscles of the exercising athlete. These can be treated with oral rehydration, stretching and ice on the sideline, and generally are a minor nuisance. After the cramps have stopped, return to play may be allowed.

b. **Heat exhaustion** is a more severe form of heat injury. This typically occurs because of hypovolemia. Athletes with heat exhaustion will show a slight increase in their core temperature (but less than 104°F). Typically, these athletes are sweating profusely and appear flushed. They often demonstrate orthostatic syncope. Treatment of athletes with heat exhaustion involves removing them from competition and placing them in a ***cool environment*** in the shade. Effective cooling can be accomplished with *cool water mist and fans*. Oral *hydration* with cold water is usually all that is necessary. More severe forms may need IV hydration and even brief hospitalization.

c. **Heat stroke** is the most severe form of heat injury. This occurs when there is thermo-regulatory failure. These individuals have extremely high temperatures above 104°F. Often there is no sweating and their skin can appear very hot and dry, though sweating does not preclude the diagnosis of heat stroke. The hallmark of heat stroke is mental status changes, as well as coma and even seizures. Eventually, individuals with heat stroke progress on to multisystem organ failure. Heat stroke has a high mortality, especially if the temperature is above 107°F (42°C) or if coma lasts longer than two hours. The key to treatment of athletes with heat stroke is a *rapid cooling*. This can be accomplished with *cool water mist and fans*, as well as placing *ice packs* over the major vessels in the axilla, groin and neck. Athletes with heat stroke should be transported immediately to a hospital where the administration of cooled intravenous fluids can also be helpful to lower the core body temperature. Often times these athletes need oxygen and mechanical ventilation and intensive treatment of other organ system failures.

d. The key to treating heat related illness is *prevention*. Physicians must be aware of athletes who are at particularly high risk. Various precautions can be taken to decrease the risk of heat related illness:
   (1) Athletes should wear light colored clothing which breathes well.
   (2) It is important that athletes be gradually acclimatized to the heat before vigorous exercise is undertaken. Generally, this period should include 10–14 days of increasing levels of exercise in the heat prior to prolonged participation.
   (3) Most important is that athletes be encouraged to drink water. They need to hydrate, before, during and after their exercise.
   (4) Athletes undertaking daily exercise in the heat should monitor their weight. Athletes whose weight is not returning to the previous day's level should not be allowed to continue participation.
   (5) Finally, athletes should be encouraged to get themselves in good physical condition prior to beginning strenuous practices in a high heat stress environment. Athletes who are in poor condition and attempt to exercise in hot and humid conditions are much more likely to have problems.

K. Other (MI, Bleeding)

1. **Suspected Myocardial Infarction**
   a. More likely to effect older athletes or spectators with risk factors of hypertension, diabetes mellitus, previously diagnosed heart disease, smoking, hyperlipidemia, lack of regular exercise, positive family history of coronary artery disease.
   b. Symptoms include chest pain or tightness, diaphoresis, nausea, dyspnea, and feeling of impending doom.

c. Early access to emergency department care is essential in decreasing morbidity and mortality in myocardial infarction.
d. Immediate electrocardiographic monitoring, early use of aspirin (162 to 325 mg chewed), oxygen at high flow, nitroglycerin, and rapid transport to the emergency department.

2. **Bleeding**
   a. Bleeding must be controlled with attention to preventing blood contamination of other athletic personnel and the physician.
   b. Direct pressure over the wound using sterile gauze held in gloved hand is usually sufficient to stop bleeding.
   c. Excessive bleeding or arterial bleeding, may require emergency department transportation to control bleeding or, in extreme circumstances, blood transfusion.
   d. The blood-contaminated materials must be disposed of following universal precautions.

Suggested Readings

Mellion MB, Walsh WM, Shelton GL (Eds.): *The Team Physician's Handbook, 2nd Edition*. Hanley and Belfus, Philadelphia, 1997.

Sallis R, Massimino F (Eds.): *ACSM"s Essentials of Sports Medicine*. Mosby, St. Louis, 1997.

Cantu RC (Ed.): Neurologic Athletic Head and Neck Injuries. *Clinics in Sports Medicine* 17(1). W. B. Saunders, Jan, 1998.

Fadale PD, Hulstyn MJ (Eds.): Primary care of the injured athlete (Part I and II), *Clinics in Sports Medicine* 16(3 and 4). W. B. Saunders, Jul and Oct, 1997.

6. EVENT COVERAGE

William O. Roberts

I. Medical Team and Prevention Planning

A. Mass-participation events have an inherent risk for medical casualties and should be approached as planned disasters.
   1. The *primary purpose* of the medical team is to ensure competitor safety.
   2. A secondary purpose of the medical team is to prevent emergency room overload.
   3. The risks for different event types are unique, although the general strategy for injury prevention and care is shared from event to event.
   4. The weather, condition of participants, and exact field and course conditions cannot always be predicted and will account for many of the event-to-event differences in injury.

B. The medical operations planning and services can be divided into three phases.
   1. *Pre-event phase* prevention strategies
      a. Develop primary prevention strategies to keep the risk of an event to a minimum for the competitors.
      b. Develop secondary prevention protocols to decrease severity of injury.
   2. During the *event*, implement secondary prevention strategies to halt progression of injury or illness associated with the activity.
   3. After the *event*, analyze the outcomes of the prevention strategies and implement new strategies for the future.

C. Event physicians are not always covered by "Good Samaritan" laws.
   1. Members of the medical team should inform their malpractice carriers.
   2. Event insurance should extend coverage to the medical providers.

II. Preparation for Injury Care at Mass Participation Events

A. Anticipate and prepare for the common problems and the uncommon catastrophes associated with the event type from literature descriptions and from data collection at each specific event.

B. The *predicted incidence* of injury during an event is used to project the needs for staff, supplies, and equipment and can be estimated by the equation: (Anticipated number of participants) × (casualty incidence).
   1. The event-specific variables
      a. can be calculated after 2 to 3 years of experience.
      b. Based on literature ranges as follows:
         (1) Running (41 km), 1% to 20%
         (2) Running (<21 km), 1% to 5%
         (3) Triathlon (225 km), 15% to 30%
         (4) Nordic skiing (55 km), 5%
         (5) Triathlon (51 km), 2% to 5%
         (6) Cycling (variable), 5%
         (7) Nordic skiing (55 km), 5%
   2. The risk of sudden cardiac death in marathoning is in the range of 1:50,000 to 1:100,000 entrants.

C. Casualty types in an endurance event include
   1. Exercise-associated collapse.
      a. Hyperthermic
      b. Normothermic
      c. Hypothermic
   2. Trauma
      a. Macrotrauma is common in collision and contact sports and in high-velocity endurance events.

   b. Microtrauma is common in all repetitive activities and affects the tissues most frequently used.
   c. Skin trauma is common in areas of friction and during falls.
3. Random medical emergencies of low incidence but high public visibility, such as cardiac arrest, insulin shock, asthma, and anaphylaxis are life-threatening and should be considered in the medical plan.
4. Drowning and near-drowning are risks in water events.

D. *Medical protocols* should be agreed upon in advance to speed the diagnosis and treatment of multiple casualties. Some standard intervention protocols include.

1. Exercise-associated collapse
   a. Symptoms include exhaustion, fatigue, nausea, stomach cramps, lightheadedness, headache, leg cramps, and palpitations.
   b. Signs include abnormal rectal temperature, unconsciousness, altered mental status, central nervous system (CNS) changes, inability to walk unassisted, leg muscle spasms, tachycardia, vomiting, and diarrhea.
   c. The classification scheme is outlined in Table 6-1.
   d. The management protocol
      (1) Diagnosis and documentation
         (a) Initiating the medical record
            i) Presenting symptoms
            ii) Medical history
            iii) Vital signs, including rectal temperature, blood pressure, pulse, and respiration
            iv) Mental status and orientation
            v) Walking status
            vi) Other physical examination findings
      (2) Fluid replacement and redistribution
         (a) Ambulation to promote the muscle pump in mild casualties
         (b) Supine position if person unable to ambulate
         (c) Elevation of legs and buttocks to restore pooled blood to the circulation
         (d) Oral fluid intake is the preferred method of rehydration in all mild cases and in moderate cases (persons who can tolerate oral intake)
         (e) Intravenous fluids are administered when patient unable to tolerate oral fluids.
            i) Hyponatremia has been shown to occur in marathon and longer races.
               - May be a reason for poor response to treatment
               - May be a reason to transfer a casualty who is not responding to the usual treatment protocol

Table 6-1. Exercise-associated collapse

Parameter	Mild	Moderate	Severe
Hyperthermic	T≥103°F (39.5°C)	T≥105°F(40.5°C)	T≥106°F (41°C)
Normothermic	97°F≤T≤ 103°F	97°F≤T≤103°F	97°F≤T≤ 103°F
Hypothermic	T≤97°F(36°C)	T≤95°F (35°C)	T≤90°F (32°C)
Key symptoms and signs	No specific symptoms or signs; walk with or without assistance	Inadequate oral intake, extra fluid loss, unable to walk, severe muscle spasm	CNS changes Unconsciousness

CNS, central nervous system.

ii) Avoid administration of intravenous (I.V.) K^+ until the serum K^+ is known.
iii) Lactate should not be used in hypothermic casualties.

(3) Temperature correction and maintenance
(a) Hyperthermic exercise-associated collapse (EAC)
i) Stop exercise.
ii) Move to cool or shaded area.
iii) Remove excess clothing.
iv) Institute active cooling (temperature > 105°F) protocols: (see Chapter 11) until cooled to 102°F.
v) Control continued muscle contractions with diazepam 1 to 5 mg by slow i.v. push.
vi) Monitor temperature every 5 to 10 minutes to assess efficacy of treatment and avoid overcooling.

(b) Hypothermic EAC
i) Handle gently.
ii) Move to warm area.
iii) Remove wet clothing.
iv) Dry skin.
v) Insulate with blankets.
vi) Begin warming protocols (Chapter 12).
vii) Monitor temperature at regular intervals.

(c) Normothermic EAC
i) Maintain temperature.
ii) Monitor temperature if not improving.

(4) Fuel supply for energy replacement
(a) Oral glucose solutions
(b) Intravenous (I.V.) glucose solutions with 5% dextrose
(c) Dextrose 50% in water (D50W) 50 ml by I.V. push
(d) Blood glucose which can be measured from the great toe or ear lobe before using a home glucose monitor

(5) Disposition
(a) Transfer to an emergency facility should be considered if
i) a casualty is not responding to usual treatment.
ii) a severe casualty is not responding rapidly.
iii) automatic transfers criteria are met.
(b) When clinically stable and normothermic, an athlete can be discharged from the medical facility.
(c) Discharge instructions
i) Fluid and energy replacement
ii) Criteria for reevaluation
iii) Follow-up recommendations for severe casualties

2. Leg cramp protocol
a. A neural etiology is suggested by recent evidence
b. Fluid and fuel replacement.
c. Assisted walking
d. Avoidance of massage until athlete is well hydrated.
e. Medications
(1) Consider diazepam.
(a) 1 to 5-mg IV push
(2) Consider Mg^{++} sulfate.
(a) 5-g. i.v. loading dose

3. Advanced cardiac life support
a. If *cardiac arrest* occurs,
(1) the chances of survival are low in the marathon, especially in the last 15 km of the race.
(2) cardioversion should be attempted as soon as the cardiac rhythm is determined.
(3) consider the following *modifications to the ACLS protocol* early in the resuscitation effort:

(a) substrate repletion with 50% dextrose in water.
(b) high-dose intravenous epinephrine (5 to 10 mg).
(c) sodium bicarbonate.

4. Anaphylaxis
   a. Subcutaneous epinephrine
   b. Intramuscular diphenhydramine (50 mg)
5. Insulin shock and/or hypoglycemia
   a. Concentrated oral glucose solutions
   b. Dextrose 50% in water (D50W) 50 ml by i.v. push
   c. Subcutaneous glucagon
6. Advanced trauma life support.
   a. For closed head injury and concussion in sports in which helmets, are used, casualties should be transported with the athlete's helmet on if the airway is open and breathing is adequate.

E. Transfer protocols should be determined in advance.
   1. Participants with suspected cardiac chest pain should be transported to a hospital emergency facility rather than delayed by evaluation in the medical facility at the race.
   2. "Automatic transfers" at the Twin Cities Marathon include cardiac arrest, respiratory arrest, hyperthermia with seizure, rectal temperature less than 94°F, and shock.

F. Integrate all protocols into the Emergency Medical Services system.

III. Protecting the Athletes and Volunteers From Injury

A. Define *hazardous conditions* that will require the event administration to alter, postpone, or cancel the activity.
   1. The usual behavioral adaptations that an individual would follow in normal circumstances are relinquished to the medical team during athletic contests.
   2. Common conditions such as lightning, combined high heat and humidity, cold stress, traction, wind speed, and air pollution can pose risk to life and limb.
   3. Consider the possibilities in advance and decide how the safety plan will be implemented if conditions are deemed hazardous.
      a. The safety plan should include an evacuation alternative and adequate shelter or protection for participants and volunteers.
      b. The protocol should be published in advance.
      c. Risks of the event in the current conditions should be announced at the start.
      d. Volunteer safety should be considered in the event planning.
   4. Heat and cold recommendations
      a. The risk of heat illness increases above 65°F (18°C) or 50% relative humidity.
      b. The American College of Sports Medicine has suggested a temperature cascade for risk modification in endurance running events utilizing the wet bulb globe temperature (WBGT), which measures the combined thermal stress from the wet bulb, dry bulb, and radiant energy or black globe thermometers (WBT, DBT, BGT).
         (1) The WBGT = 0.7 WBT + 0.2 BGT + 0.1 DBT.
         (2) A WBGT thermometer can be purchased from Metrosonics, Rochester, NY (1-716-334-7300).
         (3) A WBGT can be calculated with the following tools:
            (a) a sling psychrometer for dry and wet bulb temperatures.
            (b) a copper toilet bulb painted flat black with an air conditioning thermometer positioned so that the sensor is in the center of the globe for black globe temperature.
      c. A colored-flag system can be used to signal visually the thermal injury risk of current weather conditions to competitors.
         (1) The flags can be displayed at the start and at predetermined sites along the course.

(2) In conditions that are not expected to change the start may be the only site where the flag is displayed.

d. The modified American College of Sports Medicine *color-coded flags* based on WBGT to indicate the risk of thermal stress are:

(1) *Black flag:* Extreme risk—WBGT is above 28°C (82°F).

(a) Races should be canceled, postponed, or modified if conditions exceed this level at starting time.

(b) If the event cannot be cancelled, it may be prudent to advise the participants of the risks and advise no competition.

(2) *Red flag:* High risk. WBGT is 23° to 28°C (73° to 82°F).

(a) This signal indicates that all runners should be aware that heat injury is possible and any person particularly sensitive to heat or humidity should probably not run.

(b) Advise participants to slow pace and stress hydration.

(3) *Yellow flag:* Moderate risk. WBGT is 18° to 23°C (65° to 73°F).

(a) The air temperature and radiant heat load will increase during the course of the race if conducted in the morning or early afternoon.

(4) *Green flag:* Low risk. WBGT is 10° to 18°C (50° to 65°F).

(a) This does not guarantee that heat injury will not occur—only that the risk is low.

(b) Both hyperthermia and hypothermia can easily occur in this temperature range.

(5) *White flag:* Lower risk for hyperthermia, but increasing risk for hypothermia. WBGT is below 10°C. (50°F).

(a) Hypothermia may occur, especially in slow runners during long races, and in wet and windy conditions.

(6) *Blue flag:* Increased risk for frostbite and hypothermia, especially in fast—moving activities. Ambient temperature less than 20°C (–4°F).

(a) Consider cancellation or postponement.

(b) Advise added layers of clothing.

B. An *impaired competitor policy* should be developed and published prior the event to allow the medical staff the opportunity to intervene in cases of suspected heat, cold illness, or suspected cardiovascular compromise.

1. No competitor should be disqualified for medical evaluation.
2. At the Twin Cities Marathon, to proceed in the race, an athlete must
   a. be oriented to person, place, and time.
   b. progress with straight-line movement toward the finish.
   c. maintain a good competitive posture.
   d. look clinically fit.

C. Notify local hospital emergency rooms of the event date, location, start and finish times, and the anticipated casualty types and numbers.

D. Preparticipation screening is probably not cost effective

1. It is useful to have a space on the back of the race bib for name, emergency contact, health problems, allergies, and medications.

E. Education for competitors and volunteers

1. Competitor education should include safety measures and risks for the competitors, recommended fitness levels, hydration recommendations, and medical volunteer identification.
2. Medical volunteers should
   a. "first do no harm."
   b. stay within the limits of training for medical services and licensure.
   c. for recurrent events, use standard colors or uniforms.
   d. be readily available.

F. Race scheduling should be based on the geographic location and anticipated environmental conditions.

1. The event should be planned with the safety of all the athletes given the highest priority during a safe season of the year.

2. Particular emphasis should be directed to the start and finish times, which can markedly alter the injury rates for heat and cold stress.
   a. In potentially hot, humid conditions it is best to start in the early morning hours, that the race will be completed before the temperatures rise into high-risk ranges.

G. Course considerations
   1. The *start* should be located away from steep downhill areas, especially if wheelchair athletes are to participate.
      a. Some variations that may decrease the risk of injury due to crowding at the start include wave (sequential) and split starts.
   2. The *course* should be assessed for hills, turns, and immovable objects, traffic control, altitude changes, and open water, which may increase the risk to the athletes.
   3. The type and location of *course aid stations* should be established.
      a. The options include major aid stations that provide full medical care and minor aid stations that provide comfort care, fluids, and first aid.
      b. Aid stations should be located every 15 to 20 minutes according to the average race pace along the course, i.e., at intervals corresponding to about 15 or 20 minutes of race time. The interval may need to be shortened for very large fields to improve access.
         (1) An alternative to a fixed aid station are mobile medical aid teams in buses or vans supplied with medical equipment.
      c. First-response teams on motorcycles or bicycles equipped with an automatic defibrillator can decrease the time to defibrillation in cases of cardiac arrest.
      d. Some form of shelter for participants who drop out will be necessary in inclement weather.
         (1) School buses can be used for drop outs who are well
         (2) A stationary ambulance or tent provides shelter for drop outs who are ill.
   4. The finish area should be equipped and staffed as a major medical station or field hospital.
      a. The medical area can be subdivided into triage, intensive medical, intensive trauma, minor medical, minor trauma, and skin areas (or tents).
         (1) A medical records coordinator and crew is useful to improve collection of medical data.
      b. The medical team will also be responsible for triage in the finish line chute and postchute areas.
         (1) Sweep teams should patrol the remaining finish areas for casualties.
      c. An advanced life support ambulance should be available for immediate transport to the nearest hospital emergency facility.
      d. Shelter should be available for finishers who are well.
      e. A *dry clothes shuttle* should be provided from the start to the finish area to ensure that warm dry clothing is available to the participants at the finish.
         (1) In cold conditions, a portable clothes dryer will allow casualties to dry sweaty clothing and to leave the medical area when immediate access to dry clothing is not available.

H. Transportation for competitors who cannot finish the event.
   1. Competitors who drop out, even if well will need some form of transportation to the finish area.
      a. 10% to 40% of entrants may drop out.
   2. Ill or injured competitors will have to be transported to prevent progression of illness or injury.
   3. In the finish area, wheelchairs, litters, and stretchers are used to transport casualties who are unable to walk with assistance.

I. A *bloodborne pathogens policy* should be implemented, using modified universal precautions as a minimum standard.
   1. Sharps and contaminated waste disposal should be provided.

J. If a death or other *adverse medical event* occurs a protocol should be in place to inform the relatives and the news media.

IV. Supplies, Equipment, and Staffing for a Mass Participation Event

A. Fluids and foods should be available at the start, finish, and transition areas, and at every fluid station along the course.
   1. Fluid stations should be located at every 15–20 minutes (of the race pace) and every 10 minutes of the race pace for very large fields (more than 15,000).
   2. Fluid quantities
      a. Provide 6 to 12 ounces of each fluid for each competitor at each location.
         (1) Double the fluid amounts for the start, finish, and transition areas.
   3. Fluid types
      a. Water will suffice for shorter races.
      b. Carbohydrate-electrolyte solutions can improve performance for events lasting longer than 50 minutes and may be safer for running distances greater than 42 km.
         (1) Decrease the risk of water overload and hyponatremia.
   4. Cups
      a. Provide three cups per entrant per aid station.
      b. Provide six per entrant at start, finish, and transition areas.
   5. High carbohydrate foods and fruits should be available at the finish and along the course for longer events.
      a. Select foods based on the preferences of the competitors.
   6. The fluid and food types and course locations should be published in advance of the event so that the competitors can use the same fluids in training.

B. The equipment and medical supplies for a major aid station are shown in Tables 6-2 to 6-4, those for minor aid stations are shown in Table 6-5.
   1. Intravenous fluids recommended for events are as follows:
      a. less than 4 hours—$D_5{}^1/_2$ NS or D_5 NS.
      b. more than 4 hours—D_5 NS
      c. It is prudent to avoid fluids containing K^+ until a serum K^+ has been measured.
   2. Medications that have proven useful at the Twin Cities Marathon and other races include
      a. Advanced cardiac life support (ACLS) drug kits with epinephrine, atropine, lidocaine, procainamide, bretylium, verapamil, Na bicarbonate, morphine, $D_{50\%}W$.
      b. $D_{50\%}W$.
      c. Albuterol MDI and nebulizer.
      d. Epinephrine (Epi-pen).
      e. Antihistamine.
      f. Valium.
      g. Acetominophen.

C. Staffing the medical team
   1. Physicians, acute care nurses, paramedics, emergency medical technicians, certified athletic trainers, persons trained in first aid, and nonmedical assistants form the medical team.
   2. Common sources of medical volunteers apart from the hospital and clinic staff include the American Red Cross, Explorer Scouts, community ambulance services, National Ski Patrol, Civil Bicycle Patrol, Civil Defense, and the National Guard or Armed Services Reserves.

Table 6-2. Medical supplies for an event[a]

Equipment

- Bandage scissors
- Batteries
- Blue light
- Coins
- Cotton tip applicators
- Cups
- Emesis bags (airline type)
- Emesis basin
- Examination gloves
- Eye patch pads
- Flashlight
- Fluorescence stain strips
- Measuring tape
- Moist towelettes (individual)
- Oto-ophthalmoscope
- Paper
- Paper bags (lunch size)
- Pen
- Plastic bags (Ziploc)
- Red bag
- Reflex hammer
- Safety pins
- Sharps box
- Slings
- Sphygmomanometer
- Stethoscope suction machine
- Thermometer (rectal):
  - Clinical
  - High temperature
  - Low temperature
- Tin snips
- Tongue blades
- Urinals
- Water jug

For trauma

- Aluminum padded splint
- Back board
- Blankets
- Cast padding (3″, 4″, 6″ rolls)
- Cervical collar (hard)
- Cervical collar (soft)
- Crutches
- Elastic bandage (2″, 3″, 4″, 6″ rolls)
- Garbage bags
- Ice
- Ice chest
- Knee immobilizer
- Plastic bags
- Sand bags
- Screwdriver
- Splints
  - cardboard
  - inflatable
- Stretcher
- Turkey baster (suction bulb)

For skin and wound care

- Lidocaine 1%
- Alcohol swabs
- Bacitracin ointment
- Band-Aids
- Benzoin adherent
- Elastic bandage (4″ & 6″)
- Forceps
- Irrigation syringe or bag
- Kling gauze
- Nasal packing
- Needle holder
- Needles (30, 25, 22, and 18 gauge)
- Normal saline for irrigation (250 mL to 1,000 mL)
- Petroleum jelly
- Provodine iodine rolls)
- Scalpel (#10, #15, #11)
- Scissors
- Silvadene cream
- Soap (small can shave cream)
- Steri-strips
- Sterile gloves
- Sterile barrier (full and fenestrated)
- Sterile dressing (2″×2″, 4″×4″, 8″×7½″)
- Sterile basin
- Suture (3-0,4-0, and 5-0 nylon)
- Suture kits
- Syringes (10 cc, 5 cc, and 3 cc)
- Tape
  - Adhesive (½″, 1″, 2″)
  - Paper (½″, 1″ rolls)

For airway & ALCS

- Bulb suction or turkey baster
- Cricothyrotomy kit
- Defibrillator and monitor
- Endotracheal tubes (3 mm, 5 mm, 7 mm)
- Laryngoscope (plastic—adult and pediatric size)
- Mouth-to-mouth mask
- Nasal pharyngeal airway (three sizes)
- Oral airway (three sizes)
- Oxygen tank and administration set
- Ventilation bag, mask, and reservoir with $C0_2$ whipple

Intravenous fluid

- Butterfly catheter (18, 22, and 25 gauge)
- D5% ½ NS (or D5%NS) – 500 mL
- Intravenous administration sets
- Tourniquet
- Vein catheters (16, 18, and 22 gauge)

Medications

- Acetaminophen
- Albuterol nebs
- Albuterol MDI
- Atropine
  - Cardiac
- $D_{50}W$ (50 mL)
- Demerol
- Diazepam
- Diphenhydramine
- Epinephrine 1:10,000
- Epinephrine 1:1,000
- Lidocaine (Local)
- Morphine
- Sodium bicarbonate
- Naloxone
- Nitroglycerin SL
- Opthaine
- Propranolol

Table 6-3. Equipment for mass participation endurance events at major aid stations[a]

Air conditioner
Ambulance: advanced cardiac life support (1)[b]
Blankets, wool or synthetic (150)
Chairs (12)
Clothes dryer, portable
Cots (50)
Extension cords (3)
Fans
Flashlights (6)
Heater (1 propane gas with fuel for 8 hours)
Ice (6 bags, large)
Lights (trouble or clamp) (12)
Massage towels (100)
Mylar-aluminum or plastic blankets (6,000)
Plug strips (3)
Portable toilet (1 at finish tent)
Portable electric generator (1)
Portable telephone (1)
Respiratory humidifier (2)
Security fencing (400 feet)
Shelter
Tents (1—30 × 50 in finish area)[c]
Vehicles
Buildings
Stretchers
Tables (6)
Tubs for immersion cooling
Wash stand (1 at finish tent)
Wheelchairs (10)

[a]See Table 1.
[b]Twin Cities Marathon numbers for 6,500 participants and an injury rate of 1.8 per 1,000 entrants.
[c]Larger size required for higher injury rates.

Table 6-4. Medical supplies for mass participation endurance events at major aid stations[a]

#11 scalpel blades (100)[b]
1/8″ cord (100 feet)[c]
Advance cardiac life support kits (3)
Autolet (1)
Blood glucose sticks (1 box)
Clipboards (50)
Contaminated waste container bag (2)
$D_{50}W$, 50-mL preloads (50)
Defibrillator-monitor pack (1)
Diaper pins (3 dozen)
Examination gloves (3 boxes)
Facial tissue (6 boxes)
Home glucose monitor (1)
Intravenous set-ups (50)

Table 6-4. (*continued*)

Intravenous fluids 500-mL bags
  D5 NS for events >4 hours
  D5 ½NS for events <4 hours (50)
Medical record forms (200)
Oxygen tanks with regulators and masks (2)
Pens (50)
Physician's kit (see Chapter 5A)
Sharp instrument disposal container (2)
Thermometer covers (200)
Thermometers (rectal)
  High-temperature range–110°F (1)
  Clinical (200)
  Low-temperature range–70°F (10)
Wet wipes (6 boxes)

NS, normal saline.
[a]Estimate numbers for expected casualties.
[b]Twin Cities Marathon numbers for 6,500 participants and an injury rate of 1.8 per 1000 entrants.
[c]To hang intravenous bags.

Table 6-5. Minor aid station supplies

#11 scapel blades
4×4 gauze pads
Albuterol MDI
Alcohol or betadine preps
Automatic defibrillator
Bacitracin ointment
Band-Aids
Chairs
Clinical rectal thermometer
Clipboard
Cots
Elastic wrap
Emesis bags
Facial tissue
Garbage bags[a]
Handi-wipes
Ice
Medical record forms
Moleskin
Mylar or plastic "blankets"
Non-sterile tongue blades
Paper towels
Pen
Penlight
Pocket ventimask
Tape (adhesive) ½″ and 1″
Vaseline, 1# jars (3–6)
Wool blankets

[a]Cut head and arm holes to make windbreaker.

Table 6-6. Injury record form[a]

(side 1)
MARATHON MEDICAL RECORD - CONFIDENTIAL 19___
Race # ______ Location: Finish / Aid Station Mile __________ Arrival time _______
Name ______________________________________ Discharge time ______
Age _______ Gender M / F Finish Time __________ Best previous time _______
Previous marathons: Entered ______ Finished ______
Weekly Mileage _________ Pre-race injury/illness Y / N Describe: __________

Skin, Bones, & Joints
Complaint: Pain Blister Abrasion Bleeding Cramps Swelling
Other ________________________
Tissue: Skin Muscle Tendon Ligament Bone
Other ______________________________________

Location:

Toe	R / L	Knee	R / L
Foot	R / L	Thigh	R / L
Ankle	R / L	Hip	R / L
Calf	R / L	Back	R / L

Other ______________________________________

Diagnosis:

Blister	Tendinitis
Sprain	Abrasion
Strain	Cramps
Bursitis	Stress Fx (suspected)
Fasciitis	

Other ______________________________________

Notes:

(side 2)
Medical Problems Arrival time _______
Race # _________ Discharge time _____
Symptoms & Signs

Exhaustion	Lightheaded	Stomach cramps
Fatigue	Confused	Leg cramps
Hot or Fever	Headache	Rapid heart rate
Vomiting	Nausea	Palpitations
Unconscious	CNS changes	Muscle spasms

Other ______________________________________
Mental Status: Alert or Responds to: Voice / Touch / Pain
Orientation: Person/Place/Time
Walking Status: Alone / With assistance / Unable
Other ______________________________________

Time	Temp (rectal)	BP	Pulse	IV fluids	Meds/Rx

Notes:

Diagnosis

EAC	Other _________	IV fluid	Y / N
Hyperthermic: mild / mod/severe	_________	$D_{50}W$	Y / N
Normothermic: mild / mod/severe	_________	ER transfer	Y / N
Hypothermic: mild / mod / severe	_________	Discharge home	Y / N

[a]This form can be printed on two sides of a 8 1/2" x 5 1/2" heavy paper card.

D. *Communications systems* should be developed for the medical team to converse with spotters and medical personnel on the course and at the aid stations.
   1. Such systems can be achieved with portable or hard-wire phones or hand-held radios.
   2. Communications can be coordinated through a central dispatcher located in the medical area at the finish.
   3. The emergency phones access system with 911 can be used in urban areas by any volunteer to summon an ambulance.

E. *Medical and race records* should be kept to document care, calculate incidence of casualties, project future needs, research injury rates and trends, and document environmental conditions. An example is shown in Table 6-6.

V. Postrace Review

Conduct a postrace review to determine what went right and what went wrong and to develop proposed changes to improve the medical delivery system.

VI. Summary

A. Competitor safety is the primary goal of the medical team.
   1. Prevent injuries by not permitting unsafe activity.
   2. Stop the progression of injury once it has occurred.
   3. Relieve the emergency rooms of minor casualties.

Suggested Readings

American College of Sports Medicine. Position statement on the prevention of thermal injuries during distance running. *Med Sci Sports Exerc* 1985; 17:9–14, (to be reissued in 1996).

Elias S, Roberts WO, Thorson DC. Team sports in hot weather: guidelines for modifying youth soccer. *Physician Sportsmed* 1991; 19:67–80.

Jones BH, WO Roberts. Medical management of endurance events, In: *Guidelines for the team physician.* Cantu RC, Michell LJ, eds. Philadelphia: Lea & Febiger, 1991:Ch. 28 in ACSM.

Laird RH. Medical care at ultra endurance triathlons. *Med Sci Sports Exerc* 1989; 21 (suppl 5):222–5 1989.

Roberts WO. Exercise associated collapse in endurance events: a classification system. *Physician Sports Med* 1989; 17:49–55.

Robertson J. *Sports medicine manual for long distance running.* Indianapolis: The Athletics Congress/USA. 1986.

II. CONDITIONING

7. BUILDING AEROBIC POWER

Carl Foster and Curtis Brackenbury

Whether an athlete is simply beginning systematic training for an upcoming season or is recovering from some particular illness or injury, the term "get in shape" will almost invariably be used. Other than applying to some ultraspecialized athletes (e.g., competitive weight lifters), the term "get into shape" almost invariably implies improving aerobic power. Even athletes in sports that are largely anaerobic in terms of the specific energy systems used during competition (football, baseball) find that preseason improvements in aerobic power allow better recovery during subsequent sport specific practices. Therefore, with very few exceptions, building aerobic power is a conditioning factor common to all athletic participants.

Assessment

Except in older persons, those with known cardiovascular, respiratory, or metabolic disease or risk factors for developing these diseases, there are few contraindications to aerobic exercise training that are not otherwise included in the preparticipation physical or under the term "good clinical judgment." Accordingly, diagnostic testing is probably not indicated for most patients likely to be treated by "sports medicine" physicians. However, many of the same techniques that are used with diagnostic graded exercise testing can be useful in terms of assessing exercise capacity and providing advice regarding exercise training. Common to most exercise capacity tests is evaluation of the maximum oxygen uptake ($\dot{V}_{O_2max}$), which is regarded as the best single index of aerobic power. $\dot{V}_{O_2max}$ can be expressed in a variety of ways. Most common are: (1) the gross value (L/min), (2) the value normalized for body size (ml/min/kg body weight), (3) the value normalized for body size and an assumed average resting metabolic rate (METs), or (4) normalized as percentages of age- and sex-associated norms. All have their place. In ordinary clinical practice (without the availability of gas exchange technology necessary for the direct measurement of $\dot{V}_{O_2max}$), the use of either METs or percentage predicted values is probably most useful.

The Bruce treadmill protocol is the exercise test most commonly used in the United States and can serve equally well for diagnostic studies or for simple exercise capacity assessment (Table 7-1). With either a portable heart rate (HR) monitor or electrocardiogram (ECG), the maximal HR can be determined. Because much of exercise prescription is based on HR and because the individual maximal HR is widely variable in relation to norms, advice about how to train effectively is best given based on a measured maximal HR. Under ideal conditions, the exercise protocol will be completed without use of handrail support. However, a large percentage of athletes will feel compelled to use the handrails during their exercise test. Because equations for estimating $\dot{V}_{O_2max}$ are available for both nonhandrail-supported and handrail-supported exercise (Table 7-1), whether the patient uses handrail support or not is not critical. If it is inconvenient to use the Bruce treadmill protocol, recent data suggest that $\dot{V}_{O_2max}$ can be estimated from the estimated V_{O_2} requirement of the last treadmill exercise stage completed without reference to a specific exercise protocol on the basis of the following equations:

$$\dot{V}_{O_2max} = 0.69 * (\dot{V}_{O_2}\text{ requirement}) + 3.3 \text{ (handrail support allowed).}$$

$$\dot{V}_{O_2max} = 0.87 * (\dot{V}_{O_2}\text{ requirement}) - 7.1 \text{ (no handrail support allowed).}$$

A calibrated cycle ergometer can be used just as effectively as treadmill testing to assess exercise capacity The exercise capacity must be corrected for body size since large unfit persons will still have a fairly high absolute exercise capacity measured in watts. On the basis of an exercise protocol that increases 25 W/min, METs can be estimated from the Watts of the last completed stage and body weight shown in Table 7-2.

Table 7-1. Treadmill exercise protocols

Bruce

Time (min)	Speed (mph)	Grade (%)	METs achieved	
			No HRS	With HRS
1	1.7	10	1.8	1.7
2	1.7	10	3.0	2.9
3	1.7	10	4.6	4.4
4	2.5	12	5.2	5.0
5	2.5	12	6.0	5.6
6	2.5	12	6.6	6.4
7	3.4	14	7.3	6.9
8	3.4	14	8.2	7.5
9	3.4	14	8.6	8.3
10	4.2	16	9.7	9.0
11	4.2	16	11.0	9.6
12	4.2	16	12.1	10.3
13	5.0	18	13.3	11.0
14	5.0	18	14.5	11.6
15	5.0	18	15.7	12.2
16	5.5	20	16.8	12.9
17	5.5	20	17.9	13.6
18	5.5	20	18.9	14.2

Modified Bruce

Time (min)	Speed (mph)	Grade (%)	METs achieved	
			No HRS	With HRS
1	1.4	0	1.8	1.7
2	1.7	5	3.0	2.9
3	1.7	10	4.6	4.4
4	2.0	11	5.2	5.0
5	2.4	11	6.0	5.6
6	2.5	12	6.6	6.4
7	2.8	14	7.3	6.9
8	3.2	14	8.2	7.5
9	3.4	14	8.6	8.3
10	3.6	16	9.7	9.0
11	3.8	16	11.0	9.6
12	4.2	16	12.1	10.3
13	4.2	18	13.3	11.0
14	4.6	18	14.5	11.6
15	5.0	18	15.7	12.2
16	5.0	20	16.8	12.9
17	5.3	20	17.9	13.6
18	5.5	20	18.9	14.2

Table 7-2. Calculation of functional capacity (METs) during cycle ergometry

	Body Weight (lbs)												
Watts	120	130	140	150	160	170	180	190	200	210	220	230	240	250
10.000	2.200	2.000	1.900	1.800	1.700	1.600	1.500	1.400	1.300	1.300	1.200	1.200	1.100	1.100
20.000	2.900	2.600	2.500	2.300	2.100	2.000	1.900	1.800	1.700	1.600	1.600	1.500	1.400	1.400
30.000	3.500	3.200	3.000	2.800	2.600	2.500	2.300	2.200	2.100	2.000	1.900	1.800	1.800	1.700
40.000	4.100	3.800	3.600	3.300	3.100	2.900	2.800	2.600	2.500	2.400	2.300	2.200	2.100	2.000
50.000	4.800	4.400	4.100	3.800	3.600	3.400	3.200	3.000	2.900	2.700	2.600	2.500	2.400	2.300
60.000	5.400	5.000	4.700	4.300	4.100	3.800	3.600	3.400	3.300	3.100	3.000	2.800	2.700	2.600
70.000	6.100	5.600	5.200	4.900	4.600	4.300	4.000	3.800	3.600	3.500	3.300	3.200	3.000	2.900
80.000	6.700	6.200	5.800	5.400	5.000	4.700	4.500	4.200	4.000	3.800	3.700	3.500	3.400	3.200
90.000	7.400	6.800	6.300	5.900	5.500	5.200	4.900	4.600	4.400	4.200	4.000	3.800	3.700	3.500
100.000	8.000	7.400	6.900	6.400	6.000	5.600	5.300	5.100	4.800	4.600	4.400	4.200	4.000	3.800
110.000	8.600	8.000	7.400	6.900	6.500	6.100	5.800	5.500	5.200	4.900	4.700	4.500	4.300	4.100
120.000	9.300	8.600	8.000	7.400	7.000	6.600	6.200	5.900	5.600	5.300	5.100	4.800	4.600	4.500
130.000	9.900	9.200	8.500	7.900	7.400	7.000	6.600	6.300	6.000	5.700	5.400	5.200	5.000	4.800
140.000	10.600	9.800	9.100	8.500	7.900	7.500	7.000	6.700	6.300	6.000	5.800	5.500	5.300	5.100
150.000	11.200	10.400	9.600	9.000	8.400	7.900	7.500	7.100	6.700	6.400	6.100	5.900	5.600	5.400
160.000	11.900	10.900	10.200	9.500	8.900	8.400	7.900	7.500	7.100	6.800	6.500	6.200	5.900	5.700
170.000	12.500	11.500	10.700	10.000	9.400	8.800	8.300	7.900	7.500	7.100	6.800	6.500	6.200	6.000
180.000	13.100	12.100	11.300	10.500	9.900	9.300	8.800	8.300	7.900	7.500	7.200	6.900	6.600	6.300
190.000	13.800	12.700	11.800	11.000	10.300	9.700	9.200	8.700	8.300	7.900	7.500	7.200	6.900	6.600

Table 7-2. *(continued)*

	Body Weight (lbs)													
Watts	120	130	140	150	160	170	180	190	200	210	220	230	240	250
200.000	14.400	13.300	12.400	11.500	10.800	10.200	9.600	9.100	8.700	8.200	7.900	7.500	7.200	6.900
210.000	15.100	13.900	12.900	12.100	11.300	10.600	10.000	9.500	9.000	8.600	8.200	7.900	7.500	7.200
220.000	15.700	14.500	13.500	12.600	11.800	11.100	10.500	9.900	9.400	9.000	8.600	8.200	7.900	7.500
230.000	16.400	15.100	14.000	13.100	12.300	11.500	10.900	10.300	9.800	9.300	8.900	8.500	8.200	7.900
240.000	17.000	15.700	14.600	13.600	12.700	12.000	11.300	10.700	10.200	9.700	9.300	8.900	8.500	8.200
250.000	17.600	16.300	15.100	14.100	13.200	12.500	11.800	11.100	10.600	10.100	9.600	9.200	8.800	8.500
260.000	18.300	16.900	15.700	14.600	13.700	12.900	12.200	11.500	11.000	10.400	10.000	9.500	9.100	8.800
270.000	18.900	17.500	16.200	15.100	14.200	13.400	12.600	12.000	11.400	10.800	10.300	9.900	9.500	9.100
280.000	19.600	18.100	16.800	15.700	14.700	13.800	13.000	12.400	11.700	11.200	10.700	10.200	9.800	9.400
290.000	20.200	18.700	17.300	16.200	15.200	14.300	13.500	12.800	12.100	11.500	11.000	10.500	10.100	9.700
300.000	20.900	19.200	17.900	16.700	15.600	14.700	13.900	13.200	12.500	11.900	11.400	10.900	10.400	10.000
310.000	21.500	19.800	18.400	17.200	16.100	15.200	14.300	13.600	12.900	12.300	11.700	11.200	10.700	10.300
320.000	22.100	20.400	19.000	17.700	16.600	15.600	14.800	14.000	13.300	12.700	12.100	11.600	11.100	10.600
330.000	22.800	21.000	19.500	18.200	17.100	16.100	15.200	14.400	13.700	13.000	12.400	11.900	11.400	10.900
340.000	23.400	21.600	20.100	18.700	17.600	16.500	15.600	14.800	14.100	13.400	12.800	12.200	11.700	11.200
350.000	24.100	22.200	20.600	19.300	18.000	17.000	16.000	15.200	14.400	13.800	13.100	12.600	12.000	11.600
360.000	24.700	22.800	21.200	19.800	18.500	17.400	16.500	15.600	14.800	14.100	13.500	12.900	12.400	11.900
370.000	25.400	23.400	21.700	20.300	19.000	17.900	16.900	16.000	15.200	14.500	13.800	13.200	12.700	12.200
380.000	26.000	24.000	22.300	20.800	19.500	18.300	17.300	16.400	15.600	14.900	14.200	13.600	13.000	12.500
390.000	26.600	24.600	22.800	21.300	20.000	18.800	17.800	16.800	16.000	15.200	14.500	13.900	13.300	12.800
400.000	27.300	25.200	23.400	21.800	20.500	19.300	18.200	17.200	16.400	15.600	14.900	14.200	13.600	13.100

METs, average resting metabolic rate.

Table 7-3. Predicted values

Age	Max HR	Male Treadmill METs	Female Treadmill METs	Male Cycle METs	Female Cycle METs
20.000	200.000	14.000	11.600	12.150	9.750
22.000	198.000	13.700	11.400	11.850	9.550
24.000	196.000	13.400	11.200	11.550	9.350
26.000	194.000	13.100	11.000	11.250	9.150
28.000	192.000	12.700	10.800	10.850	8.950
30.000	190.000	12.400	10.500	10.550	8.650
32.000	188.000	12.100	10.300	10.250	8.450
34.000	186.000	11.800	10.100	9.950	8.250
36.000	184.000	11.500	9.900	9.650	8.050
38.000	182.000	11.200	9.700	9.350	7.850
40.000	180.000	10.900	9.500	9.050	7.650
42.000	178.000	10.500	9.300	8.650	7.450
44.000	176.000	10.200	9.100	8.350	7.250
46.000	174.000	9.900	8.900	8.050	7.050
48.000	172.000	9.600	8.600	7.750	6.750
50.000	170.000	9.300	8.400	7.450	6.550
52.000	168.000	9.000	8.200	7.150	6.350
54.000	166.000	8.700	8.000	6.850	6.150
56.000	164.000	8.300	7.800	6.450	5.950
58.000	162.000	8.000	7.600	6.150	5.750
60.000	160.000	7.700	7.400	5.850	5.550
62.000	158.000	7.400	7.200	5.550	5.350
64.000	156.000	7.100	6.900	5.250	5.050
66.000	154.000	6.800	6.700	4.950	4.850
68.000	152.000	6.500	6.500	4.650	4.650
70.000	150.000	6.100	6.300	4.250	4.450
72.000	148.000	5.800	6.100	3.950	4.250
74.000	146.000	5.500	5.900	3.650	4.050
76.000	144.000	5.200	5.700	3.350	3.850
78.000	142.000	4.900	5.500	3.050	3.650
80.000	140.000	4.600	5.300	2.750	3.450
82.000	138.000	4.300	5.100	2.450	3.250

METs, average resting metabolic rate; HR, heart rate.

Normative values for METs during both treadmill and cycle ergometer exercise tests in relation to age and sex are shown in Table 7-3. These normative values are based on sedentary North American populations, with a "normal" range of variation of 85% to 115% predicted. Accordingly, in most sports medicine applications (e.g., preseason evaluations) exercise capacities in excess of 115% of predicted values probably represent minimal levels of fitness and 130% of predicted values represents more desireable levels of aerobic power.

There are a variety of field tests for $\dot{V}_{O_2max}$. For younger and/or more athletic persons, the best currently available test is based on the relationship between $\dot{V}_{O_2max}$ and performance in a 1-mile run/walk, modified by age, sex, and body mass index (BMI). The full equation is:

$$\dot{V}_{O_2max}\ (\text{ml} * \text{kg}^{-1}) = 108.94 - 8.41*(\text{Mile}) + 0.34(\text{mile})^2 + 0.21(\text{Age} * \text{Sex}) - 0.84(\text{BMI}),$$

where Mile is 1 mile run/walk time in minutes, sex = 0 if female and 1 if male, and BMI = kg/m^2.

In the last few years, the use of portable enzyme-based blood lactate analyzers has had significant impact on the assessment of exercise capacity for several reasons:

(1) Blood lactate may be a more accurate marker of sustainable exercise capacity than $\dot{V}_{O_2max}$, (2) maximal testing may not be required, (3) HR targets for exercise training can be developed on the basis of the blood lactate response to exercise, (4) the portability of HR monitors and blood lactate analyzers facilitate field evaluation. Normative data have been less systematically collected for blood lactate responses to exercise than for $\dot{V}_{O_2max}$. At present, evaluation of exercise capacity using blood lactate technology is, like gas exchange technology, beyond the scope of most clinical settings and requires the support of appropriately trained exercise physiologists.

Training Guidelines

Exercise works in much the same dose–effect/dose–side effect way as most drugs. The components of exercise dose are the frequency, intensity, and time (FIT) of the exercise session. Frequency and time of training are fairly easy to assess. In many sports medicine applications (e.g., general fitness), training frequencies of three to four times weekly for 20 to 40 minutes produce excellent results. Obviously, in athletes who are particularly dependent on endurance, greater total amounts of training are indicated. However, even the most serious endurance athletes rarely perform more than three to five "heavy" training sessions per week. Generally, increases in $\dot{V}_{O_2max}$ of about 20% are possible in previously sedentary individuals in 6 months of training. Generally, the fitter the person at the beginning of the training period, the less improvement will be observed. Although more difficult to obtain, blood lactate-based methods of assessment will be more revealing of changes occurring in already athletic persons than of changes in $\dot{V}_{O_2max}$ or incremental exercise test performance.

Most of the "art" of prescribing exercise is related to intensity, which may be assessed in relation to % $\dot{V}_{O_2max}$, % HR_{max}, %HR reserve (difference between resting and maximal HR), or HR in relation to blood lactate. At the same time, intensity is the factor most potent relative to the development of basic endurance and the most difficult to manage relative to side effects. The more rapidly a person wishes to achieve desired levels of fitness, the more important is intensity. With fairly intense training, very good progress may be evident in as little as a few weeks. We have observed increases of 5% to 10% in $\dot{V}_{O_2max}$ (L/min) in speed skaters and ice hockey players (who are quite fit even during vacation periods) over the course of 10 weeks of summer training. However, intense training is generally less comfortable and requires a relatively well-motivated person.

General guidelines for exercise prescription are shown in Table 7-4. For serious endurance athletes, the training plan is usually based on %HR_{max} zones. The relative proportion of training time with the HR in defined zones is the subject of intense debate. Most authorities recommend that no more than 25% of the total training time should be performed at loads exceeding the aerobic–anaerobic threshold (blood lactate ≥ 4.0 m*M* or HR ≥ 80% max). A simpler method of estimating exercise intensity is the rating of perceived exertion (RPE), developed by Gunnar Borg of Sweden. This method links quantitative indices of perceived exercise intensity and verbal anchors (Table 7-5). For most purposes, RPE values of 3 to 4 relate to 60% to 70%HR_{max} and an RPE of 5 is approximately equivalent to 80%HR_{max}.

Interval Training

Many athletes prefer to use interval training (alternating hard and easy periods) to allow development of both speed and endurance simultaneously. Interval training is usually described in terms of the intensity of hard and easy segments, the duration of the hard segment, and the ratio of hard to easy segments. For general conditioning, an intensity that approximates the greatest achieved load during a maximal graded exercise test, the average pace for a 1-mile run/walk, or 120% of the workload at a blood lactate concentration of 4 m*M* represents a convenient intensity. For aerobic training, fairly brief (10–20 seconds) hard segments with a ratio of 1:1 may be very satisfactory. For young male athletes, this might be represented by 80- to 100-m runs at about 1-mile pace with a new one beginning every 30 seconds. Continued for 15 to 20 minutes, such practice provides both aerobic training and fairly high muscular loading. If the duration of the hard segments becomes greater than about 20 seconds, the ratio of hard to easy must increase (often into the range of 1:2 to 1:4) and the

Table 7-4. General guidelines for exercise training

Parameter	General fitness	Preseason fitness	Endurance
Frequency	3–4 times weekly	3–5 times weekly	6–10 times weekly (2–4 hard sessions)
Intensity			
$\%HR_{max}$	60%–75%	70%–80%	60–70%, 25% 70–80%, 50% 80–90%, 15% >90%, 10%
Time	20–40 min	30–45 min	30–120 min (weekly total ≥ 2.5 race duration)

anaerobic contribution to the exercise bout increases. With specialist endurance athletes, the intensity of the hard segment is often reduced into the range of 90% of HR_{max} or to the HR associated with a blood lactate concentration of 4 m*M*. The duration is often increased into the range of 3 to 5 minutes and the ratio of hard to easy may be 2:1 to 5:1.

Cross-Training

Many athletes prefer to use so-called cross-training either to meet general fitness goals or to continue training despite injuries preventing sport specific training. If muscularly similiar training (e.g., cycling, stairclimbing, or water running by runners) is used, the training value of cross-training, on a minute-by-minute basis, is probably 75% of specific training. If this contributes to greater regularity of training, minimizes the risk of injury in athletes making a comeback, or allows maintenance of fitness during injuries, it is certainly worthwhile. If some sport-specific training can still be performed, even muscularly dissimiliar training (e.g., swimming by runners) probably has 50% of the value of sport-specific training on a minute-by-minute basis.

Progression of Training

One of the hallmarks of aerobic training is its progressive nature. This is comparable to upward titration of various pharmacologic agents. The general rule of thumb is that the total training load should not progress more rapidly than about 10% a week. More rapid progression of the training load is frequently associated with injuries. For young athletes beginning preparation from "ground zero" before an athletic "season,"

Table 7-5. Rating of perceived exertion scale (Borg Scale)

Rating	Verbal description
0	Rest
1	Very easy
2	Easy
3	Moderate
4	Somewhat hard
5	Hard
6	
7	Very hard
8	
9	Very, very hard
10	Maximal

it is probably reasonable to start at about 15 minutes at an appropriate effort (70% to 80% HR_{max}), three times weekly. Because this represents 45 minutes of effort weekly, the ordinary progression would be about 4.5 minutes a week. Rounded, this would suggest 20 minutes three times weekly in the second week, 20 minutes four times weekly in the third week, and 25 minutes four times weekly in the fourth week, progressing to 30 minutes four to five times weekly in 10 weeks. For older or more orthopedically fragile persons, the rate of progression might be slowed somewhat and/or cross-training might be used to minimize the likelihood of orthopedic side effects.

Suggested Readings

American College of Sports Medicine. *ACSM's guidelines for exercise testing and prescription,* (5th ed.) Baltimore: Williams & Wilkins, 1995.

Cureton KJ, Sloniger MA, O'Bannon JP, Black DM, McCormack WP. A generalized equation for prediction of VO2 peak from 1-mile run/walk performance. *Med Sci Sports Exerc* 1995;27:445–51.

Edwards S. *The heart rate monitor book.* Sacramento: Fleet Feet Press, 1992.

Foster C, Lemberger K, Thompson NN. Functional translation of exercise responses from graded exercise testing to exercise prescription. *Am Heart J* 1986;112: 1309–16.

Foster C, Crowe AJ, Daines E, et al. Predicting functional capacity during treadmill testing independent of exercise protocol. *Med Sci Sports Exerc* 1996;28:752–76.

Maud PJ, Foster C, eds. *Physiological assessment of human fitness.* Champaign, IL: Human Kinetics, 1995.

McConnell TR, Foster C, Conlin NC, Thompson NN. Prediction of functional capacity during treadmill testing: effect of handrail support. *J Cardiopulmonary Rehabil* 1991;11:255–60.

8. BUILDING STRENGTH

William J. Kraemer and Fred S. Harman

Exercise Stimulus and Program Design

In the past 25 years, strength training has gained widespread acceptability as an important component of a physical conditioning program for purposes ranging from sport preparation to improving physical fitness and health. Strength is only one performance variable of human skeletal muscle that can be improved using methods involving external resistance universally known as resistance training.

The primary objectives in resistance exercise training programs are to prescribe specific acute and chronic exercise regimens that result in improvements in muscular strength, power, hypertrophy, and/or local muscular endurance. The types of programs customized for specific attainment of these goals yield a variety of workout designs (Table 8-1). The effectiveness of these prescriptions is dependent on the configuration of the exercise stimulus so that chronic application of the exercise sessions specifically dictates the body's adaptational response. The program specificity is thus defined by the frequency of exercise. The body's adaptation to the frequency of training is influenced by several factors regardless of the program design. These factors include (1) individual genetic predisposition to exercise stimulus, (2) the pretraining fitness level, and (3) age. The genetic "ceiling" is the primary basis for the absolute level and/or magnitude of training adaptations. Pretraining fitness levels and age determine the type of initial training program that can be tolerated and percentage of improvement that will be observed. As a person progresses from an untrained to a trained state, the magnitude of strength increases will be larger for untrained persons than for highly strength-trained athletes. It is important that the design of the resistance training program be tempered by realistic goals for training expectations.

Variables That Influence Training Adaptations

Training Specificity

Exercise specificity is defined as the training adaptations achieved by training one muscle group that are not realized in other muscle groups. For example, training adaptations resulting from training the thigh muscles are not realized by the muscles in the arms. Exercise adaptations are specifically related to the mode, velocity, and metabolic demands of exercise and to the joint angles used. Muscle that is not recruited will not realize any training adaptations.

Type of Resistance Exercise

Resistance exercise training is the general heading that encompasses several types of training modalities.

1. **Isometrics.** Isometrics or static resistance training refers to a muscular action in which no change occurs in length of the muscle. The generation of muscular force is insufficient to move the mass. This type of resistance training is performed against an immovable object such as a wall, a barbell, or a weight that exceeds the maximal concentric strength capacity of the person. Visual feedback has been shown to enhance isometric training results. Isometrics can be performed with weak muscle groups working against stronger anatomically opposed muscle groups. Increases in strength from isometric training are related to the number of contractions performed, the duration of the contractions, the type contractions (submaximal or maximal), and the frequency of training. Because in most studies involving this type of training several of these variables are manipulated simultaneously, it is difficult to measure any one variable. In addition, this type of training is highly joint angle specific in that strength increases occur at the joint angle trained and not necessarily at the remaining untrained angles. A carryover effect of about ± 20 degrees around the joint angle at which training is directed.

Table 8-1. Specific characteristics of workouts needed to attain optimal training objectives[a]

One repetition maximum strength

TRAINING OBJECTIVE

Program characteristics

In choice of exercise, the specific types of muscle actions (e.g., concentric or isometric etc.) and movement patterns needed are emphasized.

Exercises to be emphasized (e.g., large muscle groups) are performed earlier than assistance exercises in a training session.

High-intensity (typically less than 10 RM) resistances are varied over time (periodized) 1 to 5 RM (heavy); 6 to 10 RM (moderate); more than 10 RM (light).

A moderate to long duration of rest periods (2 to 7 minutes) are used, especially when heavier resistances are lifted.

A moderate to a high number of sets (3 to 8 sets) is performed for major muscle groups [a low to moderate number of sets is used for assistance exercises (1 to 3 sets)].

POWER

Program characteristics

In choice of exercise, the specific movement patterns for power development are typically related to multijoint total body movements (e.g., Olympic-type exercises such as power cleans, hang pulls and so on) when no momentum ends in a joint when using free weights, eccentric actions are typically deemphasized.

Isokinetic, pneumatic, or hydraulic modalities are used for isolated joint high-speed movements (e.g., bench press), so that deceleration of the mass is not inappropriately promoted.

Exercises to be emphasized are performed earlier than assistance exercises in a training session.

High-intensity (typically less than 10 RM) resistances are varied over the training cycle [(periodized) 1 to 5 RM (90% to 100% of 1 RM) (heavy); 6 to 10 RM (80% to 90% of 1 RM) (moderate); more than 12 RM (less than 80% of 1 RM) (light)], yet rarely is a set of repetitions performed for more than five repetitions in a set, whether a heavy, moderate, or light load is used. Power development lags behind strength as to the load used. Therefore, in a specific set, the number of repetitions performed will be slightly lower than the number in the RM load.

Duration of rest periods is moderate to long (more than 2 to 7 minutes); the heavier the resistance the longer the length duration of the rest period.

A moderate to high number of exercise sets (3 to 6) is used. A low to moderate number of sets is used for assistance exercises (1 to 3).

MUSCLE HYPERTROPHY

Program characteristics

The greatest possible variety of exercise choice or movement patterns, is used, including a large amount of isolation exercises, along with use of concentric and eccentric muscle actions.

A great variety of exercise orders is used; muscles to be emphasized being exercised earlier in a session.

Moderate to high intensity (6 to 12 RM) is used; even greater numbers of repetitions sometimes result when the intensity is lowered at the end of set and additional repetitions are completed. Variation in loads with training is employed.

The rest period is brief (less than 1.5 minutes).

A multiple number of sets is performed per muscle group, including warmup sets (3 to 10).

Table 8-1. *(continued)*

One repetition maximum strength
LOCAL MUSCULAR ENDURANCE
Program characteristics
In choice of exercise, the specific movement patterns and types of muscle actions needed are emphasized.
Muscles to be emphasized in training are exercised earlier in a workout.
Intensity is low (more than 12 RM)
Rest periods are moderately long depending on the number of repetitions in the set (more than 2 minutes).
A low to moderate number of sets is performed per exercise (2–4).

RM, repetition maximum.
[a]Each of the RM load ranges and rest period time ranges (approximate zones) shown implies the use of various narrower ranges within it, the zone depending on the training status of the trainee and the phase of the training cycle.

2. **Dynamic constant external resistance.** Also inappropriately termed "isotonic" training, dynamic constant resistance training refers to training in which force is generated using a constant external load over the full range of motion (ROM). Free weights and stack plate machines are the most common types of equipment. However, the force generated by a muscle or muscles during the performance of these exercises is not constant through the full ROM, but varies with the mechanical advantage of the involved joint (i.e., strength curves).
3. **Concentric and eccentric.** Dynamic muscle actions can be performed with two types of muscle actions. Concentric (muscle shortening) and eccentric (muscle lengthening) actions constitute the two forms of a resistance exercise. The generation of muscular force is higher during the maximal eccentric muscle actions than it is during maximal isometric or maximal concentric muscle actions. Training with eccentric loads greater than 100% of the concentric 1 repetition maximum (RM) has been shown to result in delayed muscle soreness, especially in untrained persons at the start of a resistance training program.
4. **Variable resistance.** Variable resistance exercise incorporates use of equipment with a mechanical device (e.g., lever arm, cam, or pulley) that alters the resistance throughout the ROM of the exercise in an attempt to match the increases and decreases in strength (strength curves) throughout the ROM of the exercise. Studies have demonstrated that although theoretically attractive, due to variations in limb length, point of attachment of the muscle's tendon to the bones, and body size, the construct of one mechanical arrangement that would match the strength curve of all persons for each particular exercise is difficult to conceive.
5. **Isokinetics/hydraulics/pneumatics.** Isokinetics refers to a muscular action performed at a constant angular limb velocity. Unlike in other types of resistance training, there is no set resistance to meet in isokinetics; rather, the velocity of movement is controlled. The resistance offered by the isokinetic apparatus cannot be accelerated; any force applied against the apparatus results in an equal reaction force. Isokinetic, hydraulic, and pneumatic resistances allow rapid movements with resistance but without development of a momentum curve because there is no acceleration of a significant mass. Power development of isolated joints appears to be most effective using these types of equipment.

Development of a Single Workout

Several variables describe each resistance training session, and the combination of variables in a training program determines the type of exercise stimulus presented to the body and, subsequently with training, the body's adaptations. Five basic variables describe a resistance training session: (1) choice of exercises, (2) order of exercises, (3) intensity or load, (4) length of rest periods between sets and exercises, and (5) number of sets. These are termed "acute program variables" and can be used to describe any type of resistance exercise protocol. An infinite number of possible variable combinations in an resistance exercise session may be implemented. Defining exactly what is being done for each acute program variable during a training session enables deliberate modifications in that program based on the adaptive responses of the trainee to a known exercise prescription. A solid history of the needs of the trainee (needs and goal analysis) helps in this process as it relates to the injury prevention, biomechanical requirements of the sport being trained for, and sports metabolic demands. Changes in the exercise prescription are based on the alterations in the acute program variables. Clinical judgment based on testing and achieving training goals provides a quantitative rationale for changes in a resistance training program.

Choice of Exercise

The choice of exercise is related to the specific muscle actions that require training. These decisions can be facilitated by an appropriate biomechanical analysis of the sport and/or injury site profile performed in the needs analysis of the resistance exercise program design process. Changes in the angle of the exercise functionally alters the neuromuscular recruitment patter for the exercise. The type of muscle action (i.e., concentric, eccentric, or isometric) used will affect such variables as strength gains made over the ROM and the spatial orientation of the exercise [i.e., two-dimensional control in resistance exercise equipment (fixed-form movements) versus multidimensional control in the use of free weights (free-form movements)]. Because the prescription of exercise is based on the specific needs of the athlete, no one type of muscle action is superior in every situation; the selection of exercise depends on good clinical judgment. For example, isometric exercise may be indicated in a rehabilitation program in which movement is limited. Conversely, dynamic concentric/eccentric exercises may be necessary during training for a sport. Major considerations must be given to the biomechanical specificity, safety of the exercise at the angle chosen, and the ability of the method to provide appropriate recruitment of muscle fibers.

Order of Exercise

Conventional selection of exercises in resistance training programs has proceeded from large to small muscle groups. In the past 20 years, some competitive lifters have used "preexhaustion" methods in which the opposite sequence pattern of exercises is used. Nevertheless, for maximum intensity to be achieved, large muscles are usually exercised first in an exercise session when strength/power development is the primary concern. Other methods of ordering the exercise include performance of the more complex exercises first, pairing push/pull movements, and pairing exercises for agonist/antagonist muscles. In circuit weight training, order should proceed from arm to leg or arm-arm to leg-leg as the exercises move from station to station. This order selection is related primarily to the pretraining fitness level of the individual. The greater the experience level, the higher the tolerance for consecutive exercises performed per muscle group. Because the resistance commonly used in circuit training is much lighter (40–60% of the 1 RM), this probably becomes more of a concern if the resistance is increased or if the rest periods are reduced to less than 1 minute. The order of exercise will dictate the degree of continuous stress placed on the muscle or muscle group. For example, executing consecutive exercises for the pectorals using the bench press, incline press, and dumbbell flys places an increased duration of stress on the muscles of the chest than does use of the bench press, leg press, and shoulder press.

Exercise Intensity

In resistance training, the intensity of the exercise is determined by the objectives of the program (strength, hypertrophy, power, or local muscular endurance) and the associated masses to be lifted. These resistances are commonly identified as the load of the exercises depending on the method of opposing force created by the exercise equipment. The load is the acute program variable most studied because it is perceived to be the primary component that elicits training adaptations. The basic strategy used to achieve training adaptations as well as provide a framework for decisions regarding intensity is the RM, which is the mass that permits the performance to exhaustion of a chosen number of repetitions without sacrifice of safe exercise form. The RM is a continuum of training zones such as strength/power that is divided by repetition number. Implied in this number is the load that will permit completion of a selected RM (e.g., 10 RM) or completion within an RM zone (e.g., 3 to 5 RM). Also disclosed by the RM is the associated level of strength of the individual (e.g., 1 RM equals maximal force production for slow velocities). From an administrative viewpoint prescribing RM zones is much easier because one knows what the athlete is achieving during each training session. However, some exercises (e.g. Power exercises) still need to be prescribed by % of IRM as they cannot be performed to extreme fatigue. It is important not to go to complete failure to limit joint stress even when using RM zones!

Length of Rest Periods
In resistance training, the amount of rest allowed between sets and exercises must be specified in the program design. This variable appears to be related to the development of high-intensity muscular endurance and muscle hypertrophy. High volume (sets × repetitions) with moderate intensity (e.g., 8 to 10 RM) and short rest periods appears to be the primary configuration of the stimulus for development of exceptional muscle hypertrophy. Toleration of short rest workouts is vital because handling of moderately heavy loads (e.g., 10 RM) together with short rest period lengths (1 minute) can produce disruption in the acid/base system, as indicated by blood lactate levels ranging from 8 to 20 m*M* in young healthy adults. Circuit weight training, in which short rest periods and light loads are used, has not demonstrated large increases in muscle hypertrophy, but high lactate levels have been observed (10 to 14 m*M*/L). The associated moderately heavier loads (e.g., 10 RM) handled for sufficient duration by moderately to highly trained athletes under such low rest conditions may interact with more optimal muscle tissue remodeling mechanisms in the development of greater hypertrophy. Manipulation of the rest period length allows metabolic configuration of the resistance training workout and will have impact on the loads that can be handled for a given set of an exercise. Typically, in programs designed for optimal development of strength and power, longer rest periods are used (more than 2 minutes) allow greater recovery and the ability to lift heavier loads in each set of an exercise. The creative use of rest period length in a training session can save time and can also be a potent tool to stimulate physiologic adaptation specific to the bioenergetics of the sport and physical demands placed on the muscle.

Number of Sets
The number of sets performed for a given exercise has been another acute program variable of considerable interest for 45 years or more. The use of multiple sets for an exercise still appears to be the most effective method of producing more rapid and greater absolute gains in strength, power, and muscle hypertrophy. In untrained persons, few differences are observed in the first 8 to 12 weeks of training with regard to the number of sets as exercise toleration improves. As longer (more than 3 months) programs continue, the volume (sets × repetitions) of exercise becomes more influential if improvements are still desired. Furthermore, the effects of higher volumes of total work influence changes beyond strength, such as body composition, caloric expenditure, and local muscular endurance. The optimal number of sets depends on the specific goal of the program for that muscle or muscle group and on the training level of the athlete. For example, early in a training program, due to the low level of strength fitness, a person may not need much of a stimulus to create an adaptational change. Therefore, performing only one or two sets of an exercise may be more than enough to stimulate the initial training adaptations. Furthermore, some "assistance" exercises may not require as many sets as the "core" or primary

(text continued on p. 83)

Table 8-2. Sample program guidelines using periodization concepts

General Prepreparation phase. Six to 8 weeks used for general strength conditioning to allow the individual to gain toleration of performing a strength training program. Teaching of exercise technique should be stressed with light resistance. Start at a low intensity that allows the trainee to perform at least 12 to 15 repetitions with resistance. Start with a low volume of exercise by using only one or two sets and a low number of exercises. Add exercises as the trainee learns how to perform the exercises properly. The key is to introduce the trainee to the concept of a strength training workout. Usually large muscle group exercises are periodized and small muscle group exercises (e.g., arm curls, leg curls) are performed with a moderate intensity (8 to 10 RM). Nevertheless, these exercises can be periodized like the large muscle group exercises. The number of times that the training cycle phases are performed will be determined by the amount of time available before the season begins. Several shorter cycles are believed to better than one long one; therefore, the duration of each phase has been typically reduced to as little as 2-week cycles. Typically, a minimum of 6 weeks is allowed for the three cycle phases to be completed. Children (prepubescent) and older adults usually train two to three times a week to ensure proper recovery.

Preparation phase. A cycle length of 2 to 4 weeks is chosen that will be used for all of the following lift cycles. This phase formally starts a training cycle because the number of exercises and initial toleration should already be established from the prior cycle. Two to three sets of each exercise should be performed at an intensity that allows 12 to 15 repetitions. This will create a high-volume, low intensity stimulus. A rest period of 1 to 2 minutes is allowed between sets and exercises.

Power phase. Using the same cycle length of 2 to 4 weeks, the trainee uses a resistance that allows only 8 to 10 repetitions and performs two to three sets of each exercise. Rest periods of 1.5 to 2 minutes are allowed between sets and exercises. Again technique is stressed together with progression in the resistance that can be used for the repetitions performed. Sets of 5 with 8–10 RM (70–85% of IRM) can be used.

Strength phase. Using the same cycle length of two to four weeks and using a resistance (children use a different resistance that allows 6–8 repetitions) that allows only three to five repetitions. Trainees perform two to three sets of each exercise. Rest periods of 2 to 2.5 minutes are used between sets and exercises. Again technique is stressed together with progression in the resistance that can be used for the repetitions performed.

Transition phase. As the competitive sport season begins an "in season" program is initiated. The in-season program may vary the workout between heavy, light, and moderate intensities as used below in the method of periodized training. The key is to maintain strength and power but, due to the sport season, to reduce the total amount of exercise

NONLINEAR PERIODIZED TRAINING

1. Initially, a general prepreparation phase identical to that described is used.
2. In the nonlinear periodizing training method, 8- to 12- week cycles of training are used: On different days, the trainee uses a light (12 to 15 RM, 2 to 3 sets, 1 to 2 minutes of rest) day; heavy (3 to 5 RM, 2 to 3 sets, 2 to 3 minutes of rest) day or a moderate (8 to 10 RM, 2 to 3 sets, 1.2 to 2 minutes of rest) day.

   The rationale is that varying the workout within the week allows the athlete with adequate recovery and variation. At the end of a training cycle, the athlete enters an in-season program using the same method of intensity variation but a reduced number of exercises or sets to decrease the volume of training.

exercises for a particular muscle group. Therefore, the acute program variable of the number of sets is a potent tool in development of the exercise volume in a resistance training program. Not all exercises in a workout have to be performed for the same number of sets.

Periodization (Variation in Training)

The primary value of periodization is the manipulation of training variables such as the number of repetitions performed per set, the number of exercises performed, and the rest periods between sets to provide for variation in training and optimize the exercise stimulus. The key to the modern concept of progressive overload is variation and recovery from training. The body needs variation in the exercise stimulus and rest to enhance tissue remodeling. Periodized training has been shown to be superior to single and constant set (e.g., three sets of 6 RM) training in building strength, power, and muscle size. The benefits realized from these variable manipulations include the controlled culmination of a peak athletic performance; larger gains in strength, power, and muscular size; prevention of overuse injuries; prevention of overtraining; and less boredom from training. Resistance training has one of the lowest injury rates (children to adults) per exposure time if the rate of progression is not too fast and, most important, if proper exercise and spotting techniques are used. As adaptation to resistance exercise begins, the volume of exercise can be increased by modifying the program variables, such as intensity. Increases must be gradual and should match an individual's ability to tolerate the exercise stress.

Premature increases in an exercise program can lead to undue cardiovascular and musculoskeletal stress and possible injury. Yet without adequate overload, physiologic adaptation of skeletal muscle does not occur. Therefore a balancing strategy is in effect whereby the exercise stress should be sufficient to elicit physiological adaptation without causing injury. This condition is of special concern when resistance exercise programs are designed for sedentary persons and the elderly. The success of achieving the desired objectives of the resistance training program is dependent on the balanced emphasis of low injury incidence and appropriate degree of physiologic stressor regardless of the type of exercise regimen or equipment used. This balance and the effectiveness of the program is achieved by periodic evaluation through testing, and changes should be made when necessary. Table 8-2 provides some example program guidelines for resistance training using basic periodization concepts.

Suggested Readings

Fleck SJ, Kraemer WJ. *Designing resistance training programs,* 2nd ed. Champaign, IL: Human Kinetics Publishers, 1997.

Fleck SJ, Kraemer WJ. *Periodization breakthrough.* Ronkonkoma, NY: Advanced Research Press, 1996.

Kraemer WJ, Baechle TR. Development of a strength training program. In: *Sports medicine,* 2nd ed. Allman FL, Ryan AJ, eds. Orlando, FL: Academic Press. 1989: 113–27.

Kraemer WJ, Fleck SJ. *Strength training for young athletes.* Champaign, IL: Human Kinetics Publishers, 1993.

Kraemer WJ. Koziris LP. Muscle strength training: techniques and considerations. *Phys Ther Pract,* 1992;2:54–68.

Newton RU, Kraemer WJ. Developing explosive muscular power: implications for a mixed methods training strategy. *J Strength Condition* 1994;16:20.

9. **FLEXIBILITY**

Karl Anthony Salesi

Flexibility may be defined as the range of motion (ROM) possible at a given joint or group of joints. It is therefore incorrect to say that someone is flexible, as the person may be flexible only at a specific joint or joints and have limited motion at other joints, which may limit the person's ability to function normally. Lack of flexibility or hypermobility both may result in awkward patterns of movement and may predispose an athlete to muscular injury. Flexibility may be essential to achieving desired fitness goals but, this idea is often based primarily on observation rather than research.

I. Neurophysiologic Basis

A. Muscle receptors are required for proper muscle function, as they provide continuous information from each muscle to the nervous system.

1. The receptors provide information regarding muscle length and muscle tension and how rapidly length or tension is changing.
2. Receptors that provide this information are muscle spindles, which are found in the muscle belly and provide information on muscle length and the rate of change of length.
3. The Golgi tendon organs in the musculotendinous junctions provide information on muscle tension and information on the rate of change in tension.

II. Types of Responses

A. Static response. The response of both the primary and secondary ending is to provide information to the central nervous system (CNS) regarding length. The muscle spindle is stretched slowly, and the neural impulses generated from this deformation are transmitted from both the primary and secondary endings. The impulse increases in direct proportion to the degree of the stretch. These impulses are transmitted as long as the receptor remains stretched; the nuclear chain fibers are believed to be responsible for this function.

B. Dynamic response. The dynamic response is a function of the primary endings, where the muscle spindle is stretched suddenly. The powerful stimulation of the primary endings results in the rapid rate of change in length and causes extreme activity. The primary receptor transmits this increased number of impulses only while the length is changing. When the length ceases to increase, the rate of impulse charges decreases to the original level except for a small static response. The nuclear bag fibers are believed to be responsible.

III. Stretch Reflex:

This lends itself to the stretch reflex, sometimes termed the myotatic reflex, which indicates that whenever a muscle is stretched, excitation of the spindle causes a reflex contraction of the muscle.

A. Neurocircuitry of the stretch reflex. The stretch reflex is a monosynaptic pathway in the spinal cord that originates in the muscle spindle.

B. Dynamic Stretch Reflex. The dynamic stretch reflex is elicited by strong afferent neural signals from the primary ending of the muscle spindle, where the muscle is suddenly stretched. This signal is transmitted to the spinal cord, which results in an instantaneous reflex contraction of the same muscle from the site of origin of the the signal. The function of this response is to oppose sudden changes in the length of the muscle, such as when a muscle contraction opposes the stretch. This stimulation discontinues a fraction of a second after the muscle stretches to its new length; however, a weak static stretch reflex contraction persists for a prolonged time. This continues to cause a muscle contraction as long as the muscle is maintained at its excessive length and is elicited by a continuous static receptor signal transmitted by both the primary and secondary endings.

IV. Athletic Training Application and Development of Flexibility Programs

A. Two components of a stretch reflex include a phasic or jerky type stretching and a static maintained stretching.
   1. The phasic response or the dynamic response is faster, stronger, and causes a more synchronous discharge from the muscle spindle.
   2. The static response, which is slower and weaker, causes an asynchronous discharge from the spindle.

The key to understanding flexibility is to understand the rate of response of the stretch reflex proportional to the amount and rate of stretching. An example is bouncing movements in stretching that cause the muscle to contract proportional to the vigor of the bouncing.

V. Considerations for Flexibility Program

A. Time: 15 to 20 minutes to stretch the major muscle groups in an organized manner to minimize time.
B. Location: Usually in a gym or field with utilization of all resources available.
C. Sport: With concentration on different areas of the body that may be used more frequently (Examples: Emphasis on upper-extremity flexibility exercises versus lower-extremity flexibility exercises for swimmers and soccer players, respectively).

VI. Therapeutic Methods

A. The basics of stretching require a thorough musculoskeletal examination to rule out contraindications. The procedure or type of stretching depends on type and seriousness of the injury.
   1. Passive stretching may indicate a more serious injury and may require a stretched position to be held for 2 minutes in area of soft tissue restrictions.
   2. Proprioceptive neuromuscular facilitation (PNF): Apply slight traction to the joint to ensure minimal articular movement and have the athlete contract all muscles and resist.

VII. Types of Stretching

Stretching can be defined as any therapeutic maneuver designed to lengthen (elongate) soft tissue structures and thereby increase range of motion (ROM).

A. Ballistic stretching. A rapid stretching movement is often characterized as bouncing. The bouncing method of toe touching, lateral flexion of the trunk with the arms raised overhead, and the pectoral stretch executed by flinging the arms in a transverse abducted position is often used.
   1. Rapid stretches on muscles result in a partial contraction because the stretch reflex is activated.
   2. Ballistic stretching is ineffective in enhancing flexibility, promoting full ROM of motion of a joint as well as promoting relaxation of the muscle.
B. Static stretching. Static stretching involves a slow stretch and maintenance of the position for several seconds to 1 minute.
   1. Static stretching is less likely to produce the myostatic stretch reflex.
   2. Emphasize the importance of relaxing the stretched muscle and achieving full ROM.
C. Proprioceptive neuromuscular facilitation (PNF)
   1. The muscle to be stretched is placed actively to its limited end ROM (longest position).
   2. The athlete forcefully isometrically contracts the muscle to be stretched, using a partner or a wall. This forceful isometric contraction may stimulate the Golgi receptors so that relaxation may be facilitated in the muscle immediately after the contraction. The athlete should contract in a

graded manner to the maximum tension in 2 seconds and then hold for a maximum of 4 seconds.

3. Immediately thereafter, a gentle external force is applied to the segment as the athlete contracts the muscle group opposite to the group being stretched (this stretch is maintained for 4 seconds and is then repeated).

VIII. The Optimal Method of Stretching

The purpose of stretching is to enhance the permanent lengthening and relaxation of the muscle, which ultimately will lead to an increase in flexibility.

A. Slow static stretching is recommended and involves a low application force of longer duration.
   1. Easy stage. The muscle is slowly stretched with little resistance for 20 to 30 seconds and where relaxation should occur and the stretch reflex is inhibited.
   2. Developmental state. An added stretch is used and held for 30 seconds or longer. No painful or drastic stretching should occur during this period. The muscle has time to relax, and a stretch reflex is dissipated again.
   3. There is evidence that slow static stretching causes less muscle soreness than ballistic stretching. Sudden tension is placed on the tissue during ballistic stretching, which can result in small tears in the connective tissue or muscle fibers that can lead to pain and swelling.

B. WARMUP

   Warmup should involve only a related activity that puts the muscle at a physiological advantage, i.e., the muscle actually heats up.
   1. This increases cardiovascular and pulmonary responses whereby where more oxygen is supplied to the working muscles, as a result of a more rapid dissociation between O_2 and hemoglobin at higher temperatures. Vascular responses decrease as oxygen becomes more accessible to the cells. Metabolic processing increases; therefore, muscles improve their ability to contract and relax, resulting in a more efficient and forceful contraction. As muscle viscosity diminishes, *contractions* become easier and smoother, and *more efficient* and therefore require less energy. Activity of the gamma nerve fibers decreases, in turn decreasing occurs and the sensitivity of the muscle spindle to stretching, thereby relaxing the muscle.
   2. Warmup should be intense enough to increase body temperature (5 minutes of progressive muscular exercise) while avoiding general muscular fatigue.
   3. Warmup should include some movement specific to the activity.
   4. The longer the event, generally the shorter the warmup.
   5. Warmup before stretching is not advisable in a cool or cold environment.

C. Because flexibility is specific, stretching exercises should include specific muscle groups used in the specific sport along with general flexibility exercises for each of the major areas of the body.
   1. Stretching will enhance flexibility only of the joints being stretched.
   2. Because there are individual differences in flexibility, flexibility training should not be a contest.

D. While cooling down stretching after post activity allows the following to occur:
   1. Permanent elongation
   2. Reduction in muscle spasm (relaxation)
   3. Removal of metabolic byproducts, reducing muscle soreness

IX. Stretching Application in Sports Medicine

A. Uses in rehabilitation

   Stretching is applied to specific conditions in which adaptive shortening of soft tissue around joints and the subsequent loss of ROM may result from initial injury.

1. Prolonged immobilization (e.g., casting or splinting) after a fracture or surgery, leads to long-term static conditions and often faulty positioning of joints and soft tissue.
2. Neuromuscular disease or trauma often leads to paralysis, spasticity, muscular imbalance, weakness, pain, and difficulty moving through the ROM.
3. Connective tissue and joint diseases lead to pain, muscular spasm, inflammation, and weakness and can alter the structure of soft tissue.
4. Tissue pathology resulting from trauma leads to inflammation, edema, ischemia, hemorrhage, and formation of dense fibrous tissue replacing normal soft tissue. These soft tissues lose their normal elastic and plastic properties, resulting in loss of motion.

B. Uses in injury prevention
Lack of normal flexibility (increased or decreased) potentially predisposes an athlete to injury.
1. Full ROM is necessary for successful execution of athletic skills.
2. Normal resting lengths and adequate excursion of extensibility of the muscle tendon unit may afford some protection against injury.

X. Stretching Programs and Usefulness in Injury Prevention

A. An example of injury is repeated-use injury caused by of a sport that tends to make a muscle too tight. Running increases the likelihood of developing tightness in gastrocnemius and hamstring muscles. Such tightness in the calf could interfere with normal foot function. Tightness in the hamstrings could alter the movement of the leg during the swing phase of running. Therefore, biomechanical problems of the foot or leg can be reduced by proper implementation of a stretching program. Shoulder and elbow injuries can increase the tightness of the external rotator and abductor muscle groups. Therefore, lack of full ROM of a joint as well as lack of proper mechanics could lead to overuse injuries.

B. Increased flexibility or hypermobility can also predispose an athlete to injury; e.g., increased flexibility in the ankle joint can result in inability to exert more force in some movements. However, without the proper amount of strength and coordination to bear weight, the foot can be placed in an inappropriate biomechanical position, predisposing the athlete to some type of injury.

XI. Indications and Contraindications for Stretching

A. Indications
1. When ROM is limited as a result of contracture, adhesions, and scar tissue formation, leading to shortening of muscles, ligaments, connective tissue, and skin.
2. When contractures interfere with everyday functional activities and activities of daily living (ADL).
3. When there is muscle weakness and opposing tissue tightness. Tight muscles must be stretched before weak muscles can be effectively strengthened.

B. Contraindications
1. When a bony block limits ROM.
2. After a recent fracture.
3. Whenever there is evidence of an acute inflammatory or infectious process or when heat and swelling is evident in or around joints.
4. Whenever there is sharp acute pain during joint movement or muscle elongation or when empty end feel is noted where there is no physical or mechanical endpoint; e.g., sharp unusual pain often occurs in acute bursitis during muscle stretching, because no real end of ROM is reached due to pain.
5. When a hematoma or other indications of soft tissue trauma are observed.

6. When contractures are short and soft tissues are providing increased joint stability in lieu of normal structure (or mechanical) stability or muscle strength.
7. When contractures are short and soft tissues are the bases for increased functional activities, particularly in athletes with paralysis or severe muscle weakness.
8. When the point of movement stops or occurs before a normal stop or end feel should have occurred. This may be evident in contracted ligaments or capsules in someone with rheumatoid arthritis or osteoarthritis and is termed premature end feel.
9. The point of movement occurs after a normal stop or extended end feel (frequently termed instability hypermobility).

Suggested Readings

Binder MD, Stuart DG. Responses of la and spindle group II afferents to single motor unit contractions. *Neurophysiol* 1980;43:621–9.

Brady WD, Irion JM. The effect of time on static stretch on the flexibility of the hamstring muscles. *Phys Ther* 1994;74:845–50.

Halbertsma JP, Goeken LN. Stretching exercises: effect on passive extensibility and stiffness in short hamstrings of healthy subjects. *Arch Phys Med Rehabil* 1994;75:976–81.

Sady SP, Wortman M, Blake D. Flexibility training: ballistic, static, or proprioceptive neuromuscular facilitation. *Arch Phys Med Rehabil* 1982;63:261–3.

Smith CA. The warm up procedure: to stretch or not to stretch. *J Orthop Sport Phys Ther* 1994;19:12–7.

III. ENVIRONMENTAL CONCERNS

10. THERMOREGULATION

Peter B. Raven

Because human energy generation for movement is only 25% efficient, 75% of our metabolic energy production is added to the body as heat. When we perform prolonged exercise in ambient environments with temperatures above 22°C (71.6°F), exercise capacity is reduced. More important, when we exercise in excessive heat (more than 30°C or 86°F) or high humidity (i.e., relative humidity above 50%; the higher the humidity, the greater the danger), serious illness or death may occur if adequate care is not taken. Heat illness (or injury) occurs as *thermoregulatory mechanisms* fail to cope with the competing processes of external heat loss and metabolically produced heat. When this occurs, the body's core temperature continues to rise and heat illness may occur, especially if rectal temperature exceeds 39.0°C or 102.2°F. Heat illness has a broad spectrum of symptom severity, ranging from heat cramps and heat-induced dehydration to heat exhaustion and heat stroke.

Thermoregulation

Thermoregulation is the physiologic process by which one's body temperature is regulated. A generalized description of the regulatory process is to consider the body as a balance. The balance point is the central temperature "set point" and is that temperature at which the body's core temperature is regulated. For this balance to be maintained, heat lost must equal heat gained. Regulation of the body's temperature is an active physiologic process; e.g., when the body is hot, it sweats. The regulated central body temperature of the adult human is accepted as 98.6°F or 37°C and ranges between 97°F (36.1°C) to 100.4°F (38.0°C). Oral temperature measurements are approximately 1°F (0.6°C) less than rectal temperature. Core temperatures have both a seasonal (hotter in summer than in winter) and a circadian or diurnal variation of approximately 1°F, lowest in the morning (4 to 6 a.m.) and highest in late afternoon (4 to 6 p.m.). Women have variations in core body temperature related to ovulation; approximately 1°F increase in core temperature at ovulation in regularly cyclic women. Besides the core temperature, the average skin temperature ($\bar{T}_{SK}$) and the average body temperature ($\bar{T}_B$) are additional ways of describing the body temperature. The skin temperature (T_{SK}) is the surface temperature and reflects the ambient environmental temperature, especially in the cold (i.e., the skin is cold in cold temperatures and hot in hot temperatures). The average body temperature ($\bar{T}_B$) is the sum of the weighted average core and skin temperatures:

$$\bar{T}_B = 0.7_{core} + 0.3\ \bar{T}_{SK}.$$

The physiologic factors that add heat to the body include metabolic heat from digestion of food, unconscious tensing of muscles, exercise, and shivering. Environmental heating of the naked body occurs at ambient temperatures above 82.4°F (28°C) and with direct solar radiant heating.

The physiologic factors that result in heat loss are evaporation of sweat (major in humans) and panting (minor in humans, except at high altitude and during helium/oxygen breathing during scuba dives, in which respiratory heat loss can be large). The environmental factors that result in heat loss of the naked body include radiant, convective, and conductive heat transfer when the temperature of the environment is less than 82.4°F (28°C).

The physiologic process of thermoregulation is an active process by which the body physiologically responds to heat loss or heat gained. Heat is gained or lost according to the thermodynamic principals, which encompass a set of physical concepts. The first law of thermodynamics (i.e., heat lost equals heat gained), can be rewritten to summate these physical concepts for humans: $M \pm W \pm K \pm C \pm R \pm E = S$, where

M is metabolism; W is Work [going uphill is positive work (+W) and going down hill is negative work (–W)]; K is conduction; C is convection; R is radiation; E is evaporation; and S is storage. Simply stated, the contracting muscles are the engine that generates heat (more heat is produced in going down hill than in going up hill) which is added to the body. The blood is the coolant which picks up the heat from the muscles and is pumped by the heart to the skin to allow cooling to occur through the physical principles of heat transfer (convection, conduction, radiation). However, because heat is only transferred from a hot to a cold environment when the human exercises in the heat, evaporation of sweat is the only means available for cooling the skin because the environment is hotter than the skin. As the blood passes within the skin it is cooled, and on its return to the working muscles the blood picks up more heat and is then pumped back to the skin to be cooled.

Heat Lost

Heat flows down a gradient, i.e., from hot to cold. All four physical avenues of heat exchanges can play a part in heat loss. The greater the body surface area to body weight ratio, the faster a person will lose or gain heat; e.g., a neonate left in a cool room (24°C) will lose heat much faster than an adult.

1. Conduction. The flow of heat that occurs when objects of two different temperature touch (the heat flows from hot to cold) is conduction. As an example, pick up a bag of ice and notice how quickly your hands become cold. The heat of your hand flows to the bag of ice. Conduction plays a relatively minor part in heat loss.
2. Convection. Heat loss is directly related to air movement across the body because it always reestablishes an optimum heat flow gradient. For any given air temperature, the loss increases with the square of the wind velocity up to 60 mph, i.e. wind chill.
3. Radiation. The rate of cooling of an object varies directly with the thermal gradient between its surface and objects in its environment. The rate of cooling is directly proportional to the fourth power of the difference between the temperatures of the two objects. Changing skin temperature by physiologic means causes the skin-to-air heat gradient to be altered. The means by which humans can change skin temperature is primarily redistribution of blood flow from the central volume circulation (heart, lungs, and splanchnic bed) to provide more blood flow to the skin. In the heat, this redistribution is not stimulated by metabolic drive but is redirected by central nervous system (CNS) innervation of the sympathetic nervous system. However, in the cold, the increased metabolism of shivering and the hormonal stimulation of metabolism by catecholamines and thyroxine provide a stimulus to increase the circulation to the muscles and reduce the circulation to the skin.
4. Evaporation. Evaporation is by far the most important avenue of heat loss in a hot environment. Evaporation of 1 liter of sweat rids the body of approximately 700 kcal. In very hot conditions, heavy exercise may result in whole body sweat rates approaching a maximum of two liters per hour. Dripping sweat is not evaporated and, therefore, does not play a role in cooling, however it does increase the rate of dehydration. As the relative humidity of the environment rises, there is less opportunity for the sweat to evaporate, and the amount of dripping sweat increases.

Heat Gained: Energy Production

1. Exercise. Humans are approximately 25% efficient; therefore, only 25% of energy is used to perform muscular work. The other 75% is added to the body as heat. At the beginning of exercise, blood flow increases to the active muscles to support metabolic demands. At the same time, blood flow to the skin increases to dissipate the enhanced heat production. This increased flow to the muscles and skin occurs because of increased cardiac output (CO) and redistribution of regional blood flow. To compensate for the redirection of blood flow, the body reduces circulation to the visceral organs through sympathetic vasoconstriction. The body's ability to balance these competing demands can be overwhelmed by exercising in conditions of

high external heat load. A high ambient temperature reduces the gradient between the air and skin, reducing effective convective cooling and sweat evaporation. The body attempts to compensate by enhancing skin blood flow and cutaneous blood volume. This peripheral shunting of blood leads to a decrease in central venous pressure, cardiac filling, and stroke volume. In these conditions, the heart rate (HR) must therefore increase to maintain the same CO at a fixed exercise intensity. If the exercise and thermal load are sufficiently severe, the HR can reach its maximum and CO will be insufficient to meet the competing demands. In these conditions, hyperthermia with resultant heat injuries and illness may occur if specific precautions are not taken.

2. During cold exposure, shivering is an involuntary mechanism by which the body adds heat to itself. Unfortunately, it is costly in terms of use of the muscles' energy substrates and is only 11% efficient; i.e., only 11% of the energy generated in producing shivering is added to the body as heat. Table 10-1 summarizes daily heat loss.

Control Theory: Central and Peripheral Integration

The central controller is a thermostat to which our body temperature is referenced is believed to be situated in the anterior preoptic hypothalamus (APH). However, other sites in the hypothalamus (such as the posterior preoptic hypothalamus) have been shown to interact with the efferent responses. In terms of control theory, the APH is the locus of the "set point" about which afferent signals generate an error signal (the error is the difference between the set point temperature and the actual temperature) and, depending on the amount of error, the efferent response occurs. Indeed, the hypothalamus can be viewed simply as a thermostat that switches the physiologic responses on and off when the body is too hot or too cold.

The body appears to be responsive not only to a central temperature change and a peripheral temperature change, but to respond more accurately to an integration of the two afferent inputs (i.e., from the core and the skin). The body's physiologic response to the error signal of being too hot or cold is to alter its shell in terms of insulation. The changes in the shell of the body are accomplished physiologically by altering blood flow to different areas of the body. The degree of response that the body makes depends on the degree of error (or difference from the set point) assessed at the APH.

Because the sweat glands are controlled by sympathetic cholinergic receptors and blood flow redistribution is controlled by sympathetic adrenergic receptors, medica-

Table 10-1. Partitioning of heat loss of a subject whose daily energy exchange is 3,000 Kcal[a]

	Cool Environment		Hot Environment	
Mechanism of loss	Kcal	%	Kcal	%
Radiation, convection, and conduction	1,950	65	—	—
Evaporation of water from skin and lungs and liberation of CO_2	900	30	3,000	100
Warming inspired air	90	1	—	—
Urine and feces (specific heat of these excreta over that of the blood and water)	60	4	—	—
Total daily heat loss	3,000	100	3,000	100

[a] Equivalent to a daily schedule that includes light work in cool environment and a hot environment.

tions affecting the sympathetic adrenergic system (e.g., α and β-adrenergic blockers) and the muscarinic receptor release of acetylcholine (ACh, e.g. atropine) compromise the body's ability to thermoregulate and should be used cautiously or not at all by anyone exercising in the heat.

Suggested Readings

Gisolfi CV, Lamb DR, Nadel ER, eds. *Exercise, heat and thermoregulation. Volume 6, Perspectives in exercise, science, and sports medicine* Wm P. Brown, Chicago, Illinois, 1993:389.

Pandolf KB, Sawka MN, Gonzalez RA, eds. *Human performance: Physiology and environmental medicine at terrestrial extremes.* Dubuque, IA: Brown & Benchmark, 1988:1–634.

11. EXERCISE IN THE HEAT AND HEAT INJURIES

James Moriarity

"The tragedy of heat stroke is that it so frequently strikes highly motivated young individuals under the discipline of work, military training and sporting endeavors. Under other circumstances, these same individuals would have rested when tired, taken liquid when thirsty, or remained at home when ill."
– S. Shibolet

I. The Spectrum of Heat Injury in Athletes

A. Heat syncope is the orthostatic collapse of an athlete during or after exercise as a consequence of decreased or insufficient venous return to the heart. It is not associated with central nervous system (CNS) symptoms or hyperthermia.

B. Heat exhaustion is the inability to continue exercising in the heat. Rectal temperature is generally less than 104°F (40°C). CNS symptoms may be present but consciousness maintained.

C. Exertional heat stroke occurs in a previously healthy person who collapses while exercising and whose rectal temperature is above 40.6°C (105°F). CNS symptoms predominate and are always present.

D. Exertional rhabdomyolosis is sudden onset of acute muscle pain occurring during or shortly after brief, often heroic, exercise. Associated with disseminated intravascular coagulation, acute renal failure, and cerebral edema.

E. Effort-induced muscle cramps are involuntary contractions of exercising muscles during or following strenuous activity in the heat.

II. The Pitfalls of Ambient Temperature, Core Temperature, and Heat Illness

A. Man's ability to thermoregulate allows exercise to progress in a wide range of climactic conditions. The addition of heat and humidity to exercise has long been known to affect both performance and sense of well-being. Thermoregulation maintains core temperature in a physiologic range. Without this adaptation, heat generated from exercising muscle would soon elevate core temperature to levels incompatible with life. Heat generated from exercising muscle is transferred to the environment by the processes of conduction, convection, radiation, and evaporation of sweat. As the ambient temperature and humidity increases, the transfer of body heat to the environment is slowed, stopped or, when ambient temperature exceeds body temperature, actually reversed.

The incidence of all forms of heat injury increases with increases in ambient temperature. Heat illness, including heat stroke, also may occur in relatively cool, dry environmental conditions. Although regard for high ambient temperature and humidity is justly important, exercise-induced heat injury may occur in comfortable climactic conditions.

B. Measuring temperature during sports activities in athletes suspected of having heat injury is not always easy. Mercury thermometers, infrared scanners to measure tympanic membrane temperature, and rectal thermistors have been used. The rectal temperature as measured with a rectal thermometer is still the gold standard with which other measurements are compared and is an essential requirement for the diagnosis of heat stroke. Tympanic membrane measurements require operator training and knowledge of their limitations in evaluating exercising athletes. Rectal thermistors with a thin flexible rectally inserted probe provide continuous temperature measurement valuable in monitoring temperature in a heat-injured athlete.

One of the difficulties in evaluating heat illness in athletes is that well-acclimated athletes exercising in the heat can attain a rectal temperature of 102° to 104°F without exhibiting any signs of heat illness. The presence of increased temperature as an isolated finding in an otherwise normal athlete should not be construed as evidence of or criteria for heat illness. Rectal temperatures will remain elevated for as long as 30 minutes after cessation of exercise. Rectal temperatures less than 104°F (40°C) in the *absence* of CNS symptoms is not an indication for *aggressive* cooling techniques when less aggressive methods may be suitable. Conversely, temperatures *higher* than 104.4°F (40.2°C) *with* CNS symptoms are *always* an indication for use of aggressive cooling.

Conversely, an elevated core temperature is not a requirement for the diagnosis of serious heat illness. Many athletes who experience cardiovascular collapse and mental confusion during exercise in extreme heat have been shown to have core temperatures that are only mildly elevated or, surprisingly, below normal.

Failure to document rectal temperature in a timely interval is a common finding in cases of athletes with heat stroke. Core temperature less than 105°F (40.6°C) measured remotely in time (more than 15 to 20 minutes) in an athlete who has collapsed with symptoms of heat stroke does not rule out heat stroke as a diagnosis. In addition, core temperature may change rapidly in an athlete with heat illness necessitating frequent or continuous monitoring of rectal temperature.

C. It is tempting to view heat syncope, heat exhaustion, and heat stroke as a continuum with progression from one stage to the next occurring through the increase in core temperature. No evidence suggests that such a continuum exists. It is too simplistic to think that heat illness in athletes can be prevented by frequent measurement of core temperature and by cessation of activity as the core temperature rises. It is equally misguided to categorize heat illness as syncope, exhaustion, or heat stroke based solely on core temperature measurements.

III. Exercise-Associated Collapse (EAC) in the Heat: Initial Evaluation

A. Athletes do not present with a diagnosis, they present with symptoms. One of the most common symptoms noted in strenuous exercise lasting more than a few minutes is EAC, a clinical term used to describe the phenomenon of an athlete collapsing during or after a competitive event or practice. Because EAC occurs most often in road races, many of which are held during the summer months, heat injury is often the diagnosis made in collapsed athletes.

The etiology of EAC and syncope is multifactorial, including heat illness, hypoglycemia, hypothermia, arrhythmia, volume depletion, and others. EAC during race events is more common in athletes who have concurrent illness or faster race times and in those who have previously experienced heat illness. Collapse *during* activity is more often associated with significant physical findings than is collapse at the *end* of an activity.

B. Because collapse of an athlete from heat is such an alarming event, physicians and trainers who must treat such athletes on the practice field or roadside must make an initial assessment that will expeditiously eliminate conditions that demand immediate intervention and action. Once life-threatening diagnoses are considered and dismissed, a less urgent evaluation can be made to assess the various forms of heat illness. Table 11-1 shows points to be considered in the initial assessment of athletes who collapse from heat.

Table 11-1. Initial evaluation of an athlete who collapses in the heat

Remove athlete from harm's way (i.e., water, traffic).
Assess and initiate the ABCs of life support if required.
Measure temperature.
Assess level of consciousness.
Determine whether emergency cooling is necessary and, if so, implement it.
Make initial diagnoses and remove the athlete from heat, evaluate and treat.

In the following discussions of treatment of heat injury, it is assumed that such an initial evaluation has been made.

IV. Pathophysiology of Heat Injury

A. Heat syncope

1. Heat syncope is **defined** as collapse of an athlete on cessation of active exercise due to insufficient cardiac output (CO) to the brain.
2. Heat syncope **results from** rapid decrease in central venous blood return as muscle "pumping" of blood decreases the conclusion of exercise. Dehydration is also a critical factor. High ambient temperature and humidity contribute to an increased incidence of heat syncope since blood volume must be "borrowed" from the central circulation and redirected to the peripheral circulation to aid in thermoregulation. Loss of body fluids through sweating, respiratory-insensible water loss, diarrhea, or lack of access to fluids may contribute to dehydration.
3. The **clinical presentation** of an athlete with heat syncope is one of lightheadedness, orthostasis, dizziness, nausea, or frank syncope. Other signs of heat injury such as confusion, disorientation, loss of consciousness (LOC), and acute muscle pain are not evident. Core temperature may or may not be elevated. Sweating is generally evident. The pulse is elevated, and blood pressure (BP) is low. Athletes with heat syncope generally become symptomatic at the conclusion of a race or between episodes of vigorous exertion. Heat syncope occurs most often during exercise on days 1 to 5 of heat acclimation. During this time, the athlete has not yet achieved maximal plasma volume and renal salt conservation.
4. To **treat** heat syncope and ensure rapid recovery, have the athlete assume a recumbent position and initiate simple cooling procedures such as fanning, shading from the sun, and oral rehydration. Athletes who experience one episode of heat syncope on a given day are at great risk of recurrence and should not be permitted to practice for the remainder of the day.

B. Heat exhaustion

1. Heat exhaustion is **defined** as the inability of an athlete to continue exercise in the heat. Whereas heat syncope is a specific diagnosis, heat exhaustion may be better categorized as a syndrome with a constellation of symptoms and presentations. It is the most prevalent heat-related condition.
2. The **etiology** of heat exhaustion is the effect of hyperthermia on CNS (Central Nervous System) function and/or the sustained, compromising demands that thermoregulation places on the body's organ systems. Eventually, the failure of an essential organ, usually the cardiovascular system or the CNS, renders the athlete incapable of further effort. Failure may occur at the cellular level, the organ level, or both.
3. The **clinical presentation** of heat exhaustion is characterized by weakness, lassitude, confusion, memory impairment, headache, orthostasis, frank syncope, muscle cramping, and decreased performance. Temperature measurements are generally elevated, in the range of 37° to 40°C. Hypothermia in the range of 35° to 36°C is not rare and should alert the physician to the possibility of hypoglycemia. Pulse is rapid, respirations are elevated at rest, and blood pressure (BP) measurement shows a narrowed pulse pressure. Sweating is generally present. Signs and symptoms of dehydration are often evident. Symptoms that are predominantly those of the CNS should alert health care providers to the possibility of impending heat stroke and the necessity for core temperature monitoring and rapid cooling.

   Heat exhaustion is more common in the young, the elderly, those who are not acclimated, the obese, those who are less fit or sleep deprived, and those with recent or intercurrent illness. Like that of heat syncope, the incidence of heat exhaustion varies directly with ambient temperature, sun exposure, and humidity. Although heat syncope is characterized as a transient, single event (usually at the end of exercise) with rapid recovery, heat exhaustion may begin insidiously or abruptly at any time during the exercise and with more prolonged duration of symptoms.

Attempts have been made to subcategorize heat exhaustion into water-depletion and salt-depletion models. Clinically, the two are difficult to distinguish. During exercise lasting less than 1 to 2 hours when fluid intake has balanced fluid loss, when weight loss is apparent, and when the patient demonstrates cardiovascular orthostasis, volume depletion undoubtedly is the critical factor in the development of heat exhaustion. In longer endurance events or during cumulative, intense practice sessions for several days if adequate fluid sources are available and weight has been maintained, consideration of salt depletion and tissue hyponatremia is more pressing. In such circumstances, the choice of fluid to be infused (if necessary) is more controversial.

Currently, controversy exists over the proper fluid treatment for marathon runners who collapse and are diagnosed with heat exhaustion. Traditionally, EAC in marathon runners was presumed to be the result of hypernatremic dehydration (water-depletion model) from loss of hypotonic fluid during the race. Some clinicians maintain that dilutional hyponatremic dehydration, resulting from excessive consumption of hypotonic fluids (salt-depletion model) is more common.

Also relevant to evaluation of heat exhaustion and fluid and salt status is knowledge of an athlete's relative state of acclimation. Athletes are more likely to require salt-containing fluids and foods early in the course of acclimation than later.

4. In **treatment** of heat stroke the initial assessment of an athlete is the same as that outlined in the section on evaluation of EAC. A diagnosis of heat exhaustion mandates careful temperature monitoring to ensure that critical hyperthermia does not develop. The athlete should be moved to a shady or cool location, lying recumbent with the legs and pelvis elevated, with vital signs monitored. Equipment such as shoulder pads, helmets, and other padding should be removed. Cooling with fans, iced towels, and plenty of cool liquids is indicated. In an athlete who manifests orthostatis or tachycardia, administration of intravenous fluids may be necessary.

   Asking the athlete about recent illness, weight loss from sweating, acclimation, sleep deprivation, gastrointestinal (GI) upset, previous heat problems, and current medications may provide a clue to causality. Athletes with core temperatures that continue to rise despite active cooling measures should be transported to a medical facility. If the athlete's core temperature is subnormal, hypoglycemia may exist.

   Preferred fluid replacement treatment for athletes clearly demonstrating signs of heat exhaustion with findings of orthostasis, weight loss evident on weigh-ins and weigh-outs, reduced urine amount, and increased specific gravity is rapid infusion with normal saline or Ringer's lactate until urine output is established. For athletes with symptoms of heat exhaustion but normal weights, a history of relatively clear urine, and no orthostatic changes, a slower and more conservative approach that permits ad libitum oral fluid intake, a longer time away from practice, and time for the kidney to regulate fluid and electrolyte imbalance is advocated.

5. **Return to competition** should be based on severity of symptoms, particularly with regard to CNS status, core temperature, and ability to self-hydrate. Many athletes will manifest signs of heat exhaustion that respond quickly to simple cooling measures and to "time out" for 15 to 30 minutes. An athlete with normal temperature and mental status can resume activity, but should do so with caution and under close observa-

tion. Athletes who exhibit confusion, irritability, or lethargy should not be allowed to return to play for that day and should be screened carefully the following morning for consideration of further activity. Athletes with severe heat exhaustion including syncope, temperatures as high as 39°C, and CNS symptoms are at greater risk of heat stroke and recurrence of heat exhaustion. These athletes should be restricted from high-intensity workout for a minimum of 48 hours and gradually reintroduced to intense workouts. Frequent monitoring of temperature during workouts is advised.

C. Heat stroke

1. Exertional heat stroke is **defined** as collapse of a previously healthy exercising athlete who exhibits severe neurologic impairment (most commonly unconsciousness) and has a rectal temperature higher than 40.6°C (105°F). As distinct from heat exhaustion, which is a failure of *performance,* exertional heat stroke is a failure of *homeostasis* and threatens the survival of the athlete. Once initiated, heat stroke sets off a series of cascading pathologic events that, left untreated, may be fatal.

   The incidence of exertional heat stroke is difficult to determine. Approximately 175 deaths yearly in the United States are reported to be heat related. Among amateur football athletes, 84 deaths due to heat stroke were recorded for the years 1955 to 1990. The mortality of heat stroke is 10% to 25% and is directly correlated with the duration of elevated temperature and duration of coma.

2. The precise **etiology** of heat stroke is not known. Current theory suggests an "energy-depletion" model in which hyperthermia alters cellular ability to produce energy and maintain cell membrane integrity. Cellular swelling is characteristic of heat stroke. The brain is especially susceptible to hyperthermia, and CNS impairment is also characteristic of heatstroke.

   Exertional heat stroke, like all heat illness, is more likely to occur in athletes who are not acclimatized or who are unfit. Some persons may demonstrate a persistent inability to tolerate exercise in the heat. Medications may also interfere with themoregulation (Table 11-2).

3. Heat stroke is **diagnosed** in an athlete who collapses in the heat and who exhibits neurologic impairment and a body temperature of 40.6°C (105°F) or higher. Twenty-five percent of heat stroke victims will have prodromal symptoms and 75% will not; all will have neurologic symptoms, including coma. The frequency of some clinical characteristics of heat stroke are shown in Table 11-3.

Table 11-2. Medications affecting thermoregulation

Beta-blockers
Laxatives
Antihistamines
Monoamine oxidase inhibitors
Phenothiazines
Alcohol
Diuretics
Anticholinergics
Methyldopa
Tricyclics
Vasoconstrictors
Drugs of abuse

Table 11-3. Clinical characteristics associated with heat stroke

Characteristic	%
Coma	100
Convulsions	72
Confusion/agitation	100
Hypotension (systolic BP <90)	35
Dry skin	26
Rectal temperature >41°C	55
Vomiting	71
Diarrhea	44

Adapted from Epstein Y, Sohar E, Shapiro Y. Exertional heatstroke: a preventable condition. *Isr J Med Sci* 1995;31:454–462.

Central nervous symptom dysfunction is the result of thermal injury to the brain. Core temperatures above 40.6°C (105°F) are considered to initiate brain cellular edema in humans. Fatality rates of heat stroke are directly related to the duration of coma.

The clinical progression of heat stroke has three phases.

a. In the acute phase, CNS symptoms predominate. Delirium, confusion, coma, ataxia, dysarthria are present, along with GI dysfunction, hyperventilation, and lactic acidosis.
b. In the hematologic/enzymatic phase, there is leukocytosis of 20,000 to 30,000 WBC cells/deciliter, hemorrhagic diathesis with bleeding from venipuncture sites, hemoptysis, purpura, melena, hypofibrinogenemia, prolonged prothrombin time (PT), increased FDP (fibrin degradation products), and decreased platelets. Muscle enzymes characteristically are very high with, creatine phosphokinase (CPK) peaking at 24-48 hours.
c. In the late phase of heat stroke, disturbances in renal and hepatic function begin. Bilirubin and hepatic enzymes are elevated. Blood urea nitrogen (BUN) and creatinine levels begin to increase. Twenty-five percent to 30% of persons with heat stroke have acute renal failure.

4. Heat stroke is a true medical emergency and must be treated as such. Once a diagnosis of heat stroke is made the victim must be cooled aggressively and immediately and then evacuated to a medical facility. A treatment plan for persons diagnosed with heat stroke is shown in Table 11-4.

   What constitutes the best method of aggressive, emergency cooling is controversial. Techniques using cool (not iced) water immersion and spray mist with fan cooling have been shown to lower core temperature rapidly without inducing shivering. For someone with heat stroke who cannot be transported quickly to a cooling site, continuous bathing with copious amounts of tap water, removal of clothing, fanning, and relocation to the shade is a suitable emergency procedure to lower dangerously high temperatures.

   Aggressive cooling techniques should be discontinued when rectal temperature decreases to 38.5°C (101.3°F). Because rectal temperature decreases slowly, one can "overshoot" the mark and induce hypothermia and unnecessary shivering.
5. Return-to-play criteria for an athlete with heat stroke mandate that the athlete be fully recovered from any complications of heat stroke and be evaluated for heat tolerance. The term heat tolerance, or acclimation to heat, implies that the athlete is able to adapt physiologically to exercise in the heat. After an athlete recovers from heat stroke, acclimation may

Table 11-4. Emergency treatment for athletes with heatstroke

1. Regard situation as a medical emergency.
2. Energetic, aggressive cooling: ice bath, ice packs, copious water bathing with fanning
3. Rectal temperature monitoring with rectal thermistor
4. Airway management
5. Oxygen 6 L/min by mask
6. Establish intravenous (i.v.) line
7. Diazepam to control seizure activity if present
8. Fluid resuscitation with normal saline or Ringer's lactate; 2 L in first hour, followed by rate in accordance with hydration
9. Minimize shivering if possible, administer chlorpromazine 50 mg i.v. or diazepam i.v.
10. Cardiac monitoring
11. Urine flow measurement with catheter: if CVP adequate mannitol may be administered at dose of 0.25 mg/kg or furosemide 1 mg/kg to maintain urine output
12. Sodium bicarbonate may be considered in cases of rhabdomyolosis
13. Anuria, uremia, and hyperkalemia may require dialysis
14. Frequent measurement of serum chemistries, enzymes, and coagulation factors
15. Treat with fresh frozen plasma, cryoprecipitate, and platelets if necessary

Adapted from Epstein Y, Sohar E, Shapiron Y., *Isr J Med Sci* Exertional heatstroke: a preventable condition. 1995;31:454–462.

occur in as little as 2 months and as long as one year. Heat tolerance is evaluated by measuring rectal temperature response and heart rate (HR) response to controlled exercise for a 6-day period (Armstrong et al.).

E. Muscle cramps

1. Muscle cramps are involuntary contractions of exercising muscle and most commonly occur in athletes exercising in the heat.
2. The prevailing theory regarding the etiology of muscle cramps is that they occur secondary to a generalized deficiency of sodium and chloride as a consequence of sweat loss and dehydration. Their exact cause is unknown. Other proposed etiologies include deficiencies of magnesium, potassium, calcium, or glucose and accumulation of hydrogen ions and lactic acid. Myoneural theories describe alterations in stretch receptors, synaptic irritability, and failure of Na/K-ATPase–dependent pumps. Although muscle cramps occur more commonly in hot and humid conditions in fluid-depleted athletes, in cool weather athletes with full bladders may experience severe cramping. Severe muscle cramping in athletes has been associated with malignant hyperthermia, which affects muscle function.
3. Muscle cramps commonly present during activity and mimic an acute extremity injury. They may not become evident until after exercise has ceased and the athlete is leaving the practice field. Muscle cramps may be a component of heat exhaustion or heat stroke. Cramps, especially if generalized, are excruciatingly painful and possibly dangerous if the athlete is operating a vehicle or swimming. Once cramping becomes generalized, it is exceedingly difficult to arrest.

   Although muscle cramps often have rapid onset, many athletes describe initial tightness followed by muscle fibrillation and fasciculation with a progressive crescendo to a painful contraction. Muscles susceptible to cramping include all those of the extremities, gluteals, abdominals, and back.

4. The classic sideline treatment for heat cramps is stretching of the affected muscle. Massaging the muscle after the cramp has subsided may be helpful. Ice may be applied. For lower extremity cramping of agonist/antagonist muscle groups, a squatting position will stretch of the quadriceps, upper hamstrings, and calves. Another technique useful for agonist/antagonist cramping that does not respond to stretching is tight circumferential wrapping of the muscle groups with prewrap and 3-inch Elasticon or Conform tape. For severe generalized cramping of the extremities, abdomen, and back, intravenous fluid therapy with normal saline may be useful. Judicious use of diazepam or meperidine to provide pain relief and muscle relaxation may be necessary.

   Although a variety of electrolyte products are available (including calcium, salt tablets, potassium, magnesium, and phosphorus) to help prevent muscle cramps, none have been shown to prevent cramping in electrolyte-stable individuals. Neither has quinine. Vigorous stretching programs decrease the incidence of cramping in athletes. Athletes should be evaluated for serum abnormalities of sodium, potassium, calcium, for thyroid function, and for glucose levels, but such abnormalities are rare causes of muscle cramps. Early in heat acclimation, sodium loss in sweat and urine is greater and extra salt should be added to the athlete's diet.

   Maintaining hydration is essential in lessening the incidence of heat cramps. Athletes should be instructed to "prehydrate" before participating in competition and practice. The type of fluid to be used during competition or practice to counter the loss of sodium in sweat depends on duration of activity. Electrolyte-containing beverages are useful in countering the loss of sodium in sweat during exercises of prolonged duration. Daily weigh-in and weigh-out is a useful tool to ensure that athletes are adequately rehydrated.

5. The athlete's ability to return to competition is based on the severity of the cramping episode and the intensity level of the anticipated exercise. With minor cramps of one muscle group, the athlete can resume activity immediately after resolution of the cramp. When cramps are severe, walking and stretching on resolution of the cramping episode, followed by biking or jogging the next day and gradual introduction of more vigorous exercise in the next 24 to 48 hours will reduce recurrence of cramps.

V. Prevention of Heat Illness

A. Acclimation

1. Although high-intensity exercise in the heat can cause heat illness in any athlete, heat acclimation reduces the signs, symptoms, and incidence of most heat illness. The incidence of heat cramps, heat syncope, and heat exhaustion decreases after athletes exercise for 1 week in the heat. Heat stroke incidence and heat acclimation have no clear relationship. Table 11-5 shows the physiologic changes that accompany acclimation.
2. For maximum acclimation, exercise intensity should exceed 50% VO_{2max}, fluid status should be optimal, and sleep deprivation should be avoided. Heat acclimation is rapidly lost after a few days to weeks of inactivity. Athletes maximally trained in cool environments will not be able to reproduce high-intensity workouts in hot environments without becoming acclimatized. Exposure to heat without exercise in the heat will not produce acclimation.
3. The minimal ambient temperature necessary to achieve acclimation is not known. The incidence of heat injury increases as ambient conditions exceed 21°C/50%humidity. Vigorous exercise in wet bulb globe temperature (WBGT) above 28°C (82.4°F) is not recommended by the American College of Sports Medicine. Likewise, ambient temperatures above 32°C with minimal wind and bright sun essentially cause "shut down" of conductive, convective, and radiant heat loss. Evaporative heat loss is greatly impaired when humidity is greater than 70% or if restrictive,

Table 11-5. Physiological change of heat acclimation

Parameter	Days
Heart rate decrease	3 to 6
Plasma volume increase	3 to 6
Rectal temperature decrease	5 to 8
Perceived exertion improvement	3 to 6
Sweat Na and Cl concentation decreases	5 to 10
Sweat rate increases	8 to 14
Urine Na and Cl concentration decrease	3 to 8

Adapted from Armstrong L, Maresh C. *Sports Med* 1991;12:302–312.

sweat-soaked clothing is worn. Therefore, exercise must take place in an ambient temperature above 21°C and in 50% humidity, preferably with a WBGT reading below 28°C.

B. Environmental factors

1. Environmental conditions obviously affect the likelihood of incurring heat injury. One of the major methods of preventing heat injury is avoidance of exercise during extremes of heat and humidity. Although simple in theory it is difficult in practice. Outdoor practice early and late in the day are generally less extreme than other time periods.
2. The WGBT index is used as a risk indicator for exercise in the heat (Table 11-6). WBGT measurements take into account the relative contributions of radiant heat, humidity, and ambient temperature in the formula: WBGT = 0.7(wet bulb) + 0.2(black bulb) + 0.1(dry bulb). WBGT devices can be easily assembled from thermometers, clamps, and stands available in a general chemistry laboratory and a toilet bowl float (metal) painted black (available from a hardware store). Alternatively, dry bulb and wet bulb readings can be obtained from a sling psychrometer and a black bulb reading taken from a thermometer placed in a black toilet bowl float.

   Heat index is a measurement that combines only ambient temperature and humidity, without the important contribution of radiant sun energy. Heat index can be obtained from a sling psychrometer. In general, the combination of ambient temperature above 85°F (29°C) and relative humidity above 60% places the heat index in the danger zone.
3. If exercise activity in extreme heat is unavoidable, liquids should be readily available, as should shade. More frequent rest periods should be allowed and, if possible, workouts should be less intense and practice shorter. Heat injuries should be anticipated. Physicians with institu-

Table 11-6. WBGT index for heat stress

WBGT (°C)	Recommendation
<10	Low risk of hyperthermia; some risk of hypothermia
<18	Low risk of heat injury
18–23	Moderate risk of heat injury
23–28	High risk of heat injury
>28	Extreme risk of heat injury

WBGT, Wet bulb globe temperature.

Table 11-7. Coaching strategies for safe exercise in the heat

"Heat education" of athletes, coaches, and training staff
Consideration of age, acclimation, and fitness level of the athlete
High regard for ambient temperature and humidity
Scheduling of practice times in the cooler part of the day or evening
Loose fitting "breathable" clothing
Maintenance of hydration: 1–2 cups of fluid every 15 minutes
Rest periods (preferably in the shade) every 30 minutes
Availability of cooling devices: shade, fans, ice, immersion tanks
Availability of trained medical personnel

tional responsibility for the health and well-being of athletic participants must have direct input into the conduct of practice and race events, fully realizing that published medical standards regarding the safety of exercise in the heat often go against prevailing custom. Physicians and coaches should also be aware that minors may not be of legal age of consent and that parents may not waive the legal rights of their children. Suggestions for coaches and players to achieve successful and safe practice in extreme heat are shown in Tables 11-7 and 11-8.

C. Hydration

1. Hydration has a direct affect on the athlete's ability to thermoregulate and maintain performance. As plasma volume decreases, less blood is available for transport of heat to the periphery for dissipation. Fluid loss in the heat occurs primarily through sweating, which can attain a level of 1 to 3 L per hour. Sweat is hypotonic, with a $Na+$ concentration of 40 to 60 mEq/L. Gastric emptying is slowed by the presence of fat, greater caloric content, higher temperature, and more acidic content. Gastric emptying is speeded by cooler liquid temperature, decreased osmolality, and greater volume of stomach distention. Maximum gastric emptying ranges from 500 to 100 ml/h, obviously, therefore, some athletes will find it impossible to maintain adequate hydration during periods of prolonged exercise.
2. The choice of best fluid replacement is controversial. Cool water is the most efficiently absorbed liquid and will help absorb heat in the body cavity. The addition of carbohydrate has been shown to delay fatigue but slow gastric absorption. Salt in the solution will have little effect on electrolyte balance in the acclimatized athlete but may be a cofactor in the absorption of glucose and water.

Table 11-8. Team member strategies for safe exercise in the heat

Understand the impact of heat on performance and health.
Prepare for the season: achieve peak conditioning.
Prepare for the heat: train in the temperature and humidity you will practice in.
Delay exercise if you are ill; take no medication unless advised to do so.
Minimize unnecessary clothing, bracing, and tape.
Drink 16 ounces (2 cups) of fluid before and 8–16 ounces every 15 minutes during practice.
Replenish fluids after practice (2 cups of liquid for every pound lost).
Replenish muscle energy by eating a high-carbohydrate diet.
Salt your food.
Sleep is essential; get 8 hours of sleep each night.

Table 11-9. Contents of a heat bag

Rectal thermometers	Lubricant
Blood pressure cuffs	Stethoscopes
Oral airways	Tongue blades
Flashlight and batteries	Alcohol wipes
Antiseptic scrub	Dressings
Syringes and needles	Venipuncture supplies
Intravenous catheters and tubing	Normal saline (2L)
D_{50} solution	Parenteral diazepam
Tape	Band-aids
Tape cutters	Scissors
Disposable gloves	Sterile gloves
Optional	
Rectal thermistor thermometer	Tympanic membrane thermometer
Sling psycohometer	Glucometer

3. A recommendation for fluid replacement in exercising athletes is pre-exercise hydration with 16 ounces of fluid 15 to 20 minutes before exercise and 8 ounces of fluid every 15 minutes during exercise. Postexercise consumption of fluids should be adequate to produce dilute urine.
4. Athletes in heavy training regimens involving multiple daily workouts as is common in late summer football, soccer, and cross-country programs, are at greater risk for cumulative salt, carbohydrate, and water deficit. Athletes with large amounts of lean muscle mass may lose significant hepatic and muscle glycogen. Water is stored with glycogen at a rate of 2.6 g (ml)/g glycogen. Consumption of diets high in carbohydrate with liberal added salt will facilitate water absorption and help maintain hydration.

D. Medical preparation for exercise in the heat
   1. Anticipation of heat injury by medical personnel implies that necessary provisions for treatment of heat injury are in place. Table 11-9 describes the contents of a heat bag that should be readily available on the practice field, race tent, or other medical location for emergency treatment of athletes with heat injury.
   2. On-site equipment needed to treat heat-injured athletes adequately are immersion tanks filled with cool or iced water, large cooling fans, hoses, cots, and a tent or building to provide shade. Access for emergency vehicles and personnel should be considered in choosing a practice site.

Suggested Readings

Wilmore J, Costill D. *Physiology of sport and exercise.* Springfield, IL: Human Kinetics Publishers, 1994.

Epstein Y, Sohar E, Shapiro Y. Exertional heatstroke: a preventable condition. *Isr J Med Sci* 1995;31:454–62.

Armstrong LE, Maresh C. The induction and decay of heat acclimation in trained athletes. *Sports Med* 1991;12:303–12.

Armstrong LE, DeLuco JP, Hubbard RW. Clinical symposium on heatstroke. *Med Sci Sports Exerc* Feb 1990;22:36–48.

Selected articles on heat injury in athletes in *Physician and Sports Medicine,* May and June 1989, December 1990, May and July 1991, May and June 1992, July 1993, August 1994, and July 1995.

12. EXERCISE IN THE COLD AND COLD INJURIES

Wayne K. Gersoff

Cold-related problems for the athlete represent one of the most common athletic environmental hazards. Although cold-related problems are usually associated with winter sports, like skiing, skating, mountaineering, and snowshoeing, there is risk too in other sports, including running, cycling, swimming, and hiking.

I. Cold-Weather Physiology

A. Body requirements. Core temperature (37.6°C or 99.6°F) must be maintained within a narrow range (4°C or about 12°F).

B. Heat production. Body heat is generated by four mechanisms.

1. Basal heat production. Heat is produced by normal metabolic processes and is adequate under resting conditions but inadequate for colder environments.
2. Muscular thermoregulatory heat. The heat that is produced by shivering increases body heat three to five times basal level but also uses large amounts of energy.
3. High-intensity exercise-induced heat. The heat produced during various activities involving increased muscular activity generates 10 times basal heat production but can only be maintained for several minutes.
4. Mild to moderate exercise-induced heat. Because of its lower rate and intensity this heat only produces an approximate five times basal heat generation, but it can be maintained for a longer time.

C. Heat conservation

1. Constriction of peripheral vasculature. When the body is exposed to cold, blood flow is shunted away from the surface area of the body to the core.
2. Body insulation. The layer of subcutaneous fat helps conserve heat.
3. External heat sources. Clothing and other external heat sources aid heat conservation.

D. Heat loss. Heat production must be balanced by heat loss. Most heat produced by the body is lost through the skin. The body loses heat by four methods.

1. Conduction. Direct heat loss occurs from contact with materials that conduct heat better than air. Immersion in water increases the cooling rate 100 times faster than air.
2. Convection. Loss of heat is caused by the motion of air or water across the body surface; heat is lost in relation to the velocity of the air or water.
3. Evaporation. The best way to control heat loss is to prevent evaporation. When water evaporates, heat is lost. One third of evaporation occurs through the lungs and two thirds occurs through the skin.
4. Radiation. From 55% to 65% of the body's heat loss is caused by radiation; the loss is related to the mass of the body and its surface area.

II. Specific Cold Injuries

A. Local versus systemic. Local injuries occur when the shell temperature is exposed to freezing temperatures but the core temperature is maintained. These include *frostnip, chilblains, and frostbite*. If the cold induces a drop not only in the peripheral temperature but also in the core temperature, then hypothermia can be produced.

B. Frostnip. A condition that develops slowy and results in blanching of the skin, frostnip is associated with reversible ice crystal formation on the skin's surface. It will affect the tips of the ears, nose, cheeks, fingertips, chin and toes. Frostnip is often confused with frostbite. Treatment is to provide gradual warming of the tissue by the contact of a warm hand, by blowing hot breath on the body part, or by holding the injured body part in the axilla or groin area. Do not rub the skin with snow. As the tissue gradually warms, the color returns and there may be tingling in the body part.

C. Chilblains, trench foot, and immersion foot. These are commonly grouped together because they all result from repeated exposure of bare skin to cold water or from repeated exposure of an extremity for prolonged periods of time, usually at temperatures around freezing. Chilblains can occur on the hands and feet. The lesions are localized, erythematous, or cyanotic, and are often raised as plaques or nodes. This injury initially results in red, hot, swollen, and tender skin. The first symptoms are tingling, burning, numbness, and coldness. In most cases, there is almost complete recovery. Treatment involves gradual rewarming in an appropriate environment. If this environment is not available then the limb is at risk for re-exposure and further injury from the cold and wet environment. Immersion foot and trench foot share a similar pathophysiologic basis. Both are secondary to an extremity exposed to a cold wet environment for an extended period of time. While immersion foot is associated with immersion of the extremity in cold water, trench foot is caused by cold, wet exposure on land. Diagnosis of this injury is strongly based on history and physical examination. While different treatment plans have been suggested, little of therapeutic value occurs from these treatments. Most important to treatment are elevation of the leg and prevention of systemic infections. Most often, observation and pain control should be carried out until the extent of injury declares itself, and then, if necessary, surgical debridement or amputation is performed.

D. Frostbite. One of the worst local cold-related injuries, frostbite is caused by actual freezing of the skin. Body areas commonly involved in frostbite injury are the fingertips, earlobes, tip of the nose, toes, and any exposed areas of the skin. Frostbite can be classified into various stages based on the degree of injury. *First-degree frostbite* usually is associated with local pain and discomfort. There is usually a numbness, redness, or swelling of the affected area. *Second-degree frostbite* displays all of the prior symptoms along with the development of a superficial serous blistering. *Third-degree frostbite* brings on development of deep hemoserous blistering. *Fourth-degree frostbite* involves the deep soft tissue. This includes bone and may result in possible mummification of the tissues, requiring amputation. Several factors increase the risk of frostbite. These include constricting clothing, smoking, atherosclerosis, arthritis, diabetes mellitus, use of vasoconstrictive drugs, previous cold injury, immobilization, and hypothermia. The affected tissue may be waxy yellow or mottled blue. If vesicles or bullae form in 6 to 24 hours, the tissue will be lost. If the area is more severely frostbitten, black, dry eschar forms in 9 to 15 days. Mummification and autoamputation occurs in 22 to 45 days. Treatment of frostbite should be directed toward prevention of any further injury to the tissue and of the necrosis of any damaged tissue. Rubbing or massaging frostbitten tissues is strongly contraindicated. The accepted therapy for frostbite is rapid rewarming; a whirlpool device is ideal. The water temperature should be 40° to 42°C (104° to 108°F). The use of dry heat, such as from a campfire, car exhaust, or radiator is contraindicated, because these types of heating are slow and not equally distributed. In addition, because of numbness, the skin could be burned. If out in the field, the frostbitten part should not be thawed unless there is a mechanism available to keep it thawed. If the frostbitten part is thawed and allowed to refreeze there is a greater risk of more extensive damage. During the rewarming process, the victim will experience pain relative to the degree of frostbite. The victim may require analgesic support and should be instructed that the pain is not a dangerous sign but is, rather, a part of the natural process of rewarming. Hospitalization is generally recommended for those with frostbite injuries greater than first-degree.

E. Hypothermia is a systemic injury. It will occur when the body's core temperature decreases to less than 95°F or 35°C. Hypothermia causes 500 to 700 deaths per year in the United States. It can occur at almost any altitude and in any temperature lower than body core temperature. Individuals at increased risk for hypothermia include accident and trauma victims, the very young and the very old, people with chronic metabolic disease, people with acute or chronic alcoholism and/or acute intoxication or drug overdose, and those who are mentally impaired.

1. Classification
   a. Mild hypothermia occurs when the rectal core temperature (RCT) is greater than 95°F but less than 98.6°F.
   b. Moderate hypothermia occurs when the RCT is greater than 90°F but less than 95°F.
   c. Severe hypothermia occurs when the RCT drops to below 90°F.
2. Mild hypothermia. In this most common stage of hypothermia, symptoms include cold fingers and toes, shivering and chills. The person will develop increased pulse and respiratory rates, and may experience mild incoordination and urinary urgency. Early recognition of symptoms prevents an increase in severity. The person usually can be rewarmed by external means: The athlete should be placed in a protective shelter, kept dry, rested, and insulated, to prevent further bodily heat loss. Complete recovery usually will occur.
3. Moderate hypothermia. In this stage, the person will develop increased fatigue, an increase in muscular incoordination, and loss of the shivering mechanism. He or she will experience numbing of fingers and toes, with actual functional loss and an altered mental status and as such are poor reporters of their state. Physiologically, the person commonly shows hypotension, hypoventilation, and cardiac arrhythmias, including sinus bradycardia and atrial fibrillation. Moderate hypothermia requires immediate treatment. The suspicion of moderate hypothermia should be considered when a person shows decreased signs of shivering, slow reactions, or any other altered state of mental capacity, and appropriate treatment begun. The victim should be warmed and protected from the environment. Attention should be directed first toward rewarming of the body core rather than the extremities. Water immersion rewarming is extremely dangerous, secondary to rewarming shock, where blood is rapidly shunted to the extremities and skin from the core. If a water bath is the only available means then the extremities should be left out of the water and only the trunk immersed. If there is alteration of mental state, the person should not be given fluids or food by mouth, to avoid the possibility of aspiration.
4. Severe hypothermia. Severe hypothermia results in a complete loss of shivering, marked confusion, inappropriate behavior, and visual disturbances as well as changing levels of consciousness. This person is at high risk of death. The victim's blood pressure, pulse, and respiratory rate are markedly depressed. Pulmonary edema may develop. Indeed, these individuals may appear clinically dead. Severe danger of cardiac arrhythmias exists, and electrocardiographic monitoring must be performed. Monitoring in a medical facility is mandatory. Because the body core temperature is lowered, the hypothermia can actually be protective, like a metabolic icebox. The victim may not require a high pulse or blood pressure to support life. Performing cardiopulmonary resuscitation (CPR) prematurely may cause arrhythmias because of the fragile nature of the cardiac muscle. Rewarming the patient is an active process and has been accomplished by airway warming, warmed IV fluids, warmed peritoneal dialysis, and cardiopulmonary bypass.
5. Prevention. Hypothermia is potentially life-threatening; its prevention is of the utmost importance. Preparation probably is the best way to prevent hypothermia, by preparing appropriately for the worst conditions: arranging appropriate food supplements for duration of outdoor exposure, ensuring appropriate fluid intake to prevent dehydration, providing appropriate clothing that can be worn in layers (clothing that is

windproof, well insulated, and allows for water evaporation), and avoiding getting wet, abstaining from alcoholic beverages, recognizing high-risk situations, knowing when one is at risk, and using common sense.

III. Cold and Athletic Performance

Cold environments reduce a person's exercise efficiency. Endurance athletes must use additional energy for thermogenesis, which can adversely affect performance. Anaerobic activity can also be affected. Muscle function generally is decreased and nerve conduction can be slowed. During exercise, an individual is protected by increase in body temperature. However, when the energy reserves used during exercise are depleted, the exhausted athlete is at increased risk for hypothermia. This applies to exposure to cold in water as well. It is estimated that the average swimmer in 50°F (10°C) can swim only about one km before experiencing hypothermia.

IV. Medical Problems Stimulated By Cold Exposure

A. Cold urticaria (see Chapter 29)

B. Cold-induced asthma or bronchioconstriction (see Chapter 27)

C. Raynaud's phenomenon: Raynaud's phenomenon represents an abnormal constriction of the peripheral small arteries and arterioles of the hands and feet. It is very commonly associated with exposure to cold but can also be triggered by emotional stress. Although it can occur at any age, it is more common after puberty and before age 40 years. Women are affected more frequently than men are. Clinically, on exposure to cold, the fingers of both hands will demonstrate demarcated blanching, which can then be followed by cyanosis. During recovery, the cyanosis is replaced by hyperemia. In the initial ischemic phase, the digits are cold and numb. However, in the hyperemic stage, throbbing, tingling, swelling, and an increase in temperature will be felt in the digits. In these cases that are purely related to Raynaud's phenomenon and not to an underlying disease process, treatment is aimed at reassurance, protection from cold exposure, and gradual rewarming. In rare cases, a vasodilator might be prescribed to allow an athlete to participate in a sport.

13. HIGH ALTITUDE

Robert B. Schoene

Access to high altitude for work, recreation, and habitation has increased in the past few decades. People worldwide have recognized the pleasures of venturing to such regions, and there is little evidence that the influx of people is abating.

Along with the enjoyment of mountain travel comes the inevitable physiologic stress of adapting to the hypoxia which results from the lower barometric pressure that exists at high altitude. Although the fraction of oxygen in the earth's atmosphere remains constant at 0.2093, barometric pressure decreases at higher altitudes and there is less oxygen in the air. For instance, at sea level, the barometric pressure is approximately 760 mm Hg; on the summit of Mt. Everest, it is about 250 mm Hg. Because oxygen is vital to human life, how does the body adapt?

Adaptation

The body is resourceful in optimizing transport of oxygen from the air to the blood and to the mitochondria in the cells. Several responses are invoked, immediately and over time, that facilitate transport of oxygen. The important point is that although most people adapt in a similar manner, each is slightly different, which may lead to maladaptation or altitude illnesses. Normal acclimation is summarized briefly in Table 13-1.

Maladaptation

Not everyone adapts well to high altitude, and most people will suffer to some degree if they go too high too fast. It must be emphasized that each person has his or her inherent rate at which adaptive processes proceed.

The clinical syndromes of high-altitude maladaptation can be divided into mild and severe. The mild form is acute mountain sickness (AMS); the more severe forms are high-altitude pulmonary and cerebral edemas (HAPE, HACE). These entities are probably a continuum, but it is important to separate them for practical purposes, because the latter forms are potentially fatal. Each is a manifestation of fluid leakage from intra- to extravascular spaces, especially in the brain and lung. There are more chronic forms of altitude illnesses, but they do not fall into the purview of this chapter.

Acute Mountain Sickness

AMS is a self-limited form of altitude illness which usually occurs in the first 12 to 36 hours of arrival at moderate altitude (7 to 10,000 feet). It affects 25% of lowlanders arriving at 9,000 feet. Its symptoms are headache, loss of appetite, trouble in sleeping, lethargy, nausea, and vomiting. Its signs are tachycardia and mild tachypnea. Two or more symptoms in the appropriate setting allow the diagnosis of AMS. The symptoms may be mild to severe but usually abate at the same altitude in 1 to 2 days.

Treatment

The best way to avoid AMS is by ascending at a slower rate to allow one's body time to adapt. In these days of quick access and transportation, a slower rate is not always desirable or practical, but the following guidelines provide a structure for prevention and/or treatment of AMS.

1. For rapid ascents to 10,000 feet or more, prevention with pharmacologic agents is a reasonable approach. For those who are not allergic to sulfa drugs, acetazolamide has been used to prevent AMS. The recommended dose is 125 mg twice daily (b.i.d.) which can be started as the person is ascending. Use of the drug should be continued for the first several days and then discontinued, but its use can be reinstituted if symptoms recur. The mechanism of action of acetazolamide is not clear, but probably has to do with some of its effects, which mimic normal

Table 13-1. Normal acclimation

System	Result	Time
Ventilation	Higher alveolar pO_2	Immediate and ongoing
Gas exchange	Improves V/Q, optimizes PaO_2	Immediate
Blood	Erythropoiesis to increase O_2-carrying capacity;	More than 7–10 days, ongoing
	Shifts in O_2/hemoglobin dissociation curve to facilitate O_2 loading in the lung (left shift) and unloading in tissue (right shift)	Immediate Ongoing
Tissues	Increased capillary density, increased mitochondrial density, mild atrophy of muscle cells, and optimization of oxidative enzymes—all to improve O_2 availability and utilization (controversial area)	Weeks

acclimation. For persons allergic to sulfa drugs, dexamethasone, a potent corticosteriod, is a viable alternative. It too can be started as the person ascends, in doses of 4 mg four times daily (q.i.d.). The drug does not facilitate acclimation, and symptoms may ensue or recur if its use is discontinued. Both drugs are effective in treating AMS if symptoms are noted.

2. For those who are particularly susceptible to AMS at high altitudes, it is prudent to use prophylactic pharmacologic measures. The guidelines outlined above also apply to the "susceptible" individual.
3. In travel to high altitude (more than 10,000 feet) where medical care may not be accessible (e.g., an alpine climb, or a trek to the Himalayas or the Andes), sojourners should bring medication along to use at the onset of symptoms, or a portable hyperbaric bag (a light bag the victim is placed in; with increased pressure the effective altitude is lower) should be available for more severe symptoms.

High-Altitude Pulmonary Edema

High-altitude pulmonary edema (HAPE) is a severe form of altitude illness marked by interstitial and alveolar fluid that is very high in protein and cells. The mechanism of the disease is not known, but is in part secondary to high intravascular pressures in the pulmonary vasculature, which causes leakage from the intravascular space. It usually occurs at higher altitudes than does AMS. The symptoms of dry cough, marked shortness of breath and decreased exercise tolerance have onset in 2 to 4 days, often are preceded by symptoms of AMS, and may progress to severe dyspnea, cough productive of pink frothy sputum, and death. Because of associated right-to-left shunting of blood in the lung, all cases have varying degrees of hypoxemia, which can be severe. Some individuals are predisposed to HAPE, and it can occur in people, especially children, living at high altitudes who reascend after a sojourn in low altitude. If treated soon after the onset of symptoms, all patients recover and return to normal physical function in the remarkably short period of a few days. Unless orthopedic injury occurs while patients are in remote areas, or unless severe weather prevents descent, no one should die from HAPE.

Treatment

Even more so than in AMS, especially at higher altitudes, slow, graded ascents can prevent most cases of HAPE, even in those who are susceptible. The following guidelines, however, should decrease the occurrence and/or severity of HAPE:

1. For HAPE-susceptible individuals who insist on returning to high altitudes but who will take the time to acclimate, nifedipine-XL 30 mg (q.i.d. or b.i.d.) is effective

in preventing most cases of HAPE. Presumably, the drug minimizes the degree of hypoxic pulmonary vasoconstriction and may explain why the degree of pulmonary hypertension, has been shown to be quite high in HAPE victims, thereby decreasing stress on the pulmonary microvasculature. The drug is well-tolerated.
2. Individuals with HAPE should not ascend further. If it is available, low-flow supplemental oxygen is effective in preventing worsening of symptoms, and is effective in and of itself in treating HAPE. In areas where medical care is available (i.e., recreational ski areas), when the patient's oxygen saturation can be increased to more than 90% with low-flow oxygen, and if the patient has family or friends to watch him or her, he or she can be sent home on oxygen and seen the next day in follow-up.

If the patient is more severely ill, has concomitant symptoms of HACE, cannot achieve an adequate oxygen saturation while on oxygen, then descent, if possible, is mandatory. It is important to try to effect the evacuation before the person becomes too ill to walk or to help in the descent. A decrease in altitude of from 2,000 to 3,000 feet can be remarkably effective. The patient should stay at a lower altitude until all symptoms are resolved but then may be able to reascend.

Several of drugs (morphine, diuretics, digitalis, and steroids) have been used to treat HAPE, but there are reasons that many of them may be dangerous to use, especially in the field setting. If evacuation or descent from a remote setting is not possible, the portable hyperbaric bag is effective as a temporizing measure.

High-Altitude Cerebral Edema

High-altitude cerebral edema (HACE) is the most severe form of acute altitude illness, can occur with HAPE, usually occurs at altitudes of more than 12,000 feet, is the severe end of the spectrum of AMS (i.e., brain edema), can be rapid in onset, and can be fatal. The critical difference between AMS and HACE is the evolution from moderate headache to severe headache, not relieved with analgesics, which evolves to changes in mental state (confusion, greater lethargy, stupor, coma) with accompanying hard neurologic signs (especially ataxia).

Treatment

The signs and symptoms of HACE must be recognized, and immediate descent must be undertaken. Oxygen is helpful, but its administration should not delay descent. Once a mountain climber is non-ambulatory, greater risk is incurred by those who must evacuate the climber, and the likelihood that any of the group will be saved is dramatically reduced. Dexamethasone should be administered immediately (parenterally if possible, 10 mg intramuscularly (i.m.), and then 4 mg orally (p.o.) q.i.d.), thereafter. Recovery is almost always complete, but some cases of residual neurologic deficits have been reported.

Miscellaneous

Exercise capacity decreases at high altitude but, with time for acclimation, can return to near sea level values at up to more than 8,000 feet. Above these altitudes, it is not possible to regain the same aerobic capacity that one has at sea level. The reasons for the impairment in aerobic capacity are not fully understood. The explanation that it is hypoxia does not completely explain the decrease.

Training

High-altitude training (from 6,000 to 9,000 feet), has gained much popularity, although the benefits or detriments are not clear. On the positive side are an increase in red blood cell (RBC) mass, which improves endurance (natural "blood-doping"), a possible increase in respiratory muscle strength, and the psychological advantage of training in an inspiring setting. The downsides are that the intensity of training is necessarily less (i.e., interval training must be slower), recovery time after workouts is longer, and there may be a prolonged gradual decline in overall strength and fitness. Researchers continue to try to answer many of these questions. In the meantime, the guidelines for training and competing at altitude are as follows: For events of short duration (less than 2 minutes), one should train at low altitude and arrive very close to the time of the event. For longer events, it is probably prudent to train at low altitude but to allow a week or more at the altitude of the competition, if possible, for some adaptation to occur, especially mollification of dyspnea, which may be quite limiting.

Suggested Readings

Bartsch P, Maggiorini M, Ritter M, et al. Prevention of high altitude pulmonary edema by nifedipine. *N Engl J Med* 1991;325:1284–9.

Honigman B, Theis MK, Koziol-McLain J, et al. Acute mountain sickness in a general tourist population at moderate altitude. *Ann Intern Med* 1993;118:587–92.

Schoene RB. High altitude pulmonary edema, In: Goldhaber SZ, Braunwald E, eds. *Atlas of heart disease,* vol. III, Philadelphia: C.V. Mosby, 1995: Ch. 4.

Schoene RB, Hornbein TF, Hackett PH. High altitude In: Murray JF, Nadel JA, eds. *Textbook of respiratory medicine,* 2nd ed. Philadelphia: W.B. Saunders, 1995:00–00.

Ward MP, Milledge JS, West JB. *High altitude medicine and physiology,* 2nd ed., London: Chapman and Hall Medical, 1995.

14. DIVING-RELATED ILLNESSES

Alfred A. Bove and Tom S. Neuman

The sport-diver community in the United States is estimated to number more than 3 million. In 1994, 1,164 cases of diving-related injuries were reported to the Divers Alert Network, a volunteer agency which collects diving statistics. Commercial, military, and scientific divers constitute a smaller community but are subject to greater depth and time exposure. With transportation readily available to tropical regions where sport diving is popular, diving-related disorders may occur anywhere in the United States, when a diver returns home from a distant diving site.

The weight of atmospheric gases and water on the surface of the earth or beneath the surface of the water commonly is expressed in units of pressure. The air column at the earth's surface weighs 14.7 pounds per square inch (PSI), a pressure designated as one atmosphere absolute (1 ATA). Pressure underwater increases linearly with depth. One foot of sea water weighs 0.445 PSI, thus $14.7 \div 0.445 = 33$ feet of sea water or about 10 m, which is equivalent to 1 ATA.

Underwater exposure subjects divers to increased pressure, which causes an increase in concentration of gases in blood and tissues. Because metabolic processes control the concentration of CO_2, this gas is returned to physiologic concentration in tissues, oxygen concentration increases, and attempts to normalize cellular concentration result in small increases in oxygen concentration, except under conditions of high oxygen partial pressure (e.g., more than 1 ATA oxygen). Nitrogen and other inert gases maintain an increased concentration in tissues, and will become supersaturated upon ascent from depth. Excess supersaturation will form a gas phase with consequent tissue injury. Protocols have been established for safe decompression (decompression tables) to prevent gas formation.

Barotrauma

As pressure increases, the volume of gas in deformable spaces diminishes according to Boyle's law (Pressure $*$ Volume = CONSTANT). Volume in the lungs, middle ear, paranasal sinuses, gastrointestinal tract, etc., is reduced as pressure increases. The tympanic membrane may be displaced inward and ultimately may rupture (ear squeeze). Blood in the middle ear from engorged mucous membranes can cause infection and hearing loss. Prevention is achieved by ensuring that the eustachian tube is patent and the middle ear can be equilibrated with ambient pressure before descending. Sinus squeeze occurs in a paranasal sinus with a blocked orifice, in residual air pockets beneath a dental filling (tooth squeeze), and in the air space within a diving mask (mask squeeze). All will produce tissue injury due to displacement of tissues into the diminishing air space. Treatment of ear squeeze includes use of decongestants, and use of antibiotics if blood is present in the middle ear with no diving permitted until the ear has returned to normal. A ruptured tympanic membrane usually heals without intervention if infection does not develop. Sinus squeeze may be accompanied by epistaxis, because blood exits the engorged sinus. The injury is usually self-limited, and treatment consists of administration of decongestants. If acute sinusitis occurs, the patient should be treated with antibiotics. Mask squeeze causes conjunctival hemorrhage, and engorgement of the face within the mask. The patient will show a well-delineated injury shaped by the diving mask. No specific therapy is needed. Squeeze is a common, usually minor consequence of diving. Middle ear barotrauma is the most common diving-related disorder occurring in divers.

Inner ear barotrauma may occur on descent when a diver with a blocked eustachian tube performs forceful valsalva maneuvers. The low pressure in the middle ear, combined with increased pressure in the endolymph resulting from the valsalva maneuver may cause the round window to rupture and spill endolymph into the middle ear. Symptoms include sudden onset of vertigo with nausea and vomiting, tinnitus, and loss of hearing in the affected ear. On examination the diver may exhibit nystagmus, and a sensorineural hearing loss. Treatment includes management of vertigo with medication, appropriate positioning to minimize continued endolymph leakage, and use of decongestants. Surgical repair of the ruptured round window is often necessary to restore hearing and vestibular function. Divers who sustain a rupture of the round window are advised to avoid further diving, even after surgical repair.

Pulmonary Barotrauma

Because divers breathe gas pressurized to the ambient pressure, pressure gradients from the breathing supply to the airways are minimized. A diver exposed to compressed air at depth will experience expansion of the lung volume on ascent, according to Boyle's law, because ambient pressure decreases. If the diver breathes normally and exhales the increasing gas volume, no lung injury will occur; but if the diver ascends while breath-holding, at the surface the expanding gas will damage the lung. Overpressure of 95 to 110 cm H_2O can initiate damage to the lung. During ascent, expanding lung gases may not exit from the lung because of breath-holding or local pulmonary obstructions (such as bronchospasm, pulmonary secretions, or broncholiths). There may be other characteristics of the lung which predispose to pulmonary barotrauma.

Sport-diving accident statistics suggest that both heavy physical exertion while diving and rapid ascent, are common causes of pulmonary barotrauma and arterial gas embolism (AGE), but many cases occur without obvious provocation. Symptoms usually are evident shortly after the diver surfaces, when air is injected into the pulmonary veins, and embolization of the heart, brain and other organs occurs. 50% of victims are symptomatic immediately upon surfacing, and 95% of victims demonstrate symptoms within 7 minutes of surfacing. The most commonly involved organ is the brain, where stroke-like symptoms are found within minutes of surfacing. Changes in behavior, difficulty with concentration, irritability, severe headache, and visual changes, may also be manifestations of AGE. Serum creatine kinase may be markedly elevated due to embolization to skeletal muscle. In severe cases, coronary embolization will cause ECG changes which suggest acute myocardial infarction; replacement of blood in the heart and great vessels with air usually is fatal. Gas can migrate through the perivascular sheaths of the pulmonary vasculature to cause mediastinal emphysema and pneumothorax, can dissect into the retroperitoneum, and may dissect into the subcutaneous tissues of the neck. Divers breathing compressed air at depths greater than 4 feet are susceptible; therefore, the injury can occur even in a swimming pool if a compressed air source is used. Prevention is accomplished by training. Treatment for AGE is recompression in a hyperbaric chamber (see below). Pneumothorax, mediastinal, and subcutaneous emphysema do not require recompression therapy.

Decompression Sickness

Evolution of inert gas in tissues and blood due to supersaturation following diving causes decompression sickness (DCS). Unlike AGE, DCS produces delayed symptoms after ascent from diving and, because the gas supersaturation must exceed a threshold value, DCS usually does not occur after dives to depths of less than about 26 feet. In 50% of cases, DCS is evident less than one hour after the diver surfaces. Aviators may sustain DCS when flying in unpressurized aircraft above 18,000 feet, and divers may sustain DCS when flying shortly after diving, due to the reduced barometric pressure of most pressurized commercial aircraft. DCS is classified into two forms, a mild, nonsystemic form (type 1), which involves skin and joints, and a serious form (type 2), which involves the blood and several organ systems (Table 14-1). Symptoms (Table 14-2) can mimic a variety of other disorders. DCS develops after ascent from depth when a diver does not follow established procedures to prevent effervescence of dissolved inert gas (nitrogen). Free gas entering the vascular system can traverse the veins and cause pulmonary vascular obstruction. This syndrome is manifested by chest pain, dyspnea, and cough. Bubbles and tissue injury alter vascular permeability. In severe cases, pulmonary edema, hypovolemia, plasma loss, and hemoconcentration will result. A common manifestation of DCS in divers is spinal cord dys-

Table 14-1. Classification of decompression sickness

Type I: Pain-only decompression sickness
Limb or joint pain
Itch
Skin rash
Type II: Serious decompression sickness
Central nervous system
Pulmonary (chokes)
Systemic (hypovolemic shock)
Inner ear/vestibular

function. Symptoms include paresthesias, muscle weakness, paralysis of the lower extremities, bowel or bladder incontinence, urinary retention, and sexual impotence. In cases of sudden ascent from deep or prolonged dives, cerebral and spinal neurologic symptoms and unconsciousness may accompany hypovolemic shock and pulmonary edema. A rare symptom of DCS is sudden acute neurologic hearing loss or vestibular dysfunction. Decompression sickness of this type usually is caused by deep, prolonged commercial diving exposures and may result in permanent hearing loss.

A less serious form of DCS is manifested by pain in extremities and joints, itching, or an erythematous rash. Extremity and joint pain from DCS may be confused with pain from injuries; a rash may occur from contact with marine organisms while diving, and be mistaken for DCS. Peripheral manifestations of DCS may be isolated or accompanied by systemic manifestations. To determine whether more serious systemic manifestations are present, careful neurologic examination is essential in a diver with isolated joint pain or a rash.

Treatment of Decompression Sickness and Arterial Gas Embolism

Treatment of DCS and AGE requires recompression in a hyperbaric chamber with simultaneous administration of oxygen. If recompression therapy is not immediately available, the patient should be provided 100% oxygen by tight fitting mask, and IV fluid (normal saline) to prevent hemoconcentration. Divers with joint pains or neurologic abnormalities which develop within 24 hours of a diving exposure (Table 14-3) should have recompression treatment. Divers who have symptoms immediately upon surfacing should be managed in a similar fashion. Inappropriate treatments have resulted in permanent brain and spinal cord injury because of misdiagnosis. Because there are only a few centers in the United States which can provide expert consultation in this area, it is important to identify a local treatment facility for consultation. Persons suspected of having had a diving-related accident involving neurologic

Table 14-2. Frequency of decompression sickness-symptoms in 100 cases

Symptom	Percentage of all decompression sickness symptoms
Skin itch	4
Headache	11
Fatigue/malaise	13
Bone/joint pain	54
Spinal/back pain	11
Spinal/neurological	22
Respiratory	21

Adapted from U.S. Navy Diving Manual. NAVSEA 0994-LP001-9010. Washington, D.C.; U.S. Govt. Printing Office, 1993.

Table 14-3. Time of onset of decompression sickness after diving

Cumulative percentage	Time of onset
50	30 minutes
85	1 hour
95	3 hours
99	6 hours
100	24 hours

Adapted from U.S. Navy Diving Manual. NAVSEA 0994-LP001-9010. Washington, D.C.; U.S. Govt. Printing Office, 1993.

abnormalities should not be admitted to a hospital without hyperbaric treatment facilities because prolonging the time between onset of symptoms and recompression treatment increases the risk of permanent neurologic injury.

Adjunctive therapy has been developed to counteract the secondary (i.e., non-obstructive) effects of bubbles. Persons with neurologic DCS or AGE may benefit from fluid therapy to prevent hemoconcentration, use of intravenous steroids to inhibit cerebral or spinal cord edema, and of antiplatelet agents to prevent platelet aggregation by bubble surfaces in the blood. The benefits of these interventions, however, are based primarily on animal studies, and clinical trials to determine efficacy have not been conducted. In severe DCS, disseminated intravascular coagulation (DIC) may develop and anticoagulation may be considered. Unlike traumatic cord injury or stroke, prompt treatment of neurologic injury from DCS or air embolism often results in excellent recovery of function.

It is sometimes difficult to distinguish between severe DCS and cerebral air embolism. These two conditions may coexist when a diver who has been underwater for a significant period of time ascends rapidly and develops pulmonary barotrauma. Because treatment of both injuries involves recompression in a hyperbaric chamber, hyperbaric oxygen, and adjunctive drug therapy, it is less important to make a precise diagnosis and more important to institute therapy quickly. Decompression sickness usually develops sometime after diving (Table 14-3). Symptoms may develop within minutes of ascent or may develop late, appearing 24 hours after a dive has been completed. On the other hand, pulmonary barotrauma with AGE occurs immediately upon ascending and may produce initial unconsciousness. Because subtle signs of pulmonary barotrauma may go undetected in the initial few hours after ascent, timing of symptom onset should not be the only criteria for differentiating this disorder from DCS. When pulmonary barotrauma is suspected, a chest radiograph may be helpful in ruling out pneumothorax, mediastinal emphysema, or water aspiration. If water aspiration accompanies AGE, treatment for near-drowning should also be provided. Long delays in recompression treatment in order to obtain diagnostic tests should be avoided.

Recompression therapy involves one of several available protocols for application of pressure and oxygen. Commonly used protocols are U.S. Navy Table 6 for DCS and Table 6-A for AGE. These tables describe the course of pressure and oxygen to be provided to the afflicted diver.

Inert Gas Narcosis

Inert gas narcosis (nitrogen narcosis) results from breathing air at depth greater than 100 feet (four atmospheres pressure). Symptoms increase with depth, and include loss of coarse and fine motor control and high-order cognitive skills, bizarre and inappropriate behavior, improper response to emotional stress, hostility and eventually, unconsciousness. At depths of 300 to 400 feet, the anesthetic effect of nitrogen at this pressure causes unconsciousness. Susceptibility varies; some persons may manifest severe symptoms at 130 feet. Fatigue, heavy work, and cold water can augment the narcotic effect of nitrogen. Symptoms disappear immediately upon surfacing and often there is amnesia about the events that occurred below. In deep diving, helium is used in place of nitrogen, because narcosis does not occur with helium.

Diving with Medical Disorders

Many persons with chronic medical disorders want to dive, and some disorders limit or prohibit diving. Medication-dependent seizure disorder usually is considered an absolute contraindication to diving. Some authorities also consider residual neurologic injury from a previous diving accident a relative contraindication. Pulmonary disorders which are usually considered to be incompatible with safe diving include spontaneous pneumothorax, emphysema, and severe cases of reactive airway disease, with difficult-to-control clinical asthma. Individuals with mild asthma well controlled with medication or those with a history of asthma without overt symptoms appear to have no increased risk of diving-related injury. Atrial septal defect is a contraindication due to the risk of paradoxical embolism, and patients with coronary disease should not dive if exercise tolerance or ischemic threshold is less than 10 to 12 mets (maximum oxygen consumption 35 to 42 mL/kg/min).

Some evidence indicates that a patent foramen ovale (PFO) may increase risk of decompression sickness, but screening for its presence is not recommended because of its high prevalence (about 30% of all people) and its uncertain relationship with DCS. An echocardiogram performed to detect a PFO may be useful in patients with clinical DCS, particularly when the severity of the injury is out of proportion to the diving exposure. Insulin-dependent diabetes mellitus is considered by some authorities to be an absolute contraindication, but many divers with well-controlled diabetes appear to be diving safely. In most medical disorders, the prime consideration is the need to tolerate a reasonable amount of physical exertion. Persons with exercise tolerance of 10 to 12 mets (see above) usually have the capacity to dive safely.

Drugs and Diving

There are few concerns regarding interaction of medications with the diving environment. Of greater importance is the need to understand the medical disorder that prompts the drug treatment, to ensure that the disorder itself does not prohibit diving. Because most sport divers are exposed to sunlight, drugs that produce photosensitivity should be avoided. Sedative drugs, including antihistamines, may augment the effects of nitrogen narcosis, but in the usual sport-diving depths, this is of minimal concern. Antihypertensive medications, including β-blockers, calcium channel blockers, and angiotensin-converting enzyme inhibitors, in moderate doses, do not cause problems with diving, as long as exercise tolerance is adequate (see above). Diuretics should be used with caution when divers are exposed to high ambient temperatures such as those in tropical latitudes.

Suggested Readings

Anonymous. *Report on diving accidents and fatalities.* Durham, NC: Divers Alert Network, 1996.

Anonymous. *U.S. Navy diving manual.* NAVSEA 0994-LP001-9010. Washington, D.C.; U.S. Government Printing Office, 1993.

Bennett PB, Elliott DH. *The physiology and medicine of diving.* Philadelphia: W.B. Saunders, 1993.

Bove AA, Davis JC. *Diving medicine.* Philadelphia: W.B. Saunders, 1997.

Edmonds C, Lowry C, Pennefather J. *Diving and subaquatic medicine.* Oxford: Butterworth-Heinemann, 1992.

IV. PROTECTIVE EQUIPMENT

15. PROTECTIVE EQUIPMENT

Arthur L. Boland and Shawn D. Sieler

Protective Equipment

Protective equipment functions either to prevent injury or to protect an injury from repeated trauma. Equipment may prevent injury by adding mechanical support or enhancing proprioception. Energy from collisions is distributed over a wider area and is directed away from specific body regions. There are many technological improvements in the equipment and clothing now used to protect athletes. Lighter and more durable plastics have replaced leather in helmets and pads. Air and gel cells are used in addition to foam for shock absorption in various pads, helmets, and footwear. These advances have made equipment more protective yet lighter and less cumbersome, facilitating both functional performance and athlete compliance. Despite these improvements, however, fit remains the most important factor in selection of equipment. Equipment that is too small will not protect the body region adequately, while equipment that is too large will be cumbersome and restrict full range of motion (ROM). Fancy, expensive equipment that does not fit correctly will not provide the intended protection, placing the athlete at risk of injury.

The goal of equipment manufacturers and athletic departments is to provide the lightest, least restrictive, equipment while providing maximum protection. The new and reconditioned equipment is subject to impact standards, such as helmet-testing by the National Operating Committee on Standards for Athletic Equipment (NOCSAE). This is to ensure that the equipment can withstand forces likely to be encountered during competition. The governing body of each league specifies which equipment is mandated. These bodies also ensure that equipment is designed and padded so that it may not be used as a weapon against another player.

Pads, braces, splints, and tape are among the types of protective equipment. Pads are used to distribute contact forces to prevent injuries. Pads are the type of equipment mandated for most contact sports. Braces provide mechanical support and restrict joint motion, protecting muscles and ligaments. Splints provide external protection and limit joint motion. Splints may be rigid, semirigid, or soft. The materials range from thermoplastics, soft elastomers, or polyethylene foam. Tapes are used either to hold pads inplace or to limit joint motion, similar to braces. These different equipment types all have the same ultimate goal: providing protection from injury while allowing maximum athletic performance.

The protective equipment for many common competitive and recreational sports will be described. Emphasis will be on the required equipment for each sport. For each piece of equipment, the intended purpose, design, and construction materials, as well as proper fit and maintenance, will be discussed.

Football

The following equipment is required: helmet with face-mask; chin strap; mouth guard; shoulder pads; and hip, thigh, and knee pads. The football helmet protects the head from low-velocity, high-mass collisions which may cause diffuse injuries such as concussion and diffuse axonal injury. Concussions are more than 10 times more common than focal injuries such as a catastrophic subdural hematoma. The helmet design is a firm outer shell with an inner liner of energy-absorbing pads made of foam and inflatable air cells. The helmet is fitted by matching head size to an outer shell, then varying liner thickness or adjusting inflatable air cells to tailor the fit. The helmet fit must be rechecked within a few days of the initial fit to ensure that the air cells remain properly inflated. The four-point chin strap is now mandatory because it prevents the helmet from tilting forward or backward with impact. The face mask requirement is that it must have more than one bar. Individual masks are chosen by balancing vision and facial protection, which is determined by position and personal preference. The plexiglass shields give added eye protection and are now scratch-resistant and fog-free. The mouth guard is an intraoral, upper jaw retainer, which projects to the last molar. This enables unrestricted breathing and speech while protecting the teeth and providing shock absorption from chin blows.

The shoulder pads protect the shoulder girdle and decrease the force transferred onto the lateral acromion from collisions with other athletes or the playing surface. There is soft padding under the firm outer shell, which is held away from the acromioclavicular (AC) region like a cantilever. The fit is determined by chest size, being as snug as possible without interfering with breathing. The outer pad size and shape varies with position. Additional padding may be placed underneath, with foam inserts or doughnut cutouts used to protect the AC joint. Other pads may be attached to the main shoulder pad to provide protection for adjoining body regions. The neck guard is fastened right to the shoulder pad, limiting cervical spine extension and lateral bending. Longer anterior and posterior trim lines and newer side pads are available to protect the quarterback's thoracic cage, eliminating the older bulky "flak jacket." A plethora of non-required pads and braces are used on the upper extremity. An example is the shoulder harness, which limits abduction and external rotation in players with anterior shoulder instability. There are elbow, forearm, wrist, and finger pads available to limit motion or protect bony prominences or soft tissue contusions.

The hip girdle pads protect the coccygeal area and the lateral iliac crest prominence. The pads slip into inserts sewn into the shorts so that the pads remain in the area of intended protection. The pant jersey has similar inserts for the thigh and knee pads designed to protect the leg from direct blows. They are made of a firm plastic surrounded by foam. These pads are fitted to the players' waist and leg sizes. Linemen often prefer additional protection from prophylactic knee braces. The perceived risk of injury outweighs the speed and agility impairment in that group. These braces are single or double upright off-the-shelf devices designed to prevent varus or valgus knee injuries.

External ankle support is a combination of hightop cleats, tape, and braces. The lace-up ankle brace is used frequently. The effectiveness of bracing versus taping has been studied extensively. The tape appears to have similar stabilizing properties initially, but support is lost with exercise.

Hockey

Whereas football players need protection from direct forces of the playing surface and opposing players, hockey players require additional protection from rapidly moving projectiles and sticks. The equipment requirements for ice hockey are helmet, mouth guard, shoulder pads, elbow pads, gloves, hip girdle and thigh pads, and shin pads. Professionals are not required to wear face masks, although some routinely use half shields or visors, and face-injured players may wear full masks temporarily. The visor does not protect the upper face and eyes completely. Collegiate and other nonprofessional players must always wear full-length face shields.

Hockey helmets may be suspension or foam-air combination types. The helmet is fitted to the head size, and the outer shell is adjusted with a screwdriver; some inner liners are adjustable with air inflation. The hockey helmet must protect against both high-velocity, low-mass impacts (such as a puck or swinging stick) and low-velocity, high-mass impacts (such as body to end-board contact). The helmet also protects the ear from stick and puck injury. The face mask protects the chin, mouth, nose, and eyes from bodily contact and flying projectiles. Face masks must be full length and have the approval of the sponsoring league. As scratch-resistant and anti-fog technology has advanced, the trend is toward complete plexi-glass masks or combinations, with the traditional wire cage. The chin strap is combined with a chin pad attached to the mask, providing direct protection for the chin and preventing the helmet from tilting back and exposing the face. The mouth guard also is an intraoral, upper-retainer type. Although goaltender helmets may be available in a variety of styles, all will have the mandatory throat protector.

The shoulder pads provide protection of the lateral acromion and AC joint just as in football, but are generally smaller and lighter. Longer anterior and posterior extensions protect the midsection from stick and puck contact. These pads are fitted by chest size and now extend down to the top of the hip protection. Many women hockey players prefer the standard shoulder pads developed for men; however, pads with relief for the breast area made specifically for women are readily available. Neck rolls and shoulder harnesses are optional equipment, just as they are in football. The elbow pads cover the bony prominence of the olecranon and prevent slashing stick injuries to the forearms. The gloves extend from elbow pad to the finger tips. The protection is dorsal, while the palm is thin leather, allowing for better feel while handling a stick. The palm is protected when the fingers are wrapped around the stick or when the fist is clenched. If the leather is torn, purposely or through extended wear, the exposed fingers are at significant risk for injury.

The hip girdle and cup provides firm shell and foam protection for the sacrum, iliac crests, and groin. Groin protectors specifically for women are available, and are definitely recommended to prevent pelvic injuries. The thigh and shin protection is now both anterior and posterior. The shin-knee pad combination has a raised firm plastic shell along the anterior crest of the tibia. The posterior and superior foam extension gives added protection from sticks and pucks, especially during shot-blocking. The ankle has minimal protection from this pad and, together with the foot, is lightly protected only from the skate.

Lacrosse

The requirement for men's college lacrosse is: helmet, face mask, mouth guard, shoulder pads, elbow pads and gloves. Women are required to wear only the helmet, face mask, and mouth guard. Most of the equipment has a function and design similar to that of hockey equipment. The players not only have low-velocity, high-mass impact with each other and the playing surface, they are subject to repeated contact from a stick or firm ball moving at high speeds. Most of the equipment is similar to hockey in size, shape, and function.

The helmet is sized to the head and is supposed to sit off the crown of the skull. The face mask is mounted onto a short visor, which keeps the mask slightly further from the face. This provides both additional protection and visibility. The chin strap directly protects the chin and prevents helmet motion. The shoulder pads are nearly identical to hockey pads, though even smaller and lighter. The elbow pads and gloves complete the requirement for upper-extremity protection while providing maximal feel for stick handling.

Soccer

Soccer players need protection from direct force to the anterior crest of the tibia. The contact may be from an opposing leg, foot, or shoe cleat. The tibia is protected with a light shin guard worn and taped under each sock. There are a few preferred types of splints, all made of rigid or semirigid materials. The protection derives from a single large pad or multiple vertical slats. They are based on leg size and are chosen mainly for lightness, not protective quality. The men and women use essentially the same equipment.

Field Hockey

Participants in field hockey also need protection to the lower leg. The impact comes from the other competitors, their sticks, and the firm ball. Field hockey pads are nearly identical to those used in soccer. Unlike other contact stick sports, in field hockey the hands are not well protected with specialized gloves. Instead, golf- or sailing-type gloves are used, mainly to aid with grip and to prevent blister formation.

Wrestling

Wrestling requires the use of head gear to prevent the ear from repetitive trauma. The development of "cauliflower ear" may be a lasting deformity. The firm ear protector is covered by foam to protect the other competitor and is secured by a chin strap. If the head gear is dislodged or rotated, the match will often be delayed to replace the gear correctly. Boxers and water polo participants are the other athletes who require ear protection.

Baseball

Most nonprofessional leagues require batters to wear helmets with protection for both ears. The helmet is design to absorb the shock of the fast-pitched baseball. Because an impact from the ball is a relatively rare event, low-recovery foams may be used. These foams have maximal energy-absorbing capacity. Unlike football, in which prevention of diffuse injuries is the main concern, focal injuries like acute subdural hematoma directly under the impact site are most common in baseball and are thus the main priority of prevention. It is the responsibility of the batter to turn the exposed face away from a pitch directed at the head. This self-preservation turning is a learned maneuver and requires split-second reflexes as well as appropriate coaching instruction. Some Little Leaguers are now required to have additional facial protection consisting of a face bar attached to the helmet.

The catcher wears specialized gear for protection from the swinging bat, and from the pitched baseball, which rapidly changes direction just a few feet away. Like those of hockey goalies, the helmet and face mask in baseball must provide throat protection. Serious neck and airway problems have been caused by splintered bats and foul balls. Most masks have a throat extension built onto the lower portion. The chest protector is soft foam, to lessen impact. The catching shoulder is protected by the chest pad, while the dominant shoulder is exposed so that throwing is unimpeded. A cup absolutely is needed to protect the groin area. The thighs have no pads, but are protected by the squatting posture of the catcher. The shin pads are foam under a raised firm shell. They span from the ankle, across the knee, to the lower thigh. All equipment is made to match the particular body size.

In-line Skating

In-line skating is performed on concrete and asphalt surfaces shared by bikers and motorists. This, combined with the rapid speeds attainable, puts the skaters at risk for serious head injuries. A securely strapped helmet is therefore strongly recommended. The helmet is different in design than those for football and baseball. It is designed for one massive impact at a higher velocity. The foam liner is crushable, a type that can absorb the most impact. The fiberglass outer shell is designed to self-destruct on impact, also enabling maximal force dispersion. After an accident, the helmet must never be used again. The wrist guards contain a rigid plastic longitudinal slat which deflects the impact of a fall from the outstretched hand and wrist. It is very rare for a skater to incur a wrist fracture while wearing these guards. The knee and elbow pads mainly help reduce the frequency and severity of abrasions. Similar recommendations can be made to skate-boarders.

Cycling

In many states, it is mandatory for children to wear a helmet while riding a bicycle. Helmet wear is strongly recommended for all cyclists because of the risk of preventable head injury. The helmets' design is described in the above section on in-line skating.

Summary

Protective equipment must not be heavy or cumbersome, or athletes will not comply with established recommendations. The equipment must provide the maximum protection while being least restrictive. Most equipment now is certified as meeting safety standards intended to guarantee some minimal amount of protection. The most important measure, however, is ensuring proper fit of the equipment, to ensure the maximum benefit from modern equipment design and to comply with league rules. Frequently used equipment requires regular maintenance. Finally, optional and custom pads are available which may be tailored to each athlete's particular needs.

Suggested Reading

Albright J et al. Medial collateral ligament knee sprains in college football, brace wear preferences and injury risk. *Am J Sports Med* 1994; 22:2–18.

Greene T et al. Comparison of support provided by a semirigid orthosis and adhesive taping before, during, and after exercise. *Am J Sports Med* 1990; 18:498.

Nicholas J, Hershman E. *The lower extremity and spine in sports medicine,* 2nd ed. St. Louis, C.V. Mosby, 1995.

Nicholas J, Hershman E. *The upper extremity in sports medicine.* St. Louis: C.V. Mosby, 1990.

Pappas A. Upper extremity injuries in the athlete, New York: Churchill Livingstone, 1995.

Torg J. *Athletic injuries to the head and face,* 2nd ed., St. Louis: Mosby Yearbook, 1991.

V. NUTRITION

16. NUTRITION

Ann C. Grandjean, Kristin J. Reimers, and Jaime S. Ruud

In Part I of this chapter, we outline nutrition guidelines for calories, carbohydrate, protein, and fat. In Part II, we review fluid and electrolyte concepts. In Part III, we provide information to guide athletes whose goals are fat loss, rapid weight loss, or weight gain.

PART I. ASSESSING THE TRAINING DIET

I. Energy Requirements

Energy requirements depend on many factors such as body size, demands of the sport, period of training, training conditions, age and nontraining activity level. Significant intra- and interindividual variation exists in energy requirements. Among the highest reported energy intake groups are male swimmers, cyclists, triathletes, and basketball players, with intakes as high as 6,000 kcal/day being reported. Groups with lower energy intake include female figure skaters, gymnasts, and dancers, who may consume as few as 1,200 kcal/day. Based on per kilogram of body weight (bw), the highest intakes (65 kcal/kg bw) reported are those of adolescent swimmers and the lowest (28 kcal/kg bw) are those of wrestlers during the competitive season. Examination of individual data shows an even larger range of energy intakes, from a few hundred calories to more than 7,000 calories.

A. Estimating calorie requirements is difficult due to significant day-to-day, season-to-season, and athlete-to-athlete variation. However, general estimates of calorie requirements can be derived by energy balance techniques or by equations.
   1. Energy balance techniques. In the presence of stable weight, energy intake equals energy output/requirement. Assessment of energy intake is best achieved by analyzing one or more accurate, complete 3-day food logs.
   2. Equations for estimating daily energy needs. A simple rule of thumb to estimate energy needs is to multiply the athlete's weight in pounds by one of the following factors: activity level for males, light—17, moderate—19; heavy—23; activity level for females, light—16, moderate—17, and heavy—20.

II. Carbohydrate Requirements

Carbohydrate (CHO) requirement for most situations are not known due to wide interindividual and intersport variation. In most research conducted to determine CHO requirements, runners and cyclists have been examined in laboratory settings. Data from these studies has been extrapolated to athletes in other sports because no better data currently exist. As more applicable data become available, current recommendations may change.

A. Range of requirements. Research indicates that athletes training or competing frequently at high intensities (more than 70% VO_{2max}) for prolonged periods of time (more than 60 min) have a high CHO requirement; approximately 8 to 10 g CHO/kg bw/day will maintain muscle glycogen. Examples include distance runners and triathletes. Athletes whose training and competitions consist of brief periods of high-energy output, alternating with short periods of rest, such as those of sprinters, weight lifters, and football players, have lower CHO requirements; 5 g CHO/kg bw/day will support training. Regardless of sport, 200 g CHO/day is considered the minimum requirement. Along this continuum of CHO requirements, actual intakes vary significantly. Unless a problem with performance is observed, a drastic change in CHO intake is not indicated.

III. Protein

Athletes have increased protein requirements as compared with sedentary persons. Although, in the popular press, carbohydrate is emphasized and protein deemphasized as being essential to diet, adequate protein intake is not to be assumed in all athletes.

A. Factors that increase an athlete's protein requirements include:
   1. Low-calorie diet. An important factor affecting protein requirements is the interrelationship of protein and energy (calories). Increasing energy intake improves nitrogen balance. Therefore, protein requirements increase as energy intake decreases.
   2. Vegetarianism. Because digestibility and amino acid composition of plant protein is inferior to animal protein, vegetarians require greater protein intake. The Recommended Dietary Allowance for protein intake assumes a mixed diet containing 65% to 69% of protein derived from meat, poultry, fish, milk, milk products and/or eggs with the remaining 31% to 35% derived from plants. As the percentage of protein derived from plant protein increases above 35% of total protein intake, the amount of total protein needed on a basis of gram per kilogram of body weight also increases.
   3. Endurance or strength training. Utilization of protein (primarily leucine, isoleucine, and valine) as an energy substrate increases during endurance events. The amount utilized is variable based on glycogen stores and/or carbohydrate consumption.
   4. Resistance training. Resistance training and the muscular hypertrophy it produces increases protein requirements. The increased need appears to vary with degree of effort and phase of training.
   5. High muscle:fat ratio. A higher percentage of muscle tissue at a given weight will increase protein on a gram-per-kilogram basis.
   6. Growth. Growth in young athletes increases protein requirement.

B. Protein requirement (assuming adequate calorie intake and a representative American diet containing both animal and plant proteins) for endurance athletes is 0.9 g to 1.4 g/kg bw/day; for strength athletes, it is as much as 1.8 g/kg bw/day. Because many athletes do not fall neatly into either category, as a rule of thumb, most athletes are assured adequate protein requirements by consuming 1.5 to 2.0 g/kg bw/day.

IV. Fat

Fat is a concentrated source of energy. It functions as a carrier of fat-soluble vitamins, adds palatability to the diet, and has a protein-sparing effect. The dietary fat intakes of athletes vary considerably; intakes well above and below the commonly recommended 30% of total calories are common. Because dietary fat intake has not been shown to be ergogenic or ergolytic, if protein and carbohydrate intakes are appropriate, dietary fat manipulation is not indicated unless there is medical indication.

PART II. FLUIDS AND ELECTROLYTES

I. Fluid Replacement

Fluid replacement is critical to athletic performance. Consumption of fluids in sufficient amounts is essential for normal body function and, of particular concern to athletes, for thermal regulation. Failure to replace fluid loss results in dehydration, which can not only impair performance but can also be life-threatening. Unfortunately, deaths of athletes as a result of medical problems related to excessive heat stress during practice or game continue to be reported.

II. Total Body Water

Total body water is determined largely by body composition; water constitutes 65% to 75% of the weight of muscle and less than 25% of the weight of fat. Approximately two thirds of total body water is intracellular.

A. Water requirements. Requirement for water is approximately 1 ml/kcal energy expenditure for adults under normal conditions of energy expenditure and environmental exposure. This recommendation is increased to 1.5 ml/kcal to cover variations in activity level and sweating. Extreme or prolonged conditions, as well as individual variations, must be considered.

B. Water balance. Under normal conditions, fluid balance is achieved by regulation of fluid intake induced through changes in thirst sensations and regulation of loss through the kidneys (Table 16-1). However, during periods of physiologic stress, thirst is not an adequate regulator of water requirements. See section V on monitoring hydration status.

III. Temperature Regulation

The core temperature regulatory center is in the preoptic area of the anterior hypothalamus and performs an important role in maintaining thermal balance. When the blood bathing the hypothalamus exceeds 37°C (98.6°F), a reflex response (Benzinger reflex) dilates skin blood vessels and causes sympathetic cholinergic stimulation of eccrine sweat glands.

A. Heat gain. Heat is gained directly from the reactions of energy metabolism, especially in conversion of biochemical energy into mechanical work. During vigorous exercise, the metabolic rate can increase as much as 20 to 25 times basal level, producing a theoretical increase in core temperature of 1°C every 5 minutes. Heat may also be gained directly from the environment through radiation, conduction, and convection when the ambient temperature is greater than skin temperature. Dark clothing absorbs light and adds to radiant heat gain. In response to exercise in the heat, skin blood vessels dilate and blood is shunted from the visceral organs to working muscles and skin. Total peripheral resistance decreases and pulse pressure increases. Heart rate (HR) and stroke volume increase, improving cardiac output (CO) to meet the increased demands on the circulatory system.

B. Heat loss. As ambient temperature rises, the body must rely more on sweat evaporation for heat loss. Sweat evaporation lessens in high humidity. Heat loss in high humidity depends on (1) the surface exposed to the environment,

Table 16-1. Average daily water balance in adults

Water	Milliliters
Intake	
Liquids	1,100–1,200
Food	500–1,000
Water of oxidation	300–400
Total	1,900–2,600
Output	
Urine	900–1,400
Insensible loss via skin and lungs	800–1,000
Feces	200
Total	1,900–2,600

(2) the temperature and relative humidity of the ambient air, and (3) the convection air currents around the body. Athletes exposed to high temperature, high humidity, and sunlight can experience sizable fluid losses: 2 to 3 L of sweat per hour to as much as 15 L/day. If fluid lost from sweat is not replaced, strength, power, endurance, and aerobic capacity will decrease.

In conditions that allow rapid evaporation (including cloud cover, steady breezes, and low humidity), daily cooling capacity from sweating is several thousand calories per day. As sweat in contact with skin evaporates, the heat transferred by conduction from the skin to the sweat is transferred to the environment, which has a cooling effect on the skin. The cooled skin subsequently cools the blood that has been shunted from the interior to the periphery.

IV. Dehydration and Thermoregulation

The ability of the thermoregulatory and circulatory systems to meet the thermal and metabolic stress of exercise is markedly reduced in the volume-depleted state. A lowered blood volume in the dehydrated state results in decreased blood flow to the skin and hinders heat loss. A fluid loss of as little as 1% of total body weight is associated with a significant increase in core temperature during exercise. When dehydration becomes extreme, the body stops sweating in an attempt to conserve remaining blood volume. In this state, core temperatures can rise to lethal levels.

A. Adverse effects of dehydration. Fluid loss equal to 1% of body weight impairs thermoregulation; at 3% to 5%, rectal temperature and HR increase and CO decreases; and, at 7% loss, collapse is likely.

B. Involuntary dehydration. Humans will not maintain euhydration during periods of physiologic/thermal stress when fluid is consumed ad libitum. Experience shows that most athletes will voluntarily replace only two thirds of body water lost as sweat during exercise. Thirst is not an adequate indicator of fluid requirements during exercise, because an athlete is already 1% dehydrated when thirst is sensed.

Dehydration can be acute or chronic in nature. Acute dehydration can occur in a matter of 2 to 3 hours. Chronic dehydration is less visible and potentially more dangerous than acute dehydration. It usually results from several days of cumulative dehydration and, in athletes commonly occurs during early fall football or soccer practice.

V. Monitoring Hydration Status

Hydration status is best monitored by weighing before and after exercise while nude and dry. A decrease in body weight after exercise represents fluid loss from sweating; a pound of weight lost is equal to 16 ounces (480 ml) of water. This fluid should be replaced and weight should be normalized before the athlete participates in the next training episode or competition. Other signs of volume depletion include increased urine specific gravity, resting tachycardia, and prolonged muscle soreness.

Although less accurate, hydration status can also be assessed by the volume and color of urine. An adult produces a urine volume of about 1.2 quarts every 24 hours. Therefore, infrequent urination can be an indication of dehydration.

VI. Fluid Replacement

The primary goal of fluid replacement is to maintain plasma volume so that circulation and sweating are not compromised. An adequate fluid replacement schedule is critical. Failure to replace fluids during exercise can result in impaired heat dissipation, which can elevate body core temperature to levels above 104°F.

A. Absorption. The amount of ingested fluid that enters the circulatory blood depends on specific factors that influence gastric emptying and subsequent intestinal absorption of ingested fluids. Gastric emptying rate is influenced by the volume, temperature, and composition of the ingested fluids. Gastric emptying increases in proportion to the amount of fluid consumed, with a maximal rate of emptying achieved at a volume of approximately 600 ml. Maintaining a relatively large gastric fluid volume is beneficial when sweat rate is high.

B. Fluid type and amount will depend on the athlete, the duration and intensity of exercise, and the environmental temperature. In addition to normal daily fluid requirements (approximately 64 ounces), athletes should consume enough fluid to normalize weight after each training session or competition. Until the athlete determines that amount, a starting guideline is consumption of 2 cups (16 ounces) of fluid 2 hours before exercise followed by another 2 cups 15 to 20 minutes before exercise and 4 to 6 ounces of fluid every 10 to 15 minutes during exercise.

Cool water (between 59°F and 72°F) is an ideal fluid replacement. The addition of carbohydrate and/or electrolytes (e.g., sport drinks) can enhance fluid intake and absorption and delay fatigue in endurance exercise lasting more than 60 minutes. A 6% to 8% carbohydrate solution in the form of glucose, glucose polymer, or sucrose is absorbed rapidly and helps maintain blood glucose levels and enhance carbohydrate oxidation during exercise. Fructose is not actively absorbed and, when consumed in large quantities, can cause gastro-intestinal (GI) distress. After activity, flavored fluids can be more palatable than water and thereby will promote fluid replacement, as can food intake.

VII. Electrolytes

The role of electrolytes includes regulation of body water distribution between various fluid compartments, muscle and nerve contraction, and enzymatic control of cellular reactions.

A. Sodium is the mineral most affected by physical exercise; a deficiency can impair athletic performance. The concentration of sodium in sweat averages approximately 50 mmol$\cdot L^{-1}$ (1,150 mg/L) but can range from 20 to 100 mmol$\cdot$ L^{-1} (460 to 2,300 mg/L) depending on the state of heat acclimation, diet and hydration. In most cases, sodium lost in sweat can be replaced by normal dietary intake. Some athletes may need to increase intake of foods higher in sodium (i.e., pizza, ham, salted snack foods, and so on), and/or salt their food at the table.

1. Heat cramps due to sodium depletion may occur under extreme conditions in athletes who sweat excessively, who are not acclimated to the heat, and/or who have low sodium intakes (less than 2 to 4 g/day).

B. Potassium plays an essential role in muscular contraction and nerve conduction and helps in the transport of glucose across cell membranes and in the storage of glucose. More than 90% of ingested potassium is absorbed from the GI tract but, due to the kidney's regulatory role in potassium balance, higher and lower intakes are not reflected in fluctuations in plasma potassium. The most frequent cause of potassium deficiency is excess loss, usually through the kidney or alimentary tract such as during prolonged diuretic use, severe vomiting, chronic diarrhea, or laxative abuse. Signs and symptoms include fatigue, neuromuscular disturbances, and/or GI disorders. For most athletes, potassium replacement is not a major concern because losses are minimal relative to normal intake. Potassium lost in sweat can generally be replaced with a balanced diet providing approximately 1,875 to 5,625 mg/day. The average U.S. intake is 2,000 to 4,000 mg/day. Potassium requirements for an athlete who sweats profusely can usually be met by increasing potassium-rich foods such as citrus fruits and juices, meat, melon, strawberries, tomatoes, bananas, potatoes, and milk. Potassium supplements and/or electrolyte beverages containing potassium usually are not necessary. Table 16-2 lists potassium-rich foods.

Table 16-2. Foods that provide 5.0 mEq (200 mg) or more of potassium per average serving

Cereals	Carrots, raw
All Bran	Celery, boiled
100% Bran	Lentils and legumes
Bran Buds	Parsnips
Bran Chex	Kale, boiled
Meat	Potato
Beef	Pumpkin
Lamb	Spinach
Pork (except bacon)	Squash, winter
Turkey	Tomato
Veal	Zucchini, boiled
Fish	Fruits
Bass	Apricots, raw
Carp	Avocado
Catfish	Banana
Cod	Cantaloupe
Flounder	Honeydew melon
Haddock	Kiwi
Halibut	Mango
Herring	Orange
Perch	Pear, fresh
Pile	Pineapple
Pollack	Prunes
Red snapper	Raisins
Salmon	Rhubarb
Sole	Strawberries
Tuna	Tangelos
Dairy	Peach
Milk	Nuts/seeds
Buttermilk	Almonds
Cottage cheese (2% fat)	Chestnuts
Yogurt	Peanut butter
Vegetables	Pistachios
Broccoli, boiled	Soybean nuts
Brussels sprouts	Sunflower seeds

PART III. ISSUES OF WEIGHT AND BODY COMPOSITION

Athletes commonly seek out nutritional advice for three reasons: to reduce body fat, reduce body weight rapidly, or increase lean body mass. Assessment and guidelines are covered.

I. Body Fat Loss

Body fat loss can be ergogenic for athletes who are required to carry their mass through space at a high rate of horizontal or vertical velocity, e.g., high jumpers, sprinters, and pole vaulters. Body fat loss may also be ergogenic for athletes whose speed, endurance, agility, and jumping height would be enhanced through body fat loss, e.g., distance runners; road cyclists; and football, basketball, volleyball, baseball, softball, and soccer players. Likewise, athletes who participate in sports in which scoring is influenced by appearance attempt to maintain low body fat levels (e.g., those who participate in artistic and rhythmic gymnastics, figure skating, dancing, and bodybuilding). As these examples indicate, athletes who seek to lose body fat may be very lean or moderately "fat."

A. Assessment includes body composition assessment, weight change history, food intake and eating habits, and family weight history to determine genetic influence. Menstrual history in female athletes will help determine the health status of a lean female athlete. If amenorrhea exists, further calorie restriction is contraindicated.

   1. Determining minimum body fat levels depends on the athlete's genetic predisposition, development, sex, and performance. Some athletes naturally have levels of body fat considered subminimal and remain healthy and competitive. Others have body fat levels considered "high" as compared with those of their teammates, but below those which performance and health suffers. Determining optimal percent body fat on a case-by-case, trial-and-error basis appears to be the most useful method.

      If a lean female athlete is trying to achieve prepubescent body fat level, expect that fat loss will be difficult to achieve. If menses cease, if energy level/performance diminishes, or if weight/fat loss ceases despite continued calorie restriction, reassess and determine whether body fat loss efforts should continue. The ability to achieve and maintain minimal body fat levels is largely genetic. Some athletes will be able to do so while maintaining health and performance. Others will experience health and performance problems (e.g., recurrent illness or injury, amenorrhea, diminished strength and endurance). The clinician must be aware that athletes who can not easily achieve low body fat levels may try more extreme methods. Sometimes an athlete's acceptance that he or she has "matured out of" a sport or weight class requires counseling and support from the clinician.

B. Guidelines. Body fat loss is best achieved during the off-season and/or early preseason. Lean athletes can expect a rate of loss of less than or equal to $1/2$ lb/week. Athletes with excess body fat can lose as much as 2 pounds of body fat or 1% body weight per week.

   Creating a negative calorie balance by dietary modification and physical activity is the cornerstone of body fat loss. Based on the athletes' ability to modify diet (determined by such factors as training schedule, food availability, financial constraints, likelihood of compliance, and others), consider recommending methods such as establishing a regular eating schedule consisting of at least three meals a day, substituting fruits and vegetables for higher-calorie snacks, substituting low-fat foods for foods with higher fat content, and restricting alcohol, beer, and wine. Maintenance of food logs by the athlete is a valuable tool to increase awareness of consumption. Because a lean athlete's food intake typically is not excessive, reducing calorie intake by 200 to 300 calories a day is significant/maximal.

   For some athletes, physical activity/training is already at maximum. However, for others, aerobic activity can be increased to enhance calorie expenditure. Cross-training can enhance calorie expenditure in athletes who have become efficient in the primary training activities.

II. Rapid Weight Loss

Rapid weight loss (primarily fluid loss) is commonplace in sports with weight classifications, e.g., wrestling, judo, crew, weight lifting, or boxing. The process of rapid weight loss, often referred to as "cutting," is typically accomplished by restricting food and fluids and increasing sweating for 3 to 10 days before competition. Methods used include fluid and food restriction, exercise, and use of rubberized sweat suit, sauna, diuretics, and laxatives. After precompetition dieting/dehydration, athletes "refeed" and rehydrate after weighing in. The practice is repeated with each competition of the season.

Many professionals in the areas of science and medicine believe that cutting weight is ergolytic and detrimental to health. However, research does not confirm or negate this belief. Despite potential thermoregulatory dangers posed by dehydration, high-power performance lasting less than 30 seconds may not be affected if weight loss through dehydration is less than 5% of body weight. Seasoned athletes practice cutting weight with no apparent adverse consequences. Athletes who experience problems (e.g., frequent infections, heat illness, inability to make the weight class) are usually those who attempt to lose too much weight or to stay at the lower weight instead of refeeding and rehydrating. Investigators have claimed that cutting weight will increase the incidence of eating disorders, growth failure, and renal compromise is increasing, but no data either support or discount these claims. Earlier claims about reduction in resting metabolic rates in wrestlers who weight-cycle (i.e. rapidly lose and gain weight repeatedly during the season) have been refuted; no long-term change in metabolic rate has been observed.

A. Assessment. Although it is conventional (and often indicated) for health professionals to advise against cutting weight, most athletes will cut weight with or without professional guidance. Based on their personal philosophy and the specific situation, to help minimize or to avoid complications, clinicians may find it suitable to offer guidance to athletes who are cutting weight.

B. Risks. The risks of rapid weight loss should be reviewed with the athlete. These include fatigue, weakness, dizziness, decreased concentration, irritability, muscle cramps, muscle loss, glycogen loss, inability to restore fluid-electrolyte balance between weigh-in and competition, and diarrhea, nausea, and vomiting during the refeeding phase. Those most susceptible to complications are young inexperienced athletes who cut significant weight (e.g., more than 5% of body weight) and try to maintain a chronic state of dehydration and food restriction.

C. Guidelines. The schedule of competitions, tolerance to dehydration and refeeding, age, experience, and competitive status will have impact on the weight-cutting routine and guide the clinician who chooses to work together with the athlete to establish a routine that "works" for the athlete in terms of health and performance. The following guidelines will help an athlete develop a weight-cutting routine.

1. If competitions are spaced a week apart, do *not* restrict food and fluid during the first 2 to 3 days of the week. This will only prolong the state of dehydration.
2. Reduce bulk-forming foods (high-fiber cereal, raw fruits and vegetables, milk and cheese) in the diet a few days before weigh-in.
3. Twenty-four to 48 hours before weigh-in, decrease food and fluid and increase exercise. The safest routine allows the athlete to achieve the desired weight for the shortest time possible.
4. Immediately after weigh-in, rehydrate with a carbohydrate-electrolyte replacement beverage or water. Consume more concentrated food or fluid as tolerated. Liquid meal replacements may be better tolerated by athletes who are significantly dehydrated than will a traditional meal.
5. Recording weight-loss methods, refeeding techniques (what is drunk and eaten and how much), and performance outcome will help the athlete develop a routine that is suitable and help determine the viability of cutting weight.

III. Weight/Strength Gain

The key to gaining lean muscle mass is progressive resistance training (i.e., systematic weight-lifting program) and adequate diet. However, genetic predisposition, somatotype, maturity level, and compliance will determine the progress of an athlete.

A. Strength training program. The appropriate progressive, resistance-training program is the basic impetus to create lean tissue rather than fat tissue. Without training, fat mass will increase.

B. Nutrition program
   1. Meal/snack frequency. Five to nine meals/snacks daily normally are required. Skipping breakfast will impede progress. Continuous availability of food allows the athlete to eat whenever hungry or on the predetermined schedule.
   2. Diet composition. If the athlete's food volume is maximum, the goal is to increase calories without adding bulk. This can be accomplished by adding butter, margarine, peanut butter, sauces, salad dressing, syrup, jam, jelly, sugar, cheese, or powdered milk to the diet.
   3. High-calorie supplements in the form of shakes, canned beverages, or bars are beneficial when an athlete is unable to increase calories by consuming traditional meals and snacks and when conventional foods are not convenient. The primary goal is increased caloric intake; therefore, the supplement chosen is appropriately determined by the athlete's preference, product availability, and financial resources.
   4. Protein. Muscle hypertrophy increases protein requirements. Although the typical protein intake of many athletes will meet this increased requirement, that of others will not. Protein intake is often deemphasized by health professionals, but protein intake is a priority (real or perceived) for most weight-training athletes. Use of protein powders and amino acid supplements remains prevalent. Although such supplements usually are not a significant or necessary source of protein during weight gain, the psychological benefit derived from their use can be significant. Athlete's questions regarding supplements or other weight-gain aids deserve adequate attention, from the team physician or trainer because they can indicate a curiosity about other anabolic alternatives.

Suggested Readings

American College of Sports Medicine. Position stand: exercise and fluid replacement. *Med Sci Sports Exerc* 1996; 28:i–vii.

Fogelholm GM, Koskinen R, Laakso J, et al. Gradual and rapid weight loss: effects on nutrition and performance in male athletes. *Med Sci Sports Exerc* 1993;25:371–7.

Gisolfi CV, Duchman, SM. Guidelines for optimal replacement beverages for different athletic events. *Med Sci Sports Exerc* 1992;24:679.

Greenleaf JE. Problem: thirst, drinking behavior, and involuntary dehydration. *Med Sci Sports Exerc* 1992;25:645–56.

Lemon PWR. Protein and amino acid needs of the strength athlete. *Int J Sports Nutri* 1991;1:127–45.

Reimers KJ, Ruud JS, Grandjean AC. Sports nutrition. In: Mellion MB, ed. *Office sports medicine,* 2nd ed. Philadelphia: Hanley & Belfus, 1996.

Sawka MN. Physiological consequences of hypohydration: exercise performance and thermoregulation. *Med Sci Sports Exerc* 1992;24:657.

Tarnopolsky MA, Atkinson SA, MacDougall JD, et al. Evaluation of protein requirements for trained strength athletes. *J Appl Physiol* 1992;73:1986–95.

VI. **PHARMACOLOGY**

17. PERFORMANCE ENHANCERS

John A. Lombardo

I. Background

Performance enhancers are drugs, supplements, or procedures used to advance an athlete's performance from a "normal" level to a "supranormal" level. A supranormal level is one that is not attainable at any point without the use of the drug or procedure. If an athlete develops a tolerance for the drug or procedure, he or she is taken from a subnormal level, when not using the drug or procedure to a normal level, when one is used.

There are four types of performance enhancers.

1. Anabolic agents
2. Stimulants
3. Enhancers of oxygenation
4. Relaxants

When one evaluates a drug or procedure in this area, five questions must be answered:

1. What is the pattern of use?
2. Does it give the desired benefit (is it efficacious)?
3. What are the adverse effects?
4. What are the moral and legal implications of use?
5. Can it be detected by drug testing?

A. Pattern of Use. The information for patterns of use is obtained through:

1. Surveys—there are inherent problems with surveys but these give the best information about drug use patterns.
2. Drug testing results—the only information obtained from these results is the number of athletes that test positive, not the number of athletes that use the drugs.
3. Anecdotal reports—any statements or reports based on unscientific experiments or hearsay.
4. Legal infractions—like the drug testing results, these report only individuals who have had legal problems.
5. Beware the "Guesstimates of experts"—certain persons often are portrayed as experts by the media but have a limited frame of reference and inaccurate information.

B. Efficacy. The information for efficacy is obtained through:

1. Scientific data—results of research are difficult to evaluate because studies are few and do not replicate the environment in which the drugs or procedures are used.
2. Anecdotal reports—like unscientific information, anecdotal reports of success with a drug or procedure are fraught with confounding biases as well as the unknown influence of the "placebo effect."

C. Adverse effects. The information on adverse effects is dependent on:

1. Large series of individuals using the drugs—these series generally are found in the original research performed in preparation of the drug for FDA approval; there have been few large series done on athletes who have problems associated with drug use (these would be difficult to gather because drug use is not readily admitted and also because there is a large percentage of counterfeit drugs distributed, making it questionable whether the drug use is real or perceived).
2. Case reports, either individual or a series—as with any clinical entity, patients are seen by busy clinicians and are underreported for a number of reasons.
3. Anecdotal reports—anecdotal reports are still an inaccurate mechanism through which to reach conclusions (although they must be considered).

D. Moral or ethical implications. Performance enhancers are coercive drugs that result in an uneven playing field and limit the choices for the athlete who wants to be successful but does not want to use drugs.
E. Legal implications. Many of these drugs are controlled substances and possession and their distribution is illegal.
   1. In many states, medical licenses can be suspended or revoked for prescribing some of these drugs for performance enhancement.

II. Performance Enhancers

A. Anabolic Agents
   1. Androgens
      a. Testosterone and synthetic anabolic steroids
         (1) Oral and injectable synthetics have been popular in the past. However, with the advent of drug testing, these agents are now used predominantely by high-school athletes or those who either compete in an activity in which testing is not performed or are not involved in competition but simply take the drugs to "look good."
            (a) Dimethyltestosterone—potent, short half-life
         (2) Testosterone had been only available in long and short acting injectable forms. Now scrotal patches are available which deliver steady levels of testosterone.
      b. Efficacy
         (1) Lean mass increases when a high dose of androgen is used regardless of exercise, or when high-intensity exercise and proper diet and a moderate dose of androgen are used.
         (2) Strength increases with high-intensity exercise and proper diet and the use of androgens.
         (3) Recovery from high-intensity work is facilitated by the use of androgens. The mechanism for this effect is unknown but is believed to be related to the levels of catabolic corticosteroids and anabolic androgens combined with high-intensity work.
         (4) A rapid recovery can result in a higher level of work and can lead to increased speed and endurance.
      c. Adverse effects. Most of the adverse effects of androgens are reversible when the drugs are removed. Those that are irreversible are indicated by an asterisk (*).
         (1) Cardiovascular
            (a) Increased blood pressure
            (b) Decreased high density lipoprotein cholesterol (HDL-C)
            (c) Increased risk of cardiovascular accident (CVA) and myocardial infarction (MI)
            (d) Possible association with cardiomyopathy
         (2) Carcinogen–associated with an increased risk of developing cancer*—possibly through alterations in immune function
            (a) Liver
            (b) Kidney
            (c) Prostate
            (d) Testicular
         (3) Musculoskeletal—weakening of connective tissue through possible changes in collagen structure leading to increased incidence of injury
         (4) Psychological/behavioral—associated with psychosocial changes, including
            (a) Psychoses
            (b) Depression
            (c) Aggressive behavior
            (d) Mood swings
            (e) Libido changes—increase or decrease

- (5) Other
  - (a) Masculinization in women* including lowering of voice, skin, and hair pattern changes and associated with hirsutism, enlargement of the clitoris, and decrease in breast tissues.
  - (b) Premature closure of growth plates* with an unknown mechanism and an uncommon but real occurrence
  - (c) Immune system changes
  - (d) Human immunodeficiency virus (HIV) transmission with needle use*
  - (e) Acne
  - (f) Gynecomastia*
  - (g) Prostatic hypertrophy
  - (h) Impotence
  - (i) Decrease in number and function of sperm
- d. Drug testing
  - (1) Sensitive and specific for synthetics
  - (2) T/E ratio for testosterone, with a ratio of 6:1 being positive Approximately 2 in 1,000 have a ratio naturally greater than 6:1.
  - (3) DMT can be identified but has short half life.
  - (4) Profiling key for future

2. Human growth hormone (HGH) and insulin growth factor 1 (IGF-1)
   - a. Short half-life, structure identical to naturally occurring HGH and IGF-1
   - b. Not a controlled substance
   - c. Believed to be "Fountain of Youth"
   - d. Increasing availability
     - (1) Efficacy. No research has been done on IGF-1 efficacy and study of HGH is limited.
       - (a) HGH enhances strength and lean mass in HGH-deficiency states
       - (b) Studies on strength in those without HGH deficiency mixed
       - (c) No studies on IGF-1
     - (2) Adverse effects
       - (a) Acromegaly
       - (b) Diabetogenic
     - (3) Drug testing
       - (a) Short half-life
       - (b) Same structure as naturally occurring
3. Human chorionic gonadotropin (HCG)
   - a. Analogue of luteinizing hormone (LH) stimulates testes to produce testosterone
   - b. Efficacy
     - (1) Anecdotal reports: positive effects
   - c. Adverse effects
     - (1) Gynecomastia—increase in estrogen
     - (2) Fluid retention
     - (3) Changes in libido
     - (4) Blood pressure increases
   - d. Drug testing
     - (1) Can be identified by gas chromatography/mass spectrometry (GC/MS)
4. β-Sympathomimetics
   - a. Shown to have anabolic qualities when taken orally, but no anabolic effect when inhaled
   - b. Efficacy
     - (1) Moderate to strong anecdotal evidence of strength increases
     - (2) Increases in lean mass shown in animal studies and anecdotally

c. Adverse effects
   (1) Tachyarrhythmias
   (2) Anxiety, tremors, insomnia
   (3) Anorexia, nausea, vomiting
d. Drug testing
   (1) Sensitive and specific urine test

5. Amino acids
   a. Lysine, ornithine, and arginine believed to be building blocks for muscle and stimulants of HGH release
   b. Efficacy
      (1) Weak anecdotal reports
   c. Adverse Effects
      (1) Renal and hepatic overload
      (2) Purity of substance (if it is classified as food it is not as controlled by the FDA as drugs are).
   d. Drug testing
      (1) No test used
6. Creatine
   a. Ninety-five percent of total body creatine found in skeletal muscle
   b. Functions in the cellular energy system
   c. Efficacy
      (1) Early studies show enhancement of strength and performance in high-intensity exercise
      (2) No improvement in endurance exercise
   d. Adverse effects
      (1) No known adverse effects with short-term supplementation
      (2) No studies or reports on effects of high-dose, long-term supplementation
   e. Drug testing
      (1) Creatine is neither banned nor are tests conducted for use.
7. Natural Steroids
   a. Yohimbe, Smilax, γ-oryzanol
   b. Efficacy
      (1) Weak anecdotal reports
   c. Adverse effects
      (1) Purity
   d. Drug testing
      (1) No test used

B. Stimulants
   1. Amphetamines
      a. Indirect sympathomimetics
      b. Once very popular; popularity decreased because of adverse effect profile and testing
      c. Efficacy
         (1) Increased performance in a fatigued state
         (2) Mixed results in a rested state
      d. Adverse effects
         (1) Atrial and ventricular arrhythmias
         (2) Sudden death
         (3) Anxiety, tremors, insomnia
         (4) Dependency
         (5) Anorexia, nausea, vomiting
      e. Drug testing
         (1) Sensitive and specific test
         (2) Short half-life
   2. Caffeine
      a. A methylxanthine, found in many foods and drinks (coffee, colas, tea)

b. Efficacy
   (1) Increases alertness in fatigued state
   (2) Increases skeletal muscle contraction
   (3) Increases utilization of free fatty acids in endurance event
c. Adverse effects
   (1) Atrial arrhythmias
   (2) Vascular headaches
   (3) Diuresis
   (4) Anorexia, diarrhea
   (5) Anxiety, tremors, insomnia
   (6) Dependency
d. Drug testing
   (1) Banned by U.S. Olympic Committee (USOC) and International Olympic Committee (IOC) at a level of 12 μg/dL level
   (2) Not banned by professional leagues or National Collegiate Athletic Association (NCAA)

3. α-sympathomimetics
   a. Ephedrine and pseudoephedrine, both sold over the counter as an energy and power producers
   b. Efficacy
      (1) Increases alertness in fatigued state
   c. Adverse effects
      (1) Tachyarrhythmias
      (2) Anxiety, tremors, insomnia
      (3) Anorexia, nausea, vomiting
      (4) Dependency
   d. Drug testing
      (1) Specific and sensitive urine test
      (2) Banned by USOC and IOC
      (3) Therapeutic drugs and therefore not banned by professional leagues and NCAA
4. Nicotine
   a. Strong stimulant used by athletes mostly in the form of chewing tobacco
   b. Efficacy
      (1) No studies and only weak anecdotal evidence
   c. Adverse effects
      (1) Oral leukoplakia and oropharyngeal cancers
      (2) Dependence
      (3) Deleterious changes in lipid profile
      (4) Anxiety, tremors, insomnia
      (5) Anorexia, nausea, vomiting
   d. Drug testing
      (1) Not tested
      (2) Banned by NCAA at championship events

C. Enhancers of oxygenation
   1. Erythropoietin (Epo)
      a. Hormone used to stimulate the bone marrow to produce red blood cells (RBC)
      b. When given exogenously, overrides the body's natural controls
      c. Efficacy
         (1) Effective in raising circulating RBC and enhancing performance in endurance events
      d. Adverse effects
         (1) Polycythemia with sludging of RBCs and multiorgan failure
         (2) Death
      e. Drug testing
         (1) Reportedly urine test exists which may be effective

2. Blood doping
    a. Removal of 1 to 2 units of blood, stored as packed RBC and reinfused before an event to increase the circulating RBC and increase oxygen-carrying capacity and performance in endurance events
    b. Decreased in popularity with introduction of Epo
    c. Efficacy
        (1) Increases circulating RBCs and enhances performance in endurance events
    d. Adverse effects
        (1) Transfusion reaction
        (2) Blood-borne infection
        (3) Polycythemia with sledging and multiorgan failure
        (4) Death
    e. Drug testing
        (1) No sensitive urine test

D. Relaxants
1. Used by archers and rifle and pistol shooters to calm themselves and to remove their body tremors before they shoot.
2. Efficacy
    a. Low doses of both β-blockers and EtchOH have been shown to be effective in reducing tremor and enhancing performance in these events.
3. Adverse effects
    a. There are minimal adverse effects at the low levels used.
4. Drug testing
    a. There are sensitive and specific tests for these drugs.
    b. They are banned by the USOC and IOC in archery, riflery, and pistol shooting.

III. Addressing the Problem

A. What is needed?
1. Program
    a. Policy
    b. Education about:
        (1) Drugs
        (2) Program for
            (a) Athletes
            (b) Parents
            (c) Coaches
            (d) Administration
            (e) Public
        (3) Types of testing
            (a) Event
            (b) Cause
            (c) Random
            (d) As a result of a positive test
        (4) Discipline
        (5) Evaluation and treatment
2. High school program
    a. Include parents, students, teachers, administration, school board and local drug experts in planning.
    b. Education of all groups is key.
    c. Discipline should be realistic and enforced.
    d. Testing is rarely affordable or acceptable to all.
3. Research
4. Values
    a. If winning is the main goal, the environment is ripe for use of performance enhancers.

b. Our society exhibits a bottom-line mentality which, when applied to sports, can result in a disregard for rules as the winning or the result becomes the only important part of the program.

Suggested Reading

Balsam PD, Soderlund K, Ekblom B. Creatine in humans with special reference to creatine supplementation. *Sports Med* 1994;18:268–280.

Dodd SL, Herb RA, Powers SK. Caffeine and exercise performance. *Sports Med* 1993;15:14–23.

Kreider RB, Miriel V, Bertun E. Amino acid supplementation and exercise performance. Analysis of the proposed ergogenic value. *Sports Med* 1993;16:190–209.

Lombardo JA, Hickson RC, Lamb DR. Anabolic/androgenic steroids and growth hormone. In: Lamb DR, Williams MH, eds. *Perspectives in exercise science and sports medicine. Vol. 4: ergogenics: enhancement and performance and exercise in sport.* Brown and Benchmark, 1991.

Melchert RB, Welder AA. Cardiovascular effects of androgenic-anabolic steroids. *Med Sci Sports Exerc* 1995;27:1252–62.

Prather ID, Brown DE, North P, Wilson JR. Clenbuterol: a substitute for anabolic steroids. *Med Sci Sports Exerc* 1995;27:1118–21.

Spangler JG, Salisbury PL. Smokeless tobacco: Epidemiology, health effects and cessation strategies. *AFP* 1995;52:1421–30.

18. RECREATIONAL DRUGS

Gary I. Wadler

Although most discussions of drug abuse in sports focus on performance-enhancing drugs, abuse of so-called recreational or social drugs by athletes continues to be a significant problem. Whereas the use of ergogenic drugs is limited to a relatively small and well-defined group of athletes, the use of recreational drugs (e.g., illicit drugs, alcohol, nicotine) must be viewed within a much broader societal context. According to the National Institute on Drug Abuse, an estimated 74 million Americans have used at least one illicit substance in their lifetime; 13 million have used an illicit substance in the past month.

Substance use and abuse, including use and abuse of alcohol and nicotine, is the number one health problem in the United States, placing an enormous burden on the nation's health care system. It has been estimated that more deaths, illnesses, and disabilities result from substance abuse than from any other preventable health condition. Twenty-five percent of the 2 million deaths in the United States are attributable to the use of alcohol, illicit drugs, or tobacco.

Many diverse pathways lead to drug abuse. Factors contributing to recreational drug abuse include age, genetics, family influences, peer pressure, education, personality, and an array of mental health factors, including stress and underlying psychopathology. Athletes are not immune to these factors.

For some athletes, participation in competitive athletics may be an unusually anxiety-producing experience, thus representing yet another risk factor for substance abuse. The stress of failing to make a junior or senior high school team was rated in one study, as greater than that associated with the death of a grandparent, suspension from school, or the loss of a job by a parent. In such circumstances, drug and alcohol abuse can be a destructive coping mechanism. Two groups of young people who are most likely to experience repeated failure and suffer psychological trauma from competitive athletics are (1) those who demonstrate a low level of competence, relative to their peer group, due to inexperience, a lack of innate ability, or late maturation; and (2) those who perceive that they are not meeting the expectations of their peer group, coaches, or parents.

Forman's study of more than 1,000 male athletes in high school-sponsored athletic programs in the Chicagoland and Northwest Indiana areas, provides insight into the substance abuse patterns of high school male athletes. All 19 drugs studied were shown to have a lower prevalence of use among athletes in their senior year of high school than by nonathletes. The serial studies of Anderson et al. in 1985, 1989, and 1993 of the drug abuse habits of approximately 2,000 male and female college athletes participating in 10 different sports in NCAA Division I, II, and III schools have shed light on the patterns of use of both ergogenic and recreational drugs by college athletes.

No comparable studies, particularly with respect to recreational drugs, have been made of the incidence and prevalence of such drug use by professional athletes, although beginning in the 1980s, the media has contained numerous anecdotal stories of recreational drug abuse by high-profile elite athletes. Four factors—fame, fortune, free time, and a feeling of invincibility—seem to contribute in varying degrees to recreational drug abuse by professional athletes, particularly those involved in baseball, football, basketball and hockey. Great variations exist in the sociology, psychology, and physical demands of each sport which may have impact on the potential for recreational drug abuse within a given sport. Except for the concerted effort of the National Football League (NFL) to eliminate anabolic-androgenic steroids from the NFL, the principal focus in professional sports has been to eliminate recreational drug abuse, most notably, alcohol and cocaine abuse.

Some measure of the prevalence of recreational drug use by elite athletes might be deduced from the drug testing data of the National Collegiate Athlete Association (NCAA), the International Olympic Committee (IOC), the U.S. Olympic Committee

(USOC), the various National Governing Bodies (NGBs), and related organizations, as well as from those of the professional sports leagues. However, these data are confidential, which limits our ability to understand the qualitative and quantitative nature of the problem.

Alcohol

General

Alcohol is the most widely used and abused drug throughout the world; its consumption has waxed and waned over the centuries. In the United States, alcohol is consumed regularly by more than half the adult population; as many as 15 to 20 million people are alcoholics. Alcoholism and the 100,000 lives that are lost annually to alcoholism occurs at a cost of more than $100 billion. Persons who die of alcohol-related causes are estimated to lose, on the average, 26 years of their normal life expectancy. In the past decade, a slight decline in alcohol consumption appears to coincide with two factors: (1) the raising of the minimum drinking age to 21 years in all 50 states to counter the large number of fatal automobile accidents involving alcohol and teenagers, and (2) the shift from consumption of distilled spirits to consumption of beer and wine (which generally have a lower ethanol content). Coincident with the decline in alcohol consumption, there has been a significant decrease in alcohol-related traffic fatalities, particularly among young drivers.

In the early 1990s, researchers had estimated that by the time 70% of young people reach the eighth grade they had tried alcohol; 92% of high-school seniors had used alcohol; 5 percent were daily drinkers, and 38% periodically drank five or more drinks in a row. It has been conservatively estimated that the average American college student drinks more than 34 gallons of alcohol yearly. Beer is the predominant alcoholic beverage consumed by college students; the annual beer consumption of American college students is just short of 4 billion cans. This number of cans stacked end to end would extend 70,000 miles beyond the moon.

Alcohol remains by far the drug most commonly used by college athletes, with approximately 89% having reported alcohol use in the past 12 months in the studies of Anderson et al.

Although no firm data are available regarding the prevalence of alcohol use and abuse by professional athletes, three facts are clear: alcohol is the drug most abused by professional athletes; problems associated with alcohol abuse, e.g., driving while intoxicated (DWI) are far too commonplace; and a long-standing association exists between professional sports and the marketing of alcoholic beverages.

Physiology and Clinical Pharmacology

Alcohol (ethanol), a simple two-carbon structure, is a central nervous system (CNS) depressant. In general, its effects are proportional to its concentration in the blood, correlating best with rapid increases in blood concentration. Chronic ingestion leads to tolerance and physical dependence. Alcohol is rapidly absorbed from the gastrointestinal (GI) tract and is widely distributed to all organs and fluid compartments of the body, readily crossing the blood–brain barrier (BBB). More than 90% is completely oxidized to acetaldehyde; the remainder is excreted unchanged in the urine. In a person whose stomach is empty, peak alcohol blood levels may be reached within 45 minutes. In nonalcoholics, impairment of sensory perception, cognitive functions, and motor coordination occur with ethanol concentrations of 31 to 65 mg/dL. Intoxication occurs with blood concentrations of 50 to 100 mg/dL. Legal intoxication, in most states, is defined as ethanol concentrations greater than 100 mg/dL (0.1%).

On the average, "one drink" (1 ounce of 50% hard liquor, 50 proof), 12 ounces of 4% beer, or 3 ounces of wine will result in the same maximum blood concentration of 20 mg/dL. Blood ethanol levels decline at an average rate of 10 to 20 mg/dL/h irrespective of consumption, and the blood ethanol level is greatly, and inversely, influenced by body weight.

Effects on Performance

Alcohol is generally not considered performance enhancing and has been shown to have numerous deleterious effects on performance. It adversely effects balance and steadiness, reaction time, fine and complex motor skills, information processing and, inconsistently, may cause some decrease in anaerobic strength. Endurance, as reflected by aerobic capacity, $\dot{V}_{O2max}$, and oxygen consumption is not affected by alcohol. Poorly appreciated is the fact that athletes who consume alcohol the evening after practice or competition may subsequently perform significantly worse in tasks requiring attention and visuo-motor coordination skills for as long as 14 hours after ingestion of alcohol sufficient to raise their blood alcohol to 100 to 125 mg/dL. The anxiolytic effects associated with low-dose alcohol ingestion, hypothetically might improve athletic performance, particularly by controlling postural essential tremor. Alcohol may impair temperature regulation during prolonged exercise in the cold, and in the heat its diuretic effect may lead to dehydration.

Adverse Effects

The acute and chronic adverse effects of alcohol are numerous, and are well known and are not described herein.

Drug Testing

Alcohol is banned by the NCAA in rifle sports as well as in the modern pentathlon. Although alcohol is not specifically banned by the IOC, individual federations or NGBs may request testing for alcohol use.

Cocaine

General

Cocaine abuse has reached epidemic proportions in the United States. Once a drug for the affluent, its use cuts across all class lines. More than 30% of men and 20% of women aged 26 to 34 years have used cocaine at least once. Five million Americans use cocaine regularly. By 1986, cocaine had become the most common illicit drug of abuse in patients presenting to emergency rooms; in great measure the increase in use paralleling the appearance of "crack" cocaine. Chest pain was the most common complaint of patients presenting to emergency rooms with cocaine-related medical problems.

The abuse of cocaine moved center stage in sports with the 1986 deaths of Len Bias and Don Rogers. The serial studies of collegiate sports of Anderson et al. have shown an encouraging trend: The use of cocaine/crack decreased dramatically, 17.0% (1985), 5.4% (1989), 1.1% (1993). A large percentage of users had begun using cocaine in high school or earlier. Epidemiologic data on cocaine use patterns among elite amateur and professional athletes are almost nonexistent, but news stories of cocaine abuse by athletes are too common.

Physiology and Clinical Pharmacology

Cocaine is an ecgonine alkaloid derived from the leaf of the coca plant. Esterification of the base, ecgonine, produces the water-soluble product, cocaine hydrochloride, the form of cocaine that is either inhaled or injected. Cocaine hydrochloride readily decomposes when heated. By contrast, free base cocaine (requiring a volatile solvent in its preparation), and "crack" cocaine (not requiring a volatile solvent in its preparation) are heat stable and thus are smoked. Cocaine has a complex physiologic effect on the brain and shares similarities in this respect with amphetamine. Centrally, much of cocaine's effects are related to the blocking of neuronal reuptake of dopamine and excitatory amino acids, in turn increasing neurotransmitter concentrations. Peripherally, cocaine produces its sympathomimetic effect by inhibiting the reuptake of epinephrine and norepinephrine while stimulating the presynaptic release of norepinephrine.

Cocaine administration produces stimulation of the sympathetic nervous system (vasoconstriction, tachycardia, mydriasis, and hyperthermia), CNS stimulation (increased alertness, energy, loquaciousness, repetitive behavior, loss of appetite, and altered sexual behavior), and psychological stimulation (intense euphoria). Cocaine gains access to the cerebral circulation fastest when it is smoked. Inhalation of cocaine results in euphoria in 3 to 5 minutes, with blood concentrations rapidly increasing for 20 minutes and peaking at 60 minutes; levels of the drug are measurable for as long as 3 hours afterward. Increasing doses of the vaporized cocaine leads to increasingly intense euphoric internal sensations and increased social withdrawal and to cocaine binging (as often as every 10 minutes).

The biologic half-life ($t^{1/2}$) of cocaine in blood is approximately 1 hour. It is primarily metabolized to benzoyl ecgonine and ecgonine methyl ester, which have biologic half-lives of about 6 and 4 hours, respectively.

Effects on Performance

Aside from Freud's 1884 observation that within minutes of inhalation, cocaine transiently increased strength (as measured with a hand dynamometer), and increased reaction time, the few studies of the effects of cocaine on exercise suggest that little to no performance gains are incurred from cocaine use. Despite the amphetamine-like properties of cocaine, no evidence suggests that cocaine enhances athletic performance in a sustained way. Reporting late or early for practice, missing practices, and fighting with teammates may be clues indicating an athlete's use of cocaine.

Adverse Effects

The adverse effects associated with cocaine abuse are innumerable, but some of them are of particular concern when athletes abuse: cardiac death and other sudden death.

The sudden cardiac death of Len Bias is illustrative of the lethality associated with cocaine abuse by athletes. The mechanisms considered causative of myocardial ischemia associated with cocaine abuse include increased myocardial oxygen demand, coronary vasoconstriction, in situ thrombus formation (enhanced platelet aggregation), premature atherosclerosis, and biventricular hypertrophy. Because of the nature of the symptoms that may be associated with cocaine abuse (i.e., palpitations, anxiety, dyspnea, and nausea), physicians are obligated to evaluate a cocaine abuser with chest pain for possible myocardial infarction. However, in some studies, the percentage of actual infarctions was quite low, approximating 6% in two prospective studies. Of note is the increased association of actual infarction with cigarette smoking, presumably related to the induction of coronary artery vasospasm mediated though the α-adrenergic system, similar to that of cocaine. In some studies, approximately one third of the patients who sustained cocaine-related myocardial infarctions had angiographically normal coronary arteries. Because the physiology of cocaine-induced myocardial ischemia differs from that of more typical myocardial ischemia, Hollander has suggested a treatment paradigm that takes these physiologic considerations into account.

Sudden death has been associated with cocaine use. The blood levels of cocaine in these cases have varied widely. Various mechanisms of sudden death have been postulated and include arrhythmias, status epilepticus, respiratory arrest, and intracerebral hemorrhage. The arrhythmias associated with cocaine use include ventricular fibrillation, asystole, and accelerated ventricular arrhythmias.

Drug Testing

Because of the very short serum half-life of cocaine—1 hour—measurements of blood levels will detect only very recent usage. The detection window of cocaine's urinary metabolites, benzoyl ecgonine and ecgonine methyl ester, is determined by the amount of cocaine used and the sensitivity of the drug assay. Immunoassays (enzyme-linked immunosorbent assay) are used for screening, and gas chromatography/mass spectrometry (GC/MS) is used for confirmation. Screening immunoassays for benzoyl ecgonine have a threshold of 300 ng/mL, whereas GC/MS can detect concentrations of 1 to 10 ng/mL. Accordingly, the approximate detection window is 1 to 2 days if an immunoassay is used and 5 to 6 days if GC/MS is used. With long-term cocaine use, the metabolite can be detected as long as 22 days after the last cocaine use.

Smokeless Tobacco

Cigarette smoking, uncommon in 1900, peaked in 1964, according to the Surgeon General's Report, when 44% of all adult Americans smoked. With the decline in cigarette smoking, the use of smokeless tobacco increased, almost tripling in the past 20 years. Smokeless tobacco, an extremely addictive substance, has a particularly high incidence of use in certain demographic groups, particularly adolescents and Native Americans. Smokeless tobacco is available as chewing tobacco or as snuff. Between approximately 1980 and 1990, while chewing tobacco sales in the United States declined 12% from 72.3 million pounds to 63.5 million pounds, moist snuff sales increased 57% from 26.7 million pounds to 49.5 million pounds. Currently, three quarters of a billion tins of snuff are sold annually; more than 12 million Americans use smokeless tobacco, and 50% use it regularly. The greatest increase in smokeless tobacco use in the past two decades has occurred among adolescents, with as many as 24% of white male high school students identifying themselves as current users. The highest use of smokeless tobacco is among white males between age 18 to 24 years.

Associations that correlate positively with continued smokeless tobacco use include male sex; smoking; use of other substances, particularly alcohol; use by family member or peers; and initiation of use between the ages of 6 and 8 years. Loose-leaf smokeless tobacco is typically sold in pouches; moist or dry powdered tobacco (snuff) is usually sold in small round cans. When loose-leaf tobacco is "chewed" a golf ball-sized amount is placed between the cheek and lower gum and is either sucked or chewed. "Dipping" is leaving a pinch of tobacco (snuff) between the cheek or lip and the lower gum. A wad of tobacco may be left in the mouth for as long as 30 minutes. Twenty-five percent of users may use as many as 10 wads a day.

Smokeless tobacco has long been used by athletes. Its association with baseball is well known; 100 years ago it was reputed to have been used in baseball in an attempt to keep the players' mouths moist during play in dusty parks. Its widespread presence and influence in the sports world are indisputable. The studies of Anderson et al. showed that the use of smokeless tobacco increased greatly from 19.8% in 1985 to 27.6% in 1989 and appeared to level off at 26.9% in 1993. There was a steady increase in reported use of smokeless tobacco by women during the 8-year study period, except among softball players, among whom the use remained relatively high.

Twenty-one percent of these student athletes had begun using smokeless tobacco in junior high school or before, and 54% did so in high school. Despite the common belief that the use of smokeless tobacco is more common in certain parts of the country, its use was shown to occur evenly across all regions. Furthermore, the studies showed that although use of smokeless tobacco was particularly prevalent among baseball players, it was also widespread among football players as well as among male tennis players and male track athletes. As many as 9% of female softball players reported using smokeless tobacco.

The studies of Anderson et al. also provide some insight into athletes' motivations for using smokeless tobacco: 62% used it for recreational reasons, 28% used it because it made them feel good, and 1.3% used it in an attempt to improve performance.

Various organizational strategies have been devised to halt the widespread use of smokeless tobacco. In major league baseball all tobacco products have been banned throughout the minor league system, from the Rookie League to Triple A. This ban on tobacco use applies to players, managers, coaches, and umpires. Major League Baseball is offering counseling and assistance to those who wish to quit and many teams have banned free samples from their clubhouses. The NCAA has banned use of all tobacco products by athletes, coaches, and officials during practices and games. The American College of Sports Medicine released a Current Comment denouncing the use of smokeless tobacco by athletes as well as tobacco sponsorship of athletic events.

Physiology and Clinical Pharmacology

Nicotine, a potent alkaloid found in smoking and smokeless tobacco, is responsible for the pharmacologic effects of tobacco use. Its physiologic effects are dose related and biphasic, leading to a variety of clinical responses. The plasma nicotine levels in smokers and smokeless tobacco users are similar. Prolonged use leads to tolerance which permits an increase in dose without the resultant unpleasant side effects observed in nicotine-naive individuals. As with cigarette use, physical dependence develops with smokeless tobacco use and withdrawal may be manifested by craving, irritability, restlessness, anxiety, changes in appetite, and GI complaints.

Conitine is the major metabolite of nicotine and has a much longer half-life than nicotine. Accordingly, conitine is widely used as a biochemical marker of average daily nicotine use.

Effects on Performance

The effects of nicotine on performance are of doubtful significance. While there is some calming effect, some enhancement of alerting mechanisms, and some improvement in information processing, there is also some performance decrements during sustained vigilance tasks. Despite some athlete claims to the contrary, no improvement in reaction time or movement time has been noted with smokeless tobacco.

Adverse Effects

The adverse effects of smokeless tobacco, aside from its addictive quality, principally relate to its dental and oral effects and to its systemic effects.

The dental sequelae of smokeless tobacco include gingival recession and the loss of periodontal attachments. These effects are particularly evident at the site in the oral cavity where the snuff is typically placed. Although caries do not appear to be more common in users, there is staining and abrading of the teeth. Halitosis is common.

Oral leukoplakia is frequently associated with smokeless tobacco use. A white or yellowish brown, wrinkled lesion is apparent in at least 50% of regular snuff users. The lesion may be irreversible and may be associated with a 3% to 6% transformation rate to squamous cell carcinoma over time. These smokeless tobacco-related cancers appear to be particularly aggressive, with a 5 year survival rate of less than 50%.

The systemic effects of smokeless tobacco correlate with the amount of nicotine delivered systemically. Smokeless tobacco generally has very high levels of nicotine as compared with cigarettes. A typical single dose of nicotine in snuff is almost twice the dose of nicotine in cigarettes, and the typical single dose of nicotine in chewing tobacco is more than 15 times the dose in cigarettes. Although smokeless tobacco use has not been demonstrated to potentiate atherosclerosis, short-term adverse effects of smokeless tobacco on heart rate, diastolic blood pressure (DBP), total and high-density lipoprotein (HDL) cholesterol have been reported. Platelet aggregation appears to be enhanced through nicotine's inhibitory affect on prostacyclin synthesis. The increase in gastroesophageal reflux and peptic ulcer disease is a function of nicotine's cholinergic agonist activity.

Marijuana

Marijuana's history and knowledge of its properties dates back almost 5,000 years, beginning with the cultivation of hemp, *Cannabis sativa,* in mainland China. Currently, marijuana is the most widely used and abused illicit psychoactive substance in America and probably the world, with 1 billion people worldwide having used the drug. Beginning in the 1950s, the use of marijuana exploded. Forty to 45 million Americans are estimated to have tried marijuana; 15 to 20 million are regular users. The sequential studies of college athletes of Anderson et al. show a gradual decline in usage of marijuana/hashish between 1985 and 1993, from 35.3% to 21.4%, paralleled by sizable decline in heavy users (40 or more times a year). Fifty-nine percent of users began using marijuana/hashish in high school and 15% did so in junior high school or earlier. No recent data are available regarding marijuana use by professional athletes.

Marijuana is considered a gateway drug, like alcohol and cigarettes; research has shown that young people are unlikely to use marijuana if they have not already used alcohol and cigarettes; they are even less likely to use hard drugs if they have not already used marijuana.

Physiology and Clinical Pharmacology

The principal active ingredient of marijuana is delta-9-tetrahydrocannabinol (delta-9-THC), which influences diverse neurochemical pathways in the CNS. Marijuana differs from many other drugs in that it produces both CNS excitation and depression, expressed both behaviorally and neurophysiologically. Chronic use is associated with tolerance, and users may tend to increase both the dose and frequency of use, potentially leading to both psychological and physical dependence.

The marijuana that is used illicitly is typically derived from the female plant and is a mixture of dried hemp flowers, seeds, leaves, and small stems. The stems and seeds are discarded before the marijuana is smoked. Hashish is derived from the resin of the female flowers. Within minutes of inhalation of either form, blood levels of THC are achieved, with peak physiologic and subjective effects occurring in 20 to 30 minutes and subjective effects lasting 2 to 4 hours. Because of the lipid solubility of marijuana, blood levels decrease very rapidly and reach 5% to 10% of their initial levels in 1 hour. However, because of redistribution, the terminal half-life of marijuana in the blood is about 20 hours.

In recent years, the potency of marijuana has increased 5 to 10 times or more. An understanding of the pharmacology of illicit marijuana use is complicated by the variations in dosages used as well as by the presence of numerous adulterants, including phencyclidine (PCP).

Marijuana is typically smoked in the form of cigarettes termed "joints" or from a water pipe termed a "bong." Hashish is smoked alone or is mixed with tobacco or marijuana. It may be eaten as well (e.g., mixed in brownies).

Effects on Performance

Many of the acute effects of marijuana are deleterious to athletic performance. It impairs eye-hand coordination and fast reaction time and reduces motor coordination, tracking ability, and perceptual accuracy. Time appears to move more slowly, and impaired concentration and dreamlike states are common. Although these acute effects may last as long as 4 hours, skill impairment may persist for as long as 24 h after marijuana intoxication. As with alcohol, social use of marijuana the night before a practice or a game may impair performance. Marijuana reduces maximal exercise performance, and $\dot{V}_{O2max}$ is achieved prematurely. No ergogenic effect has been attributed to marijuana usage.

Adverse Effects

For a detailed review of the adverse effects of marijuana, see Hollister's *Health aspects of Cannabis.* With respect to athletes, several adverse effects associated with marijuana use and abuse are noteworthy. Acute behavioral manifestations may include paranoia, panic attacks, and delirium and psychoses. An "amotivational syndrome," though controversial, has been attributed to chronic marijuana use and includes apathy, impaired judgment, loss of ambition, and inability to carry out long-term plans.

Tachycardia, mediated primarily through changes in vagal tone, and orthostatic hypotension may occur after acute use of marijuana, but tolerance to these effects may develop with chronic use. Carboxyhemoglobin saturation increases nearly threefold when marijuana is smoked, 5 times the increase that cause by smoking of a single filter-tipped tobacco cigarette. Impaired sweating ability may lead to increases in core temperature.

Particularly bothersome may be the appearance of rhinitis, pharyngitis, bronchitis, and bronchospasm, as well as an increase in gastric emptying time and a decrease in GI motility.

Drug Testing

Whereas marijuana is not specifically banned by the IOC, it may be banned by the NGBs, and it is banned by the NCAA. The biologic half-life of delta-9-THC varies greatly among individuals, ranging from 56 hours in acute users to 28 hours in chronic users. Delta-9-THC is rapidly transformed into urinary metabolites, whereas the metabolite THCA may be detected in acute users for 4 to 6 days and in chronic users for 20 to 30 days by GC/MS.

Suggested Reading

Anderson WA, Albrecht RR, McKeag DB. Second replication of a national study of the substance use and abuse habits of college student-athletes. Presented to the National Collegiate Athletic Association, Overland Park, Kansas, July 30, 1993.

Forman ES, Dekker AH, Javors JR, Davison DT. High-risk behaviors in teenage male athletes. *Clin J Sport Med,* 1995;5:36.
Hollander JE. The management of cocaine-associated myocardial ischemia. *N. Engl J Med* 1995;333:1267.
Holister L. Health aspects of cannabis. *Pharmacol Rev* 1986;38:1
Wadler GI. Sports organizations. In: Coombs RH, Ziedonis D, eds. *Handbook of drug abuse prevention,* Boston: Allyn and Bacon, 1995:197–216.
Wadler GI, Hainline B. *Drugs and the athlete.* Philadelphia, F.A. Davis, 1989.

19. DRUG TESTING

Christopher A. McGrew

I. Introduction and Overview

A. In the United States, a variety of mandatory drug-testing programs affect many athletes.
   1. These programs include drug testing for the United States Olympic Committee (USOC) and associated national governing bodies (NGBs), the National Collegiate Athletic Association (NCAA), certain high school districts, and professional sports leagues.
   2. It is imperative that physicians treating competitive athletes be familiar with these programs, including their testing procedures and potential ramifications.

B. In the United States, there are two primary drug-testing programs for "amateur" athletes. These programs are the focus of this chapter.
   1. The NCAA drug-testing program began in 1986 and has jurisdiction over all NCAA athletes.
   2. The USOC drug-testing program began in 1985 (although drug testing started in the Olympics in 1968), and has jurisdiction over Americans competing in the PanAm Games, the United States Olympic Festival, and the Olympic Games.
   3. The basic goal for both programs is to promote the health of athletes and fair competition.
   4. There are some minor differences in the programs because of specific characteristics of the organizations and variance among interpretations of limited scientific data concerning several substances (e.g., caffeine, over-the-counter decongestants). In general, their similarities are far greater than their differences.

II. Informed Consent

A. In the NCAA athletic program, all athletes sign an annual consent form indicating their understanding of and compliance with NCAA rules and regulations including those of the NCAA drug-testing program. An athlete who fails to sign the consent is ineligible until they do so.

B. In the USOC program, each athletic NGB also obtains and forwards signed athlete consent forms to the USOC.
   1. Only athletes who have agreed to submit to testing may compete in USOC-sanctioned events.
   2. The consent forms are required for selection to national teams and participation in international competitions.
   3. Because these events vary in frequency, consent forms are not necessarily obtained on an annual basis as they are for the NCAA.

III. Types of Testing

A. Championship/in-competition testing
   1. In the NCAA, participants in all championship events, tournaments, and so on, are subject to drug testing from year to year, although all are not tested in any given year.
   2. The substances tested for include those listed for year-round testing (anabolic steroids and related masking agents), along with stimulants (including caffeine in high concentrations (see Appendix 3) and street drugs.
   3. In riflery, alcohol and β-blockers are included in the banned substance list. (See Appendix 3.)
   4. The USOC and NGBs may test for drugs at any camp or competition they sponsor.

5. The drug list for their testing includes stimulants, certain narcotics and pain killers, anabolic agents, diuretics, peptide and glycoprotein hormones, and tranquilizers and sedatives (in certain sports). (See Appendix 3).
6. In addition, alcohol, β-blockers, and marijuana may be tested for in certain sports. (See Appendix 3).
7. Certain local anesthetics, corticosteroids, and β_2-agonist asthma inhalers are restricted, meaning that they can be used only under specific and circumscribed conditions.
8. Caffeine in concentrations greater than 12 μg/mL is prohibited by USOC, >15 μg/ml for NCAA.

B. "Off-season"/out-of-competition/year-round testing
1. In the NCAA, for Divisions IA and IAA and Division II Football and for Division I Women's and Men's Track and Field teams, the NCAA drug testing program is in effect throughout the academic year (August to June) for anabolic steroids and related masking agents. (See appendix 3.) (Individual schools are free to conduct additional drug testing of their student athletes throughout the academic year, but these are not reported to the NCAA, nor are they subject to NCAA sanctions.)
2. In the USOC out-of-competition program, athletes are subject to testing at any time during the year, (also known as "short-notice" testing). Only designated "high-risk" sports are required to participate in this program. Substances tested for in this program include anabolic agents, diuretics, manipulative/masking agents, and peptide glycoprotein hormones (and analogues). (See Appendix 3.)

IV. Selection for Testing

A. The NCAA method
1. The NCAA method for selecting a specific student athlete for testing at a particular championship or individual institution (during year-round testing) is recommended and modified by the NCAA Competitive Safeguards Committee and is approved by the NCAA Executive Committee.
2. The year-round selection for testing is either entirely random or may be based on a variety of factors, including playing time, position, and financial-aid status.
3. In championship events, the selection for testing may include the first-, second-, and third-place finishers (or in the case of team sports, playing time) as well as other randomly selected athletes from the remaining field.

B. The USOC method
1. The USOC method follows a prescribed protocol (established by the USOC's Division of Drug Control Administration) of randomly selecting athletes to be tested at competitions, including those participating in USOC established events (e.g., sport festivals, Pan American Games trials, Winter and Summer Olympic Games trials, Olympic Training Center camps, and so on).
2. All members of the Olympic team, including alternate members, are tested 30 to 90 days before the Olympic Games.
3. Athletes are selected for testing in a manner mutually agreed on by the responsible authorities (e.g., the NGB, USOC, IOC).
4. In some cases, selected medalists are chosen; testing is performed on a random basis at other events.

V. Notification for Drug Testing

A. In USOC and NCAA championship events, selected athletes are notified as soon as is reasonably possible after their event is completed.
1. They are told to report to the drug testing station within 1 hour and are observed continually from the time they are notified until they provide and verify a satisfactory specimen.

B. In the USOC year-round, out-of-competition, short-notice testing, the selection process requires short notice to the athlete, generally less than 48 hours.

1. The athlete is notified in one of three ways: telephone, direct personal contact, or return receipt correspondence.
2. It is anticipated that this program will shortly evolve to encompass "no-advance notice" testing, with athletes being required to undergo testing immediately upon being notified of their selection.

C. For NCAA out-of-competition or off-season testing, the NCAA notifies the director of athletics or their designee 2 days before the day of on-campus drug testing.
   1. The institution then notifies the student athlete of the date and time to report for testing.
   2. All student athletes from the official NCAA squad list at the school are subject to testing.

D. Both the USOC and NCAA realize that even 48 hours of "lead time" may be sufficient for some athletes to use methods to foil the test. Both groups are investigating plans to shorten this lead time.

VI. The Drug Testing Station

A. Obviously, it is difficult to describe one consistent layout for a drug-testing station since athletic facilities differ as do laboratories. In addition, the protocols are constantly updated and changed.
   1. The athlete provides identification when entering the drug-testing station (picture identification (ID) is now required for NCAA Division I year-round testing and for USOC out-of-competition testing), and the athlete is under constant observation by a testing official at all times.
   2. The athlete is asked to select a container to provide a urine sample.
   3. At this point, the USOC and the NCAA protocols are different in that the USOC protocol asks that the athlete to declare all medications that have been taken recently. The NCAA has discontinued this part of the protocol.
   4. The athlete, still under observation, then provides a urine sample. A witness of the same sex as the athlete observes the urination process. This is a key step in the testing procedure to ensure that the urine sample is genuine and is that of the athlete being tested.
   5. The athlete then chooses two laboratory specimen bottles (bottles A and B) and divides the urine sample into bottle A and bottle B for sealing and submission to the laboratory. The split urine sample is handled in strict chain-of-custody protocol. (Chain of custody is the sample handling procedure designed to prevent specimen tampering or a mixup.)
   6. The athlete then signs a statement that the above procedures have been followed strictly and leaves the testing area.

B. Athletes have as much time as they need to provide a urine sample.
   1. Nonalcoholic beverages are provided in the testing center to facilitate production of urine. Caffeinated beverages are excluded in certain test facilities: i.e. Champion Competition.
   2. The beverages are provided cost-free by the NCAA and USOC and must be in sealed containers. They must be opened and consumed only in the testing station.
   3. Food is not provided, but athletes (at their own risk) are permitted to bring their own food into the testing area.

C. At least 80 mL urine is necessary (100 mL in the USOC program) for testing.
   1. If the urine specimen is incomplete, the athlete must remain in the collection station under observation of a crew member until the sample is complete.
   2. During this period, the athlete is responsible for keeping the urine collection beaker capped and controlled.

D. Before final packaging for shipping to the testing laboratory completed, a small amount of the urine is tested for specific gravity and pH. If these values are outside stated limits, the protocol is repeated (i.e, specific gravity below 1.010 or pH greater than 7.5).

VII. Drug Analysis

A. Urine specimens are analyzed at only highly specialized laboratories that have passed a vigorous accreditation process.
   1. The USOC only uses laboratories that have International Olympic Committee (IOC) accreditation. The NCAA uses laboratories that are certified by the College of American Pathologists (CAP) for any testing. (Some laboratories have both certifications.)
   2. Specimen analysis involves two procedural phases.
      a. The first phase, screening, is an initial test that allows convenient and often rapid analysis of many samples.
      b. A positive result on the screening phase is presumptive only; these samples then undergo the second procedural phase, the confirmation test.
   3. Laboratories use specimen bottle A for all their screening and confirmation tests. A positive result is reconfirmed by at least one more sample from specimen A.
   4. Specimen bottle B is saved for use in case of an appeal by the athlete and to reverify a positive specimen A. In general, screening tests are expected to be very sensitive and confirmatory tests to be very specific for drug detection.
   5. Two phases of drug-testing analysis are required to ensure the most accurate results.
   6. The most commonly used screening procedures include immunoassay thin-layer chromatography, gas chromatography (GC), and high-performance liquid chromatography.
   7. Currently, the preferred confirmation technique is GC/mass spectrometry (GC/MS) because it provides the most specific and definitive identification possible. (A full review of the techniques used in drug screening and confirmation is beyond the scope of this chapter. Please see the selected readings at the end of the chapter for a further, more detailed review.)

VIII. Techniques Used by Athletes to Escape Detection

A. A variety of techniques have been developed in an attempt to falsify drug-testing results. Substances such as salt, vinegar, lemon juice, hand soap, bleach, Visine, Drano, and epitestosterone have all been used. Several adulterating agents are also marketed, such as Urinaid (Byrd Laboratories), which contains gluteralderhyde and causes false negatives on emit screening immunoassys. These materials must be added to the urine; therefore, closest observation of the athlete giving the specimen and constant observation of the athlete in the testing area is meant to reduce the chances of this happening. Laboratories routinely test for adulteration by visual examination of the urine specimen (color, consistency, and so on); odor detection; and measurement of pH, specific gravity, creatinine, and chloride. The laboratories also use counterdetection assays, maintain constant vigilance for new urine manipulation agents, and continually update their counterdetection procedures accordingly. Evidence of adulteration or other urine manipulation techniques can result in automatic penalties equivalent to those for a positive test result on a drug test imposed by both the NCAA and USOC.

B. Catheterization and evacuation of the bladder, followed by instillation of another person's urine, is another technique used rarely. No specific techniques for detecting this method have been developed.

IX. Other Possibilities for Drug Testing

A. Blood testing is being investigated for some drug analyses, such as those used to detect erythropoietin (EPO) and testosterone salt/esters but remains unfeasible at this time.
   1. The technology for hair analysis has not yet been perfected for testing for the more common drugs of ergogenic potential, although research continues in this area.

2. Urine is still considered the preferred specimen for drug testing.
   a. Most drugs misused by athletes are present in higher concentration in the urine than in the blood.
   b. Shipping and waste disposal are less restricted with urine than with blood.
   c. Larger specimen samples are more easily obtainable.
   d. Urine can be conveniently obtained without physical pain or potential harm to the athlete (i.e., the collection process is noninvasive).

X. Penalties

A. USOC: Sanctions may be imposed by the NGB and/or the USOC. Penalties range from 3 to 24 months for the first drug violation (depending on the drug) and from 2 years to a lifetime ban for any subsequent violation.

B. NCAA: The penalty is 1 calendar-year of ineligibility after a positive test. A second positive test can result in a penalty of another year (for street drugs) and up to lifetime expulsion.

XI. Cost/Miscellaneous

A. The NCAA conducts approximately 9,000 tests per year; approximately 1,000 are conducted at championships and the remainder are conducted during the year-round program. The budget for testing and education in the NCAA program was approximately $2.7 million for 1995/1996.

B. The USOC conducts approximately 3,500 to 4,000 tests yearly, of which 500 to 1,000 are conducted in the out-of-competition program. The USOC's annual budget, including drug testing and education, is approximately $1.5 to 2 million yearly.

Suggested Readings

Benson MT, ed. *1996–97 NCAA Drug Education and Drug Testing Program,* Overland Park, KS (1-913-337-1906).

Exom W, ed. *U.S. Olympic Committee drug education handbook 1993–1996.* One Olympic Plaza, Colorado Springs, CO (USOC Drug Hotline: 1-800-233-0393).

Fuentes R, Rosenburg J, Davis A. *Athletic drug reference '96 (Alan and Hanburys).* Glaxo, Triangle Park, NC, 1996.

VII. SPECIAL GROUPS

20. YOUNG ATHLETES

Lyle J. Micheli and Craig M. Mintzer

More than 30 million children and adolescents participate in organized sports in the United States today. This figure increases with each passing year, as does the absolute number of injuries cared for by those involved in sports medicine. In comparison with their adult counterparts, children who are athletes have an additional risk for injury due to their more vulnerable growth cartilage at the physeal plates, joint surfaces, and sites of major muscle tendon insertions. Evidence also shows that growth, in particular the adolescent growth spurt, may presdispose children to injury.

The type of injury sustained by young athletes is changing. With the rise of organized sports in North America, children are no longer participating in a variety of physical activities as they had in the past during free play. Many now perform the same activity or sport repetitively for prolonged times, increasing their risk of overuse musculoskeletal injury. Because of the growing social and economic constraints on informal sports and exercise, as well as growing concern for child safety, the trend toward organized children's sports will probably increase, as will the injuries that accompany these activities. This growth in the organization of sports for children and adolescents will provide opportunities for proper care and prevention of injury.

Aerobic Capacity

Maximal aerobic power ($\dot{V}_{O2max}$, maximum oxygen uptake) is a measure of the greatest amount of oxygen that can be used to synthesize energy in the form of adenosine triphosphate through aerobic metabolic pathways. Studies have shown that in males peak $\dot{V}_{O2}$ increases linearly from age 8 years through age 16 years, whereas in females it increases linearly until age 13 years, at which time it plateaus. Peak $\dot{V}_{O2}$ of girls is approximately 85% that of boys before puberty and 70% that of boys after puberty. This difference has been attributed to variations in hemoglobin concentrations, body composition, maturation of the pulmonary and cardiovascular systems, and biochemical and histologic differences in muscle tissue.

In adults, $\dot{V}_{O2max}$ expressed relative to body weight is a valid marker of the ability to perform endurance athletic events and an indicator of the reserve capacity of cardiopulmonary function. $\dot{V}_{O2max}$/kg has been shown to be significantly greater in well-trained prepubertal endurance athletes than in nonathletes. Children can improve $\dot{V}_{O2max}$ with aerobic training. However, use of maximal aerobic power as an indicator of cardiovascular function, endurance capacity, or response to training may not be as appropriate in prepubertal children as in adults. The association of $\dot{V}_{O2max}$ with performance in field events is weaker in children than in adults. Unlike adults, less than 50% of all children can be expected to demonstrate a $\dot{V}_{O2}$ plateau during progressive maximal testing. Values for $\dot{V}_{O2max}$ do not parallel improvements in endurance fitness during the growing years. Absolute values of $\dot{V}_{O2max}$ increase with growth, but when they are related to body mass, no increase is documented. In addition, endurance performance in children can steadily improve while $\dot{V}_{O2max}$/kg values remain unchanged. In children, endurance performance probably is dependent on factors such as progressive improvements in running efficiency submaximal economy and oxygen delivery reserve and on nonaerobic factors such as sprint speed and anaerobic capacity.

Temperature Regulation

Heat is a metabolic byproduct of energy production, and the ability to dissipate this heat is crucial to maintenance of activity. Owing to their greater surface area relative to body mass and lesser amount of subcutaneous fat, children are at a disadvantage with respect to dissipating heat and adapting to cold. Although children have a higher sweat gland density than adults, they produce less sweat than adults and therefore dissipate heat through evaporation less efficiently. Children demonstrate higher skin and rectal temperatures when subjected to heat stress. Children do not acclimate to heat as quickly as adults, nor do they perceive the work they are doing and the energy they are expending during intense exercise as adults do. Children and adults become more efficient at dissipating heat when they are exposed to periods of increased activity in the heat; however, young adults exhibit better thermoregulatory responses than children.

Tanner Staging

The Tanner classification is an aid to clinicians dealing with sports-active children. Patterns of development and associated patterns of injury can be divided into four groups: prepubescence (Tanner 1 and 2), early pubescence (Tanner 3), midpubescence (Tanner 4), and late pubescence (Tanner 5). Knowledge of the stages of maturation can lead to a greater understanding of the pattern and pathophysiology of injury in the child athlete.

Tanner stages and secondary developmental characteristics in **females**:

Stage 1: Preadolescent

The papilla is elevated in the breast; there is no pubic hair.

Stage 2: Breast bud stage

Breast and papilla are elevated as small mounds, and the areola diameter is enlarged. There is sparse growth of long slightly pigmented, downy hair, straight or ony slightly curled, appearing mainly along the labia. The mean age is 11 years.

Stage 3: Further enlargement of the breast and areola occurs, without separation of their contours.

Pubic hair is considerably darker, coarser, and more curled. The hair spreads sparsely over the junction of the pubis. Mean age is 12 years.

Stage 4: Areola and papilla project to form a secondary mound above the level of the breast.

The pubic hair is now an adult type, but the area covered is less than will be covered in adulthood. There is no spread to the medial surface of the thighs. Mean age is 13 years.

Stage 5: Mature stage. Projection only of the papilla because of recession of the areola to the general contour of the breast. The pubic hair is adult in quantity and type and is distributed as an inverse triangle. There is spread to the medial surface of the thighs. Mean age is 15 years.

Tanner stages and secondary developmental characteristics in **males**:

Stage 1: Preadolescent stage. Testes, scrotum, and penis are of about the same size and proportion as in early childhood. There is no pubic hair.

Stage 2: Scrotom and testes have enlarged and there is a change in the texture of the scrotal skin. There is some reddening of the scrotal skin. Testicular length is greater than 2 cm but less than 3.2 cm. There is sparse growth of long, slightly pigmented, downy hair which is straight or only slightly curled and appears chiefly at the base of the penis. Mean age is 12 years.

Stage 3: The penis has grown, mainly in length, but with some increase in breadth. There is further growth in the testes and scrotum. Testicular length is greater than 3.3 cm but less than 4.0 cm. The pubic hair is darker, coarser, and curlier. Hairs spreads sparsely over the pubic junction. Mean age is 13 years.

Stage 4: The penis has further enlarged (both length and breadth) with the development of the glans. The testes and scrotum have further enlarged. There is darkening of the scrotal skin. The testicular length is greater than 4.1 cm but less than 4.9 cm. The pubic hair is adult in type, but the area covered is considerably smaller than that in most adults. There is no spread of pubic hair to the medial surface of the thighs. Mean age is 14 years.

Stage 5: The genitalia are adult in size and shape. Testicular length is greater than 5 cm. Pubic hair is adult in quantity and type. There is spread to the medial surface of the thighs. Mean age is 15 years.

On the field, youths participating in organized sports are often grouped by age in an attempt to match their muscular strength, anaerobic power, aerobic capacity, and skill level. Stratification by age works well in the prepubertal period (Tanner stages 1 and 2). However, once the pubertal growth spurt is reached, there is a rapid increase in body size as well as an acceleration in strength and power. Because of the differences in the chronologic age at which these changes occur and the extent of development between individuals, matching by age alone may result in an increase in injury risk owing to mismatch in development and size.

In several individual sports, including wrestling, martial arts, and boxing, it is recognized that weight differences are associated with strength and power differences. These sports, as well as some football leagues, have devised weight classes to promote matching. Athough a weight classification is an improvement, it is not ideal. A young, obese, skeletally immature athlete may have to compete with older mature adolescents. Use of the Tanner stages, which can be assessed during the preparticipation physical examination, may be better than use of age, body weight, or grade in school in an attempt to match athletes. Progression in physical maturation, as determined by Tanner staging, is associated with increased strength, coordination, and physical skills in both boys and girls. Males at Tanner stages 4 or 5 are bigger and stronger that boys at lower stages of maturation. Additional ways to stratify participants include establishing bone age by radiograph and grip strength. Currently, there is no uniformly agreed-upon way to subdivide athletic competitors in these age groups that will ensure both fair and safe competition. However, with the ever-increasing numbers of participants in organized sports, this issue merits serious consideration by youth sports organizations.

Growth Spurts

Each person demonstrates a characteristic pattern of growth rate that to some degree is unique. However, every child goes through the same sequence of growth changes. During the first year of life, average linear growth rate is 30 cm/year. There is a rapid deceleration to 9 cm/year by age 2; by age 5, the rate of growth levels off to about 5 cm/year. This steady rate persists during the prepubescent phase (age 6 to 10 years in boys and 5 to 9 years in girls), but just before the onset of puberty it decreases further.

Puberty is marked by a rapid return to accelerated growth. The marker for this accelerated growth rate is early pubescence (Tanner 3), when secondary sexual characteristics start becoming further delineated. The stage of midpubescence corresponds to the time of peak growth velocity in the child (Tanner 4). In females, growth velocity can reach a peak of 10.5 cm/year between the ages of 10 and 12 years. In males, the skeletal growth spurt usually begins several years later. On the average, male growth acceleration begins at age 12 years and reaches a peak velocity of 12 cm/year by age 14. The rapid growth in adolescence accounts for approximately 25 cm height in females and 28 cm height in males. Late pubescence (Tanner 4), the final stage of development, corresponds to the time when the growth rate begins to decline and physeal closure ensues in the child. Skeletal maturity is usually reached by age 15 years in females and by age 17 years in males.

Weight velocity decelerates from a rate of 10 kg/year at birth to a rate of 2 kg/year by age 2. During childhood, a relative steady state of 3 kg/year of weight gain is achieved. The onset of puberty is marked by an acceleration in weight gain in females to 9 kg/year and in males to 10 kg/year. In both sexes, the peak weight velocity is followed by a rapid deceleration to less than 1 kg/year for females at approximately age 15 and for males at approximately age 17.

Flexibility Training

Flexibility decreases with age and growth, especially during the adolescent growth spurt. During the growth spurt, longitudinal growth of bones advances at a greater rate than that of the surrounding muscle tendon units. The resultant tightness can predispose children to unique injuries during this developmental stage. Athletes must be counseled during the growth spurt so that flexibility is emphasized and injury is minimized. Slow stretch technique should be taught, with a duration of 20 to 30 seconds of sustained stretch.

Clinicians should be particularly aware of the association between the growth spurt and knee pain. The most frequent symptom reported by young athletes, especially females, is the patellofemoral stress syndrome, with presentation usually during or just after the athlete's growth spurt. Anterior knee pain is aggravated by activities and relieved by rest. With the growth spurt, there is superior and lateral migration of the patella secondary to tightness in the quadriceps, iliotibial band, and hamstrings. Patella alta may be present, as may a weak vastus medialis obliquis muscle. Treatment consists of progressive resistance exercises to strengthen the medial musculature and flexibility exercises for the iliotibial band, hamstrings, and lateral quadriceps.

Strength Training

The American Orthopaedic Society for Sports Medicine (AOSSM) defines strength training as "the use of progressive resistance methods (which include using body weight, free weights, and machines) to increase one's ability to exert or resist force." Enhanced physical condition improves muscular strength, musculoskeletal flexibility, the percentage of lean body tissue, cardiovascular efficiency, body image, and confidence. Resistive weight training has been shown to benefit athletes by enhancing sports performance and by decreasing susceptibility to injury. Those involved in training young athletes, should note that progress toward adult stature in terms of height, weight, and circumferences and of rates of change in height velocity and weight velocity is not adversely affected by training. Young athletes grow at the same rate and to the same degree as young nonathletes, but body composition is influenced by strength training.

Longitudinal studies of strength measuring isometric grip strength demonstrate that males and females increase grip strength linearly throughout childhood. The increase in muscle strength with age is a product of body size and muscle mass and neuromuscular, and endocrine maturation. With the onset of puberty, the strength development of males, as measured by grip strength, accelerates rapidly as compared with that of females. In similar studies of elbow and knee flexion and extension comparisons support this divergence in strength between the sexes. Studies document a linear muscular endurance increase from 5 to 13 years of age in males which leads to a further acceleration of endurance during puberty. In females, muscular endurance increases linearly throughout childhood and adolescence, but there is no similar pubertal acceleration. Males have more muscle than females on both an absolute body weight basis and a percentage of body weight basis.

Before starting a training program, all athletes must provide a preparticipation history and undergo physical examination, which will serve to identify any preexisting health problems or physical limitations that might predispose to injury. For athletes starting a strength training program for the first time, three sessions a week with 1 day of rest is appropriate. Protein muscle synthesis occurs during rest. Training programs should consist of three basic parts to include a warmup period, the training activity, and a cool-down period.

Warmup refers to any sequence of activities undertaken before participation in more strenuous exercise that results in increased blood flow to the tissues of the body. This increased blood flow is accompanied by an increase in body temperature and enhancement of a muscle's force-generating capacity, speed of contraction, and tissue plasticity. Cardiovascular, respiratory, endocrine, and nervous systems become primed for activity during the warmup. The warmup period consists of a prestretching phase involving gentle repetitive activity such as fast walking, jogging, stationary bicycling, or other light activity. This is followed by a series of stretching exercises that targets each of the major joint and muscle areas, the shoulder girdle, back, hamstrings, quadriceps, and gastrocsoleus group. The flexibility program should include exercises to enhance the ranges of motion (ROM) required to perform the sport-specific skills. The warmup period should last approximately 15 minutes.

Strength training follows the warmup period. The training program may include isometric exercises to maintain tone and improve strength slightly. Isometric exercises do not allow change in the length of the muscle while it is under contraction. Resistance for the muscle is provided by any immovable object. For isometric exercise of a muscle, the muscle must be contracted maximally for 6 to 10 seconds. Because there is no ROM during muscle contraction, the muscle should be exercised at three or four different lengths with four contractions at each step.

Depending on the equipment available and the sport in question, a structured program of dynamic exercises can be included in the training program. In such exercises, the muscle moves a joint through a ROM and can have constant resistance, variable resistance, or accomodating resistance. Resistance may be provided by the child's own body weight, a free weight, or a machine. Resistance should be increased gradually. For young athletes, the intensity should be restricted to a lighter weight/resistance and at least 10 repetitions per set. Qualified adult supervision of the training program is mandatory.

The child must fit the equipment. The skill and technique required to perform the exercises must be properly taught, and the exercises chosen must involve major muscle groups and both agonist and antagonist muscles of the joint. Almost no data exist regarding the optimal order of exercise. Common practice is to exercise large muscle groups first and then smaller ones. Longer rest periods (2 to 5 minutes) are typically used when heavier weights are being lifted or during the learning phases of an exercise.

The training session should not exceed 1 hour. Progress should be monitored. For children, it is often best to measure improvement by measuring performance of a particular task such as the number of a particular calisthenic performed (push-ups, sit-ups, pull-ups). Such a general program can help avoid repetitive motion injuries.

Prepubescent athletes deserve special consideration. Studies have demonstrated that prepubescent children, as well as adolescent athletes, can safely benefit from strength training with a well-supervised program. The primary reason for strength training in these young athletes is to strengthen tissues and decrease the risk of injury. Enhancing sports performance is a side benefit and should be a secondary consideration. Strength training should be only a small part of the child's overall activity. The National Strength and Conditioning Association states that "50% to 80% of the prepubescent athlete's training must include a variety of different physical activitites in addition to strength training." Young children benefit from general strength conditioning and should not follow a program that is too sport-specific. Emphasis should be placed on proper technique and body position. Low weights with multiple repetitions provide the safest training programs in younger athletes.

Skills Training

Sports-specific training in youth sports has grown in intensity and sophistication in recent years with the onset of regimented training beginning at earlier ages and including increased amounts of training time. In general, systematic training is not beneficial before age 6 years. The volume and intensity of training in the young age group, as well as the rate of progress of training, should be monitored closely.

With regard to progression of training, the "10% rule" is useful: Increases in the amount of training should not exceed 10% a week. Determining the safe total volume of training per week for child athletes is difficult. Some children may experience inhibition of normal growth and development when performing as little as 10 hours of sports-specific training per week, whereas the threshold of another child in another sport may be 16 to 18 hours a week. Our ability to provide more specific guidelines in this area is confounded by the difficulty of determining intensity of exercises in a training program. The best way to guide training may be to monitor height, weight, and body composition at least every 6 months in a child involved in rigorous sports or dance training.

Injury

Two basic mechanisms of injury in sports have been described. The more familiar injury is macrotrauma, which results from a single application of force. Such injuries consist of torn ligaments, strained muscle-tendon units, and fractured bones. Because the tissues of sports-active children and adolescents differ from those of adult athletes, the patterns of such injuries also differ. Growing bone is more porous and more plastic than adult bone and can undergo a significant amount of deformation before frank fracture occurs. The physis is unique in skeletally immature athletes and responds to trauma in a particular way depending on the stage of maturation of the athlete. In prepubescent children, the physis is strong and ligamentous injuries can occur with the physis remaining intact, resulting in contusions or strains similar to those that occur in adults. During the growth spurt, physiologic changes in the physis render this region relatively weaker and more vulnerable to injury. In adolescents, trauma may result in a physeal fracture or apophyseal avulsion.

The second type of injury is microtrauma and is often classified as an overuse injury. This type includes tendinitis of muscle-tendon units, stress fractures of bone, osteochondritis dissecans, apophysitis, and direct injury to the growth plate. These injuries can result from the sport itself or the training process.

Acute Physeal Injuries

Physeal injuries in child athletes, although relatively uncommon on the field, receive much attention because of their possible long-term implications for the child. Macrotrauma in a child athlete is similar to macrotrauma in a child who is not an athlete. The Salter-Harris classification system is used to describe acute physeal and juxtaphyseal bony injuries to the immature skeleton. Fractures are divided into five groups based on the pattern of physeal injury and the increased potential for subsequent growth arrest (Fig. 20-1A–E).

A Salter I fracture (Fig. 20-1A) involves only the growth plate without propagation into the surrounding metaphysis or epiphysis. Radiographs of a nondisplaced Salter-Harris I injury will demonstrate normal bony alignment with possible soft tissue swelling. Displaced injuries require reduction.

A Salter-Harris II (Fig. 20-1B) fracture involves the physis and the metaphysis. Because the fracture propagates through the growth plate, it exits through the metaphysis. The epiphysis is spared. The triangular metaphyseal fragment that is involved in the fracture line is termed the Thurston-Holland fragment.

A Salter-Harris III (Fig. 20-1C) fracture involves the physis and the epiphysis, but spares the metaphysis. This injury results in a disruption of the joint surface as the fracture traverses the growth plate and then exits through the epiphysis and into the joint.

A Salter-Harris IV fracture (Fig. 20-1D) involves both the epiphysis and the metaphysis. This fracture does not travel along the growth plate, but instead traverses it in an oblique or vertical fashion. In these injuries, there is vertical displacement of the fracture fragment and disruption of the joint surface.

A Salter-Harris V fracture (Fig. 20-1E) is a crush injury to the growth plate that involves only the physis. Magnetic resonance imaging (MRI) may be required for proper diagnosis of such injury, which often is diagnosed in retrospect after a disturbance is identified in a growth plate.

Fractures involving the physis that are displaced should be reduced as soon as possible. Intraarticular fractures pose a great risk to normal joint mechanics. Although rare, all physeal fractures, especially fractures that cross the physis (Salter-Harris III and IV), can result in growth retardation, arrest, or angular deformity.

Overuse Injuries

Overuse injuries are the result of repetitive application of stresses to normal tissues. Normal reparative processes are overwhelmed, and an inflammatory response is triggered. Forty percent of injuries that occur in sports are directly related to overuse. As in adults, in children overuse injuries can occur in bone as stress fractures, in tendons as tendinitis, and at bone–tendon junctions as bursitis. However, in children, repetitive trauma can injure the epiphyseal plate, the articular cartilage, and the apophyses (insertion site for muscle tendon units on the bone).

In children, stress fractures most often involve the tibia, fibula, foot, and pars interarticularis of the spine. Stress fractures occur if the intensity and duration of a repetitive force applied to a bone reaches a level at which new bone formation is not adequate to repair damage created by the repetitive force. Tenderness is localized to the fractured area. Plain radiographs initially may be nondiagnostic. A bone scan can confirm diagnosis. Treatment consists of "relative rest," and avoidance of the activities that reproduce pain and incapacitation. Sufficient mechanical support, such as a brace or crutches, should be used to relieve pain without excessively limiting activity

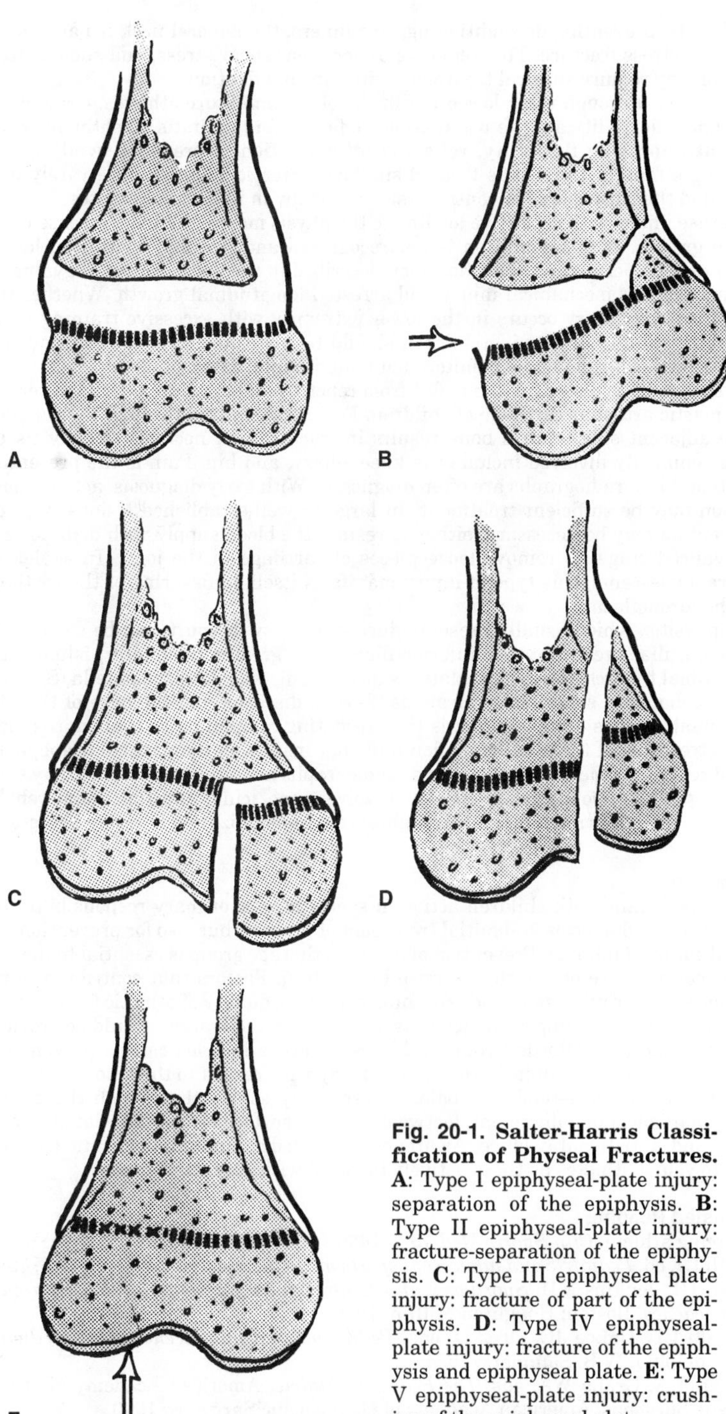

Fig. 20-1. Salter-Harris Classification of Physeal Fractures. **A**: Type I epiphyseal-plate injury: separation of the epiphysis. **B**: Type II epiphyseal-plate injury: fracture-separation of the epiphysis. **C**: Type III epiphyseal plate injury: fracture of part of the epiphysis. **D**: Type IV epiphyseal-plate injury: fracture of the epiphysis and epiphyseal plate. **E**: Type V epiphyseal-plate injury: crushing of the epiphyseal plate.

and thereby preventing deconditioning. In runners, the femoral neck is particularly subject to stress fracture. This region is under great shear stress, and such a stress fracture may require surgical treatment with internal fixation.

Tendinitis, although rare, does occur in skeletally immature athletes. Growth and resultant inflexibility are the usual etiologic factors in tendinitis. Treatment is targeted at improving flexibility, relieving inflammation, decreasing swelling, and restoring strength. Bursitis is treated similarly. Steroid injections are rarely indicated, and their use is highly controversial especially in immature athletes.

Overuse injury with repetitive loading to the physis may result in a decrease in the rate of growth. If this condition is not recognized and training continues, loss of length may be permanent. This has been described in the distal radius of gymnasts, with subsequent mechanical injury and arrested longitudinal growth. Whether this type of overuse injury occurs in the lower extremity with excessive training is not clear, but training in growing children should be instituted with caution and children's growth rate should be monitored at 6 month intervals.

Osteochondritis dissecans can result from repetitive microtrauma to the softer and more plastic articular cartilage of children. Force transmitted through the cartilage to the adjacent subchondral bone results in fracture and necrosis of bony tissue. Joints commonly involved include the knee, elbow, and hip. Pain is the presenting symptom. Plain radiographs are often diagnostic. With early diagnosis, activity modification may be sufficient treatment. In large or well-established lesions, surgical intervention may be necessary, either to restore the blood supply with drill holes or in advanced stage, to remove loose pieces of cartilage in the joint. In skeletally mature adolescents, this type of injury manifests itself as fissuring of the cartilage and chondromalacia.

Apophysitis, which usually presents during the growth spurt, can be seen in the olecranon, iliac crest, anterior inferior iliac spine, greater trochanter, ishial tuberosity, tibial tubercle (Osgood-Schlatter's disease), distal pole of the patella (Sinding-Larsen-Johansson syndrome), calcaneus (Sever's disease), and the base of the fifth metatarsal (Iselin's disease). Pain is the presenting complaint. To confirm the diagnosis, stretching of the muscle–tendon unit that inserts on the particular apophysis should reproduce the child's symptoms. Radiographs are often normal, but may show widening of the apophysis. Treatment involves rest, icing, and functional rehabilitation to include stretching and strenghtening. Immobilization is rarely necessary.

Prevention

Clinicians dealing with children active in sports have a primary responsibility not only for proper diagnosis and initial treatment of injuries, but also for prevention and rehabilitation of injuries. Prevention of injury in this age group is essential to the continued performance of healthy exercise by children. Factors that contribute to the incidence of macrotrauma include coaching expertise, quality of athletic facilities and equipment, and matching of participants. Guidance in these areas should be provided as part of the care afforded young athletes. Overuse injuries can be prevented if attention is paid to training "error," particularly with regard to the amount of training per week; muscle–tendon imbalance, especially as associated with the growth spurt; anatomical malalignment; footwear; playing surface issues; associated disease states, and nutritional balance. Awareness, knowledge, and guidance must be provided to young athletes by those actively involved with organized sports.

Suggested Reading

The young athlete. *Clin Sports Med* 1995;14:3.

Micheli LJ, ed. *Pediatric and adolescent sports medicine.* Boston: Little, Brown, 1984.

Micheli LJ, Jenkins MD. *Sportwise: an essential guide for young athletes, parents, and coaches.* Boston: Houghton Mifflin, 1990.

Stanitski CL, DeLee JC, Drez D, eds. *Pediatrics and adolescent sports medicine.* Philadelphia: W.B. Saunders, 1994.

Sullivan J A, Grana WA, eds. *The Pediatric Athlete.* American Academy of Orthopaedic Surgeons, American Academy of Orthopaedic Surgeons, 1990.

21. SPECIAL CONCERNS OF THE FEMALE ATHLETE

Aurelia Nattiv and Mary Lloyd Ireland

I. Introduction

A. History of women in sports

1. For centuries, women participated very little in sports and athletic competition. In fact, in the early 1900s women were excluded from the modern Olympic games because participation in sports was thought to be too stressful for them.
2. The adoption of Title IX to the Education Amendments Act in 1972 led to a dramatic increase in female sports participation and had a great impact on women in sport. Title IX states that men and women should have the same opportunities for participation in sports and exercise.

II. Physiologic Differences in Females and Males

A. Pre- and postpubertal differences

1. There is no significant difference in the physical capabilities of prepubertal boys and girls (controlling for body size and composition).
2. With puberty, girls show a relative increase in body fat and boys a relative increase in lean body mass (mostly due to hormonal influences). This inequality of muscle mass after puberty in women is reflected in their decreased muscle strength, power, and speed, as compared with that of men.

B. Muscle strength

1. Strength differences between women and men are more apparent in the upper extremity. Upper extremity strength in women averages 40% to 75% that of men, while lower extremity strength in women averages 60% to 80% that of men. However, women have the same capacity for strength gains as do men (controlling for body composition and size). This is because strength gains are the result of both neuromuscular recruitment and muscle hypertrophy. Women do not experience the same degree of increased muscle hypertrophy as men, primarily because their testosterone levels are lower.

C. Aerobic capacity: Maximum oxygen uptake ($\dot{V}_{O2MAX}$)

1. Women have a lower maximal level of aerobic capacity (after puberty) than men, due to several factors: lower oxygen-carrying capacity, lower hemoglobin content, lower blood volume (relative to lean body mass), smaller hearts (relative to lean body mass), lower stroke volume, higher percentage of body fat, and smaller muscle fiber area.
2. Athletic training programs produce similar increases in aerobic capacity in males and females (controlling for body composition and size).

D. Endurance performance

1. Endurance performance is 6% to 15% lower in women in most endurance events. This can be partially explained by the larger muscle fibers in men (both fast- and slow-twitch muscle fibers), although the actual muscle fiber composition is similar in men and women.
2. Athletic training programs (interval and continuous) produce similar improvements in endurance performance in men and women.

E. Menstrual cycle and performance

1. Although there is a lack of research regarding menstrual cycle and performance, most studies have shown no significant difference in athletic performance in females during the different phases of the cycle. Similarly, most studies report no significant benefit or detriment to athletic performance in women taking oral contraceptive pills.

III. Musculoskeletal Considerations

A. Common musculoskeletal problems

1. Injury rates

a. Few true epidemiologic studies have compared male and female injury rates. The rates of injury documented by the military studies are about equal.

b. Each year, the National Collegiate Athletic Association (NCAA) sends injury surveys to its member institutions. There are two true sex-comparable sports, basketball and soccer. The additional women's sports included in the injury surveys are gymnastics, volleyball, softball, lacrosse and field hockey. Men's sports included in the injury survey are ice hockey, wrestling, gymnastics, lacrosse, spring football, baseball and football.

(1) A comparison of the rates of injury with number of injuries per 1,000 athletic contests, averaged over a 3-year period, demonstrated that there was no significant change in the rate of injuries in each sport in the 3 years.

c. More studies comparing differences in injury patterns need to be conducted at many levels.

2. Specific sport demands

a. In female sports, there are fewer traumatic collision mechanisms and more repetitive axial loading microtraumatic overuse problems.

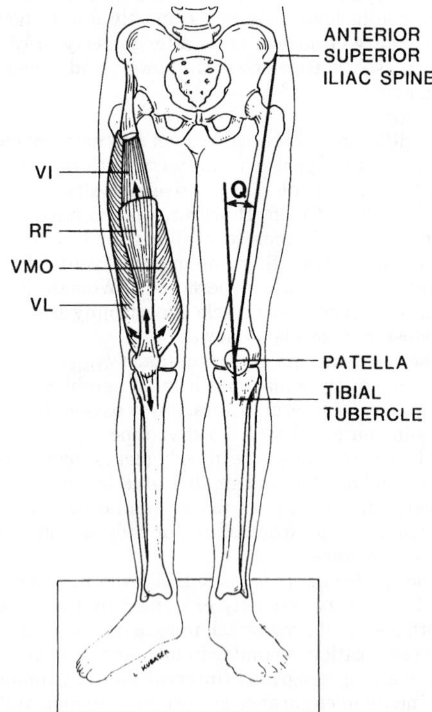

Fig. 21-1. Lower-extremity alignment: Q-angle is a measure of patellofemoral alignment. It is measured as the angle formed by the intersection of a line from the anterior superior iliac spine to the center of the patella and a line from the center of the patella to the tibial tubercle. Normal is less than 12 degrees. Quadriceps muscles are labeled with their force vectors (VI, vastus intermedius; RF, rectus femoris; VMO, vastus medialis obliqus; VL, vastus lateralis).

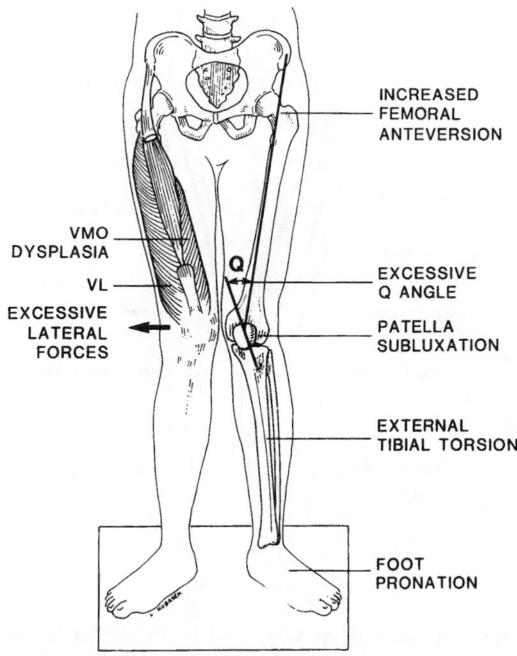

Fig. 21-2. Lower extremity alignment of miserable malalignment syndrome: Changes in patellar alignment and muscle force vectors are shown in miserable malalignment syndrome. Increased femoral anteversion, external tibial torsion, and foot pronation, along with the increased Q-angle and VMO hypoplasia/dysplasia, all create forces that laterally subluxate and tilt the patella (VL, vastus lateralis; VMO, vastus medialis obliqus).

b. Lower extremity
   (1) In running and dance sports, lower-extremity tendinitis or stress fractures are most common. To prevent injury, three assessments must be made: the sport's biomechanics, footwear and orthotic equipment and duration of training.

c. Upper extremity
   (1) Upper-extremity weakness and physiologic multidirectional laxity can result in shoulder overuse injury patterns. In the younger athlete, the primary problem is usually laxity or instability, rather than rotator cuff dysfunction. Repetitive overload results in entire upper-extremity dysfunction.
   (2) Sports can be divided into two types: axial loading (compression) and distraction (the glenohumeral joint and rotator cuff), or into a combination of both. Tennis and softball are distraction sports. Diving and cheerleading are more axial loading sports, whereas basketball and swimming are a combination of both types. Specific prevention programs for strengthening should be used in each case.
   (3) The pitcher in softball, fast-pitch underhand style, is more likely to be injured by contact with the ball than to develop an overuse shoulder problem or labral tear. Swimming rarely results in labral tears; more often, the laxity leads to rotator cuff dysfunction.

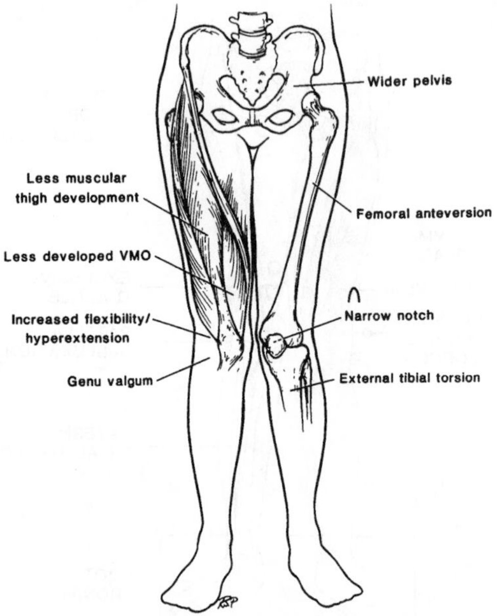

Fig. 21-3. Female lower extremity: Wider pelvis, increased femoral anteversion, external tibial torsion, pes planus, less thigh development, less developed VMO along with increased flexibility, range of motion, genu valgum, and narrow notch make women's knees more "ligament dominant." (VMO, vastus medialis obliqus)

d. Unique and female-only apparatuses are used in gymnastics: balance beam and uneven parallel bars. Varying injury patterns can occur when athletes perform on the unique equipment.

3. Stress fractures (see Chapter 37)
   a. Overall rate: the military rates of stress fractures have equalized with changes in training during the last 10 years. Stress fractures appear to occur more often in the female athlete as compared to her male counterpart. The etiology of the stress fracture whether from insufficiency or over training, must be determined. One must suspect an underlying nutritional disorder or hormonal insufficiency: amenorrhea or oligomenorrhea.
   b. Factors contributing to stress fractures
      (1) Anatomic and biomechanical factors
         (a) Training errors
         (b) Biomechanics
         (c) Low bone density
         (d) Bone geometry
      (2) Hormonal influence
         (a) Hypoestrogenic amenorrhea
         (b) Oligomenorrhea
      (3) Nutritional factors
         (a) Inadequate calories
            i) Calcium
            ii) Mineral
         (b) Disordered eating
            i) Anorexia nervosa
            ii) Bulimia
            iii) Single or combined

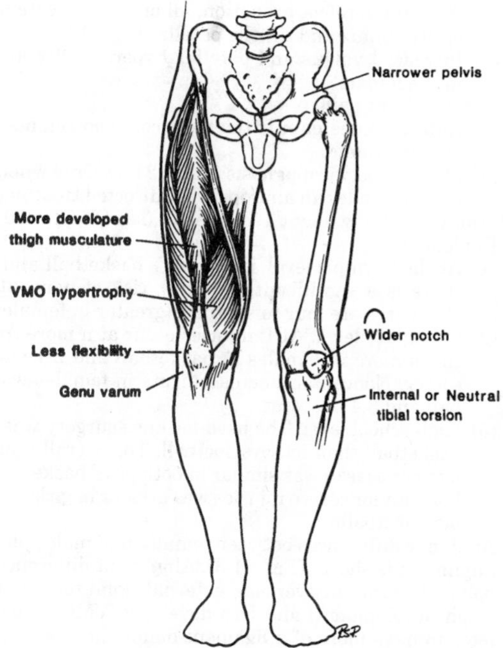

Fig. 21-4. Male lower extremity: More narrow pelvis, less femoral anteversion, wider femoral notch, neutral (to slight internal) tibial torsion, genu varum, more thigh musculature development, VMO hypertophy, and less flexibility result in a muscle dominant/less ligament-dominant knee. (VMO, vastus medialis obliqus).

c. Assess level of risk of completion of fracture
   (1) Stress fracture at risk of progression
      (a) More aggressive treatment
      (b) *At-risk location*
         i) Hip–Distraction side superior femoral neck.
         ii) Tibia–Anterior tibial cortex–dreaded black line.
         iii) Tarsal navicular
         iv) Fifth metatarsal–Jones' type
         v) Proximal second metatarsal
         vi) Sesamoids–great toe
         vii) Intraarticular fracture—unusual
   (2) Not at risk of progression
      (a) Medial tibial
      (b) Fibular fracture
      (c) Metatarsal
         i) Non-Jones
         ii) Nonproximal second metatarsal

d. After second stress fracture, bone density study should be considered.

4. Patellofemoral disorders (PF) (see Chapter 53)
   a. Anatomic alignment
      (1) The Q angle is measured by line from anterior superior iliac spine to patella and line from patella to tibial tubercle. The normal is less than 12 degrees (Fig. 21-1).
      (2) Miserable malalignment syndrome refers to lower-extremity alignment of increased femoral anteversion, vastus medialis obliquus (VMO) dysplasia, excessive Q angle, external tibial tor-

sion, and forefoot pronation, all of which create forces which laterally sublux and tilt the patella (Fig. 21-2).

(3) Increased valgus and patellar hypermobility are more common in the female.

b. Anterior knee pain

(1) Anterior knee pain is the most common complaint of the young female athlete.

(2) Make a specific diagnosis (Table 21-1). Only when a specific diagnosis is made can appropriately directed treatment be instituted.

5. Anterior cruciate ligament Tears (ACL) (see Chapter 50)

a. Epidemiology

(1) At the Olympic level, in women's basketball and team handball, there is a significantly greater risk of noncontact ACL tears. Estimates are four to six times greater in females.

(2) Collegiate level: ACL injuries occur at a more frequent rate: 4.1 times more in females in basketball and 2.4 more in women in soccer. Noncontact increased rate in females was 5.3 in basketball and 3.4 in soccer.

(3) High school level: The need for knee surgery was greater in girls' basketball than in boys' football. The overall injury rate per athlete per season was similar in both girls' basketball and boys' football, but for severe injuries was greater in girls' basketball than in boys' football.

b. Anatomic differences between females and males play a role. Female alignment is shown (Fig. 21-3). Alignment differences include wider pelvis, femoral anteversion, external tibial torsion, pes planus, less thigh development, and less developed VMO, causing female athletes to have more of a ligament-dominant knee; increased flexibility, range of motion (ROM), and genu valgum are more common in female athletes. In male athletes, alignment of a more narrow pelvis, less femoral anteversion, wider femoral notch, internal or neutral tibial torsion, and genu varum are common, as are a more muscle-dominant structure of more developed thigh musculature, VMO

Table 21-1. Differential diagnosis of anterior knee pain[a]

Mechanical	Inflammatory	Other
Patella	Bursitis	Reflex sympathetic dystrophy
Subluxation	Prepatellar	Tumor
Dislocation	Retropatellar	
Fracture	Semimembranosus	
Stress	Tendinitis	
Acute (transverse)	Patellar	
Bipartite	Pes anserinus	
Fibrous nonunion	Semimembranosus	
Acute fracture	Synovitis	
Quadriceps rupture	Arthritis	
Patella tendon rupture		
Inferior avulsion		
Interstitial		
Patellofemoral stress syndrome		
Pathologic plica		
Osteochondral fracture		
Trochlear groove		
Patella		
Loose bodies		
Osteochondritis dissecans		

[a] From Hutchinson MR, Ireland ML. Knee injuries in female athletes. *Sports Med* 1995; 19:288–302.

hypertrophy. Less flexibility results in a muscle-dominant, less ligament-dominant knee in males (Fig. 21-4).

c. Factors contributing to ACL injuries
   (1) Intrinsic factors
      (a) Physiologic rotatory laxity
      (b) Size of ACL
      (c) Valgus alignment
      (d) Hyperextension
      (e) Proprioception
      (f) Neuromuscular firing order
      (g) Hormonal influences
   (2) Extrinsic factors
      (a) Strength
      (b) Conditioning
      (c) Shoes
      (d) Motivation
      (e) Deceleration forces
   (3) Both
      (a) Skill
      (b) Coordination
   (4) The most important factors in the increased incidence of non-contact injuries in the female athlete are physiologic rotatory laxity, proprioception and neuromuscular firing patterns. Improvement is needed in the level of youth physical education and movement patterns, strength, and balance. Teaching a basketball athlete to land on both feet and to use posterior directed forces should help. Screening for high-risk factors should reduce incidence of injury.

IV. Female Athlete Triad: Disordered Eating, Amenorrhea, and Osteoporosis

A. Definition of the triad
   1. The female athlete triad represents the interrelationship and often co-existence of disordered eating patterns, amenorrhea, and osteoporosis. These problems represent a growing concern in sports medicine. Each component of the triad is defined in sections V and VI. The constant focus on achieving and/or maintaining an "ideal" body weight and/or "optimal" body fat often is the underlying theme.

B. Prevalence of the triad in athletes
   1. The true prevalence of the female athlete triad is unknown and difficult to determine, but a triad profile has become apparent. The female athlete triad appears to be more prevalent among athletes competing in appearance or endurance sports: gymnasts, figure skaters, dancers, runners (distance), and swimmers, although athletes of all sports are potentially at risk. It is also more common in adolescent and young adult age groups.
   2. The prevalence of amenorrhea and disordered eating in athletes is noted in sections V. B. and VI. B. The prevalence of osteoporosis in young female athletes is unknown.

C. Health consequences of the female athlete triad
   1. The potential exists for short- and long-term health consequences as well as psychological, medical, and orthopaedic repercussions of disordered eating, amenorrhea, and premature osteoporosis. (Refer to sections V. C and VI. D.)

V. Menstrual Dysfunction and Bone Concerns in the Female Athlete

A. Introduction
   1. Hormonal status has a significant effect on bone in young as well as in older persons who exercise. The various types of menstrual dysfunction most common in premenopausal female athletes and their effects on bone are summarized below:
      a. Luteal phase dysfunction: Inadequate levels of progesterone; normal or shortened cycle length; may be an adaptive response to exercise. Effect on bone mass is still controversial.

b. Oligomenorrhea: Menstrual cycle greater than 36 days; may be anovulatory; associated with bone loss due to low estrogen (primarily) and progesterone.
c. Primary amenorrhea: The lack of menarche by 16 years of age; may be associated with significant decrease in bone density and skeletal development if due to low estrogen state; may contribute to an increased incidence of stress fractures and scoliosis.
d. Secondary amenorrhea: Absence of three to six consecutive menstrual cycles or less than three cycles per year in a woman who has previously had her menarche. Significant negative effect on bone mineral density can be seen in axial and appendicular skeletal sites.

2. Definition of osteoporosis: Premature bone loss and inadequate bone formation, resulting in low bone mass, microarchitectural deterioration of bone tissue, and increased bone fragility, resulting in an increased risk of fracture.

B. Prevalence of menstrual dysfunction and bone concerns
1. The prevalence of menstrual dysfunction in the female athlete varies among sports and intensity of training, although other factors are involved. In general, there is an increased prevalence of oligomenorrhea and amenorrhea among athletic women, with prevalence rates of secondary amenorrhea between 3.4 and 66% (as compared with the rates of amenorrhea in the general female population of 2% to 5%).
2. The prevalence of premature osteoporosis in the premenopausal female athlete is uncertain, but is a significant medical concern in athletic women with a history of oligomenorrhea, amenorrhea and/or disorders of eating.

C. Potential complications of menstrual dysfunction in athletes
1. There are a number of potential complications of menstrual dysfunction in the athletic setting. Problems of some concern that may develop in this setting are those of premature osteoporosis and an increased prevalence of stress fractures and pathologic fractures (due to a hypoestrogenic state). Infertility is a potential complication if the athlete is anovulatory, but this is believed to be reversible if it is exercise related.
2. There are other theoretical risks of menstrual dysfunction in the athletic woman which include an increased risk of cardiovascular disease and a negative effect on lipid profiles (possibly due to low estrogen). Other possible risks include endometrial hyperplasia with an increased risk of adenocarcinoma of the uterus (if a woman is anovulatory and there is an unopposed estrogen state). Future research is needed to assess these potential risk factors in women with athletic-associated menstrual dysfunction who exercise.

D. Contributory variables associated with menstrual dysfunction in athletes
1. Although the etiology and pathophysiology of menstrual dysfunction in athletes is not known, several contributory variables appear to be associated with menstrual dysfunction. These include previous menstrual history (delayed menarche, irregular menses, nulliparity), increased exercise intensity, dietary factors, disordered eating patterns, abrupt changes in body composition, stress (psychological and physical), and certain high-risk sports (gymnastics, distance running, ballet, figure skating, swimming).

E. Proposed mechanisms of athletic amenorrhea
1. There are many theories relating to the mechanisms involved in athletic amenorrhea. The most popular current theories involve an inhibition of the hypothalamic gonadotropin-releasing hormone (GnRH) pulse and reduction in lutenizing hormone (LH) pulse frequency. Low energy availability may disrupt the GnRH pulse. Caloric intake may not be sufficient for the amount of energy being expended in exercise training. A state of negative energy balance exists, resulting in an energy drain manifested by amenorrhea.

F. Decreased bone mineral content in amenorrheic athletes
1. Although exercise can increase bone mineral density in healthy, normally menstruating, women, there appears to be a point of diminishing return

in women who overtrain and develop athletic-associated amenorrhea and oligomenorrhea. Multiple studies have shown that decreased bone mineral density often is a consequence of amenorrhea and oligomenorrhea in athletes. This decrease in bone mineral density is generalized throughout the skeleton and can be quite severe. The majority of studies have not shown gain in bone density in the premenopausal female athlete, despite estrogen replacement and calcium. Therefore, prevention is important.

2. Low bone density can predispose athletes to stress fractures and potentially devastating osteoporotic fractures later in life. When assessing risk factors for stress fractures, researchers have shown that athletes with stress fractures have lower bone mineral density, calcium intake, and menstrual irregularity, and use fewer oral contraceptives.

G. Stress fractures (See Chapter 37)

H. Clinical evaluation of menstrual dysfunction

1. A detailed history is important to identify potential risk factors for athletic-associated amenorrhea and to differentiate athletic-associated amenorrhea from amenorrhea due to other causes. Risk factors for athletic-associated menstrual dysfunction include a previous history of delayed menarche and irregular menses, excessive training, disordered eating behaviors, abrupt changes in body composition, and stressors. It is important to assess for other apparent etiologies of menstrual dysfunction. Medication history and history of possible associated symptoms (i.e., galactorrhea) are important, as are family history of endocrine disorders or other medical problems.
2. The diagnosis of athletic-associated amenorrhea is a diagnosis of exclusion. A thorough physical examination and pelvic examination are indicated in most instances. A work up for delayed menarche is indicated if menstruation has not begun by age 16 (or by age 14 if there are no secondary sexual characteristics) For females less than 18 years of age, a pelvic examination may be deferred if not sexually active. Vital signs, physical examination, and assessment of development of secondary sexual characteristics are important. An increase in weight or development of hirsutism, and/or acne may suggest polycystic ovarian syndrome.
3. Laboratory testing may be important to establish the diagnosis of athletic-associated menstrual dysfunction and to rule out other causes. A pregnancy test is essential in sexually active individuals. A thyroid-stimulating hormone (TSH) test to assess for underlying thyroid disease, a follicle-stimulating hormone (FSH) test to assess hormonal function, and a prolactin level to assess for a pituitary adenoma, are important screening tests. If individuals complain of hirsutism and acne, or if these findings are noted on examination, assessment of LH and FSH, dihydroandosterone sulfate (DHEA-S), and free testosterone may help in establishing whether polycystic ovarian syndrome exists or androgen-excess due to ovarin or adrenal tumors. Indirect testing includes a progesterone challenge with medroxy-progesterone acetate (Provera) 10 mg/day for 7 to 10 days. Lack of vaginal bleeding suggests a hypoestrogenic state, an obstructed outflow tract, or pregnancy.

I. Treatment and prevention of menstrual dysfunction in athletes

1. The treatment of menstrual dysfunction in female athletes varies somewhat based on the degree of menstrual dysfunction (see section V.A.). Adequate caloric intake and avoidance of disorders in eating patterns are often key components in the prevention and treatment of menstrual dysfunction. Adequate calcium intake and healthy eating patterns can help prevent the potential negative effects of athletic amenorrhea and oligomenorrhea on bone health. Specific preventive and treatment strategies are outlined, based on the hormonal milieu and type of problem. It must be remembered that the same individual may experience significant hormonal changes throughout her exercising and athletic career and treatment may vary during these times. Luteal-phase dysfunction, oligomenorrhea and amenorrhea in the athletic setting may

occur on a spectrum (see section V.I. for definitions of menstrual dysfunction common in athletes).

2. For luteal-phase dysfunction, an effect on bone is not certain. Treatment includes assessment of energy needs and optimal nutrition, calories and calcium intake. Hormonal therapy may be beneficial.
3. Treatment of oligomenorrhea may vary depending on the person's estrogen status. If the athlete is euestrogenic, oral contraceptives may be used if she is sexually active or monthly progestin may be used to protect the endometrium (medroxyprogesterone acetate 10 mg/day for seven to 10 days). Optimal nutrition and calcium intake—1,200 to 1,500 mg/day calcium—is recommended.
4. The hypoestrogenic amenorrheic woman presents the greatest challenge. A multidisciplinary approach is needed to address the many issues that may be contributory: Use of oral contraceptives or cyclic estrogen/progestin are recommended to prevent further bone loss and possibly to reduce the risk for stress injury. Decreasing exercise training intensity and/or duration should be considered. To optimize nutrition, calories and/or weight can be increased if indicated, and calcium intake can be increase to 1,500 mg/day (supplement if indicated). Disordered eating patterns can be treated by considering psychological and nutritional counseling and stress reduction techniques. Bone density testing should be considered if amenorrhea has been manifest for more than 6 months. The importance of education, counseling, and a multidisciplinary team approach must be emphasized and is essential.

VI. Disordered Eating

A. Definition of terms

1. In the athletic setting, a spectrum of eating patterns exists: from normal eating habits to disordered eating, and to development of an eating disorder. Disordered eating represents abnormal eating behaviors in persons who do not necessarily fit the psychiatric criteria for anorexia or bulimia nervosa. At the extremes of the disordered eating spectrum lie the frank eating disorders of anorexia and bulimia nervosa, which have strict (DSM IV) psychiatric criteria. Many athletes who have poor nutritional habits are at an intermediate point on the spectrum of disordered eating. These athletes are still at risk for developing serious endocrine, skeletal, and psychiatric disorders.
2. Features of anorexia nervosa include weight 15% below expected weight, feeling fat when really thin, an intense fear of becoming overweight, and amenorrhea. Features of bulimia nervosa include secretive binges two times a week for more than three months, lack of control over eating, purging behavior (laxative use, diuretic use, self-induced vomiting, overexercising), and overriding concern with body shape.
3. Anorexia (restrictive eating) and bulimia (binge/purge behaviors) often coexist. Many athletes exhibiting these behavior patterns do not fit the DSM IV criteria for an eating disorder, but may have some of the features of anorexia and bulimia and are still at risk for significant health problems. The DSM IV classification of Eating Disorders Not Otherwise Specified is sometimes used in these situations.

B. Prevalence of disordered eating in female athletes

1. The true prevalance of disordered eating in athletes is unknown. Based on a series of small studies there is a reported 15% to 62% prevalence in female athletes. A higher prevalence of disordered eating is often noted among participants in certain sports; sports in which subjective judging and aesthetics are important (gymnastics, dance, figure skating, diving), sports in which peak performance is associated with low body fat (running—especially distance running— and swimming).
2. The prevalence of anorexia and bulimia in the general female population is an estimated 3% to 5% for bulimia, and 1% to 3% for anorexia.

C. Contributory factors for disordered eating in athletes

1. Although the etiology and pathophysiology of disordered eating is not known, there are some known contributory factors, including the desire

to achieve or maintain an ideal body weight and/or optimal body fat, extreme pressure to excel in sport, pressure from coaches (weight standards, unrealistic expectations), pressure from parents, school, organization, society, self, low self-esteem, and poor body image. Athletes in sports in which appearance or endurance is important are often at higher risk. A family history of disordered eating or substance abuse and family dysfunction may also be an underlying factor, as might a history of sexual abuse. Puberty, adolescence, and young adulthood are vulnerable stages of development and it is in these periods of time when most disordered eating problems manifest.

D. Health consequences
   1. The health consequences of disordered eating are often lifelong. Psychological health consequences include the potential for significant morbidity and even mortality with anorexia and bulemia, as well as with disordered eating. Endocrine problems may involve menstrual dysfunction, premature osteoporosis, and growth and development effects. Nutritional problems often include pathologic weight-control techniques, malnutrition, and a starvation state, which can lead to a multitude of problems. Multiorgan problems of the cardiovascular and gastrointestinal (GI) systems can occur and in the more severe cases these can have a potential negative effect on every organ system.

E. Clinical evaluation
   1. History. One must maintain increased awareness of the female athlete triad and potential high-risk groups when screening for these important and often secretive problems. The preparticipation physical examination (PPE) is often an ideal time to screen and intervene for health issues of concern. Questions assessing nutritional history, menstrual history and exercise training are important. A 24-hour diet recall, highest and lowest weight in the past 12 months, a list of forbidden foods, and assessment of the athlete's sense of body satisfaction are important. A past or present history should be obtained of laxative use, use of diet pills or of self-induced vomiting. If a problem is identified, the athlete should be referred for a more detailed assessment and a physical examination can be scheduled at another office visit.
   2. Physical examination. A complete physical examination and pelvic examination (if there is menstrual dysfunction) is warranted if there is concern about disordered eating. Some signs/symptoms on physical examination that may be helpful are decreased body temperature, bradycardia, orthostatic hypotension, lanugo development (anorexia), decreased concentration, swollen parotid glands (bulimia), erosion of tooth enamel (bulimia), face and extremity edema, esophageal tears (bulimia), cardiac arrhythmias, abdominal pain, and delayed gastric emptying, in addition to other problems.
   3. Laboratory testing may be helpful in some instances. Tests obtained depend on clinical assessment of risk. Patterns that may be seen with disordered eating patterns include a complete blood count with a low white blood cell (WBC) count, low platelets; a chemistry panel with elevated LFTs (liver function tests), elevated cholesterol level; thyroid function tests with a low T3 and normal TSH; and electrolytes with low K, Na, Cl, Mg, PO4, Ca; and urine analysis to assess for ketonuria, pyuria, and hematuria. A ferritin level may be helpful to assess for iron deficiency.
   4. An electrocardiogram (ECG) should be obtained in athletes with more significant restrictive eating (anorexia) prior to clearing for sport participation. Assess for prolonged QT interval or other abnormalities if disordered eating is significant or if clinically indicated. (Prolonged QT interval and other ventricular arrhythmias have been noted as causes of death in severely ill patients with anorexia nervosa.)

F. Treatment and prevention
   1. The treatment for disordered eating should emphasize prevention. A multidisciplinary team (psychologist, nutritionist, physician, others) is essential in both preventive and treatment efforts. Medication may be

indicated in some cases (SSRIs are promising) along with individual and group therapy. A support network is important. Increasing self-esteem often is the focus of therapy sessions. The physician should emphasize optimal health, not disease. Follow/treat the patient if there is menstrual dysfunction [e.g., with ERT, calcium, etc.] for prevention of osteoporosis (dietary approaches, appropriate exercise, possible ERT, or other intervention).

2. Redefining athletic goals is important if appropriate and removal of an at-risk athlete from competition can be considered if medically indicated. Hospitalization may be indicated in some cases.

VII. Nutritional Concerns in the Female Athlete

A. Nutrient requirements

1. Female athletes have nutrient requirements similar to those of male athletes, with two exceptions: calcium and iron.

B. Calcium

1. For hypoestrogenic amenorrheic women, calcium 1,500 mg/day is needed to maintain calcium balance. For euestrogenic women, calcium 1,200 to 1,500 mg/day is needed. Dietary calcium is preferred to supplements.

C. Iron

1. Approximately 20% to 30% of female adolescent and young adults (athletes and nonathletes) may be iron deficient. It is important to differentiate iron deficiency anemia from pseudoanemia, which occurs in some athletes (see Chapter 28). Sources of iron loss include menstruation, diet, GI blood loss, sweat, urine and foot strike hemolysis.
2. It is not cost-effective to screen all female athletes for iron deficiency. Screening high-risk athletes (endurance athletes and others, based on clinical assessment) or those with a previous history of iron deficiency, may be beneficial. Serum ferritin is the most sensitive diagnostic test (more than 12 mg/dL is diagnostic). Because ferritin is an acute-phase reactant, obtaining serum iron studies may be helpful. Iron level is decreased and TIBC level is increased in iron deficiency. Decreased hemoglobin and hematocrit levels may be deceiving and can also be a finding with pseudoanemia of athletes (a physiologic dilutional effect).
3. The effect of anemia on athlete performance is controversial. Mild anemia decreases performance, whereas low ferritin without anemia probably does not.
4. The treatment of iron-deficiency anemia includes iron supplementation (varying dose depending on severity) and dietary counseling. In iron deficiency without anemia, iron supplementation is controversial. Prevention of anemia through dietary counseling is recommended and following the athlete to detect development of anemia is suggested. In athletes with normal iron stores, routine iron supplementation is not warranted. Prevention through dietary counseling is recommended.

VIII. Stress Urinary Incontinence in the Female Athlete

A. Stress urinary incontinence is experienced as involuntary loss of urine during physical exertion by some athletes.

B. The mechanism involves increased intraabdominal pressure during exercise.

C. At risk are athletes in running and jumping sports (gymnasts, runners, jumpers), hypoestrogenic amenorrheic/oligomenorrheic females, multiparous females, and those with anatomic defects.

D. Treatment includes avoiding excessive fluid ingestion for 2 to 3 hours before an event (tailored to sport and weather conditions to avoid dehydration) and use of a tampon or small sanitary napkin during an event and/or kegel exercises to strengthen muscles of the pelvic floor. Biofeedback, and other forms of behavioral therapy may prove beneficial. Physicians should assess such problems and correct menstrual dysfunction if it exists, especially hypoestrogenic state, which may contribute to stress urinary incontinence (e.g., hormone replacement may beneficial). Assess and correct for anatomic defects, such as in the posterior urethrovesical angle.

IX. Prevention of Medical and Orthopaedic Problems in the Female Athlete

A. Screening

1. The PPE is required for many athletes before they participate in organized sports and provides an ideal opportunity to screen athletes and to educate and counsel them. A thorough history is important—be specific in questions and maintain a high index of suspicion for the special concerns of the female athlete. A physical examination should be tailored to the needs of female athletes.
2. Physician office visits should be used to follow individuals when necessary for identified problems or to provide athletic training room opportunities for the physician who is also following an athletic team in a high school, college, or professional setting.

B. Education and counseling

1. Medical concerns, including endocrine, nutritional, and psychological problems, must be monitored if the athlete is to exercise in a safe and healthy manner.
2. Orthopaedic concerns include injury prevention—strength and flexibility, correction of biomechanical imbalances, appropriate footwear, and year-round training.

C. Multidisciplinary team

1. The importance of a multidisciplinary team approach cannot be overemphasized. The primary care physicians ideally should have consultants available in the areas of nutrition, psychology, orthopaedics, and physical therapy/athletic training to assist in medical care of the female athlete when needed.

Suggested Readings

ACSM Position Stand on the Female Athlete Triad. *Med Sci Sports Exerc* 1997;29:i–ix

Agostini R ed. The athletic woman. *Clin Sports Med* 1994;13.

Agostini R. *Medical and orthopaedic issues of active athletic women.* Philadelphia: Hanley and Belfus, 1994.

Arendt E, Dick R. Knee injury patterns among men and women in collegiate basketball and soccer: NCAA data and review of the literature. *Am J Sports Med* 1995;23:694–701.

Brownell KD, Rodin J, Wilmore JH, eds. *Eating, body weight, and performance in athletes: disorders of modern society.* Philadelphia: Lea & Febiger, 1992.

Drinkwater BL, Nilson K, Chestnut CH, et al. Bone mineral content of amenorrheic and eumenorrheic athletes. *N Engl J Med* 1984;311:277–81.

Ireland ML. Special concerns of the female athlete. In: Fu FH, Stone DA, eds. *Sports injuries: mechanism, prevention, and treatment,* 2nd ed. Baltimore: Williams & Wilkins, 1994:153–87.

Ireland ML, Gaudette M, Crook S. ACL injuries in the female athlete. *J Sports Rehab* 1997;6:97–110.

Johnson MD. Tailoring the preparticipation exam to female athletes. *Physician Sports Med* 1992;20:61–72.

Loucks AB, Horvath SM. Athletic amenorrhea: a review. *Med Sci Sports Exerc* 1985;17:56–72.

Nattiv A, Agostini R, Drinkwater B, et al. The female athlete triad: The interrelatedness of disordered eating, amenorrhea, and osteoporosis. *Clin Sports Med* 1994;13:405–18.

Shangold MM, Mirkin G. *Women and exercise–physiology and sports medicine.* Philadelphia: F.A. Davis, 1988.

Yeager, KK, Agostini R, Nattiv A, Drinkwater B. The Female Athlete Triad. *Med Sci Sports Exerc* 1993;25;775–77.

22. ACTIVITY FOR OLDER PERSONS AND MATURE ATHLETES

Henry C. Barry

I. Introduction

A. Epidemiologic Aspects of Aging. The average expected remaining years of life for American men and women aged more than 65 years is 14.7 years and 18.6 years, respectively. In general, the elderly are living longer, although some have a degree of impairment. Some elderly people have high functional capacities (including the capability of competing at the Master's level) and others have significant impairments.

B. Exercise, Aging and Inactivity

1. The Aging Process. Aging is marked by progressive impairment of mechanisms that control normal physiologic function. Ultimately, these alterations result in structural changes and functional decline involving all organ systems. The most important alterations, from a functional perspective, are the changes that occur in the cardiorespiratory, musculoskeletal, and the central nervous systems. Table 22-1 summarizes these changes.
2. Exercise Benefits. Many age-related changes may be prevented or ameliorated by physical activity. When people exercise habitually, blood pressure decreases, atherosclerosis slows, and muscle mass and strength increases. However, whether the relationship between an active lifestyle and good health is due to self-selection or genetic vigor or whether protection truly is afforded by being active is not clear. Many of the benefits of habitual activity are summarized in Table 22-2.
3. Aging and Inactivity. Among people aged more than 65 years about one third exercise regularly, but less than 10% exercise vigorously. The role of inactivity is a risk factor for many conditions (coronary artery disease, osteoporosis, obesity, diabetes, and others). Table 22-3 summarizes many of the changes associated with inactivity. Comparison of Table 22-1 and Table 22-3 should raise questions about parallel processes, so that one might postulate that some of the changes associated with aging may actually be due to being sedentary.
4. An Integrated Model of Aging. In this model, one would observe a vicious cycle wherein aging is associated with a reduction in physical activity, which in turn results in deconditioning, weakness, and fatigue. When disease, disability, and injury are included, the tendency to inactivity is greater, resulting in further physical decline. As the person declines physically there may be both a concomitant deterioration in the sense of wellness, and psychologic changes which lead to poor motivation and a further reduction in physical activity.

C. Hazards of Exercise. Generally, exercise may be considered either preventive or therapeutic. For example, a program of flexibility and strength may *prevent* falls. Exercise may have *therapeutic* benefit in persons with arthritis and in the rehabilitation of fractures and strokes. There are some risks to exercise, and the risk of injury is an important barrier to participation. The increased frequency of musculoskeletal impairment and cardiovascular disease makes it difficult for the elderly to return to activity after an injury.

II. General Considerations

A. Goals. Improved quality of life functional status, sense of well-being) should be the ultimate goal of an exercise routine. Enjoyment and socialization are key components of this. Compliance with exercise requirements increases when it is shared with others. The social interactions that accompany the

Table 22-1. Functional signs associated with age

Cardiovascular
Decreased cardiac output
Elevated systolic and diastolic blood pressure
Decreased maximum heart rate
Respiratory
Decreased vital capacity
Increased functional residual capacity
Musculoskeletal
Loss of muscle mass and strength
Osteoporosis
Reduced elasticity in connective tissue
Central nervous system
Reduced nerve conduction
Impaired motor responses
Decreased brain mass
Miscellaneous
Loss of subcutaneous fat
Impaired thirst sensation
Impaired thermoregulation

Table 22-2. Adaptations to exercise

Cardiovascular
Improved work capacity
Decreased resting heart rate
Increased HDL-C
Reduced blood pressure
Improved maximum oxygen consumption ($\dot{V}_{O2max}$)
Respiratory
Improved minute ventilation
Musculoskeletal
Increased bone density
Improved flexibility and range of motion
Increased muscle tone and strength
Improved coordination
Miscellaneous
Improved mental outlook
Reduced symptoms of depression and anxiety
Improved fat and carbohydrate metabolism
Increased insulin receptor sensitivity
Improved weight control

HDL-C, high density lipoprotein cholesterol.

Table 22-3. Adaptations to inactivity or immobilization

Reduced aerobic fitness
Loss of postural reflexes
Altered lipid metabolism
Negative nitrogen balance
Loss of muscle mass
Calcium extraction (osteopenia)

exercise routine provide mental and intellectual stimulation that is often missing in daily interactions of the elderly.

B. Cost. A key issue for many older patients is to limit financial expense. Many have limited financial reserves for recreational purposes. However, patients with specific rehabilitation potential may be eligible for Medicare reimbursement for therapeutic exercise programs with a physical therapist. For most ambulatory elderly, *walking is probably the single most important form of physical activity* and one that can be engaged in regularly in most locations. Little equipment is needed except for a pair of shoes that fit well, and for some, an assistive device (canes, walkers). Public television often has midday exercise shows emphasizing flexibility and low-impact aerobic exercises, well suited for many active elderly. Many senior citizen centers have similar programs at little or no cost. Frequently, the local Office on Aging will have lists of programs.

C. Safety. Safety is of prime importance for all who exercise, but the elderly present some unique challenges.

1. Fluids. The elderly are less able to adapt to changes in temperature, and total body water also is decreased in the elderly. These factors contribute to an increased propensity to dehydration and hyperthermia. The elderly should consume at least 8 ounces of fluid 1 hour before performing vigorous exercise and should take regularly scheduled water breaks while exercising rather than rely on a potentially impaired thirst mechanism to tell them when to drink. An additional 8 ounces of fluid should be consumed after every hour of exercise. The amounts should be increased by 50% if the weather is hot and humid.
2. Temperature. The elderly are more susceptible to cold injuries because of their decreased ability to perceive ambient air temperatures and react appropriately. This may be related to factors including loss of subcutaneous fat, decreased muscle mass, inadequate vasoconstriction, autonomic dysfunction, altered shivering mechanism, peripheral vascular disease, and the effects of medications (e.g., phenothiazines, tricyclic antidepressants, benzodiazepines, alcohol, nicotine). Appropriate dress must be emphasized. Clothing should be layered to allow adjustment to different temperatures and reflector garments should be worn when exercise is performed near roadways.
3. Feet. Because of impaired sensation, many elderly have a decreased ability to detect blister formation or friction injuries. Use of appropriate stockings and footwear that fits properly will prevent this. Frequent inspection of the feet and careful drying will help prevent serious blistering. This is especially important for persons with diabetes.
4. Environment. The elderly must monitor carefully for extreme environmental conditions (temperature, humidity, and air quality). They should exercise in well-lit places. With decreased sensory abilities (i.e., proprioception, eyesight, balance), there is an increased chance of injury. Because poor air quality may exacerbate COPD or asthma, exercise next to busy roadways or near traffic should be discouraged. The elderly should be especially cautious in summer, when air quality may deteriorate. In such circumstances, performing exercise indoors may be helpful. For instance, many indoor shopping malls have distances marked out and allow entry exercise indoors before the shops open.

D. Strength. The elderly can derive many benefits from resistance training. They can achieve increases in muscle strength and mass, improvements in gait speed, and increased functional mobility. Proper lifting techniques with an emphasis on proper breathing is critical. Valsalva lifting can be disastrous in the elderly.

E. Motivation. Motivating the elderly to begin or to maintain an exercise program can be as problematic as mobilizing sedentary adolescents. Conditions such as depression and dementia can impair interest in engaging in or maintaining activity. Treatment of depression and reversible causes of dementia should be key components of any attempt to manage activity among seniors.

1. Goal Identification. The spectrum of desired activity is wide: Some may want to play with their grandchildren, others to compete at the master's level; some may wish merely to be independent in toileting or other self-care activities. Goals should be realistic and attainable. Frequently, intermediate goals must be identified. Education about the benefits of exercise begins with the initial physician–patient meeting, and should be reinforced with each visit. The benefits that are likely to generate the greatest interest are those that help patients achieve their own goals. Several strategies, including use of films and videos, educational handouts, booklets, and group sessions, may help motivate the elderly. Meetings with peers or with influential role models may have even more impact.
2. Rewards. Failure to achieve goals is a common source of frustration and increases the probability of dropout. This is not unique to the elderly. If such failure occurs, goals should be reassessed. Use of an exercise diary, charts, or graphs should be encouraged, so that progress can be plotted. Praise and encouragement should be offered frequently. Positive reinforcement must be genuine and consistent. Rewards or public recognition for goal achievement will further reinforce compliance. Setbacks or plateaus should be explained as normal or anticipated occurrences.
3. Variety. To prevent boredom, types of activities ought to be rotated regularly. By alternating between different activities, older people will continue to develop skill and derive benefit, and by wise selection of activities, the problem of overuse-injuries can be minimized. In a population that already has a great propensity to become sedentary, avoidance of injury is extremely important.

III. Medication Use and Exercise

The elderly are the greatest users of medications. Frequently, seniors use multiple prescription drugs. When these are added to their use of a number of nonprescription drugs (vitamins, laxatives, analgesics, others) significant problems are more likely to occur. Polypharmacy is often a problem. Many of the more commonly used drugs present special problems for the elderly and for their activity levels.

A. Orthostatic Hypotension. Orthostatic hypotension, which may cause falls among the elderly, is a common side effect associated with several commonly prescribed drugs, including antidepressants, major tranquilizers, diuretics, antihypertensive agents, and a variety of cardiovascular medications. This problem may be worsened by reduced thirst sensation, diminished fluid replacement, or excessive fluid loss as may occur with use of antidepressants, major tranquilizers, and diuretics. Muscle cramping or myalgias may be caused by electrolyte disturbances from diuretics.

B. β-Blockers. β-Blockers may reduce exercise tolerance by decreasing cardiac output and resting rate, and blunt the increase in heart rate (HR) during exercise. This class of drugs may also impair glucose uptake by exercising muscle. This potentially limits availability of substrate for aerobic metabolism resulting in lactic acid production and muscle soreness. Any of these adverse side effects may make it difficult to maintain an exercise regimen.

C. General Guidelines for Medication Use. In general, medication use by the elderly should be minimized. When medications are required, a low initial dose should be used and small incremental adjustments made when needed. Certain classes of drugs should be avoided. For instance, the psychotropic drugs may alter further the already impaired thermoregulatory functions of the elderly, increasing the likelihood of hyperthermia and dehydration. Finally, the entire drug regimen should be periodically reassessed.

IV. Coronary Artery Disease

Coronary artery disease is one of the most prevalent chronic illnesses in the elderly. Unfortunately, coronary disease can develop even among habitual exercisers. Those with heart disease or those who plan to exercise vigorously should undergo periodic exercise tolerance tests to monitor performance and to guide safe levels of exertion. Asymptomatic persons whose exercise regimen will be low intensity do not need stress testing. Those individuals with heart disease should be instructed in common symptoms of exercise intolerance. Antianginal therapy should be monitored carefully. Keep in mind that β-blockers can present some problems in active people. (See Chapter 26)

V. Chronic Lung Disease

Many elderly patients have chronic obstructive pulmonary disease (COPD), which causes marked decrease in exercise endurance. Irritants, such as cigarette smoke or environmental pollutants, cause production of excess mucus and loss of elasticity in the alveoli. Exercise capacity is limited in COPD patients, secondary to decreased respiratory reserve, but exercise can improve overall conditioning and prevent further deterioration. It can improve diaphragmatic breathing and reduce reliance on the accessory muscles. Pretreatment with bronchodilators, inhaled steroids or cromolyn sulfate, and use of supplemental oxygen will enhance the individual's exercise tolerance.

VI. Arthritis

Osteoarthritis should no longer be considered an inevitable consequence of aging. It should be considered as *related* to aging and not an *effect* of aging. The common perception that osteoarthritis is caused by aging derives from the observation that many elderly are afflicted with osteoarthritis. Osteoarthritis is a multifactorial condition which may be caused by the interaction of weight, hereditary factors, congenital abnormalities, gender (women generally are affected earlier in life), bone density, hyperuricemia, altered joint alignment, and trauma.

A. General Considerations. Exercise can be prescribed as a treatment for osteoarthritis because it is associated with weight reduction, improved muscle tone, and reduced atrophy, increased flexibility, and improved biomechanics. A person who has arthritis should focus on exercises that are tolerated well. These are generally low-impact, low-intensity activities which emphasize flexibility and strength. Aquatic exercise is becoming more popular because the buoyancy of the body in water places less stress on the joints. There are many different types of exercise machines available for home use or at health clubs. Many strength machines have limits which allow the person with arthritis to perform strengthening exercises within a comfortable ROM. Exercise machines, however, may place stress across joints. For instance, the popular cross-country ski machines, while easier on the knees, feet, and ankles, may place more stress on the hips or low back. Table 22-4 summarizes the potential for joint stress associated with some popular exercise devices.

B. Acute Arthritis. When acute inflammation is present, exercise involving the affected joint can be detrimental. During an acute flair of arthritis, the joint should be protected by using splints. Once the acute phase has resolved, initial rehabilitation should emphasize improving ROM, and increase strength later.

Table 22-4. Exercise equipment and the stress across selected joints

Equipment	Hip	Knee	Ankle	Shoulder	Spine
Bicycle	++	++	+	–	+
Rowing machine	–	–	–	++	++
Cross-country ski	+	±	±	±	+
Step machine	++	++	++	+	+

VII. Master's Athletes

A. Common injuries in this group are similar to those that occur in younger athletes, such as overuse syndromes (although compounded by concomitant arthritis), sprains and strains. Age-associated loss of water in the cartilage can precipitate cartilaginous injuries.

B. Management of most injuries is similar to that for younger athletes, with relative rest, ice, compression, and elevation as the foundation. The healing rate is more variable among the elderly, but is generally slower than that of younger athletes. It is interesting that master's athletes tend to be retired and thus have more time to spend on rehabilitation. Because they are usually highly motivated, their recovery is facilitated.

VIII. Summary

The elderly present a number of challenges; the most important centers on the declining functional capacity associated with aging. The degree to which these changes are related to the interactions among aging, disease, illness, injury, lifestyle, genetics, and other variables remains unclear. However, it is evident that a well-designed exercise program of low to moderate intensity may be the single most cost-effective means of maintaining function. The exercise program must be goal oriented and consistent with the person's goals, but it must be individualized to account for existing impairments. No matter what their functional capacity, the elderly present some unique considerations. The primary emphasis of any regimen should be on quality-of-life issues, such as improving flexibility, strength, and mobility.

Suggested Readings

Barry HC, Eathorne SW. Exercise and aging: issues for the practitioner. *Med Clin North Am* 1994;78:357–76.

Elward K. Larson EB. Benefits of exercise for older adults: a review of existing evidence and current recommendations for the general population. *Clin Geriatr Med* 1992;8:35–50.

Fiatarone MA, Marks EC, Ryan ND, et al. High-intensity strength training in nonagenarians: effects on skeletal muscle. *JAMA* 1990;263:3029–34.

Kavanagh T, Shephard RJ. Can regular sports participation slow the aging process? Data on master's athletes. *Physician Sports Med* 1990;18:94–103.

Lane NE. Does running cause degenerative joint disease? *J Musculoskel Med* 1987;4:17–24.

Lipsitz LA, Goldberger AL. Loss of 'complexity' and aging: potential application of fractals and chaos theory to senescence. *JAMA* 1992;267:1806.

Stamford B. Exercise and chronic airway obstruction. *Physician Sports Med* 1991;19:189–90.

Stones MJ, Kozma A. Physical activity, age, and cognitive/motor performance. In: Howe ML, Brainerd CJ (eds): *Cognitive Development in Adulthood: Progress in Cognitive Development Research.* New York, Springer-Verlag, 1988, 273–321.

23. THE ATHLETE WITH A DISABILITY

Brian C. Halpern and Dennis A. Cardone

Athletes with disabilities participate in sports and represent a rapidly growing population of sports enthusiasts. This growth is fueled by recent federal legislation mandating equal access and equal opportunity for persons with disabilities, including access to physical education and sports, as well as extraordinary accomplishments of disabled athletes. Sports participation is valuable for the disabled for the same reasons as for the able-bodied: health benefits, enjoyment, and the satisfaction derived from participation and competition.

The Americans with Disabilities Act defines a person with a "disability" as an individual who has a physical or mental impairment that substantially limits one or more of his or her major life activities. Types of disabilities include cerebral palsy, blindness, deafness, paralysis, mental retardation, and amputation. Others include athletes with locomotor disabilities such as arthritis, muscular dystrophy, and multiple sclerosis. More than 3 million athletes with physical and mental disabilities are involved annually in athletic competitions in the United States; an even greater number are involved in recreational and leisure sports. Approximately 8% of Americans between the age of 16 to 64 have some type of mobility limitation.

Psychological benefits of sports and exercise for the disabled include an improvement of mood state and perceived health, a reduction of anxiety and depression, and an increase of self-esteem and satisfaction. Sports allow the participant to be part of a team, develop skills, meet new challenges, and achieve goals.

The Special Olympics and the Paralympic Games provide organized sports events for disabled athletes. The Special Olympics promote exercise and participation in sports for mentally retarded individuals 8 years of age and older. Competitions are arranged on local, state, and international levels. The Paralympic Games provide competitions for athletes with physical disabilities. They are held every Olympic year, usually in the same country hosting the Olympic Games.

I. The Preparticipation Physical Examination (PPPE)

Physicians should be aware of common problems associated with different disabilities and be able to diagnose abnormalities that may endanger the athlete. They should provide support, encourage physical activity and healthy lifestyle, and recognize the special needs of disabled athletes.

The PPPE has traditionally been performed annually. The Special Olympics require athletes to be medically cleared before participating in Special Olympics events. The "station method" of examination should be avoided because of the decreased mobility of some athletes with a disability. The PPPE should be performed by physicians who have provided longitudinal care and know the baseline status of the athlete.

A. **History.** The history should include a detailed summary of previous injuries and illnesses, risk factors for injuries and illnesses, and current medications. Does the athlete have a history of seizures? Cardiopulmonary disease? Renal disease? Atlantoaxial instability (in athletes with Down's syndrome)? Has the athlete had previous heat stroke or heat exhaustion? Fractures or dislocations? What prosthetic devices or special equipment does the athlete use during sports participation? At what levels of competition has the athlete previously participated? In certain cases the history may need to be obtained from a family member or other person familiar with the athlete.

B. **Physical Examination.** This should include blood pressure, visual acuity, and complete cardiovascular, musculoskeletal, and neurological examinations.

C. **Tests.** Laboratory tests and radiographs are usually not necessary but must be considered on an individual basis. Screening cervical radiographs in athletes with Down's syndrome is discussed in a later section.

II. Wheelchair Athletes

A. **Classification.** The classification of wheelchair athletes is by severity of disability. In the United States there are two commonly used classification systems: those of the National Wheelchair Athletic Association (NWAA) and the National Wheelchair Basketball Association (NWBA). These are based on the level of spinal injury and the extent of injury. They provide for competition between athletes with a similar degree of disability.

B. **Exercise Physiology.** Wheelchair athletes depend upon their upper bodies for exercise and exhibit physiologic responses different from that of able-bodied athletes.

1. **Aerobic and Anaerobic Capacity.** With proper training, wheelchair athletes can improve their maximal aerobic capacity. Maximal oxygen uptake ($\dot{V}_{O2max}$) has been shown to increase with activity levels and training. Differences in peak power output and aerobic power exist across classes of wheelchair athletes. Those with lower spinal cord lesions and more available functional muscle mass have more peak power output and aerobic power during exhaustive exercise.
2. **Cardiovascular response to exercise.** In wheelchair athletes, cardiac output (CO) is reduced 10% to 25% and stroke volume is 15% to 30% lower than in able-bodied athletes performing similar upper body exercise. In wheelchair athletes, multiple factors may affect the physiologic limit of the upper body's peak aerobic power and cardiac response.
   a. **Hypokinetic Circulation.** Below the level of the spinal cord lesion there is no active muscle pumping, which leads to venous pooling. Venous return of blood flow to the heart and cardiac output are reduced during exercise as compared with able-bodied individuals.
   b. **Disrupted Autonomic Reflexes.** Reduced sympathetic nerve outflow in spinal cord injured athletes reduces maximal cardiac output. Quadriplegics have a significantly lower maximal heart rate compared with paraplegics and able-bodied persons. Maximal heart rates for paraplegics and able-bodied persons are similar.
   c. **Thermoregulatory Dysfunction.** In athletes with spinal cord injuries, a lack of neural control of skin blood flow leads to increased blood collecting in the skin to compensate for heat loss during exercise. This increased skin blood volume results in decreased stroke volume during prolonged physical activity.
3. **Pulmonary Function.** Tidal Volume (TV), forced expiratory volume in 1 sec (FEV_1), and forced vital capacity (FVC) are slightly lower in paraplegic athletes than able-bodied athletes. Quadriplegics have significantly lower values than both groups for all pulmonary function variables except FEV/FVC.
4. **Mechanical Efficiency.** Wheelchair athletes require a greater energy output than cyclists. The muscles of the upper body are much less efficient than the muscles of the lower limb. For example, the efficiency of a cycle ergometer, arm crank ergometer, and wheelchair ergometer are 23%, 18%, and 8%, respectively.

C. **Injuries.** Wheelchair athletes are involved in a range of recreational and competitive sports. The five highest-injury risk sports for wheelchair athletes, in descending order of risk, are track, basketball, road racing, tennis, and field events. Most injuries in wheelchair athletes are minor. The upper extremity, particularly the shoulder and wrist, is most frequently involved, followed by the lower extremity and then the head and spine. The types of injuries found in a year-long survey of elite wheelchair athletes were strains (48%), abrasions (22%), contusions (10%), blisters (6%), fractures (6%), sprains (4%), lacerations (2%), and illnesses (2%).

The most common mechanisms of injury are overuse and falls from either direct impact with another chair or other objects. Wheelchair athletes have the same types and frequencies of injuries as able-bodied athletes. However, recovery time as a result of injury is greater for disabled athletes.

Explainations include a delayed healing process associated with the spinal cord injury or a more conservative rehabilitation program.

1. **Skin Injuries**
   a. **Abrasions/Lacerations.** These are most commonly seen on the upper extremities as a result of contact with other chairs, wheelchair brakes, or sharp edges of the wheelchair.
      (1) **Prevention.** Filing off sharp edges from the chair, wearing protective pads or clothing, and cambering wheels, especially for sports like basketball.
   b. **Blisters.** Blisters of the fingers and hands are quite common and are caused by friction, shear, and irritation from repeated contact with the wheelchair push rim. Blisters may also form on the skin of the back due to friction with the seat posts.
      (1) **Prevention.** Taping of the hands and fingers or protective gloves prevent blister formation of the fingers and hands. Using padded seat posts and wearing dry shirts help prevent blister formation on the back.
      (2) **Treatment.** The blister may be drained with a sterile needle. The roof of the blister is preserved to act as a barrier to infection and trauma. Petroleum jelly and a tape or gauze dressing can prevent further irritation.
   c. **Pressure Sores.** Pressure sores are primarily a problem of athletes with spinal cord injuries. These athletes have elevated skin pressures over the sacrum and ischial tuberosities for extended periods during training, competition, and normal daily activity. Sports wheelchairs are designed with the knees being higher than the buttocks, resulting in increased pressure over the sacrum and ischial tuberosities. The triad of pressure, shear, and moisture during sports participation leads to pressure sore formation.
      (1) **Prevention.** Preventive measures include adequate cushioning padding for the buttocks and other bony prominences, frequent pressure relief, good nutrition and hygiene, and wearing clothing that absorbs moisture and decreases friction. Frequent skin checks need to be made by coaches, trainers, and medical staff.
      (2) **Treatment.** Wheelchair athletes should not compete with open pressure sores. Training should be modified to prevent additional pressure damage and to allow healing. Local wound care includes relief of pressure at the site and occlusive dressings.
2. **Soft Tissue Injuries.** Wheelchair athletes have an increased incidence of soft tissue injuries of the upper extremity. Injuries include strains, sprains, bursitis, and tendinitis.
   a. **Etiology.** Soft tissue injuries are usually the result of overuse, improper training technique, or direct trauma.
      (1) **Muscle-Tendon Imbalance.** Wheelchair athletes predominantly use the extensor muscle groups of the upper extremity in wheelchair locomotion. These muscles increase in strength and size disproportionately to opposing groups. The result is muscle imbalance and decreased flexibility.
      (2) **Improper Push Technique.** Results in overuse syndromes of the wrist and elbow and acute sprains and strains of the soft tissue around these joints.
      (3) **Contact with the Wheelchair Push Rim or Tire.** This can result in sprains of the interphalangeal joints and the metacarpophalangeal joint of the thumb. The hands also are subject to direct trauma resulting from wheelchair collisions.
      (4) **Altered Body Mechanics.** Wheelchair athletes compensate for their disabilities by altering normal body mechanics. This causes unusual stress to joints, tendons, and muscles.

b. **Prevention.** Preventive measures include routine stretching with a warm-up and cool-down period for each workout, a slowly progressive strengthening and conditioning program, preventive taping and gloves, and proper technique. Competitors, coaching staff, and medical personnel should be educated as to the unique problems encountered by wheelchair athletes.

c. **Treatment.** The treatment of soft tissue injuries in wheelchair athletes involves the same principles and practices as in able-bodied athletes.

3. **Rotator-Cuff Impingement Syndrome.** Wheelchair athletes place constant demand on their shoulders for propulsion and weight bearing. This leads to a high incidence of shoulder injuries, especially rotator-cuff impingement syndrome.

   a. **Etiologies**

      (1) **Muscle Imbalance.** As compared with able-bodied athletes, wheelchair athletes have a significantly higher ratio of shoulder abduction to adduction strength. The ratio becomes even greater in wheelchair athletes with impingement syndrome. This imbalance allows the humeral head to migrate cephalad, causing impingement in the acromiohumeral space. Weak scapulothoracic stabilizers can also contribute to the problem.

      (2) **Chronic Overuse.** Training and activities of daily living lead to overuse syndromes. Wheelchair-dependent individuals repetitively load their shoulders in the weight-bearing, overhead position for transferring. Also, because of their low setting in the wheelchair, many of their daily tasks must be performed in the overhead impingement positions.

      (3) **Posture.** Many wheelchair athletes maintain a position of shoulder internal rotation and scapular protraction during extensive wheeling activity and while at rest. This can predispose to impingement.

   b. **Diagnosis and Evaluation**

      (1) **History and Physical Examination.** Patients usually have an insidious onset of pain, aggravated with overhead movements. Examination reveals positive impingement signs, weak shoulder adductors and internal/external rotators, tenderness over the coracoacromial ligament, a painful arc, and possible atrophy of involved muscles.

      (2) **Shoulder Radiographs.** X-rays may show subacromial spurring, a curved acromion, an enlarged coracoid, subacromial calcification, and a superior migration of the humeral head.

   c. **Treatment.** Strengthening of shoulder adductors, internal/external rotators and scapulothoracic stabilizers; modification of training program and daily activities to minimize shoulder impingement positions; posture training; ice; nonsteroidal anti-inflammatory drugs; corticosteroid injection to subacromial space.

4. **Peripheral Nerve Entrapments.** Nerve entrapment syndromes of the upper extremities are seen in more than 20% of wheelchair athletes.

   a. **Types**

      (1) **Carpal Tunnel Syndrome.** This is the most common peripheral nerve entrapment of the upper extremity in wheelchair athletes.

         (a) **Etiology.** Wrist extension posturing during wheeling and transferring, and isometric and isotonic contractions of the finger flexors that travel within the carpal tunnel result in increased carpal tunnel pressures. Also, repetitive pressure from the wheelchair on the volar soft tissues overlying the carpal tunnel contributes to carpal tunnel syndrome.

(2) **Ulnar Neuropathy.** This is most prevalent at the wrist (Guyon's canal) and less commonly noted at the distal aspect of the cubital tunnel (deep forearm flexor pronator aponeurosis).

(a) **Etiology.** Ulnar neuropathy at Guyon's canal is due to prolonged compressive forces from the wheelchair in this region. Entrapment of the ulnar nerve at the distal aspect of the cubital tunnel is caused by the repetitive contractions of the flexor carpi ulnaris muscle required by a wheelchair athlete, prolonged elbow flexion, and repetitive pressure on this area when the forearm rests against the wheelchair arm rest.

5. **Thermoregulatory Dysfunction.** Thermoregulation in athletes with spinal cord injuries is impaired because of skeletal muscular paralysis and a loss of autonomic nervous system control. The higher and more complete the spinal cord injury, the greater the thermoregulatory impairment. Individuals with spinal cord injuries have a higher core temperature in the heat and lower core temperatures in the cold.

a. **Hyperthermia.** The risk of hyperthermia and its consequences is great in wheelchair athletes who perform strenuous exercise in a hot environment. Normal autonomic responses for heat dissipation—including sweat gland secretion, redistribution of cardiac output, and vasodilation in cutaneous vessels—are impaired. Also, reduced skeletal muscle activity of the lower extremities results in decreased venous return and cardiac output. For the same reasons, dehydration is a significant problem in wheelchair athletes. Many medications used for pain, depression, allergy, bladder dysfunction, hypertension and other disorders can interfere with the normal sweat response.

(1) **Prevention.** Minimizing exposure to the heat, planning training and competition in the early morning or evening hours, replacement of fluid, acclimatization, use of appropriate clothing, and use of cooling towels or spraying water over the body surfaces to assist with heat convection.

(2) **Treatment.** See Chapter 11 for evaluation and treatment.

b. **Hypothermia.** Athletes with spinal cord injuries are also more susceptible to hypothermia. These athletes have a loss of normal autonomic regulatory responses to cold, an impaired circulation because of reduced skeletal muscle activity, and an inability to shiver. They may also fail to recognize early signs of hypothermia, like cold extremities, because of lack of sensation below the level of the neurological lesion. Certain medications and medical conditions can also predispose the athlete to problems with temperature regulation in the cold. These athletes can develop hypothermia when exercising in air temperatures as high as 50°F.

(1) **Prevention.** This includes use of appropriate clothing, drinking adequate fluids, replacing wet clothing with dry after training or competition, and using insulated blankets.

(2) **Treatment.** See Chapter 12 for evaluation and treatment.

6. **Bladder Dysfunction.** Athletes with spinal cord injuries or other neurological disorders often have bladder dysfunction or neurogenic bladders. These athletes frequently use indwelling catheters or intermittent catheterization and are at increased risk of infection. Preventive measures include adequate hydration, ensuring regular bladder emptying, and using proper antiseptic techniques with catheters.

7. **Autonomic Hyperreflexia.** This is an acute generalized sympathetic hyperactivity response seen in athletes with spinal cord injuries with lesions above the midthoracic level. Precipitating circumstance include bladder distention, catheterization, urinary tract infection, bowel or bladder obstruction, exposure to cold or hot temperatures, pressure sores, sunburn, and thrombophlebitis. The classic syndrome of autonomic hyperreflexia is characterized by paroxysmal hypertension, anxiety, sweating, headache, and bradycardia. Treatment involves removing

the athlete from physical activity, monitoring blood pressure, emptying bowel and bladder, and immediate transfer to a medical facility.

III. Down Syndrome

Musculoskeletal disorders are present in individuals with Down syndrome. Ligamentous laxity and hypermobility are prominent features. There is a high incidence of patellar instability, pes planus, metatarsus primus varus, scoliosis, hip dysplasia, and increased atlantoaxial mobility. Congenital cardiac disorders including heart murmurs, ventricular septal defects, and endocardial cushion defects are seen in 40% to 60% of Down syndrome patients. These musculoskeletal and cardiac abnormalities should be screened for in the preparticipation evaluation.

A. **Cervical Spine Abnormalities.** Structural abnormalities of the cervical spine are seen more commonly in people with Down syndrome. However, it is rare for these abnormalities to be a source of disability or death.

1. **Atlantoaxial Instability.** Approximately 15% of children with Down syndrome have atlantoaxial instability. Serious injury can result if the neck is forcibly flexed or axially loaded, causing the vertebrae to shift or compress the spinal cord. There is not, however, an increased incidence of serious cervical spine injuries in athletes with Down syndrome as compared with other athletic populations. Atlantoaxial instability is directly related to the magnitude of laxity of the transverse ligament of the atlas. A very small number of children with Down syndrome do develop signs and symptoms of cervical cord myelopathy. These children are typically girls, less than 10 years old, with significant ligamentous laxity and chronic signs and symptoms of cervical cord myelopathy prior to any catastrophic dislocation of C1-C2. Acute atlantoaxial slippage is exceedingly rare.

a. **Diagnosis and Evaluation**

(1) **History** is often difficult to obtain because the patient's complaints are frequently misunderstood or dismissed. Patients may be asymptomatic or may complain of neck pain, limited neck mobility, numbness, weakness, or paresthesias in the upper extremities.

(2) **Physical examination** must include a complete neurological evaluation. The neurological manifestations of symptomatic atlantoaxial instability include easy fatigability, abnormal gait, limited neck range of motion, torticollis or head tilt, incoordination and clumsiness, sensory deficits, spasticity, hyperreflexia, clonus, and other upper motor neuron and posterior column signs and symptoms.

(3) Radiographs of the cervical spine, including lateral views in neutral, flexion, and extension, must be done. In some cases MRI or CT scan may be necessary. The atlantodens interval is a space between the odontoid process of the axis and the anterior arch of the atlas. Normal for a preadolescent child is up to 4.5-5.0 millimeters. An atlantodens interval greater than this is significant for atlantoaxial instability

b. **Screening**

(1) Preparticipation examination with a complete neurological evaluation.

(2) Radiographs. Uncertainty exists concerning the value of cervical spine radiographs in screening for possible catastrophic neck injury in athletes with Down syndrome. The American Academy of Pediatrics recently retired their 1984 policy statement that recommended: obtaining lateral neck radiographs in athletes with Down syndrome before participating in the Special Olympics; and restricting certain activities in individuals with radiographic evidence of instability. Further research needs to be done before more definitive recommendations can be made. If screening radiographs are performed and are normal, it is not necessary to routinely repeat the screening, unless required to do so for parti-

cipation in an athletic event. If the initial films are abnormal, follow up radiographs should be performed every two to three years.

c. **Participation.** Patients with atlantoaxial instability have been prohibited from participating in sports that place excessive pressure on the head or neck muscles. These sports include gymnastics, diving, tumbling, high jump, soccer, butterfly stroke, decathlon and horseback riding. As more research becomes available these participation restrictions may be removed.

d. **Treatment.** Only patients with an increased atlantodens interval and an accompanying myelopathy require treatment. These patients will require a posterior atlantoaxial fusion.

2. **Other cervical abnormalities** seen in people with Down syndrome:
   a. Occiput-C1 instability
   b. Malformations of the odontoid process
   c. Hypoplasia of the posterior arch of C1
   d. Spondylolysis and spondylolisthesis of the midcervical vertebrae
   e. Early arthritic changes of C4-C6

B. **Hip abnormalities** seen in children with Down syndrome include acute dislocation, habitual dislocation, slipped capital femoral epiphysis, and progressive subluxation associated with acetabular dysplasia.

C. **Exercise Physiology in Down Syndrome Athletes.** Aerobic capacity has been demonstrated to be substantially lower in individuals with mental retardation than in those without mental retardation. However, with exercise training, individuals with mental retardation but without Down syndrome can significantly improve their aerobic capacity. Down syndrome athletes have not shown the same increase in aerobic capacity. This may in part be explained by a physiologic limitation related to a reduction in sympathetic response. Exercise testing of Down syndrome athletes shows lower maximal heart rates, lower maximal values of catecholamines, lower postexercise blood lactate levels and lower maximal oxygen uptake values ($\dot{V}_{O2max}$) as compared with individuals without Down syndrome.

IV. Cerebral Palsy (CP)

CP is a neuromuscular condition with muscular involvement ranging from severe spasticity and disability to slight speech impairment. The most prevalent form of CP is spastic diplegia, characterized by motor incoordination primarily in the lower extremities. Spastic syndromes represent approximately 70% of cases. One-half of all CP athletes compete in wheelchairs, and about half are ambulatory. In addition to movement disorders, athletes with CP may have other associated disorders including perceptual motor problems, learning disabilities, seizures, visual dysfunction, deafness, and mental retardation.

A. **Exercise Physiology.** CP athletes have lower aerobic capacity ($\dot{V}_{O2max}$), equivalent blood lactate concentrations, reduced mechanical efficiency, higher energy requirements, similar maximal heart rates, and similar cardio-respiratory responses as compared with able-bodied athletes. An increased displacement of the center of gravity caused by poor motor control, decreased range of motion, and loss of balance is partly responsible for the reduced mechanical efficiency and increased energy requirements.

B. **Musculoskeletal.** CP athletes with spasticity have increased muscle tone, a loss of selective muscle control, and a muscle imbalance across the joints, especially of the lower extremities. This creates excessive stress on the musculotendinous units and joints. These athletes are at increased risk for strains, sprains, and overuse syndromes.

1. **Patellofemoral pain** is common and frequently leads to chondromalacia in CP athletes. Progressive tightening of the hamstrings and quadriceps muscles leads to a shortened stride length and increased forces across the patellofemoral joint. The condition is more resistant to treatment than in able-bodied athletes. Chronic proximal patellar tendinitis is also common because of the tension on the quadriceps mechanism.

2. **Hip abnormalities** are common. Muscle tightness and imbalances across the hip can lead to the development of coxa valga and acetabular dysplasia. In more severe cases, hip subluxation and dislocation occur. The CP athlete may initially present with hip pain when running or jumping.
3. **Stress fractures,** especially of the lower extremities, may develop because of muscle and stress imbalances, and inappropriate training. They are more likely to occur at sites proximal to a brace or prosthesis.
4. **Ankle and foot deformities** seen in patients with CP include equinus deformity, equinovarus deformity, and valgus deformity. Frequently, these require surgical repair or bracing. If left untreated, metatarsalgia, ankle instability, callosities, and pressure sores may result.
5. **Prevention of musculoskeletal injuries** includes an aggressive stretching program, a warm-up and cool-down period for each workout, strength training programs, adaptive equipment, well-fitting and functioning braces when needed, and educating athletes, coaching staff, and medical staff to the unique problems encountered by athletes with CP.

C. **Coordination and Balance.** CP athletes frequently have inadequate motor control and lack of coordination and balance. Hand-to-eye coordination is impaired. Catching, throwing, and controlling necessary equipment such as racquets, bats, and golf clubs are difficult. A variety of ball games can contribute to improvements in coordination. Protective gear, such as helmets for athletes with impaired balance, should be used when appropriate.

V. Injury and illness surveillance of an around-the-world bicycle ride for disabled athletes.

Disabilities seen in these athletes included spinal cord injuries, cerebral palsy, limb amputation, mental retardation, hearing and vision impairment and muscular dystrophy. Physicians covered the entire ride and recorded injury data. The injuries and illnesses reported in order of frequency were as follows:

High:	**Moderate:**	**Low:**
Abrasions	Tinea cruris/pedis	Lacerations
Pressure sores	Bronchitis	Urinary tract infections
Gastroenteritis	Contusions	Sunburn
Strains/sprains	Muscle spasms	Fractures
Tendinitis/Bursitis		Hemorrhoids
Upper respiratory infection		Dehydration
		Concussion
		Hyperthermia/Hypothermia
		Exercise-induced bronchospasm
		Allergic rhinitis
		Contact dermatitis
		Conjunctival irritation
		Callosities/blisters
		Cellulitis

VI. Other Disabilities

A. **Deafness.** Communication is the primary problem for deaf athletes. Colored lights, light dimmers, touch, and hand signals facilitate sports participation. In some cases the vestibular apparatus is involved, affecting balance and coordination. Activities requiring sharp turns, spins, cuts, or balance can be difficult.

B. **Visual Impairment.** There is a broad spectrum of vision impairment. Some athletes are completely blind, while others may perceive light, dark, and shadows. The International Blind Sports Association (IBSA) utilizes functional classifications based upon usable vision. A wide range of sports activities are available to the blind athlete, utilizing companions, clap sticks, beeping balls, and guide rails.

C. **Limb Amputation.** These athletes compete with various assistive devices, orthoses, and prostheses. Team physicians need to be aware of regulations concerning their use in different sports. In track events, for example, prostheses are permitted while crutches and canes are prohibited.
   1. **Low Back Pain.** Lower extremity amputee athletes often develop low back pain. Excessive lumbar spine lateral flexion and extension compensate for the lack of lower extremity joint flexion at prosthetic sites. This results in an imbalance in back musculature and a functional scoliosis. Specific muscle stretching and strengthening programs are preventative and therapeutic.
   2. **Skin Trauma.** Prostheses can cause skin breakdown, abrasions, blistering, and skin rashes. Prevention includes adjustment of prosthetic fit and alignment and protective pads.
   3. **Bursitis.** Amputees may develop bursitis as a result of socket irritation. Common sites include the prepatellar, infrapatellar, or pretibial bursae in below-knee amputees and the ischial and trochanteric bursae in above-knee amputees. Treatment involves modifying the prosthesis.
   4. **Knee Injuries.** Hyperextension knee injuries can result from the body's forward momentum moving over a fixed prosthesis and residual limb.
   5. **Impact Injuries.** For example, bruising over bony prominences, can result from forces transmitted through the prosthesis to the residual limb.
   6. **Injuries to the Sound Limb.** Amputee runners place unusual stresses, including added weight, on the sound limb. Injuries include plantar fasciitis, stress fractures, and overpronation of the foot. Altered hip flexion leads to chronic hamstring injuries in both lower extremities.

D. **The Athlete with Multiple Sclerosis (MS).** MS is a progressive demyelinating disease that affects approximately 300,000 Americans. Physical symptoms range in severity and include ataxia, muscular weakness, fatigue, spasticity, sensory dysfunction, and hypersensitivity to temperature increases. Muscle performance and aerobic capacity can improve with exercise training and are influenced by the level of neurological impairment.

E. Other disabilities in athletes can include organ transplants as well as neurological, musculoskeletal, respiratory, cardiovascular, reproductive, digestive, genitourinary, hematologic and lymphatic, skin, endocrine, psychological, and learning disorders.

Suggested Reading

Bielak K. The handicapped athlete. In: *The Hughston clinic sports medicine book.* Baltimore: Williams & Wilkins 1995:106–111.

Burnham RS, May L, Nelson E, et al. Shoulder pain in wheelchair athletes. *Am J Sports Med* 1993;21:238–242.

Madorsky JG, Curtis KA. Wheelchair sports medicine. *Am J Sports Med* 1984; 12:128–132.

Schaeffer RS, Proffer DS. Sports medicine for wheelchair athletes. *Am Fam Physician* 1989;39:239–245.

VIII. MEDICAL PROBLEMS

24. INFECTIONS IN ATHLETES

Thomas L. Sevier and Matthew B. Roush

Infection and Exercise

The relationship between infection and exercise has been a misunderstood area of sports medicine. Because of this confusion, many erroneous assumptions are reported as fact by coaches, players, and medical personnel. One of these assumptions is that exercise prevents acute infections. There are no conclusive studies to indicate that exercise prevents infections. There is a paucity of research in this area. In fact, several studies support the contention that severe exertion can place an athlete at increased risk for an infection. It is well established that various measures of physical performance are reduced during an infectious episode. A mild common cold has shown a decrease in athletic performance and function. Even exercise-related sudden death, due to myocarditis, has been reported. This chapter focuses on common infections encountered in the care of athletes. Practical approaches and strategies for treatment are covered. Return-to-play considerations, ways to minimize an athlete's risk of exposure, as well as ways to prevent the spread of disease are emphasized based on current knowledge.

Infectious Mononucleosis

Infectious mononucleosis (IM) is most frequently caused by the Epstein-Barr virus (EBV). It is estimated that between 1% and 3% of college athletes and 1% and 2% of high school athletes are infected by EBV per year. The effects of the virus can last from 2 to 8 weeks. Although the athlete appears to recover more quickly than the nonathlete infected with IM, the athlete may not be able to compete or return to a preillness level of fitness for as long as 3 months.

EBV is transmitted through oral secretions; following the acute infection, it is excreted in the saliva continuously or intermittently for months. IM most often occurs between the ages of 15 and 25, with 25% to 50% of these infected individuals developing the classic syndrome. The incubation period for primary EBV infection is about 30 to 45 days.

History / Physical Examination

The prodromal period tends to last 3 to 5 days, with symptoms of headache, fatigue, anorexia, malaise, and myalgias. In the following 5- to 15-day period, the clinical manifestations include moderate to severe sore throat, with tonsillar enlargement, moderate fever, enlarged tender posterior cervical lymph nodes with lymphadenopathy often generalized, petechiae on the soft palate, and a palpable enlarged spleen by the second week in 50% to 70% of patients. Hepatomegaly occurs in about 35% of cases; less than 15% present with clinical jaundice.

Diagnostic Tests

Hematologic abnormalities most often noted are modest leukocytosis (10,000 to 20,000 mm^3) during the first week of the illness, lymphocytosis with many atypical lymphocytes (10% to 20% of all leukocytes, greater than 1,000/mm^3). A mild reduction in platelet count (<140,000/mm^3) is present in about 50% of patients. By the second week of illness, about 85% of patients with IM show abnormalities in liver function tests that reflect mild hepatitis. By the fourth to fifth week, hematologic and liver function tests return to normal.

EBV can be confirmed serologically with a rapid slide test, such as the Monospot (Ortho Diagnostic Systems, Raritan, NJ). It is extremely sensitive for detection of EBV-induced IM, but repeat testing may be needed because only 60% of patients will have abnormal tests by the second week of illness. This test is also not very sensitive in children younger than 5 years of age. If the heterophil test is negative, confirmation of IM requires an EBV-specific antibody study. The cytomegalovirus (CMV) and *Toxoplasma gondii* are also causes of heterophil-negative IM.

Natural History / Prevention

Life-threatening complications of IM are rare. The most serious include splenic rupture and airway obstruction. The prevalence of splenic rupture is less than 0.2%. Nearly all ruptures occur between day 4 and 21 of symptomatic illness. Most ruptures do not occur during athletic participation but rather during daily activities. Pain from splenic rupture begins suddenly in the left upper quadrant of the abdomen, is usually worse with inspiration, and may radiate toward the left shoulder (Kehr's sign). These symptoms may be followed by generalized abdominal pain and shock. Ultrasound and computed tomography (CT) are useful in diagnosing both splenomegaly and splenic rupture.

Airway obstruction due to massive enlargement of tonsils and adenoids has occurred and may require emergency nasotracheal intubation. Other complications include streptococcal pharyngitis, which occurs 5% to 30% of the time, and Guillain-Barré syndrome, which occurs in less than 1% of patients. Very rare complications include pneumonitis, autoimmune hemolytic anemia, severe thrombocytopenia or granulocytopenia, myocarditis, and pericarditis.

Treatment Options

Treatment for IM is supportive for the most part, consisting of rest, fluids, and analgesics. Acetaminophen is recommended for fever, headache, and muscle pain, along with lozenges, or viscous lidocaine for sore throat. Occasionally codeine is prescribed for refractory pain. Stool softeners should be used when codeine is being taken or when splenomegaly is present in order to decrease constipation and associated straining with defecation, which could lead to splenic rupture. Corticosteroid therapy is recommended in those patients with severe complications, such as airway obstruction or autoimmune conditions.

Return to Play

The patient-athlete, the coach, and the trainer are likely to be concerned about the length of time this disease will prevent participation in training and competition. In the initial stages, when fever, pharyngitis, lymphadenopathy, and fatigue are present, even the most committed athlete will not feel like exercising strenuously. There is no need for prolonged bed rest, which can cause deconditioning and possibly slow recovery. The most important consideration in determining when return to play is permitted is the possibility of splenic rupture. Because rupture usually occurs during the second or third week of illness, athletes should be restricted until at least after the third week of illness. On initial physical examination as well as during weekly follow-up examination, the spleen's size should be noted. After the third week, when permission for return to play is being considered, noninvasive imaging, such as ultrasound or CT scanning, provides a highly accurate means of determining spleen size and should be considered. If splenomegaly is present, the athlete should be held out of activity and repeat imaging should be performed in 1 week. Resumption of training may be permitted when the athlete is asymptomatic, splenomegaly is absent, and all laboratory tests have normalized. Non-contact training such as jogging, swimming, or cycling at about 50% of maximum if tolerated for 1 week can be followed by gradual resumption of full activity.

Sexually Transmitted Diseases

Gonorrhea, caused by the gram-negative cocci *Neisseria gonorrhoeae,* can cause urethritis, cervicitis, bartholinitis, proctitis, pharyngitis, salpingitis, epididymitis, and conjunctivitis. While 10% to 50% of gonococcal infections in men cause few or no symptoms, gonorrhea usually presents in *men* as purulent urethral discharge and dysuria, occasionally as testicular pain, or, in chronic cases, with a urethral stricture. The physical examination reveals a tender red urethral orifice, penis, and spermatic cord.

In *women, pelvic inflammatory disease (PID)* presents as fever, lower abdominal pain and tenderness, and sometimes metomenorrhagia or dysmenorrhea. This can

Table 24-1. Treatment options:

Medicine	Type of Syphilis
Benzathine penicillin G, 2.4 million units i.m.	Primary, secondary, and latent
Benzathine penicillin G, 2.4 million units i.m. per week for 3 weeks	Tertiary
Procaine penicillin G 2 to 4 million units with probenecid, 500 mg p.o. q.i.d. for 15 days, or Penicillin VK i.v. q 6 hours for 10 days	Neurosyphilis
Doxycycline 100 mg p.o. b.i.d. for 15 days	Alternative for 1, 2, or latent
Erythromycin 500 mg p.o. q. i. d. for 15 days	Alternative for 1, 2, or latent
Doxycycline 1000 mg p.o. b.i.d. for 30 days	Alternative for tertiary syphilis
Ceftriaxone 1 g i.v. or i. m. per day for 14 days	Alternative for neurosyphilis

lead to chronic pelvic pain and infertility. The physical examination shows a purulent endocervical discharge, with cervical motion tenderness.

In *women, PID* caused by Gonorrhea can present as a purulent vaginal discharge, dysuria, dysparunia, and fever. It is an asymptomatic cervical infection approximately 20% of the time.

In *homosexual men* and *women* who receive rectal intercourse, PID can present as a purulent to bloody rectal discharge, tenesmus, and rectal burning or itching. It also can be an asymptomatic infection in this area.

In *both sexes,* Gonorrhea can present as sore throat and exudative pharyngitis or as an eye infection with a purulent discharge, conjunctivitis, chemosis, eyelid edema, and, later, corneal ulcerations. There are also other less common presentations, such as perihepatitis, arthritis, dermatitis, endocarditis, meningitis, amniotic infection syndrome, and pneumonia.

Diagnostic Tests

Gram stain and culture of exudate with Thayer-Martin selective media, which demonstrates the gram-negative diplococci within the polymorphonuclear leukocytes (PMNs). Sensitivity tests confirm the organism's susceptibility to penicillin and tetracycline.

Natural History/Prevention

Sexual exposure to an infected individual is the leading form of transmission. A condom can provide partial protection. Avoidance of multiple sexual partners and use of an intrauterine device (IUD) will also decrease one's risk. No sexual activity should be allowed until all partners have been tested and treated.

Treatment Options

Uncomplicated gonorrheal infections: ceftriaxone (Rocephin) 250 mg i.m. or ceftizoxime 500 mg i.m., followed by doxycycline 100 mg p.o. b.i.d. or tetracycline 500 mg p.o. q.i.d. for 7 days (erythromycin 500 mg q.i.d. for 7 days for pregnant athletes) or azithromycin 1 g p.o. (four 250-mg tablets) in 1 dose. Disseminated gonoccocal infections: ceftriaxone 1 g per day i.v. for 7 days followed by cefaclor 500 mg q8h for 4 to 6 days or cefuroxime axetil 250 mg p.o. b.i.d. for 4 to 6 days or ciprofloxacin 750 mg p.o. b.i.d for 4 to 6 days.

Progression of Treatment/Recommended Treatment

Repeat cultures 1 week after treatment is complete. Surveillance of all partners to assure treatment.

Return to Play

Depending on the situation, for uncomplicated genital-anal gonorrhea, athletes can return to play once treatment has been initiated and the athlete is asymptomatic.

Chlamydial Infection

Some 30% to 50% of college-age men and women have had chlamydial infections, with asymptomatic presentations occurring more commonly in women than in men.

History / Physical Examination

Infections due to *Chlamydia trachomatis* present in males as urethritis, epididymitis, and proctitis (especially in homosexual men involved in anal intercourse) and rarely as Reiter's syndrome. In women it presents as cervicitis, urethral syndrome, bartholinitis, salpingitis or PID, and perihepatitis. Differences in comparison with gonorrheal infection are that nongonococcal urethritis (NGU) has a longer incubation period (1 to 3 weeks), less profuse and more mucoid discharge, and less symptomatic dysuria.

Chlamydial epididymitis may present with the additional symptoms of pain in the testicles and spermatic cord and pain upon ejaculation. PID (salpingitis) may be caused by *Chlamydia* and generally presents a milder clinical picture than gonorrheal salpingitis (lower fever and less pain).

Diagnostic Tests

Antigen detection by monoclonal antibody direct immunofluorescence or enzyme-linked immunosorbent assay (ELISA) is 90% to 95% sensitive; chlamydial cultures are 70% to 80% sensitive.

Natural History / Prevention

Sexual exposure to an infected individual is the leading cause of transmission. A condom can provide partial protection from the transmission of the disease. Avoidance of multiple sexual partners, and use of an IUD will decrease one's risk of contracting the disease. No sexual activity should occur until all partners tested and treated.

Treatment Options

Uncomplicated gonorrheal infections: ceftriaxone (Rocephin) 250 mg i.m. or ceftizoxime 500 mg i.m. followed by doxycyline 100 mg p.o. b.i.d. or tetracycline 500 mg p.o. q.i.d. for 7 days (erythromycin 500mg q.i.d. for 7 days for pregnant athletes); or azithromycin 1 g p.o. (four 250-mg tablets) in one dose.

Progression of Treatment / Recommended Treatment

Testing to assure resolution of the disease is not routine. If the patient remains symptomatic, it is important that all partners be treated to prevent the partners from passing the disease back and forth.

Return to Play

Depending on the situation, for uncomplicated genital-anal chlamydial infection, the athlete can return to play once treatment has been initiated and he or she is asymptomatic.

Syphilis

History / Physical Examination

Syphilis, caused by the spirochete *Treponema pallidum,* occurs in three stages; primary, secondary, and tertiary. The presentation depends on the stage of the disease.

Primary syphilis is manifest by a nontender papule that erodes into a small (less than 2 cm in diameter) ulcer called a *chancre,* which has hard edge with a yellow base. It is usually a solitary lesion but can also occur as multiple lesions. Chancres are located on the penis, genitalia, or anus. Occasionally the chancre is associated with regional inguinal lymphadenopathy. These ulcers usually occur 1 to 12 weeks after exposure. They heal spontaneously between 3 to 6 weeks.

Secondary syphilis occurs in 25% of the affected patients within 2 to 6 weeks. The rash is a "fresh ham" color, nonpruritic, and located on the hands and/or feet. Moist flat, pink, peripheral warty lesions—condyloma lata—can occur on the glans, vulva, or perianal/vulvar areas. Generalized lymphadenopathy, and flu-like symptoms can occur with the rash. Rarely nephritis, hepatitis, meningitis, and/or uveitis accompany this stage of the disease.

Between secondary syphilis and tertiary syphilis, the disease can lie dormant for years to decades. This is called *latent syphilis.* The patient in this stage is not infectious after 1 year. Twenty-five percent may relapse to the secondary stage if not treated.

Tertiary syphilis is identified particularly by lesions of the aorta, central nervous system, skin, and skeletal structures.

Diagnostic Tests

Venereal Disease Research Laboratory (VDRL) and rapid plasma reagin (RPR) are non-specific treponemal tests. They are used mainly for primary screening of syphilis. The disease is confirmed with a fluorescent treponemal antibody absorption (FTA-ABS) test. FTA-ABS test must be done in suspected patients who also have human immunodeficiency virus (HIV) infection. Lumbar puncture for cerebrospinal fluid (CSF) serologies should be done in cases of latent syphilis where penicillin therapy is planned and whenever neurological symptoms are present.

Natural History / Prevention

Early identification and treatment lead to the reduction of the frequency of this disease, which first appeared in the United States in the 1970s. Unfortunately, that trend has reversed itself in the last two decades. It is imperative that the emphasis be on primary prevention and education through discussions of abstinence, safe sex, and condom use.

All patients diagnosed with syphilis should be tested every 3 months and then yearly to assure treatment. Consider testing for other sexually transmitted diseases (STDs), such as gonorrhea, hepatitis, and HIV infection.

Return to Play

An athlete may return to play once he or she has been treated and is asymptotic.

Herpes Simplex II

Herpes simplex II is the most common cause of genital lesions in the United States. It occurs most often at ages 18 to 40, which correlates with the largest athletic population. The consequences of this disease can be recurrent and permanent.

Herpes simplex II is a DNA virus that can cause genital herpes and less commonly oral and anal herpes.

History / Physical Examination

Herpes simplex II usually appears as acute cervicitis in women and urethritis in men, with an incubation period of 3 to 5 days. The symptoms start as fever, headache, malaise, burning genital pain, dysuria, dyspareunia, inguinal adenopathy, and vesicles. The vesicles are usually small and grouped, with a variable border, bright red, serous, and superficial, lasting about 21 days. The lesions are located on the labia majora/minora, inner thighs, vaginal mucosa, cervix, or perianal area in women. In men the lesions are located on the penile glans, penile shaft, urethra, or anus. Rare complications such as meningitis and herpetic sacroradiculomyelitis can occur.

Diagnostic Tests

Viral tissue culture with a swab of the vesicle fluid is positive for the virus in 90% of those infected. A Tzanck preparation is only 40% to 50% sensitive. Acute/convalescent titers, radioimmmunoassay (RIA), and direct fluorescent assay (DFA) are also less sensitive than viral cultures.

Natural History / Prevention

Recurrence of the infection is common. The symptoms are the same as those of the primary infection except that they are less severe and do not include constitutional manifestations. The lesions also crust over more quickly—in 7 to 10 days.

Primary prevention should emphasize sexual abstinence and use of condoms/spermicide with sexual activity. Secondary prevention includes all of the items in primary prevention with the addition of prophylactic acyclovir.

Treatment Options
Primary episodes can be treated with acyclovir 400 mg 3 times a day for 7 to 10 days. Some of the newer antiviral medication can be taken with fewer daily doses. Severe local infections require 5 mg/kg i.v. t.i.d. for 7 days. Recurrent episodes are treated with 200 mg of acyclovir 5 times a day for 5 days. Chronic suppression can be treated with 400 or 200 mg two or four times a day. Acyclovir 400 mg twice a day reduces the frequency of herpes recurrences by at least 75% among patients who had had six or more recurrences a year.

Progression of Treatment/Recommended Treatment
Outpatient follow-up is advisable to detect the presence of complications.

Return to Play
An athlete may return to play once he or she has been treated and is asymptomatic.

Human Immunodeficiency Virus (HIV)
As of 1993 there were between 5 and 10 million cases of HIV infection worldwide with the number of new cases of HIV infection and acquired immunodeficiency syndrome (AIDS) continuing to increase. AIDS is the second leading cause of death among U.S. males between ages 25 and 44. Some cases of HIV and AIDS in athletes have occurred through blood or sexual contact.

HIV is a retrovirus that infects cells with CD4 receptors, usually lymphocytes. This results in decreased immune function and increased susceptibility to opportunistic infections. The virus is transmitted by certain body fluids through the skin or by sexual or perinatal contact. Cerebrospinal fluid, blood, semen, synovial fluid, amniotic fluid, and pericardial fluid all have a high or very high content of HIV. Vaginal and cervical secretions and breast milk have a moderate amount. Tears, saliva, sputum, and urine have a low amount. Sweat probably has none. The Centers for Disease Control and Prevention (CDC) state that activities such as hugging and kissing; sharing of eating utensils; sharing of towels, combs, nail clippers, and so on show no evidence of transmission. Infectivity is highest in people using intravenous drugs, engaging in unprotected sex, especially anal sex, and receiving blood products. Some 20% of patients will become HIV infected within 3 months of exposure to an adequate viral load, and nearly 100% will do so within 12 months of the exposure. Most HIV-infected patients are asymptomatic carriers.

History/Physical Examination
The first stage of the HIV infection is usually asymptomatic but infectious. Some patients will developed a mononucleosis-like syndrome, with fever, rash, myalgia, and malaise. This is a self-limited syndrome occurring during the first 6 to 8 weeks. This stage usually lasts 3 to 7 years and up to 10 years or longer. Infection with other STDs predicts a shorter first stage of infection. The second stage of HIV infection presents in patients with a variety of findings such as lymphadenopathy, fever, chills, malaise, fatigue, weight loss, and diarrhea. At this time the CD4 cell count generally decreases. The third stage of HIV infection is defined as the presence of certain opportunistic infections concurrent with severe CD4 depletion.

Diagnostic Tests
The screening test begins with an ELISA, which, if positive, should be confirmed by a second ELISA. If this is positive, an immunoblot (Western blot) test should follow.

Natural History/Prevention
Because of the lack of symptoms in those who are carrying this virus in the early stage and because of its stigma, being associated with drug use and illicit sex, it is very difficult to devise a prevention plan that will be simple, effective, and still ensure privacy for the patient and the population at large. There is no vaccine available for HIV. Organizations—including Canadian Academy of Sports Medicine, American Medical Society of Sports Medicine, and the United States Olympic Committee—have implemented guidelines to address this problem in athletics. These guidelines are based on research that helps predict the likelihood of contact

with bodily fluids and bleeding from the different types of sports. They have identified certain sports at risk:

Greatest risk: boxing, tae kwon do, wrestling
Moderate risk: basketball, field hockey, ice hockey, judo, soccer, football, team handball
Lowest-risk: other sports

Guidelines of these committees include the following:

1. All athletes must be warned of the dangers involved with sexual contact, and intravenous drug use.
2. Potentially infectious skin lesions should be covered.
3. The injured athlete should perform his or her own wound care.
4. Other athletes should not handle the injured athlete's blood.
5. Lacerations with substantial bleeding should be resolved before the athlete can return to play.
6. Clothing soaked with blood should be removed and all exposed parts washed before allowing the athlete to return to play.
7. Only disposable towels and bandages should be used.
8. Universal precautions should be taken in dealing with any athlete.
9. Disposable gloves must be worn and changed for each individual athlete.

Treatment
Treatment of HIV-positive athletes and athletes with AIDS is the same as that for nonathlete patients. Therapy is based on a combination of antiretroviral drugs consisting of nucleoside analogs, protease inhibitors and nonnucleoside reverse transcriptase inhibitors.

Return to Play
HIV is a chronic disease with a variable course. The athlete may have many years of excellent health and a productive life. There is no evidence that moderate exercise is dangerous to the HIV-positive athlete. Exercise, with appropriate monitoring, should be encouraged in these athletes. Confidentiality must be maintained at all times. The decision to continue to play must be made keeping in mind the patient's current state of health and HIV status, the type of activity, and the potential for HIV transmission to other persons associated with athlete. At the present time most governing bodies agree that HIV infection alone is insufficient to prohibit athletic competition.

Hepatitis
Hepatitis is caused by many different types of viruses (hepatitis A,B,C,D and E as well as CMV and EBV). It is most commonly caused by hepatitis A,B, or C. Hepatitis A (HAV) is a viral infection of the liver that is acute and does not have long-term sequelae. Comparatively, hepatitis B (HBV) and hepatitis C (HCV) can be chronic, cause severe disability, or be fatal. HBV and HCV are more common than HIV infections. They can pose a serious threat to the athlete's career and life.

Epidemiology
HAV causes 25% of hepatitis cases in the United States. It is more infective than HBV because it can be transmitted by the fecal-oral route. HBV is transmitted through blood products and sexual contact. HCV is also transmitted through blood exposure and much less commonly through sexual contact. Hepatitis D (HDV) can only infect a individual who is also infected with HBV. There are currently estimated to be over 1 million carriers of HBV in the United States. Although there is now a vaccine for HBV, the number of new cases continues to increase each year. Patients with HIV not uncommonly are also infected with the HBV virus.

History/Physical Examination
The presenting signs and symptoms of hepatitis include fatigue, fever, jaundice, nausea, vomiting, anorexia, light-colored stools, "Coca-Cola" colored urine, headache, and abdominal pain. The symptoms of HAV and HCV are usually less severe than the symptoms of HBV.

Diagnostic Tests

Aspartate transaminase/alanine aminotransferase (AST/ALT): marked elevation (greater than 400 to 500).

Bilirubin and alkaline phosphatase can also be elevated.

Serological markers indicate the type and severity of the infection.

Natural History

HAV is an acute disease and does not lead to a primary chronic hepatitis. HBV can continue as chronic active hepatitis with continued symptoms of hepatitis, elevated liver function tests, prolonged prothrombin time, and decreased albumin, or it continue in the chronic asymptomatic (carrier) state as chronic persistent hepatitis. Chronic hepatitis is common in HCV.

Treatment Options

Treatment includes supportive care; education to prevent infection of others; and correction of fluid, electrolyte, and acid-base imbalances as well as hypoglycemia, impaired renal function, or coagulation disorders.

Prevention

Prevention of transmission depends on the type of hepatitis and a knowledge of how it is transmitted. Proper hygiene and care around patients with HAV is imperative. HCV is prevented through proper testing and use of blood products. HBV, like HIV, is difficult to prevent because of the high-risk behaviors associated with those already infected. Many organizations have developed guidelines to avoid the transmission of HBV and HIV infections.

A vaccine (3 to 0.5 ml per dose injected intramuscularly) is available for the prevention of HBV infections. It is recommended for individuals in high-risk groups: health care workers, those receiving blood products, intravenous drug users, sexually active homosexual males, and those with household exposure, sexual exposure, or at risk for needle sticks.

Return to Play

No activity until clinical and laboratory abnormalities begin resolving. Liver function tests should be back to normal and the athlete should be clinically asymptomatic. The athlete should be negative for HBV surface antigen before returning to play. Activity shoud begin with light calisthenics with a gradual return to previous levels of exertion. Athletes persistently positive for HBV surface antigen should probably be removed from competition indefinitely.

Otitis Externa

Otitis externa, also known as swimmer's ear, is an inflammation of the external auditory canal and is typically seen among swimmers, divers, and surfers during the summer months or when the weather is hot and humid. This condition can cause considerable short-term and occasionally long-term disability in athletes. Many a swimmer or diver has been unable to compete or practice because of the effects of this condition.

Epidemiology

This condition is most commonly caused by the bacterium *Pseudomonas aeruginosa;* it has also been related to infection by a fungus, most commonly *Aspergillus*. Cerumen, which is normally present in a healthy ear canal, is water-repellent and aids in maintaining the proper acidic pH in the canal, thus preventing bacterial and fungal growth. Athletes who spend time in the water tend to have little cerumen present, causing them to lose their natural defenses to bacteria and fungus. This lack of cerumen also leads to absorption of the moisture retained in the canal after water exposure, producing a hyperhydrated and macerated canal. Other factors that contribute to the development of otitis externa are freshwater swimming, swimming in improperly chlorinated pools, scratches caused by insertion of objects to clear or relieve itching in the canal, and the degree to which the athlete's head is submerged under water.

History / Physical Examination
Patients with otitis externa present clinically with exudate, edema, and erythema in the canal along with a feeling of fullness, mild itching, and an increase in the level of pain when earlobe is pulled.

Diagnostic Tests
Cases of otitis media that do not respond to the established treatment for otitis media may be caused by a less common type of bacterium or fungus that might be resistant to conventional therapy. In those cases a bacterial and/or fungal culture of the ear canal is helpful in determining the type and susceptibility of the offending organism.

Prevention
The prevention of otitis externa is associated with keeping the ear canals as dry as possible. Suggestions include gentle towel drying of the ears after getting out of the water, avoiding scratching or touching the ear canal, the use of drying agents and antiseptics, and wearing swim caps or using silicone ear plugs.

Treatment Options
Treatment consists of cleaning the ear canal by irrigation with water or hydrogen peroxide, followed by the use of topical antibiotic drops such as polymyxin or 0.25% acetic acid solution. If excessive edema is present, insertion of a wick saturated with 50% Burow's solution may be used. Fungal infections can be treated with 1% tolnaftate solution three times per day for 7 days. Often intense itching is an annoying symptom; this can be controlled with corticosteroid drops once the infection is under control. Rare causes of otitis externa must be treated with different, specific care. For eczematous otitis externa, topical therapy could include acetic acid 2% with aluminum acetate or aluminum acetate 8%. Necrotizing otitis externa requires parenteral antistaphylococcal and antipseudomonal antibiotics.

Return to Play
After treatment has started, the athlete may return to water activities within 2 to 3 days, as long as the pain with examination, drainage, and redness has resolved.

Sinusitis

Sinusitis may be overdiagnosed or underdiagnosed. In medical care of athletes there is a large impetus to treat patients with URIs as if sinusitis were a complication with antibiotics when a firm diagnosis has not been made. On the other hand there are occasions when patients have been diagnosed with recurrent URIs, when in actuality they have sinusitis with underlying allergic rhinitis or nasal polyps.

Sinusitis is most commonly caused by a bacterial infection with pneumococci and H. influenza being the most common bacteria. Fungal infections (Aspergillus, mucomycosis) are also causes of sinus infections. Those patients with underlying seasonal allergies, and smokers appear to have a higher incidence of sinus infections. Other predisposing factors for sinusitis include immunosuppression, tooth abscess, temperature changes, and swimming in contaminated water.

History / Physical Examination
Symptoms include low grade fever, pain over the upper teeth and cheeks, eyebrows, eyes, or forehead which worsens with bending over; nasal discharge-blood tinged or purulent, nasal congestion, sinus area tenderness and pressure, malaise, sore throat, and headache. Occasionally patients will complain of cough, or worsening symptoms with air travel.

Diagnostic Tests
A CBC is performed and may show an elevated white cell count and left shift. Sinus x-rays may show air-fluid levels, thickened or cloudy sinus cavities, although many

consultants do not believe x-rays to be helpful. For a definitive diagnosis CT scan of the sinuses, or sinuscopy with biopsy and culture are the tests of choice.

Natural History / Prevention
Acute sinusitis usually resolves with appropriate treatment. Chronic sinusitis will probably linger until the offending agent (allergies, polyps, cigarette smoke, etc.) is removed. The key to prevention of sinusitis is avoiding offending agents (allergies, polyps, cigarette smoke, etc.) and treating nasal congestion prior to the occurrence of sinusitis.

Treatment Options
General conservative therapy includes avoiding smoke and other environmental irritants, steam inhalation, and if necessary, nasal irrigation. Antibiotic treatment currently recommended can include trimethoprim/sulfoxazole, amoxicillin/clavulanate, or a second generation cephalosporin for 10-21 days. Other medications commonly prescribed include analgesics, vasoconstrictors, and antihistamines. For chronic sinusitis antibiotic therapy may be required for up to 4-6 weeks.

Return to Play
Return once treatment is underway, the patient is afebrile, and the symptoms have improved. Care must be taken to avoid air travel when the acute infection has not resolved.

Pharyngitis is very common in the athletic setting and may be quite disabling unless treated. Streptococcal infections have the greatest incidence between ages 5 and 18, but the majority of the pharyngitis infections in the college age group are viral.

History / Physical Examination
Strep pharyngitis usually presents with sore throat, enlarged tonsils, pharyngeal erythema, tonsillar exudate, soft palate petechiae, cervical adenopathy, abdominal pain, headache, chills, malaise, and fever over 102 degrees F. Viral pharyngitis usually is accompanied by URI symptoms such as runny nose, cough, and sinus congestion. It does not usually, but can, cause a fever over 102 degrees F. There are virulent strains of Group A Beta Hemolytic streptococcus that cause systemic infections such as septicemia and osteomyelitis.

Diagnostic Tests
Rapid immunological screening for strep has improved over the years in sensitivity and accuracy. Currently the false negative rate is 5-8%. Blood agar throat culture from a swab is the older, established test for this condition.

Natural History / Prevention
For the prevention of rheumatic fever, antimicrobial therapy (penicillin or erythromycin) must be given.

Treatment
General supportive measures should be given to all patients. This should include increased fluids, rest, antipyretics and pain control with acetaminophen or NSAIDS. Cool-mist humidifier, and lozenges or salt water gargles. For those who have a positive rapid strep or culture test, they should receive penicillin VK 250mg tid for 10 days. Alternative medicines include erythromycin 100 mg-1200 mg for 10 days, or cephalexin 250 mg tid for 10 days. For resistant cases consider adding rifampin 10 mg/kg divided bid not to exceed 600 mg per day.

Return to Play
Return once treatment is underway, the patient is afebrile, and the symptoms have improved.

Upper Respiratory Infection (URI)

Acute URIs impose a significant burden each year in terms of days of disability, lost school or sports days, and medical costs. At the Summer and Winter Olympic games athletes have been effected by URIs more than by any other condition.

Epidemiology
Most URIs are caused by rhinoviruses, occurring year round with well-defined periods of prevalence in the fall and spring. Coronaviruses are also considered to be a major cause of winter colds and tend to be more common in the 15-19 year-old population. The enteroviruses, specifically coxsackie virus, occur mostly during the late summer and early autumn months, and even though not a common cause of URI, they are of particular significance to athletes engaged in intensive training regimens. URI's are spread from person to person by contact with respiratory secretions. Hand-to-hand contact appears to be a less common form of transmission of the virus.

History / Physical Examination
Symptoms of URI in the athlete are the same as those in the general population and may vary from case to case depending on multiple factors, such as the type of infection virus and the response of the host-immune defense mechanisms.

Common viral URI symptoms range from runny nose, sneezing, and congestion, to sore throat, hoarseness, and nonproductive cough. Patients often feel sick and occasionally have myalgias despite little or low-grade fever.

Diagnostic Tests
Not usually necessary unless the symptoms persist or unless their is a high index of suspicion that a bacterial infection could be present.

Natural History / Prevention
URI infections usually last only a couple of days to a week. The symptoms may be more severe, or prolonged, if the proper rest and conservative treatment is not undertaken. There is also a risk a secondary bacterial infection in those not taking appropriate conservative treatment steps, and in those with underlying medical conditions (asthma, diabetes, smokers, etc.). Prevention is best accomplished by avoiding others when infected and by covering the face when coughing or sneezing.

Treatment Options
Treatment is mainly supportive with rest, clear fluids, cold-mist humidifier, and pain medication being the most helpful. Decongestants and a cough suppressant may also be of benefit. Antihistamines are usually not helpful, but they are sometimes the only cold preparation allowed athletes by specific athletic governing bodies. For athletes with a URI and a non-productive cough albuterol sulfate 2 puffs q 6 hours may be of benefit in controlling bronchospasm without the sedating side-effects of a cough suppressant. It is important to check with the governing body for the athletes specific sport to assure that a prescribed medicine is not banned.

Return-to-Play Criteria
If signs and symptoms indicate that viral infection is impending, the athlete should reduce volume and intensity of training for 1 to 2 days.

If no symptoms of the common cold or constitutional symptoms occur, the athlete can safely resume play a few days after resolution of symptoms.

Mild exercise during sickness with the common cold does not appear to be contraindicated.

A useful approach is the "neck check." If symptoms (stuffy or runny nose, sneezing, or scratchy throat) are located "above the neck" and constitutional symptoms are absent, then the athlete should be allowed to proceed cautiously through a scheduled workout at reduced effort. If he or she feels better in the early stages, then the intensity can be increased and the workout completed. If the patient feels worse, he or she should rest. The athlete with "below the neck" symptoms—such as fever, aching muscles, hacking or productive cough, vomiting, or diarrhea—should not train.

If a patient has symptoms and signs of systemic involvement, up to 10 to 14 days adequate rest should be allowed before resumption of full intensive training and exhaustive exercise in order to attempt avoidance of relapse or serious complications.

Emphasize a well-balanced diet, reduction in other life stresses, and plenty of rest and sleep.

Immunizations

Guidelines for immunizations in athletes are similar to the guidelines for sedentary people.

Tetanus

Tetanus immunizations should be kept up-to-date in all adolescents and adults. A tetanus booster every 10 years will maintain immunity following a primary series. Traumatic wounds that occur in athletes who are not fully immunized should be managed according to standard guidelines.

Influenza

Influenza that occurs in a top-level athlete can mean losing valuable practice and playing time that could diminish a team's competitive edge. Immunization against influenza may be particularly beneficial for athletes who play winter sports in the snow belt. Rationales for and against immunization and factual information about specific side effects should be discussed with team coaches as well as the athletes. High-risk athletes with chronic medical problems such as asthma should all be immunized against influenza unless an egg allergy is present.

Measles

Measles vaccination is of special importance for young athletes. Besides the medical consequences for infected individuals, a measles outbreak can have deleterious effects on team sports. Team physicians can play an important role by promoting proper vaccination of their athletes. Individuals born after 1957 should receive live attenuated measles vaccine if they received measles vaccine before 15 months of age or if they received the less stable measles vaccine available before 1980. Essentially all young adults who have not had a booster since 1980 require revaccination to assure adequate immunity.

Suggested Reading

Adams GL et al. *Fundamentals of otolaryngtology,* 6th ed. Philadelphia: WB Saunders, 1989.

Alberti PW, Ruben RK eds. *Otologic medicine and surgery.* New York: Churchill Livingstone, 1988.

Astrom E, Friman G, Pilstrom L. Effects of viral and mycoplasmal infections on ultrastructure and enzyme activities in human skeletal muscle. *Acta Pathol Microbiol Scand* [A] 1976;84:113.

Atkinson WL, Hadler SC, Redd SB, et al. Measles surveillance—United States 1991. *MMWR* 1992;41:SS-6.

Berk LS, Nieman DC, Youngberg WS, et al. The effect of long endurance running on natural killer cells in marathoners. *Med Sci Sports Exerc* 1990;22:207.

Blair H, Greenberg S, Stevens P, et al. Effects of rhinovirus infection on pulmonary function of healthy human volunteers. *Am Rev Respir Dis* 1976;114:95.

Burch GE. Viral diseases of the heart. *Acta Cardiol* 1979;1:5.

Burke AP, Farb A, Virmani R, et al. Sports-related and non-sports-related sudden cardiac death in young adults. *Am Heart J* 1991;121:568.

Casey JM, Dick EC. Acute respiratory infections In: Casey JM, Foster C, Hixson EG, eds. *Winter sports medicine.* Philadelphia: FA Davis, 1990:112.

Cate T, Roberts J, Russ M, et al. Effects of common colds on pulmonary function. *Am Rev Respir Dis* 1973;108:859.

Centers for Disease Control. Measles at an international gymnastics competition—Indiana. *MMWR* 1992;32:26.

Centers for Disease Control. Sexually transmitted diseases: treatment Guidelines, 1985. *MMWR* 1985;34:94S.

Cohen S, Tyrrell DA, Smith AP. Psychological stress and susceptibility to the common cold. *N Engl J Med* 1991;325:606.

Collier A, Pimmel R, Hassellblad VC, et al. Spirometric changes in normal children with upper respiratory infections. *Am Rev Respir Dis* 1978;117:47.

Couch RB. The common cold: control? *J Infect Dis* 1984;150:167.

Dallabetta G, Hook EW. Gonoccal infections. *Infect Dis Clin North Am* 1987;25.

Daniels WL, Sharp DS, Wright JE, et al. Effects of virus infection on physical performance in man. *Mil Med* 1985;150:8.

Davis RM, Whitman ED, Orenstein WA, et al. A persistent outbreak of measles despite appropriate prevention and control measures. *Am J Epidemiol* 1987; 126:438.

Dawkins, BJ. Genital herpes simplex infections. *Primary Care Clin North Am* 1990;17:95.

Dick EC, Jennings LC, Mink KA, et al. Aerosol transmission of rhinovirus colds *J Infect Dis* 1987;156:442.

Douglas RG, Lindgren KM, Cough RB. Exposure to cold environment and rhinovirus common cold. *N Engl J Med* 1968;279:742.

Drugs for sexually transmitted diseases. *Med Lett Drugs Ther* 1991;33;119.

Eichner ER. Infection, immunity and exercise. *Phys Sportsmed* 1993;21:125.

Eichner ER. Neck check. *Runner's World* 1992;27:16.

Fitzgerald L. Exercise and the immune system. *Immunol Today* 1988;9:337.

Fitzgerald L. Overtraining increases the susceptibility to infection. *Int J Sports Med* 1991;1:S5.

Frelinger DP. The ruptured spleen in college athletes: a preliminary report. *J Am Coll Health Assoc* 1978;26:217.

Friman G. Effect of acute infectious disease on isometric muscle strength. *Scand J Clin Lab Invest* 1977;37:303.

Friman G, Wright JE, Ilback NG, et al. Does fever or myalgia indicate reduced physical performance capacity in viral infections? *Acta Med Scand* 1985;217:353.

Gatmanitan BG, Ghason JL, Lerner AM. Augmentation of the virulence of murine coxsackie virus B3 myocardiopathy by exercise. *J Exp Med* 1970;131:1121.

Graham NMH, Douglas RM, Ryan P. Stress and acute respiratory infection. *Am J Epidemiol* 1986;124:389.

Gwaltney J, Moskalski P, Hendley J. Hand-to-hand transmission of rhinovirus colds. *Ann Intern Med* 1978;88:463.

Hallee TJ, Evans AS, Neiderman JC, et al. Infectious mononucleosis at the United States Military Academy: a prospective study of a single class over four years. *Yale J Biol Med* 1974;3:182.

Hanley DF. Medical care of the US Olympic team. *JAMA* 1976;236:147.

Heath WG, Ford ES, Craven TE. Exercise and the incidence of upper respiratory tract infections. *Med Sci Sports Exerc* 1991;23:152.

Hoagland RJ, *Infectious mononucleosis.* New York: Grune & Stratton, 1967.

Inhorn, SL, Dick EC. Coronaviruses. In: Feigin RD, Cherry JD, eds. *Textbook of pediatric infectious diseases,* 2nd ed. Philadelphia: WB Saunders, 1987:1531.

Johnson CC. Do athletes need influenza vaccines? *Phys Sportsmed* 1990;18:9.

Joint Position Statement by the American Medical Society for Sports Medicine (AMSSM) and the American Academy of Sports Medicine (AASM), Human Immunodeficiency Virus (HIV) and Other Blood-Borne Pathogens in Sports.

Jokl E, McClellan JT. *Exercise and cardiac death.* Baltimore: University Park Press, 1971.

Kantor GR, Bergfeld, WF. Common and uncommon dermatologic diseases related to sports activities. *Exerc Sport Sci Rev* 1988;16:215.

Kapikian AZ, Chanock RM. Rotaviruses. In: Fields BN, Knipe DM, Chanock RM, et al, eds. *Virology,* 2nd ed. New York: Raven Press, 1990:1353.

Kapikian AZ. Viral gastroenteritis. *JAMA* 1993;269:627.

Lau RC: Coxsackie B virus infections in New Zealand patients with cardiac and noncardiac diseases. *J Med Virol* 1983;11:131.

Levinson SO, Milzer A, Lewin P. Effect of fatigue chilling and mechanical trauma on resistance to experimental poliomyelitis. *Am J Hyg* 1945;42:204.

Mackinnon LT, Chick TW, van As A, et al. The effect of exercise on secretory and natural immunity. *Adv Exp Med Biol* 1987;216A:869.

Maki DG, Reich RM. Infectious mononucleosis in the athlete: diagnosis, complications, and management. *Am J Sports Med* 1982;10:162.

Marano M. Schoenborn, CA: National Center for Health Statistics, 1988.

U.S. Public Health Service. Current estimates from the National Health Interview Survey United States, 1987. Vital and Health Statistics Series 10:166. Washington, DC: U.S. Government Printing Office.

Mardh PA, Danielsson D. In: Holmes KK, ed. *Sexually transmitted diseases,* 2nd ed. New York: McGraw-Hill, 1984.

McKeag DB, Kinderknecht J. A basketball player with infectious mononucleosis. In: Smith NJ, ed. *Common problems in pediatric sports medicine.* Chicago: Year Book, 1989:191.

Mier-Jedrzejowicz A, Brophy C, Green M. Respiratory muscle weakness during upper respiratory tract infections. *Am Rev Respir Dis* 1988;138:5.

Modlin JF. Coxsackie virus and echovirus In: Mandell GL, Douglas RG Jr, Bennett JE, eds. *Principles and practice of infectious diseases,* 2nd ed. New York: John Wiley & Sons, 1985:814.

Nehlsen-Cannarella SL, Nieman DC, Balk-Lamberton AJ, et al. The effects of moderate exercise training on immune response. *Med Sci Sports Exerc* 1991;23:64.

Nelson MA. Stopping the spread of herpes simplex: a focus on wrestlers. *Phys Sportsmed* 1992;20:117.

Niederman JC, Miller G, Pearson HA, et al. Infectious mononucleosis: Epstein-Barr virus shedding in saliva and the oropharynx. *N Engl J Med* 1984;294:1355.

Nieman DC. Exercise, immunity and respiratory infections. *Sports Sci Exch* 1992; 4:39.

Nieman DC, Johanssen LM, Lee JW. Infectious episodes in runners before and after a road race. *J Sports Med Phys Fitness* 1989;29:289.

Nieman DC, Johanssen LM, Lee JW, et al. Infectious episodes in runners before and after the Los Angeles Marathon. *J Sports Med Phys Fitness* 1990;30:316.

Nieman DC, Nehlsen-Cannarella SL. Effects of endurance exercise on immune response In: Shephart RJ Astrand PO, eds. *Endurance in sport.* Oxford, England: Blackwell, 1991.

Nieman DC, Nehlsen-Cannarella SL. The effects of acute and chronic exercise on immunoglobulins. *Sports Med* 1991;11:183.

Nieman DC, Nehlsen-Cannarella SL, Markoff PA, et al. The effects of moderate exercise training on natural killer cells and acute upper respiratory tract infections. *Int J Sports Med* 1990;11:467.

O'Connor S, Jones D, Collins J, et al. Changes in pulmonary function after naturally acquired respiratory infections in normal persons. *Am Rev Respir Dis* 1979; 120:1087.

Reyes MP, Lerner AM. Interferon and neutralizing antibody in sera of exercised mice with coxsackie virus B-3 myocarditis. *Proc Soc Exp Biol Med* 1976;151:333.

Roberts JA. Loss of form in young athletes due to viral infection. *BMJ* 1985;290:357.

Roberts JA. Viral illnesses and sports performance. *Sports Med* 1986;3:296.

Rooney JF, Straus SE, Mannix ML et al. Oral acyclovir to suppress frequently recurrent herpes labialis—a double-blind, placebo-controlled trial. *Ann Intern Med* 1993;118:268.

Ryan AJ, Dalrymple W, Dull B, et al. Round table: upper respiratory infections in sports medicine. *Phys Sportsmed* 1975;3:29.

Sawyer RN, Evans AS, Niederman JC, et al. Prospective studies of a group of Yale University freshmen: occurrence of infectious mononucleosis. *J Infect Dis* 1971;123:263.

Schelkun PH. Swimmer's ear: getting patients back in the water. *Phys Sportsmed* 1991;19:85.

Schouten WJ, Verschuur R, Kemper HCG. Physical activity and upper respiratory tract infections in a normal population of young men and women: the Amsterdam growth and health study. *Int J Sports Med* 1988;9:451.

Sharp JCM. Viruses and the athlete. *Br J Sports Med* 1989;23:47.

Simon HB. Exercise and infection. *Phys Sportsmed* 1987;15:135.

Simon HB. Immunization and chemotherapy for viral infections. In: Rubenstein, E, Federman D, eds. *Scientific American medicine.* New York: Scientific American, 1990.

Simon HB. The immunology of exercise: a brief review *JAMA* 1984;252:2735.

Smith PG, Lucente FE. Infections. In: Cummings CW, Fredrickson JM, Harker LA, et al, eds. *Otolaryngology—head and neck surgery.* St. Louis: CV Mosby, 1986.

Smith WG. Adult heart disease due to coxsackie virus group B. *Br Heart J* 1966; 28:204.

Sosin DM, Gunn RA, Ford WL, et al. An outbreak of furunculosis among high school athletes. *Am J Sports Med* 1989;17:828.

Springer GL, Shapiro ED. Fresh water swimming as a risk factor for otitis externa: a case-control study. *Arch Environ Health* 1985;40:202.

Stauffer LW. Skin disorders in athletes: identification and management. *Phys Sportsmed* 1983;11:101.

Strauss RH. *Sports medicine: exercise and sports in patients with infection.* Philadelphia: WB Saunders, 1991:109.

The Office of Disease Prevention and Health Promotion, US Public Health Service. US Department of Health and Human Services. *Disease prevention / health promotion: the facts.* Palo Alto: Bull Publishing, 1988.

Transmission of Infectious Agents During Athletic Competition, A report to all national governing bodies by the USOC Sports Medicine & Science Committee, 1991 U.S. Olympic Committee.

25. ENDOCRINOLOGY

David O. Hough and Michael J. Woods

I. Anatomy and Physiology

The anterior and posterior lobes of the pituitary gland (hypophysis) are located within the sella turcica of the sphenoid bone at the base of the skull. Its products, the pituitary trophic hormones—luteinizing hormone (LH), follicle-stimulating hormone (FSH), adrenocorticotropic hormone (ACTH), and thyroid-stimulation hormone (TSH)—act on their target tissue to influence rates of hormone synthesis and release. The resulting rates of hormone release in many cases are periodic or rhythmic, varying, for example, with circadian rhythms.

Production of most hormones is regulated directly or indirectly by the activity of the hormone through negative and positive feedback loops. Hormones produced in response to pituitary trophic hormones (cortisone, thyroxine, steroids) feed back on the hypothalamic-pituitary system to regulate rates of secretion. Parathyroid hormone and insulin are secreted in response to serum levels of calcium and glucose levels, respectively. Changes in frequency or amplitude of hormone release may characterize specific disease states.

Metabolic clearance of hormones is accomplished by several mechanisms. Most peptide hormones are inactivated by proteases in target tissues. Others are degradated in nontarget tissues such as the liver and kidneys. Hormone metabolism renders steroid and thyroid hormones soluble in urine and bile and therefore facilitates their excretion. Only a small number of hormones are excreted in urine or bile.

Endocrine disease can result from hormone deficiency or excess or from resistance to hormone action. Abnormalities in more than one endocrine system may coexist in the same individual. The disorders most commonly seen in athletic individuals—namely, diabetes mellitus and thyroid disorders—are discussed in this chapter.

II. The Role of Glucose in Muscle Metabolism

With exercise, the anaerobic breakdown of muscle glycogen, or glycogenolysis, to form lactate provides an immediate source of adenosine triphosphate (ATP). After several minutes of continued exercise, glucose is released by the liver via hepatic glycogenolysis and then gluconeogenesis, while free fatty acids (FFA) and glycerol are released from adipose tissue through lipolysis. After 30 min of continuous exercise, dietary carbohydrates become a more important energy source. After 60 to 90 min, FFA are the principal source of energy. The ability of exercising muscle to utilize glucose and FFA is improved by endurance training.

Energy utilization in exercising muscle is controlled by the influences of insulin and its counterregulatory hormones—glucagon, epinephrine, norepinephrine, cortisol, and growth hormone. Hepatic glycogenolysis, gluconeogenesis, and lipolysis are inhibited by insulin. The catecholamines and, to a lesser degree, cortisol and growth hormone counteract this insulin-mediated inhibition. Insulin secretion is suppressed in part by the alpha-adrenergic inhibition of the pancreatic beta cells to prevent hypoglycemia. Exercise also increases insulin sensitivity by enhancing the binding of insulin to receptor sites on the muscle cell. Blood glucose decreases only slightly (5 to 10 mg/dl) after long periods of strenuous exercise. This is because the uptake of glucose and fatty acid by working muscle is matched by the liver's breakdown of glycogen to form glucose and release fatty acid via lypolysis.

III. Diabetes Mellitus

A. **Pathophysiology.** Diabetes mellitus, a chronic disease characterized by relative or absolute insulin deficiency, is one of the most common endocrine disorders. The incidence in the general population is about 1 to 2%. Type I, or insulin-dependent diabetes mellitus (IDDM), is an autoimmune disorder in which there is selective destruction of the insulin-producing beta cells of the pancreas. The onset of IDDM is usually in childhood, affecting one in five hundred children less than 18 years of age.

Type II, or non-insulin-dependent diabetes mellitus (NIDDM), is almost always seen in adults. Predisposing factors include obesity and a family history of diabetes. Patients exhibit hyperinsulinemia and hyperglycemia with resistance to insulin. Approximately 20% of NIDDM patients require exogenous insulin for adequate glycemic control.

B. **Exercise in diabetes mellitus.** All types of exercise, including elite-level competitive athletics, can be performed by both type I and type II diabetics.

1. **Benefits.** Regular exercise can produce the same desirable effects with regard to weight control, cardiovascular fitness, and improved endurance in diabetics as seen in nondiabetics. Epidemiological studies have shown that regular exercise lowers blood lipids and improves the ratio of high- to low-density-lipoprotein cholesterol. These effects are more profound in NIDDM patients than in those with IDDM. In addition, NIDDM patients who moderately restrict their caloric intake and exercise regularly have improved glycemic control and will typically reduce the need for oral hypoglycemic agents or insulin. This effect is enhanced by exercise-induced weight loss and resultant improved insulin sensitivity. Aerobic exercise combined with the correct diet may even prevent the development of NIDDM in those at risk. Patients with IDDM should be encouraged to exercise regularly, but only as an adjunct to proper insulin management and proper diet. Diabetics who exercise regularly often report improvements in mood, quality of life, and anxiety level.
2. **Potential risks.** The major risks for most diabetic athletes involve complications in metabolic control. In IDDM, hypoglycemia may occur during or after exercise if insulin and caloric intake have not been properly adjusted. Delayed-onset hypoglycemia due to increased insulin sensitivity and glycogen depletion may also occur up to 30 hr after exercise.

   Development of hyperglycemia and ketosis is also a potential danger if the blood glucose level is high (greater than 250 mg/dl) prior to exercise. This is due to the influence of counterregulatory hormones causing an increase in hepatic glucose production. Exercise should be delayed until appropriate medications are taken and glucose level decreases.

   Diabetic neuropathy causing denervation and atrophy of the intrinsic foot muscles can lead to a claw-foot deformity (extension of the metatarsophalangeal joints and flexion of the interphalangeal joints), causing increased pressure on the first metatarsal head and potential tissue breakdown. This complication is most likely to occur in those with decreased or absent pain sensation.

C. **Clinical presentation**

1. **IDDM.** The clinical manifestations of diabetes mellitus vary, but most often patients, especially those with IDDM, seek medical attention for symptoms related to hyperglycemia (polyuria, polydipsia, polyphagia). IDDM usually presents before age 40, with the peak incidence in the United States around 14 years of age. Onset of symptoms may be rapid and body habitus can be normal or may reflect significant weight loss. Plasma insulin is low or not measurable and glucagon levels are elevated.
2. **NIDDM** usually begins after age 40. The patients are typically overweight; up to 80% are obese. There tends to be a more gradual onset of symptoms, and frequently an asymptomatic person is found to have elevated blood glucose on routine laboratory tests. Absolute plasma insulin levels are normal to high, but they are lower than expected relative to the level of plasma glucose. Glucagon levels are variable. Type II diabet-

ics generally do not develop ketoacidosis but are susceptible to hyperosmolar nonketotic coma.

D. **Clinical evaluation of the diabetic athlete.** A history, including frequency and severity of previous hypoglycemic or hyperglycemic episodes, should be obtained, as should a history or any other major organ system involvement (see Table 25-1). The athlete should be evaluated for existing complications of diabetes (see Table 25-1). This evaluation includes assessment of blood pressure, neurologic function, joint mobility, and skin condition as well as a recent retinal examination by an ophthalmologist. Screening laboratory evaluation for lipid abnormalities as well as diabetic nephropathy (serum creatinine and urine protein) may be indicated for adults and for younger diabetics with a family history of premature coronary artery disease, stroke, or hypertension.

Glycosylated hemoglobin (hemoglobin A_{1C}) levels are the most reliable indicators of long-term glycemic control. The athlete should have a recent acceptable level or be tested at the time of evaluation to ensure satisfactory diabetes management. In older patients, if ischemic heart disease is suspected or found on testing, a cardiac evaluation including exercise stress testing is warranted before starting a new exercise regimen.

Table 25-1. Preparticipation evaluation of the diabetic athlete

- History
  - How well is blood sugar controlled?
  - Insulin and oral hypoglycemic requirements
  - History of complications and/or coexisting problems
    - Episodes of hypoglycemia or hyperglycemia
    - Poor exercise tolerance
    - Diabetic neuropathy with skin/foot problems
    - Proliferative retinopathy
    - Nephropathy
    - Ischemic heart disease
- Family history
  - Diabetes mellitus
  - Premature coronary artery disease
  - Stroke
  - Hypertension
- Physical examination
  - Fundoscopic
  - Cardiac including blood pressure
  - Neurologic function
  - Joint mobility
  - Skin condition/feet
- Laboratory tests (as clinically indicated)
  - Serum glucose
  - Hemoglobin A_{1C}
  - Serum cholesterol
  - Lipid profile
  - Serum creatinine
  - Urine dipstick for proteinuria
- Other tests
  - Exercise stress test if ischemic heart disease is suspected
- Education
  - Selection of proper athletic activities
  - Proper glucose monitoring
  - Proper medication/insulin dosage
  - Knowledge of warning signs and treatment of hypoglycemia

E. **Management**

1. **Patient/Athlete Education**

   a. **Activity Selection.** Diabetics with either IDDM or NIDDM, especially those whose duration of disease is less than 10 years, can participate in virtually any activity. Only sports or activities in which hypoglycemia may be life-threatening—such as parachuting, scuba diving, or rock climbing—should be strongly discouraged. Diabetic patients with coexisting heart disease may also show poor exercise tolerance and generally should engage in lower-level exercise. Their specific situation should be reviewed by a cardiologist or a physician experienced in exercise recommendations for cardiac patients. Those with untreated proliferative retinopathy should also participate in low-intensity exercise, as they are at risk for retinal and vitreous hemorrhages with exercise-induced changes in blood pressure. Activities that promote aerobic conditioning and can be continued into adulthood are very beneficial, and those that require a predictable level of physical expenditure are easiest to manage.

   b. The athlete must be aware of the importance of maintaining adequate glycemic control. This can be presented in terms of optimizing performance and avoiding acute complications. He or she—as well as coaches, trainers and fellow athletes—should recognize the early warning signs of hypoglycemia (increased fatigue, excessive hunger, confusion, diaphoresis, increased heart rate, headache, nervousness, and tremor). Impaired epinephrine response to hypoglycemia, which occurs in long-standing diabetes, may reduce the usual adrenergic warning signs such as diaphoresis, weakness, tremulousness, and hunger. A Medic-Alert bracelet indicating the diabetic state is helpful.

   c. **Treatment strategies** must be in place for management of hypoglycemic episodes. This may mean that the athlete, coach, or trainer must carry hard candy or glucose tablets. Glucagon, 1 mg for subcutaneous or i.m. injection by trained personnel, should be available to treat severe hypoglycemia.

   d. Prior to starting any athletic activity, gradual introduction of a fitness program over several weeks is important. This will result in a progressive increase in insulin sensitivity and allow for proper adjustments in insulin, medication dosage, and diet. Blood glucose levels should be watched most closely during the transition from the untrained to the trained state.

2. **Diet and exercise.** Daily, rather than sporadic, exercise done at the same time each day facilitates adjustments in daily insulin dosage and diet and therefore helps avoid acute problems. This, however, may be difficult for the athlete. Insulin and diet must be adjusted to adequately cover exercise and nonexercise days. Prior to exercise, the intensity, duration, and energy expenditure of the activity should be estimated and medications and diet adjusted accordingly. As exercise after a prolonged fast should be avoided, a meal should be eaten 1 to 3 hr before exercise.

   A preexercise snack that is high in complex carbohydrates can help prevent hypoglycemia. During prolonged, strenuous exercise, 30 to 40 g of carbohydrates for adults, and 15 to 25 g for children should be taken in every 30 min. (See Table 25-2 for the carbohydrate content of common snack foods and drinks.) It is critical to replace fluids adequately to ensure control of body temperature and avoid dehydration. Symptoms of dehydration can be similar to those of hypoglycemia, including severe thirst, tachycardia, tachypnea, dizziness, confusion, irritability, and headaches. Four ounces of a cool, noncarbonated sports drink or water should be consumed every 15 min during exercise.

Table 25-2. Carbohydrate content in foods and drinks

Food group (amount)	Carbohydrates (grams)
Breads	
Bagel (1)	30
Bread (1 slice)	
White	12
Whole-wheat	11
Crackers	
Graham (3)	15
Saltines (6)	14
English muffin (1 whole)	28
Pretzels (6 three-ring)	14
Fruits	
Apple (1 medium)	22
Banana (1 small 6 in.)	22
Grapes (15 small)	16
Orange (1 medium)	18
Pear (1)	25
Fruit juice ($^1/_2$ cup)	15
Yogurt (1 cup)	16
Drinks	
Milk (8 oz)	
2%	13
Chocolate	25
All Sport (8 oz)	20
Gatorade (8 oz)	12
Powerade (8 oz)	20
Tang (8 oz)	24

Caloric intake should be increased for 12 to 24 hr after activity, based on the intensity and duration of exercise. Late-evening exercise should be avoided owing to the risk of delayed-onset hypoglycemia. A morning run is usually best tolerated if done after a small snack and before the morning insulin dose.

3. **Monitoring blood glucose level.** Blood glucose monitoring should be done before, during, and after prolonged exercise, as good metabolic control is very important. Ideally, the diabetic athlete begins exercise with glucose level between 100 and 200 mg/dL. If glucose is elevated (>250 mg/dL), hyperglycemia and possible ketosis may occur. Furthermore, hyperglycemia can cause high urine output and worsen dehydration. When glucose level is markedly elevated before exercise (e.g., greater than 250 mg/dL), especially when ketonuria is present, exercise should be deferred until urine ketones normalize and hyperglycemia is corrected. If the athlete begins exercise with a low glucose level (lower than 100 mg/dL), he or she may become hypoglycemic during or after exercise, so a preexercise snack should be taken.

   After exercise, blood sugar should be monitored if the duration or intensity of the activity is different than usual. Checking a late night or taking a 3 a.m. glucose level and adjusting insulin and diet may be necessary to avoid delayed-onset hypoglycemia, which can be severe, causing coma or seizures, and can occur with little warning.

4. **Insulin dosing.** Insulin should not be administered within 1 hr of exercise and insulin that will have its peak activity during exercise should be reduced. Insulin should not be injected into muscle or subcutaneously over a muscle that will be exercised (e.g., the thigh), as the insulin may

thus be rapidly absorbed, leading to hypoglycemia. Abdominal subcutaneous injections are optimal in those who exercise. The dosage of short-acting insulin taken before a meal may need to be adjusted to accommodate for postprandial exercise. However, intermediate- and long-acting forms of insulin have less consistent absorption patterns and therefore should not be adjusted to accommodate exercise. Instead, extra food should be eaten to avoid exercise-induced hypoglycemia. Also, insulin that will peak in the evening hours and overnight should be reduced, again based on the intensity and duration of activity.

Cold weather may slow the absorption of insulin, while very warm weather may increase it. In addition, athletes exercising in the cold expend more energy to maintain body temperature. Additional calories may therefore be necessary before winter workouts.

5. **Oral hypoglycemic agents.** Oral hypoglycemic agents may have a considerably longer duration of action than insulin. Postexercise diet and blood glucose monitoring should take this into account. Fortunately, patients with NIDDM are at much less risk for exercise-related hypoglycemia.
6. **Prolonged exercise.** The same principles noted above apply to diabetic athletes taking part in an endurance event, such as a marathon, with a few additional precautions. Good shoes are essential and any blisters or abrasions should be monitored closely.

   Morning regular insulin should be reduced by one-third to two-thirds on race day. No long-acting insulin should be taken. The athlete should eat a full breakfast and consume 30 g of carbohydrate replacement for every 30 min of exercise (see Table 25-2). Blood sugar may be checked during competition. Increasing caloric intake for 12 to 24 hr after exercise and decreasing insulin that will peak at night will help prevent late-onset hypoglycemia.
7. **Treatment of acute complications**
   a. **Hypoglycemia.** Mild hypoglycemia, with blood glucose level in the range of 50 to 70 mg/dL, may be manifest as dizziness, fatigue, hunger, or headache. The optimal treatment is readily available and rapidly absorbed carbohydrates such as fruit juices, oral glucose tablets, and candy. These foods should be supplemented with complex carbohydrates and protein to provide longer maintenance of blood glucose.

      When blood glucose is below 40 mg/dl, severe symptoms of hypoglycemia, such as alteration in consciousness, usually occur. Treatment should not be delayed while attempting to obtain a blood glucose level. If the clinical signs, symptoms, and situation suggest hypoglycemia, treatment should be initiated immediately, as a temporary elevation in blood sugar in a diabetic who is not hypoglycemic will not be harmful. The treatment of choice is glucagon 1 mg given subcutaneously or intramuscularly. Parenteral glucagon causes a rapid release of glycogen from the liver. Nothing should be given orally if the athlete's ability to protect his or her airway is in doubt. Upon regaining conciousness, athlete should be given oral carbohydrates and protein. If he or she is unable to take calories orally, intravenous glucose may be necessary.

      Hypoglycemia should be suspected in any athlete known to be diabetic who develops seizure activity. The airway should be protected and oral medications avoided. Parenteral glucagon or intravenous fluids containing glucose are the treatments of choice.

   b. **Hyperglycemia.** In addition to hypoglycemia, diabetics are at risk for two major complications of hyperglycemia. Athletes with IDDM are susceptible to diabetic ketoacidosis and those with NIDDM to hyperosmolar nonketotic coma.
      i. **Diabetic ketoacidosis** presents with anorexia, dehydration, nausea, and vomiting combined with increased urine output.

Abdominal pain may be present. If untreated, ketoacidosis may progress to alteration of consciousness and coma. Therefore, after initial on-site evaluation, immediate transport to an emergency facility is essential. Blood glucose is significantly elevated, generally in the range of 600 to 800 mg/dL. Treatment is with intravenous fluids and insulin until glucose levels begin to stabilize. Potassium supplementation is also necessary, with careful monitoring of electrolytes, urine volumes, and vital signs.

ii. **Hyperosmolar nonketotic coma** is most often seen in NIDDM. The clinical presentation is of dehydration combined with clouded sensorium, which may progress to coma. Seizure activity can also be seen. Marked elevations of blood urea nitrogen (BUN) and creatinine are characteristic. Extreme hyperglycemia, with blood sugar often above 600 mg/dl, is present, as is hyperosmolarity. Immediate transport to an emergency facility is mandatory, and treatment includes large amounts of intravenous fluids to reestablish intravascular volume while closely monitoring blood glucose. Insulin should also be given to control hyperglycemia. Again, potassium supplementation is necessary.

8. **The athlete's medications** should be reviewed as there are many medications that impair glucose tolerance, including phenytoin, estrogens, thiazide diuretics, and glucocorticoids. Beta blockers impair the sympathetic response and may mask the signs of hypoglycemia. Salicylates, ethanol, and monoamine oxidase inhibitors have also been associated with hypoglycemia.

F. **Return to sport.** As stated earlier, careful monitoring of blood glucose and proper adjustments of insulin and caloric intake allow the diabetic athlete to participate safely in almost any activity. When stabilized at an acceptable blood glucose level, with adequate hydration and proper insulin or oral hypoglycemic dosage, athletes are able to return to their previous activity.

IV. Thyroid Disorders

A. **Physiology and pathophysiology.** The thyroid gland secretes thyroxine (T4) and triiodothyronine (T3), the active thyroid hormones that influence most metabolic processes including growth and maturation, total energy expenditure, and the turnover of nearly all body substrates. Thyroid disease occurs with alterations in hormone secretion, enlargement of the thyroid (goiter), or both.

Hypothyroidism, or myxedema, is a result of insufficient hormone secretion, with decreased caloric expenditure, or hypometabolism, as its principal feature. Hyperthyroidism, due to excessive secretion of thyroid hormone, results in hypermetabolism. Enlargement of the thyroid gland may be focal or generalized and can be associated with decreased, normal, or increased hormone secretion. The incidence of thyroid disease in the general population is about 5%.

Both T4 and T3 are released into the blood from the thyroid gland, but the gland is the only source of endogenous T4. Thyroid secretion normally accounts for only about 20% of T3 production, the remainder coming from peripheral conversion of T4 to T3. These hormones negatively feed back on the anterior pituitary gland to control thyroid stimulating hormone production and the subsequent release of T4 and T3 from the thyroid gland.

B. **Hypothyroidism (myxedema)**

1. **Clinical presentation.** The hypothyroid athlete may present with complaints of decreased exercise tolerance, lethargy, constipation, cold intolerance, or weight gain. Additional symptoms may include irregular menses, dry hair and skin, or aching muscles. Hypothyroidism may also be part of a syndrome of proximal muscle weakness and fatigue, with elevated serum creatinine kinase (CK) levels. In severe cases, the condi-

tion can progress to cause a dull, expressionless face, significant hair loss, and coarse quality to the voice; however, this is unlikely in athletes and physically active individuals, for whom a significant decrease in exercise capacity usually results in presentation to medical personnel.

Cardiac manifestations of hypothyroidism include decreased cardiac output, stroke volume, pulse pressure, heart rate, and blood pressure. Additional clinical signs include cardiomegaly, bradycardia, and distant heart sounds. The electrocardiogram (ECG) may show sinus bradycardia, low voltage, prolonged QT interval, prolonged atrioventricular conduction time, and intraventricular conduction delay.

2. **Laboratory findings.** Serum thyroid-stimulating hormone (TSH) is the most useful test in evaluating conditions from subclinical to advanced hypothyroidism and should be supplemented by measurement of serum T4. The combination of elevated serum TSH and subnormal serum T4 is diagnostic for primary hypothyroidism. In secondary hypothyroidism, as from a pituitary or hypothalamic disorder, TSH may be normal or low but T4 is subnormal. This is a situation in which a thyrotropin releasing hormone (TRH) stimulation test may be helpful. A blunted TSH response to TRH identifies a pituitary disorder, while a normal response is more suggestive of a hypothalamic problem.

   Free T3 should not be used to evaluate hypothyroidism because it can often be normal and therefore misleading. The free T4 index (FT4I) can be calculated as a product of T3 resin uptake (T3RU) and total T4. Also, thyroid antimicrosomal and antithyroglobulin antibodies can be measured to confirm or rule out autoimmune disease. Elevated serum cholesterol levels may also be seen in the hypothyroid state.

3. **Management.** Hypothyroidism is treated most often with L-thyroxine (eg, Synthroid), with usual replacement doses of 100 to 125 μg, 0.1 to 0.125 mg per day. The euthyroid state is restored gradually, with initial dose of 25 to 50 μg per day. Young adults with no cardiovascular disease may be started at 100 μg per day. In older patients or those with heart disease, the usual starting dose is 25 μg in a single daily dose. This can be increased by 25-μg increments at 2- to 3-week intervals until a normal state is achieved.

   Many patients taking L-thyroxine have normal or borderline high T4 and suppressed TSH levels. Some clinicians prefer to monitor response by following free T3, while others choose to follow TSH. Ideally, TSH is brought down to normal, and T4 and T3 also normalize. At least 4 to 6 weeks should be allowed before checking TSH after a dose adjustment.

C. **Hyperthyroidism**

1. **Clinical presentation.** Common manifestations of hyperthyroidism include heat intolerance, tremors and nervousness, emotional lability, fatigue, palpitations, excessive sweating, insomnia, and frequent bowel movements. Athletes may complain of unexplained weight loss with normal or increased appetite and may report a decrease in athletic performance. Premenopausal women may experience oligomenorrhea and amenorrhea. On physical examination, the patient is usually anxious and restless, with a resting tachycardia and a wide pulse pressure. The skin is warm and moist and palmar erythema is common. Proximal muscle weakness, brisk deep tendon reflexes, and a fine tremor may also be present.
2. **Laboratory findings.** The combination of an elevated T4 and an undetectable or clearly subnormal TSH (that is, below 0.1 μU/mL) confirms a diagnosis of hyperthyroidism. The FT4I and T3RU are usually elevated also. Testing for thyroid antibodies will differentiate autoimmune diseases from others.
3. **Management.** The goal of treatment is to limit the quantity of thyroid hormone that the gland produces. The primary methods of achieving

this are antithyroid agents and surgical or radioactive ablation of thyroid tissue. The latter option may produce permanent hypothyroidism. Beta-adrenergic blockers are effective in treating the associated symptoms of tachycardia, tremor, irritability, and excessive sweating.

a. **Long-term antithyroid therapy** is recommended in children, adolescents, young adults, and during pregnancy. Most patients are successfully managed with propylthiouracil (PTU), 100 to 150 mg every 6 to 8 hr. PTU acts primarily by blocking the synthesis of T4 and has the additional advantage of inhibiting the peripheral conversion of T4 to T3. Normalization of serum T4 occurs in most cases within 6 weeks. A 12- to 20-month course of therapy followed by gradual withdrawal is usually required. The majority of relapses occur within 3 to 6 months after therapy is discontinued. Alternative treatment is recommended in those cases. Agranulocytosis is the most serious adverse effect of drug therapy.
b. **Radioactive iodine** can produce the ablative effects of surgery without perioperative complications. However, as many as 40% to 70% of patients develop hypothyroidism within 10 years of treatment. Serum T4 levels should be checked frequently for the first year and at yearly intervals thereafter. Some physicians recommend that all patients treated with high doses of radioactive iodine should also receive permanent physiologic thyroid hormone replacement once stabilized. Another potential complication is radiation thyroiditis associated with a transient increase in T4 in the period immediately following treatment.
c. **Surgery.** Subtotal thyroidectomy is used in younger patients who have failed antithyroid therapy. The incidence of recurrence postoperatively is about 10%. Therapy with radioactive iodine is used instead of operation in the case of relapse. Prior to surgery, patients should receive antithyroid agents to produce a euthyroid state. Complications include postoperative hypothyroidism, hypocalcemia, hypoparathyroidism, and damage to the recurrent laryngeal nerve.

Monitoring response to antithyroid therapy is best done by measuring serum T4, as TSH levels tend to be undetectable in many patients for long periods of time and are thus less useful.

D. **Return to sports.** As is the case with diabetes mellitus, those athletes with thyroid disease that is properly treated can fully participate in nearly all athletic endeavors. Hypothyroid patients normally respond very well to L-thyroxine therapy. Thyroid function tests return to normal quickly, followed by resolution of symptoms. Medication dosages for treatment of both hypothyroidism and hyperthyroidism should be monitored closely and adjusted appropriately.

Because of the unclear effects that exercise has on thyroid function in those with thyroid disease, guidelines for return to play have not been definitively established. Obviously, the athlete must be medically stable and able to tolerate the intensity of exercise demanded by his or her sport. This may require gradually increasing the frequency, duration, and intensity of activity, especially if the presenting symptoms included fatigue or any cardiac manifestations. Depressed cardiac contractility in older athletes may not immediately recover when the patient becomes euthyroid. It may be prudent to require several weeks of a persistent euthyroid state before allowing the athlete to resume previous levels of exercise or to progress to a more intense activity. The athlete should be followed both clinically and through laboratory testing during progression in training and competition.

Suggested Reading

Bell DSH. Exercise for patients with diabetes: benefits, risks and precautions. *Postgrad Med* 1992; 92:183–198.

Hough DO. Diabetes mellitus in sports. *Med Clin North Am* 1994; 78:423–437.

McAllister RM, Delp MD, Laughlin MH. Thyroid status and exercise tolerance: cardiovascular and metabolic considerations. *Sports Med* 1995; 20:189–198.

Ruderman NB, McCall A, Schneider S. Exercise and endocrine disorders. *Scand J Sports Sci* 1996; 8:43–50.

Taunton JE, McCargar L. Managing activity in patients who have diabetes: practical ways to incorporate exercise into lifestyle. *Phys Sportsmed* 1995; 23:41–52.

26. CARDIOLOGY

Steven P. Van Camp

Cardiovascular Examination of the Athlete

A. Sports medicine physicians are frequently involved in preparticipation physical examinations (see Chapters 2 and 3). The primary cardiology issues affecting eligibility for competition are (1) the risk of sudden death during exercise and (2) the risk of progression or deterioration of the cardiovascular condition due to the physiologic demands of exercise.

I. Eligibility for Competition

A. **Cardiovascular conditions that are absolute contraindications to vigorous exercise** (based on multiple studies reporting them to involve significant exercise-related risk):
  1. Hypertrophic cardiomyopathy (HCM)
  2. Dilated cardiomyopathy
  3. Arrhythmogenic right ventricular dysplasia (ARVD)
  4. Acute myocarditis
  5. Significant coronary artery anomalies
  6. Coronary artery disease (CAD)
  7. Marfan's syndrome
  8. Uncontrolled hypertension
  9. Congestive heart failure
  10. Coarctation of the aorta
  11. Severe valvular heart disease
  12. Idiopathic long QT syndrome
  13. Complex ventricular arrhythmias
  14. Cyanotic congenital heart disease
  15. Pulmonary hypertension

B. **Cardiovascular conditions that are relative contraindications to vigorous exercise** necessitate careful evaluation and individual recommendations prior to vigorous exercise and competition:
  1. Nonspecific cardiomyopathy
  2. Uncontrolled atrial arrhythmias, which are likely to affect cardiac performance
  3. Hemodynamically significant valvular heart disease

C. **The rationales for and extent of restriction** of athletes with these conditions are addressed in the sections in which these conditions are discussed.

D. **Screening** for these abnormalities in apparently healthy individuals requires an appreciation of their low incidences in this population, along with the limitations of the screening techniques. Nevertheless it is best accomplished through the standard history and physical examination with special attention to the following:
  1. **History**—symptoms of exercise intolerance, exertional chest discomfort, syncope, near syncope, palpitations; past history of a heart murmur or systemic hypertension.
  2. **Physical examination**—blood pressure, cardiac auscultation (in supine and standing positions), physical stigmata suggestive of Marfan's syndrome.
  3. **Family history**—premature death (sudden or otherwise) or disability due to cardiovascular disease in close relative(s) under 50 years old or history of specific conditions, including HCM, dilated cardiomyopathy, long-QT syndrome, and Marfan's syndrome.
  4. **Additional tests** are recommended if clinically indicated, including serum lipids, resting electrocardiogram (ECG), exercise stress test, echocardiogram.

E. **American Heart Association Scientific Statement:** Cardiovascular preparticipation screening of competitive athletes recommends history and physical examination before participation in organized high school (grades 9–12) and collegiate sports, repeated every 2 years with an interim history in intervening years.

F. **The assessment of athletes known to have cardiovascular conditions** may also be part of the preparticipation examination. The recommendations regarding eligibility for these athletes are made considering the type of cardiovascular abnormality, its pathophysiologic severity, and the physiologic demands of the sport in which the athlete competes (see Suggested Reading: Bethesda Conference 26: Recommendations for Determining Eligibility for Competition in Athletes With Cardiovascular Abnormalities, sponsored by the American College of Cardiology and the American College of Sports Medicine).

Individuals with selected cardiovascular conditions, while not eligible for vigorous exercise and competition, can often participate in recreational athletic activities. The decisions for such individuals must be made carefully, with emphasis on noncompetitive activities, controlled intensity, and necessity of periodic reevaluations.

II. Cardiac Murmurs

Cardiac murmurs are commonly heard in athletes and are most likely to be innocent flow murmurs (see IV. Athletic Heart Syndrome, below). A murmur, however, may be a sign of a cardiovascular condition that compromises cardiac performance and exercise capacity or places the athlete at risk for sudden death.

A. **The primary issues** in their evaluation are as follows: (1) Is the murmur functional or the result of cardiovascular pathology? (2) If due to pathology, what is the specific abnormality and its hemodynamic and pathophysiologic severity?

B. **Functional (innocent flow) murmurs** are typically early to midsystolic systolic murmurs, usually grade 1 or 2 intensity, heard best at the second or third left intercostal space at left sternal border, without ejection sounds or thrills, decreasing in intensity with Valsalva maneuver.

C. **Organic murmurs are due to cardiovascular pathology** (organic heart disease). Certain characteristics suggest specific conditions:

1. Murmurs louder than grade 2 in intensity suggest aortic stenosis, mitral regurgitation, and ventricular septal defect.
2. Diastolic murmurs suggest aortic regurgitation, pulmonic regurgitation, and mitral stenosis.
3. A continuous murmur suggests a patent ductus arteriosus.
4. A murmur that increases in intensity in response to Valsalva maneuver strongly suggests hypertrophic cardiomyopathy.

D. **Organic murmurs** include the following:

1. Midsystolic (ejection) murmurs
   a. Aortic obstructive murmurs due to supravalvular, valvular, or subvalvular (including hypertrophic cardiomyopathy) stenosis and those caused by dilatation of the ascending aorta (e.g., Marfan's syndrome)
   b. Pulmonic obstructive murmurs due to supravalvular (pulmonary arterial), valvular, and infundibular stenosis
2. Pansystolic (regurgitant) murmurs of mitral regurgitation, tricuspid regurgitation, and ventricular septal defect
3. Early diastolic murmurs of aortic and pulmonic regurgitation
4. Middiastolic murmurs of mitral stenosis, and left and right atrial tumors (e.g., myxomas)
5. Continuous murmurs (those beginning in systole, persisting without interruption into diastole) due most commonly to patent ductus arteriosus

III. Cardiovascular Adaptations to Exercise Training

All effective exercise training programs include exercise of an intensity to which the body will adapt on a chronic basis. The physiologic consequences of dynamic and resistive exercise programs differ; thus these programs are tailored to the unique physiologic demands of an athlete's sport.

A. **The cardiovascular results of exercise training,** which vary depending on intensity of training (i.e., magnitude of the stimulus), include the following:
   1. Exercise capacity—increased.
   2. Heart rate—decreased resting and submaximal exercise heart rates; no change in maximal heart rate (although peak exercise workload or capacity is increased).
   3. Blood pressure—decreased at rest in hypertensive patients and decreased risk of development of hypertension in nonhypertensives.
   4. Stroke volume—increased at rest and at all intensities of exercise.
   5. Cardiac output—increased at maximal exercise.
   6. Cardiac morphology—increased cardiac chamber dimensions in response to dynamic exercise stimulus (i.e., cardiovascular endurance exercise); increased ventricular wall thickness in response to resistance exercise programs.

B. In response to properly executed exercise training programs, cardiovascular effects occur in both sexes, at all ages, and in healthy patients as well as those with cardiac problems. Physical training has also been shown to slow the decline in exercise capacity that invariably accompanies the aging process.

C. In order to achieve significant health benefits without major risks, exercise training for adults for 30 min or more at moderate intensity—defined as equal to or greater than 6 METS (1 MET = average resting metabolic rate)—is recommended by the 1995 Centers for Disease Control and Prevention and American College of Sports Medicine statement "Physical Activity and Public Health." Training programs for most competitive athletes will require higher-intensity training.

D. The concepts of cardiovascular training and building aerobic power for athletes are addressed in greater depth in Chapter 7. The basic elements of exercise training are exercise mode, intensity, frequency, and duration, tailored for the specific physiologic demands of the athlete's sport.

IV. Athletic Heart Syndrome

A. **Definition.** In the evaluation of competitive and recreational athletes, it is important to appreciate that changes on physical exam, ECG, chest x-ray, echocardiogram, and other modes of assessment occur that reflect adaptations to training rather than cardiovascular pathology. These changes are collectively referred to as the **athletic heart syndrome.**

B. **Components:** (1) physical exam: bradycardia, gallop rhythms (S3, S4), innocent flow murmurs; (2) chest x-ray and echocardiogram: four-chamber cardiac enlargement; (3) ECG: sinus bradycardia, sinus arrhythmia, first- and second- degree (Wenckebach type) atrioventricular (AV) block, P-wave changes of right and left atrial enlargement, QRS changes of increased voltage and intraventricular delay, and resting ST-T changes of early repolarization and juvenile T-wave pattern (inverted T waves in the initial precordial leads).

V. Exercise Testing

Exercise stress tests provide significant information in evaluation of athletes. They may be performed for assessment of exercise capacity (as discussed in Chapter 7) or for diagnostic purposes. Multiple types or tests and protocols may be used. Most are multistage, continuous tests using a treadmill or bicycle ergometer, carried out until an exercise-limiting symptom (often fatigue) occurs.

A. **Information provided** by exercise testing includes (1) maximal exercise capacity, (2) exercise-limiting and related symptoms, (3) maximal heart rate, (4) maximal blood pressure, (5) arrhythmias and conduction abnormalities, and (6) ST-segment changes.

B. **Exercise stress testing should be considered before starting a vigorous exercise program** for people over age 40 and for younger individuals with multiple or severe risk factors for coronary artery disease (CAD) or exertional symptoms, as CAD must be considered potentially present in recreational and competitive athletes over 30 to 35 years of age. However, abnormal electrocardiographic ST-T responses to exercise occur commonly in healthy, well-trained athletes. Thus, in the absence of specific indications, exercise stress testing of young asymptomatic athletes other than for the purpose of exercise capacity assessment is not recommended.

Syncope

Syncope (loss of consciousness due to inadequate cerebral blood flow) may be the presenting symptom of a serious, life-threatening condition or may simply be neurally mediated (vasovagal) syncope in the absence of significant cardiac pathology. As its ultimate significance depends on the etiology of the syncope, it should be aggressively sought. Differentiation from the loss of consciousness associated with conclusive disorders is important and is addressed in Chapter 35, "The Athlete with Epilepsy."

I. Causes

Causes of syncope in the athletic population include:

1. Neurally mediated (vasovagal) syncope
2. Tachycardias, ventricular, or (less likely) supraventricular, with or without heart disease (including hypertrophic cardiomyopathy, long-QT syndrome, ARVD, Wolff-Parkinson-White syndrome, coronary artery disease, and coronary artery anomalies)
3. Bradyarrhythmias (e.g., third-degree heart block and sick sinus syndrome)
4. Obstruction to left ventricular outflow (e.g., aortic stenosis, hypertrophic cardiomyopathy)
5. Obstruction to pulmonary flow (e.g., pulmonary hypertension)
6. Orthostatic hypotension
7. Psychogenic causes

II. Evaluation. History and Physical Examination

These are directed at evidence of any of these causes and should be *supplemented as indicated by ECG, exercise stress testing,* and *echocardiography.* The first issue in the evaluation of suspected syncope is to distinguish true syncope from collapse due to exhaustive effort. The former results in loss of consciousness with quick recovery once adequate blood pressure is restored. Conversely, collapse related to exhaustive effort results in a slower recovery and a period of "being out of it" even after adequate blood pressure is restored. During this time the athlete may be able to move about, although feeling poorly.

An important aspect of the history is the activity of the athlete at the time of the syncopal episode. Syncope during exercise should be regarded as significant, suggesting a potentially life-threatening event. This is in contrast to syncope after exercise, when orthostatic hypotension, neurally mediated syncope, or syncope due to a life-threatening disorder may occur. The history should emphasize any prodrome, presence of possible arrhythmias, precipitating events or factors, prior cardiovascular problems, and family history of heart disease, syncope, or sudden death. A thorough **family history** with respect to unexplained syncope or sudden death may provide clues to the presence of important familial conditions, such as long-QT syndrome, hypertrophic cardiomyopathy, and ARVD.

III. Evaluation of Unexplained Cases

If a cause is not established after initial evaluation, it is appropriate to evaluate for the possibility of a serious arrhythmia. This evaluation requires an ECG, exercise stress test, and echocardiogram. Ambulatory ECG monitoring during routine activity may be helpful, but more often event monitors are more revealing, since they allow longer periods of monitoring and monitoring during activity that duplicates or simulates the physiologic demands of the sport. Invasive electrophysiologic studies may be considered in selected cases of unexplained syncope. Tilt-table testing adds little reliable information, as it is often positive in highly trained athletes and does not exclude more ominous causes.

Chest Pain

Chest pain in an athlete may be related to a cardiovascular condition, but often, and especially in the younger athlete, it has a noncardiovascular cause.

I. Causes of Acute and Recurrent Chest Pain in the Apparent Absence of Trauma

A. **Common causes**
   1. Bronchospasm—asthma, exercise-induced bronchospasm
   2. Musculoskeletal—chest wall pain, traumatic or nontraumatic

B. **Less common causes**
   1. Gastroesophageal reflux with or without spasm
   2. Thoracic outlet syndrome

C. **Infrequent causes**
   1. Cervical spine disease
   2. Pleurisy, pneumonia, pericarditis, pulmonary infarction
   3. Pneumothorax

D. **Rare causes**
   1. Aortic dissection
   2. Myocardial ischemia (including coronary artery anomalies) or infarction

II. Evaluation and Management

Evaluation and management of chest pain are directed toward and dictated by establishment of its cause. Although many tests are available to establish the proper diagnosis, the history will typically provide the most diagnostic information. The location, quality, duration, provocative and palliative factors, and associated symptoms often provide important information for making the proper diagnosis or narrowing the differential diagnosis.

III. The Evaluation and Management of Acute Chest Pain

This is discussed in Chapter 61, "Thoracic Injuries."

Sudden Death

Sudden death is defined as nontraumatic, unexpected death occurring instantaneously or within a few minutes of an abrupt change in a subject's clinical state. This definition generally excludes thermal injuries and drug-related deaths. However, in a sports medicine context, the issue of sudden death should also include athletic or exercise-related deaths due to thermal injuries (almost exclusively heat stroke) and deaths that do not occur immediately but rather in connection with a collapse during exercise (e.g., rhabdomyolysis). These deaths are collectively referred to as *nontraumatic sports deaths.*

I. Young Athletes

A. **Incidence.** In *young athletes (below age 30),* the incidence of sudden death is fortunately quite low. A study from the National Center for Catastrophic Sports Injury Research reported that approximately 16 nontraumatic sports deaths occur each year among approximately 3 million U.S. high school and college athletes. For unknown reasons, these occur predominately in males (10 males per 1 female, although the participation ratio in high school and college sports is 2 males per 1 female). Estimated death rates were higher among college than in high school students, but the study did not identify any sport with statistically significant higher death rates compared with rates among other athletes at the high school or college level.

B. **Causes**
   1. **Cardiovascular causes.** Structural, usually congenital heart disease is responsible for approximately three-fourths of nontraumatic sports deaths in high school and college athletics. These conditions are discussed in other sections of this chapter.
      a. Myocardial disorders
         i. Hypertrophic cardiomyopathy (HCM) is the most common cause of sudden death in young athletes, generally accounting for half of the deaths due to cardiovascular conditions.
         ii. Dilated cardiomyopathy.
         iii. Myocarditis.
         iv. ARVD.
         v. Nonspecific cardiomyopathy.

b. Coronary artery disorders
   i. Congenital coronary artery anomalies.
   ii. Atherosclerotic CAD.
c. Valvular disorders
   i. Congenital aortic stenosis.
   ii. Mitral valve prolapse (?)
d. Aortic disorders
   i. Aortic dissection and/or rupture due to Marfan's syndrome
e. Electrophysiologic disorders
   i. Wolff-Parkinson-White (WPW) syndrome
   ii. Idiopathic long-QT syndrome
   iii. Cardiac conduction system abnormalities
f. Other congenital heart diseases

2. **Noncardiovascular conditions** account for approximately one-fourth of the nontraumatic sports deaths in high school and college athletics.
   a. Exertional heat stroke (see Chapter 11)
   b. Exertional rhabdomyolysis and sickle cell trait (see Chapter 28)
   c. Status asthmaticus and exercise-induced anaphylaxis (see Chapter 27)

II. Mature and Older Athletes (above age 30)

A. **Causes**

1. **Coronary artery disease (CAD)** is the most common cause of exercise-related sudden death in persons, both athletic and nonathletic, over 30 years of age. The victims usually have abnormal risk profiles for CAD and may have prior histories of CAD. However, they may be asymptomatic individuals with high levels of cardiovascular fitness. In deciding whom to screen prior to clearance for exercise programs, it is important to remember that the absence of symptoms in a highly fit individual does not guarantee CAD-free status.
2. **Other cardiovascular conditions,** such as hypertrophic cardiac myopathy (HCM) and aortic stenosis, underlie sudden deaths in small minority of cases in this age group. Few data are available regarding exercise-related sudden deaths in women of this age range almost certainly owing to their infrequent occurrence.

III. Prevention

A. A reasonable *screening* approach prior to athletic participation is necessary but does not guarantee identification of life-threatening abnormalities. Athletes with these conditions may not have symptoms or signs of their abnormalities, which could be detected by a preparticipation physical examination (PPPE). The PPPE is discussed in Chapter 2 and eligibility for competition in the section on the cardiovascular examination of the athlete at the beginning of the present chapter.

B. **Observation** of athletes during practice and competition may identify those with serious cardiovascular conditions because of their inability to keep pace with their peers. Those unable to do so should be evaluated to determine if their difficulties are simply related to their level of fitness or due to a more significant or even life-threatening medical condition.

C. The appropriate *management of emergencies*—including life-threatening arrhythmias, exertional hyperthermia, exertional rhabdomyolysis, and status asthmaticus—is the final but critical stage in prevention of exercise-related sudden death.

Hypertension

The most common cardiovascular condition in adults, affecting an estimated 50 million in the United States systemic hypertension is also the most common cardiovascular condition in competitive athletes. The primary sports medicine issues in hypertension are (1) the effect of exercise and athletic competition on the control and progression of hypertension and (2) the acute risk of exercise and athletic competition to the athlete with hypertension.

I. Diagnosis and Classification

The diagnosis of hypertension is made by the finding of blood pressure above acceptable levels on three separate occasions, preferably over a period of weeks. Measurement of blood pressure must be made in nonstressful situations (i.e., at rest, sitting comfortably) with a blood pressure cuff of adequate size. The bladder of the cuff should be large enough to nearly encircle the arm and cover at least two-thirds of the length of the upper arm. Smaller cuffs may give inappropriately low readings.

Table 26-1 presents the classification developed by the Task Force on Systemic Hypertension for the 26th Bethesda Conference on Recommendations for Determining Eligibility for Competition in Athletes with Cardiovascular Abnormalities. This classification is taken from the Joint National Committee on the Detection, Evaluation, and Treatment of High Blood Pressure (JNC-V), and adapted from the Second Task Force on Blood Pressure Control in Children.

II. Recommendations Regarding Eligibility

A. Athletes with ***mild (stage 1) and moderate (stage 2) hypertension*** do not require restriction from athletics. Because cardiovascular endurance and resistance exercise programs have been shown to have beneficial effects on hypertension of all levels, these athletes should be encouraged to be involved in these exercise activities. Their blood pressure should be reassessed on a regular basis.

B. While there is no significant body of evidence to indicate that even severe hypertension increases the exercise-related risk of sudden death or the progression of hypertension or target organ damage, ***severe (stage 3) and very severe (stage 4) levels of hypertension*** are considered to require limitation of activity, primarily from sports with high static demands. These restrictions may be lifted (if there is no evidence of target-organ damage) when the blood pressure is controlled.

III. Evaluation

In the athletic population, just as in the general population, the presence of sustained hypertension merits evaluation for the presence of target-organ damage,

Table 26-1. Classification of hypertension[a]

	Mild (stage 1), mm Hg	Moderate (stage 2), mm Hg	Severe (stage 3), mm Hg	Very severe (stage 4), mm Hg
Adolescents age 13–15				
Systolic BP	135–139	140–149	150–159	≥160
Diastolic BP	85–89	90–94	95–99	≥100
Adolescents age 16–18				
Systolic BP	140–149	150–159	160–179	≥180
Diastolic BP	90–94	95–99	100–109	≥110
Adults above age 18				
Systolic BP	140–159	160–179	180–209	≥210
Diastolic BP	90–99	100–109	110–119	≥120

[a] Blood pressures (BP) are the average of three or more readings at two or more visits after the initial screening. When systolic and diastolic reading fall into different categories, the higher category is used for categorization.

secondary causes of hypertension, and other risk factors for subsequent development of vascular disease (e.g., hypercholesterolemia, cigarette smoking). The evaluation consists of a thorough ***history and physical examination, laboratory testing*** (blood glucose, electrolytes, creatinine, cholesterol, hematocrit, urinalysis, and ECG). ***Further testing*** should be reserved for those whose initial evaluation suggests the presence of a secondary cause. Although not generally necessary ***echocardiography*** can provide information regarding the presence of left ventricular hypertrophy, which may affect decisions regarding the initiation of pharmacologic therapy.

Exercise stress testing is best reserved for athletes over 35 years old, especially if they have other coronary risk factors. The occurrence during an exercise test of a marked increase in systolic blood pressure (BP) above 240 mm Hg or an increase in diastolic BP is considered by some investigators to be a harbinger of subsequent development of sustained hypertension, thus meriting careful follow-up and probably initiation of nonpharmacologic therapy.

IV. Management

A. **Nonpharmacologic.** Lifestyle modifications, because of their effectiveness in controlling blood pressure and in improving cardiovascular risk profiles, should be encouraged and may be sufficient to control blood pressure in nonsevere cases. These measures include weight reduction, increased physical activity, moderation of dietary sodium and alcohol intake, and avoidance of drugs of abuse (especially cocaine), anabolic-androgenic steroids, and growth hormone.

B. **Pharmacologic.** Athletes, even more than the general population, may not tolerate medications. They may feel that medications affect their performance and they often have irregular schedules, potentially resulting in significant compliance problems.

Appropriate antihypertensive therapy requires attention to the not only to a medication's efficacy but also to its potential side effects.

1. Alpha-adrenergic blocking agents, angiotensin-converting enzyme (ACE) inhibitors, and calcium channel blocking agents are efficacious, generally well-tolerated medications.
2. Diuretics may lead to hypokalemia, volume depletion, dehydration, and ultimately orthostatic hypotension, especially in endurance sports. They are also banned by some athletic organizations, including the International Olympic Committee (IOC).
3. Beta-adrenergic blocking agents may produce fatigue and decreased exercise tolerance and are also banned by some athletic organizations, including the IOC.

Arrhythmias

In the athletic population, especially among the young (below 30 years of age), arrhythmias, while ***not uncommon,*** are ***usually benign.*** However, because of recent highly publicized cardiac tragedies in apparently healthy athletes, arrhythmias and symptoms attributed to arrhythmias may cause ***great concern*** among athletes, parents, and coaches.

Arrhythmias may or may not be symptomatic. They may cause anxiety, syncope, near syncope, palpitations, decreased cardiac functioning, or even sudden death. They may be found on routine exam, ECG, exercise testing, or ambulatory monitoring, although they are typically transient and often not reproducible.

Athletes present special circumstances. They are often involved in high-intensity activities; they are usually young, healthy, and without apparent heart disease. Also, high levels of mental stress frequently accompany competition. Furthermore, we now see older "athletes" in their seventies, eighties, even nineties (groups more likely to include individuals with heart disease) involved in competitions and vigorous athletic activities.

Important factors in evaluating athletes and their arrhythmias include the type of exercise/athletic endeavor (both practice and competition) in which the athlete is involved, its intensity (high or low), its static and/or dynamic demands, and the risk of problems resulting from transient loss of consciousness (e.g., ski racing, sky diving, auto racing).

Cardiac arrhythmias of greatest significance because of the potential for cardiac arrest are those occurring in persons with structural heart disease (e.g., cardiomyopathy, congenital or valvular heart disease, coronary heart disease), left ventricular dysfunction, and/or myocardial ischemia. Also important are those that decrease cardiac output, blood pressure, and cerebral blood flow by very rapid or very slow ventricular rates. Conversely, arrhythmias—including marked sinus bradycardia, sinus pauses, first- and second- degree (Wenckebach type) AV block, and uniform premature ventricular contractions (PVCs)—occur not infrequently in healthy athletes, often as a result of their training programs.

I. Evaluation

A. **The assessment** of the athlete with an arrhythmia or symptoms suggestive of an arrhythmia should be directed toward (1) presence of structural heart disease, (2) type and complexity of arrhythmia, (3) response of the arrhythmia to exercise.

B. **The minimum evaluation** involves a history, emphasizing precipitating events or factors, prior cardiovascular problems, medication usage, and family history of heart disease, syncope, or sudden death; a cardiovascular physical examination; and a resting ECG.

C. **More extensive evaluation** (if indicated) may include chest x-ray, echocardiogram, exercise stress test, ambulatory monitor, event monitor, signal-averaged ECG, laboratory tests (serum K^+, Mg^{++}), cardiac catheterization, coronary angiography, and invasive electrophysiologic study. Tests to provoke arrhythmias and to assess therapeutic efficacy should be tailored to the athlete's specific type of activity. Also, tests may need to be repeated, as training may affect the arrhythmia.

II. Treatment

A. **General considerations.** The treatment of arrhythmias (if indicated) is directed at their prevention, and, in the case of atrial arrhythmias, control of the ventricular rate. Treatment recommendations must be consistent with those for any structural heart disease present and must recognize that compliance of athletes (amateur and professional, young and old) with medical regimens may be less than ideal. Also it must be remembered that the use of beta blockers is not permissible by certain athletic governing bodies, such as the IOC.

B. **Definitive evaluation and recommendations** for specific arrhythmias are beyond the scope of this chapter. Addressed here are two arrhythmias that sports medicine physicians may be required to manage on an emergency basis (supraventricular tachycardia and those resulting in cardiac arrest), as well as athletic eligibility for athletes with arrhythmias.

1. **Supraventricular tachycardia.** A rapid, regular tachyarrhythmia at a rate of 150 to 250 per minute is most likely to be a supraventricular tachycardia (SVT), as ventricular tachycardia is unlikely to occur in an apparently healthy athlete. If ventricular tachycardia does occur, it will almost certainly resolve spontaneously or will degenerate into ventricular fibrillation with a pulseless, apneic state and a need for the measures indicated below. Atrial fibrillation with rapid ventricular response presents with an irregularly irregular rhythm rather than a regular one.

    a. **Presentation.** SVT typically presents with an awareness of heart action inappropriately rapid for the athlete's activity and/or emotional state and possibly feelings of fatigue, near syncope, or even syncope.

    b. **Management of acute episodes.** If SVT is suspected, the athlete should assume a squatting or supine position and perform a Valsalva maneuver. If the regular tachycardia persists, consideration should be given to unilateral carotid sinus massage at the angle of the jaw for a maximum of 5 to 10 sec, with simultaneous auscultation of the heart for the resolution of the tachyarrhythmia. This technique should be performed only on persons without indications of carotid artery disease. If SVT is persistent and unresponsive to these simple measures (an unusual likelihood), ECG monitoring should be obtained and transport for further treatment arranged.

c. **Treatment to prevent recurrences of SVT** depends on multiple factors, including the occurrence of syncope or near syncope with the tachyarrhythmia, its frequency and duration, as well as the athlete's willingness to comply with medical recommendations.

2. **Arrhythmias resulting in cardiac arrest.** Any ***loss of consciousness*** requires immediate evaluation and, if the athlete is pulseless and/or apneic, immediate treatment. Cardiac arrest is usually secondary to ventricular fibrillation (rarely cardiac asystole). If this is present, basic life support measures should be instituted immediately. Simultaneously, the emergency system should be activated. A plan for both traumatic and nontraumatic (including cardiac arrest) emergencies should be developed and practiced in order to deal with such occurrences effectively.

III. Athletic Eligibility for Athletes with Arrhythmias

Table 26-2 includes a classification based on the need for participation restrictions. For any arrhythmia that occurs in the presence of structural heart disease, the final participation recommendation must also be consistent with the recommendation for athletes with the structural heart disease. See also Section I of this chapter, "Cardiovascular Examination of the Athlete" and Bethesda Conference 26 guidelines.

Table 26-2. Participation in competitive athletics—Arrhythmias[a]

Arrhythmias that do not require activity limitations	Arrhythmias that rarely require activity limitations	Arrhythmias that may require activity limitations	Arrhythmias that usually require activity limitations	Arrhythmias that almost invariably require activity limitations
Premature atrial compelexes	Sinus bradycardia	Atrial fibrillation	Atrial flutter	Ventricular tachycardia
	Sinus tachycardia	Wolff-Parkinson-White syndrome	Second-degree heart block (type II)	Long-QT syndrome
	Sinus arrhythmia	Premature ventricular contractions	Third-degree heart block	
	Sinus pause or arrest			
	Sick sinus syndrome			
	Supraventricular tachycardia			
	First-degree heart block			
	Second-degree heart block (type I)			
	Right bundle branch block			

[a] All athletes with arrhythmias require individual evaluation, specific recommendations, and periodic follow-up.

Disorders of the Myocardium

Disorders of the myocardium, while not commonly seen, have substantial importance in sports medicine as (1) they are well-recognized causes of exercise-related sudden death and (2) their manifestations may require differentiation from the cardiac morphologic changes due to athletic training.

Although few data exist regarding the risk that exercise poses to **athletes with myocardial disorders,** such individuals **are usually restricted from vigorous exercise and athletic competition.** Selected athletes with healed myocarditis and nonspecific cardiomyopathies, however, may be considered for return to full activity if cardiac evaluation establishes the absence of significant ventricular dysfunction or arrhythmias. See Bethesda Conference 26 for specific recommendations.

I. Hypertrophic Cardiomyopathy (HCM)

Hypertrophic cardiomyopathy is the most common cause of sudden death in young athletes.

A. **Genetic basis.** HCM is a genetic disorder with significant genetic heterogeneity (presently known to be caused by mutations in multiple—at least nine different—genes on chromosomes 1,3,7,11,12,14,15,19 and possibly others not yet identified). It is considered to be a ***disease of the sarcomere,*** as the proteins encoded by mutation-bearing genes thus far identified are all sarcomeric proteins: beta-myosin heavy chain, cardiac troponin T, alpha-tropomyosin, myosin-binding protein C, ventricular myosin essential and regulatory light chain and cardiac troponin I.

B. **Pathologic features.** HCM is clinically defined by the presence of a hypertrophied nondilated left ventricle in the absence of a cardiac or systemic disorder that produces left ventricular hypertrophy. Microscopically, myocardial cellular disarray and abnormally thickened intramural coronary arteries with narrowed lumens may also be present.

C. **Diagnosis** is made by echocardiography with intraventricular wall thickness equal to or greater than 15 mm. The left ventricular free wall thickness may be normal or increased. The finding of systolic anterior motion (SAM) of the mitral valve is supportive of but not required for the diagnosis of HCM.

D. **Symptoms** may include syncope, chest discomfort, and dyspnea, although many persons with HCM are asymptomatic; in fact, some may have excellent exercise capacity (despite and not because of HCM).

E. **Physical examination.** A cardiac murmur, if present, is typically a harsh, midsystolic, crescendo-decrescendo murmur heard best at the lower left sternal border or at the apex. The murmur may be labile in intensity due to functional left ventricular outflow obstruction. In these cases, the murmur will increase in intensity with increased contractility, decreased preload, and/or decreased afterload. However, HCM is typically nonobstructive and under basal conditions a murmur is either absent or soft.

II. Other Cardiomyopathies

A. **Dilated cardiomyopathy** may be seen on a familial, postviral, drug-related (alcohol, cocaine) or idiopathic basis. Diagnosis is made by the finding of ventricular systolic dysfunction, and, depending on its severity, a decrease in exercise capacity.

B. **Arrhythmogenic right ventricular dysplasia,** is characterized by fibrofatty replacement of the right and, in some cases and to a lesser extent, the left ventricle, with resultant ventricular dysfunction, ventricular arrhythmias, and risk of sudden death. It has also been identified as having a genetic basis, with the locations of disease genes mapped to chromosomes 1, 2, and 14q23-q24. Diagnosis is made by echocardiography or magnetic resonance imaging.

C. **Nonspecific cardiomyopathy.** A cardiomyopathy that cannot be classified into one of the specific diagnostic cardiomyopathy categories is defined as nonspecific cardiomyopathy. It is reported as a cause of exercise-related sudden death and may be a manifestation of a myocarditis. It is typically diagnosed by the echocardiographic finding of abnormal ventricular wall motion and may be associated with ventricular arrhythmias. The diagnosis of nonspecific cardiomyopathy should lead to an evaluation for the presence of arrhythmias, extent of left ventricular dysfunction, and exercise capacity. Consideration should also be given to the performance of an endomyocardial biopsy in an attempt to establish the presence or absence of myocarditis.

III. Myocarditis

Myocarditis (inflammation of the myocardium), usually a result of a viral infection, may be clinically difficult to detect. However, because it is a recognized cause of sudden death in athletes, it must be considered as a possible accompaniment of a severe viral illness, and the issue of restriction from athletics must be addressed. Although it is difficult in most situations to be certain of the presence or absence of myocarditis, one fairly well accepted approach is to use the "neck check"—athletes are permitted to participate if their viral symptoms are confined to the neck region and above. However, if their symptoms are also "below the neck" and involve generalized myalagias, the possibility of vital myocarditis, although small, merits activity restriction until symptoms resolve. It should also be recognized that cocaine abuse can result in a myocarditic process, with subsequent scarring and dysfunction and potential for serious arrhythmias. The diagnosis of myocarditis may require an endomyocardial biopsy; if made, it should result in restriction from vigorous exercise and athletic competition for at least 6 months.

Coronary Artery Disease

Coronary artery disease includes congenital coronary artery anomalies and acquired coronary artery disease, typically due to atherosclerosis.

I. Congenital Coronary Artery Anomalies

A. **These are the second most common cardiovascular cause of exercise-related sudden death in the under-30 age group.** In this regard the anomalies of consequence are those involving a coronary artery of abnormal origin (including acute angulation) and/or course (including passage between pulmonary artery and the aorta) of a coronary artery, which may potentially result in exercise-induced myocardial ischemia. These anomalies may produce chest discomfort or syncope or they may be asymptomatic. The most common coronary artery anomaly causing exertional sudden death is the anomalous origin of left coronary artery from the right sinus of Valsalva. Other coronary artery anomalies that are reported causes of exercise-related sudden death include anomalous origin of the right coronary artery from the left sinus of Valsalva, coronary artery hypoplasia, and anomalous origin of the left main coronary artery from the pulmonary artery. Intramural ("tunneled") coronary arteries due to myocardial bridges are reported as a cause of exertional sudden death, although their precise role is undefined and controversial.

B. **Cardiovascular evaluation** is indicated for athletes suspected or known to have congenital coronary artery anomalies. If exercise-induced myocardial ischemia is documented, athletic participation restriction is necessary, and consideration should be given to surgical repair. Athletes who have had successful surgical repair with subsequent documented absence of exercise-induced myocardial ischemia may be considered for return to competition.

II. Atherosclerotic Coronary Artery Disease (CAD)

CAD is rare in young athletes and probably occurs in this group only in presence of lipid abnormalities. However, it is more likely to be present in mature and older athletes.

A. **The most common cause of exercise-related sudden death in persons, both athletic and nonathletic, over 30 years of age.** The victims usually have abnormal risk factor profiles for CAD. They may have prior histories of CAD or may be asymptomatic individuals with high levels of cardiovascular fitness. Thus the absence of symptoms in a highly fit individual does not guarantee CAD-free status. This must be considered when deciding whom to screen prior to clearance for exercise programs (see the discussion of the cardiovascular examination of the athlete at the opening of this chapter). Athletes found to have atherosclerotic CAD are usually older, "masters"-level athletes. These athletes require individual evaluation, specific recommendations, and periodic follow-up. In general they should not engage in vigorous competitive athletics, even following successful myocardial revascularization procedures (coronary artery bypass graft surgery or coronary angioplasty). This restriction exists because of the progressive nature of the disease and the fact that even "nonhemodynamically significant lesions" may suddenly become more severe due to plaque rupture and thrombosis, leading to an acute coronary event (unstable angina, myocardial infarction, or sudden death). See Bethesda Conference 26 for specific recommendations.

B. **An increased risk of myocardial infarction** also exists during periods of vigorous exercise in those with CAD.

C. **Beneficial effects of regular dynamic, cardiovascular endurance exercise** have been demonstrated in multiple studies. These include physiologic benefits, cardiovascular disease prevention, and reduction in cardiovascular morbidity and mortality.

D. **Exercise training programs for patients with CAD.**

1. **Physiologic benefits.** In addition to the physiologic benefits obtained by all exercisers, patients with CAD and exercise-induced myocardial ischemia achieve a reduction in myocardial ischemia following periods of exercise training. This reduction is due to a decrease in myocardial oxygen demand rather than to an increase in myocardial oxygen supply. Some cardiac patients, because of their pathophysiologic abnormalities, may be limited in their ability to train and to achieve a training effect.
2. **Reduction in mortality** has been shown in metanalyses of studies evaluating the effects of exercise training programs for cardiac patients.
3. **A high level of safety** even for patients with severe cardiovascular disease has been demonstrated in studies of supervised cardiac rehabilitation programs.

Valvular Heart Disease

Acquired valvular heart disease (stenosis or regurgitation), depending upon the severity of the lesion and its hemodynamic effects, may be compatible with athletic endeavor, including competition. Sports medicine physicians need an awareness of potential seriousness of certain lesions and when referral to a specialist is appropriate. The central issues with regard to valvular heart disease are (1) What is the risk of sudden death with athletic participation? and (2) What is the risk of deterioration of left ventricular function with exercise and athletic participation?

I. The Assessment of Athletes with Valvular Heart Disease

Assessment is directed at establishing (1) the type and severity of the stenotic and/or regurgitant lesion, (2) the status of ventricular function, (3) the presence of arrhythmias, and (4) the presence of other cardiac abnormalities.

II. Recommendations for Participation

Recommendations for athletes with valvular heart disease are found in Table 26-3. Little precise information exists on which to base many recommendations, which therefore must be based on prudent judgment.

Table 26-3. Participation in competitive athletics—valvular heart disease[a]

Full participation	Selected participation	No participation
Mild aortic stenosis	Mild to moderate aortic stenosis	Severe aortic stenosis Moderate aortic stenosis with symptoms
Mild or moderate aortic regurgitation with normal or mildly increased left ventricular size	Aortic regurgitation with moderate left ventricular enlargement Mild or moderate aortic regurgitation and premature ventricular contractions at rest and with exercise	Severe aortic regurgitation Mild or moderate aortic regurgitation with symptoms Aortic regurgitation with marked dilation of proximal ascending aorta Aortic regurgitation with progressive left ventricular enlargement on serial studies
Mild mitral stenosis with sinus rhythm	Mild mitral stenosis with atrial fibrillation Moderate mitral stenosis	Severe mitral stenosis
Mitral regurgitation with normal left ventricular size and function	Mitral regurgitation with mild left ventricular enlargement but normal left ventricular function at rest	Mitral regurgitation with definite left ventricular enlargement or any left ventricular dysfunction at rest
Mitral valve prolapse without complications listed under "selected participation"	Mitral valve prolapse with moderate or marked mitral regurgitation, repetitive supraventricular tachyarrhythmias, complex ventricular arrhythmias, history of arrhythmogenic syncope, family history of sudden death associated with mitral valve prolapse, or prior embolic event Recommendations for athletes with multivalvular disorders are based on the most severe lesion Multiple lesions of moderate severity may have additive effects Postoperative athletes with a prosthetic or bioprosthetic cardiac valve	

Continued

Table 26-3. (*continued*)

Full participation	Selected participation	No participation
	Postannuloplasty or valvuloplasty mitral valve prolapse Postvalvuloplasty mitral regurgitation, mitral stenosis, and aortic stenosis depending on residual lesion severity and left ventricular function	

[a] Based on Bethesda Conference 26, all athletes with valvular heart disease require individual evaluation, specific recommendations, and periodic follow-up, especially those in the selected participation category.
Athletes taking anticoagulants should not participate in sports with a risk of bodily collision.

Congenital Heart Disease

Congenital heart disease, depending upon the severity of the lesion or lesions and their hemodynamic consequences, may be compatible with athletic endeavor, including competition. Sports medicine physicians need an awareness of the potential seriousness of certain lesions and when referral to a specialist is appropriate. The central issues with regard to congenital heart disease are (1) What is the risk of sudden death with athletic participation? and (2) What is the risk of deterioration of ventricular function and progression of pulmonary vascular disease with exercise and athletic participation?

I. Evaluation

A. **The assessment** of athletes with congenital heart disease is directed at establishing (1) the type and severity of the lesion or lesions, (2) the status of ventricular function, (3) the presence of pulmonary vascular disease, and (4) the presence of arrhythmias.
B. **Reevaluations** are especially important (at least yearly) because of the progressive nature of many of the defects and their hemodynamic effects.
C. Other than hypertrophic cardiomyopathy, dilated cardiomyopathy, and Marfan's syndrome (discussed elsewhere), the congenital heart diseases of a serious nature with respect to exercise are aortic stenosis, complex cyanotic lesions, and those with pulmonary vascular disease.

II. Recommendations for Athletic Participation

A. There is little precise information on which to base recommendations regarding athletic participation; thus they must be based primarily on prudent judgment. Recommendations for the participation of athletes with congenital heart disease are found in Table 26-4. See also Bethesda Conference 26.
B. For athletes with milder forms of congenital heart disease, most sports are permissible. Intermediate levels of sports participation may be safe for athletes with moderate forms, but careful evaluation is required. For athletes with severe forms of congenital heart disease, vigorous/strenuous exercise is likely to pose risk.
C. Inappropriate restriction must be avoided, as it can lead to adverse physical and psychological consequences.

Table 26-4. Participation in competitive Athletics—congenital heart disease[a]

Full participation	Selected participation	No participation
Atrial septal defect—small defects without pulmonary hypertension	Atrial septal defect with pulmonary hypertension and/or a right-to-left shunt Atrial septal defect with symptomatic atrial or ventricular arrhythmias or significant mitral regurgitation—based on recommendations for these abnormalities	Atrial septal defect with marked cyanosis and a large right-to-left shunt
Postoperative or post-interventional atrial septal defect without pulmonary hyper-tension, symptomatic arrhythmias, or evidence of myo-cardial dysfunction[b]	Postoperative or postinter-ventional atrial septal defect with pulmonary hypertension, symptomatic arrhythmias, or evidence of myocardial dysfunction[b]	
Ventricular septal defect—small or moderate defects	Ventricular septal defect—large defects	
Postoperative or post-interventional ventricular septal defect without symptoms, pulmonary hypertension, arrhythmias, or myocardial dysfunction[b]	Postoperative or postinter-ventional ventricular septal defect with residual moderate or large defect, significant arrhythmias, mild to moderate pulmonary hypertension, or ventricular dysfunction[b]	Postoperative or postinterventional ventricular septal defect with severe pulmonary hypertension[b]
Patent ductus arteriosus—small		Patent ductus arteriosus—moderate or large
Patent ductus arteriosus postclosure without symptoms, pulmonary hypertension, or cardiac enlargement	Patent ductus arteriosus postclosure with pulmonary hypertension	
Mild pulmonic stenosis without symptoms with normal right ventricular function	Moderate and severe pulmonic stenosis	
Postoperative or post-interventional pulmo-nic stenosis without symptoms, ventricular dysfunction, or signifi-cant residual obstruction[c]	Postoperative or postinterventional pulmonic stenosis with significant residual gradient or severe pulmonic insufficiency[c]	

Continued

Table 26-4. Participation in competitive Athletics—congenital heart disease[a]

Full participation	Selected participation	No participation
Mild aortic stenosis if symptomatic and if electrocardiogram and exercise tolerance are normal	Moderate aortic stenosis	Severe aortic stenosis
	Postoperative or postinterventional aortic stenosis patients with residual mild, moderate, or severe stenosis should be considered as above; for those with moderate or severe aortic regurgitation, see Table 26-3[b]	
	Coarctation of the aorta	
	Postoperative or postinterventional coarctation of the aorta	
	Ebstein's anomaly	

[a] Based on Bethesda Conference 26, all athletes with congenital heart disease require individual evaluation, specific recommendations, and periodic follow-up, especially those in the selected participation category.
[b] Recommendations for postoperative or postinterventional athletes are for at least 6 months after repair.
[c] Recommendations for postoperative athletes are for at least 3 months after repair and for postinterventional athletes at least 1 month after repair.
Athletes with cyanotic congenital heart disease (including tetralogy of Fallot, transposition of the great arteries, congenitally corrected transposition of the great arteries), both uncorrected and postinterventional or postoperative (palliative and corrected), require individualized evaluation and recommendation.
Athletes with elevated pulmonary resistance/pulmonary hypertension, ventricular dysfunction, residual defects, or newly created defects (e.g., regurgitant lesions) require individualized evaluation and recommendations.

Diseases of the Aorta

Aortic dissection and /or rupture due to Marfan's syndrome is the primary aortic disorder of importance in sports medicine.

I. Marfan's Syndrome

This syndrome is a genetic disorder (autosomal dominant) of connective tissue due to mutations in the fibrillin gene (chromosome 15) and one or more other genes.

II. Aortic weakening, aortic aneurysm formation with subsequent risk of life-threatening dissection or rupture may result. Other ***cardiovascular abnormalities*** include aortic insufficiency and mitral valve prolapse.

III. Characteristic Musculoskeletal Abnormalities

These abnormalities in addition to tall stature, include chest wall deformities, arachnodactyly, and an arm span greater than height.

IV. Management

Beta-adrenergic blocking agents are generally recommended to decrease the risk of aortic dilation and subsequent dissection and rupture.

V. Recommendations Regarding Eligibility for Competitive Athletics

High-intensity dynamic exercise is to be avoided, as its hemodynamic effects would counteract the beneficial effects of beta-blocker therapy. Contact or collision sports should be avoided even if aortic root dimensions are normal because of the risk of aortic dissection or rupture. Selected sports may be permissible in athletes without ARD, Mitral Regurgitation, or a family history of premature sudden death (see Bethesda 26 Conference). Echocardiographic assessment of aortic root dimensions should be performed at least every 6 months.

Suggested Reading

American College of Sports Medicine Position stand: physical activity, physical fitness, and hypertension. *Med Sci Sports Exerc* 1993;25:i-x.

Bjornstad H, Storstein L, Meen HD, Hals O. Ambulatory electrocardiographic findings in top athletes, athletic students, and control subjects. *Cardiology* 1994;84:42–50.

Cardiovascular Preparticipation Screening of Competitive Athletes: A Statement for Health Professionals from the Sudden Death Committee (Clinical Cardiology) and Congenital Cardiac Defects Committee (Cardiovascular Disease in the Young), American Heart Association. *Circulation* 1996;94:850–856.

Huston TP, Puffer JC, Rodney WM: The athletic heart syndrome. *N Engl J Med* 1985;313:24–32.

Maron BJ, Mitchell JH. Bethesda Conference 26: Recommendations for determining eligibility for competition in athletes with cardiovascular abnormalities. *J Am Coll Cardiol* 1994;24:845–899 and *Med Sci Sports Exerc* 1994;26:S223–S283.

Maron BJ, Shirani J, Poliac LC, et al. Sudden death in young competitive athletes: clinical, demographic, and pathological profiles. *JAMA* 1996;276:199–204.

Maron BJ, Thompson PD, Puffer JC, et al. Cardiovascular preparticipation screening of competitive athletes. A statement for health professionals from the Sudden Death Committee (clinical cardiology) and Congenital Cardiac Defects Committee (cardiovascular disease in the young), American Heart Association. *Circ* 1996; 94(4):850–856.

Van Camp SP. Sudden death. *Clin Sports Med* 1992;11:273–289.

Van Camp SP, Bloor C, Mueller FO, et al. Nontraumatic sports death in high school and college athletes. *Med Sci Sports Exerc* 1995;27:641–647.

Zehender MT, Meinertz T, Keul J, Just H. ECG variants and cardiac arrhythmias in athletes: clinical relevance and prognostic importance. *Am Heart J* 1990; 119:1378–1391.

Zipes DP. Specific arrhythmias: diagnosis and treatment. In: Braunwald E, ed. *Heart disease: a textbook of cardiovascular medicine.* 5th ed. Philadelphia: WB Saunders, 1996.

27. PULMONARY

Bryan W. Smith and John M. MacKnight

Asthma/exercise-induced asthma

Asthma is a chronic lung disorder with three characteristic features: (1) airway obstruction that may or may not be reversible, spontaneously or with treatment: (2) airway inflammation; and (3) airway hyperresponsiveness to a variety of stimuli such as allergens, chemical irritants, viral infections, cold air, or exercise. Airway hyperresponsiveness to exercise can result in a diffuse, progressive increase in airway resistance primarily in large airways but in small airways as well. Exercise-induced asthma (EIA) typically occurs 5 to 10 min following strenuous exercise, but it may occur during exercise, particularly in poorly conditioned persons. Characteristic of EIA is that attacks resolve spontaneously, usually in 20 to 30 min, and under most circumstances are not life-threatening. Athletic participation was discouraged for many individuals with asthma when the treatments were limited. With the exception of scuba diving, (see Chapter 14), asthma should not prohibit sports participation if adequate preventative treatments are utilized.

I. Prevalence.

Approximately 10 million individuals in the United States have asthma, and there has been a rise in the prevalence over the past 15 years. More than 90% of these individuals can have exercise-induced asthma if sufficiently provoked. There is a subset of individuals (probably underdiagnosed) who have reactive airway symptoms only with exercise. As many as 40% of individuals with allergic rhinitis have EIA. The prevalence of EIA has been reported to be approximately 10% in world-class athletes, while as many as 20% of high school athletes have been diagnosed with EIA. Undertreatment and self-selection factors are the likely explanations for the difference.

II. EIA Pathophysiology.

Due to the hyperventilation associated with intense exercise, the body is unable to warm and humidify inhaled air adequately. This results in alterations in the osmotic homeostasis of the airway fluid layer. These alterations subject irritant receptors and mast cells to physical and electro-chemical stress such that a release of chemical mediators (e.g., histamine, neutrophil chemotactic factor, and slow-reacting substance of anaphylaxis) occurs. In susceptible individuals, these substances can cause bronchospasm and subsequent inflammation. Several modulating factors play a role in determining whether an attack occurs. Air temperatures below 21°C (70°F) and relative humidities below 50% are most conducive to EIA. Airborne allergens and pollutants such as pollens and smog increase airway hyperresponsiveness. Viral, upper respiratory infections sensitize airways for up to 3 weeks. Stress and overtraining have been postulated to increase the likelihood of EIA, but this is yet to be conclusively proven.

III. Diagnosis of EIA

A. **Clinical presentation.** While wheezing can sometimes be elicited, patients typically present with nonspecific symptoms such as cough, shortness of breath, and chest tightness soon after exercise. There is a wide range of symptom severity. Rarely, ***late-phase bronchospasm*** may occur unprovoked 4 to 12 hr postexercise. This bronchospasm usually occurs in severe early responders. Many individuals with EIA assume that they are in poor physical condition. In children, chest pain and exercise intolerance or lack of energy are reported. During an attack, physical examination may reveal increased respiratory rate, prolonged expiration, decreased breath sounds, and wheezing. Severe attacks—characterized by severe respiratory distress, diaphoresis, and pulsus paradoxus—are rarely seen with EIA.

B. **Risk-factor questionnaire.** In the physician's office, many patients with EIA and no prior history of asthma have a normal physical exam and normal pulmonary function as measured by spirometry or peak flow. Therefore, clinicians have relied on the history to make a presumptive diagnosis. However, past investigators have suggested that history alone is an unreliable predictor of EIA. The United States Olympic Committee (USOC) designed a questionnaire to help identify Olympic athletes with EIA. It consisted of questions about (1) documented history of asthma; (2) documented use of bronchodilator medications; (3) formal request to the USOC for approval to use bronchodilators; and (4) positive history of chest tightness, cough, or wheeze during or following strenuous exercise. Approximately 90% of Olympic athletes with EIA were identified by positive responses to the questionnaire. Approximately 95% of high school athletes with EIA were identified in one study by using similar criteria. However, the specificity was only about 60%.

C. **Laboratory Testing**

1. **Pulmonary function tests.** Spirometry permits documentation of airway obstruction, objective measurement of the severity of the asthma attack, and objective evidence of the response to bronchodilator medications. Characteristic changes seen in asthma are reduction of forced expiratory volume in 1 sec (FEV_1), a proportionally smaller decrease in forced vital capacity (FVC), decreased FEV_1/FVC ratio, decreased forced expiratory flow between 25% and 75% of FVC ($FEF_{25-75\%}$), and decreased peak expiratory flow (PEF). If spirometry is not available, measurement of PEF can be used.
2. **Challenge Testing.** Many tests have been used to formally diagnose EIA.
   a. **Exercise** challenge is believed to be the most specific test for EIA and is the test of choice. Several modalities are available such as free running, treadmill running, and cycle ergometry, while anyone who is at risk for injury with exercise should undergo methacholine challenge. ***Free running*** is the best test for inducing EIA. It also requires less equipment and can be performed in a variety of locations. Its limitations include the inability to control the environment and absence of adequate emergency precautions for high-risk individ-uals. ***Treadmill running*** is a good method for EIA provocation but requires expensive equipment. Air temperature and relative humidity can be controlled, but it is difficult to duplicate the allergens or pollutants to which the athlete is typically exposed. ***Cycle ergometry*** is the least effective method to induce EIA owing to restricted oxygen uptake. However, this may be the best test for the high-risk or disabled individual.
   b. **Methacholine** challenge has better sensitivity than exercise testing for EIA but is far inferior with regard to specificity. The test must be conducted in a pulmonary function laboratory.
   c. **Eucapnic hyperventilation and aerosolized distilled water** are research-only protocols for inducing EIA.
3. **Exercise test protocol**
   a. **Medications.** Discontinue use of beta-agonists and anticholinergics for 8 hr, long-acting beta agonists for 24 hours, methylxanthines for 8 to 12 hr, cromolyn sodium or nedocromil for 24 hr, and leukotriene antagonists for 24 hours.
   b. **Preexercise spirometry.** Prior to challenge testing, pulmonary function tests should be at least 80% of both the subject's usual pulmonary function and predicted normal values. The best values out of three attempts for PEF, FEV_1, and $FEF_{25-75\%}$ are used as baseline values.
   c. **Exercise test.** There should be no exercise for the previous 12 hr. After a warm-up run of 30 sec to 1 min, the subject should run con-

tinuously for 5 to 8 min at 80% $\dot{V}_{O_{2max}}$ or 90% maximum heart rate. Heart rate monitoring can be via electrocardiography (ECG) or telemetry. The ambient temperature must be 21°C (70°F) or less. Ideally, the relative humidity should be 50% or less. Air pollution levels and pollen counts should be measured if warranted.

d. **Postexercise spirometry.** Pulmonary function parameters should be monitored at 0, 5, 10, 15, 20, and 30 min postexercise.

e. **EIA diagnosis**
15% or greater decrease in PEF (large- and small-airway obstruction)
15% or greater decrease in FEV_1 (large-airway obstruction)
35% or greater decrease in $FEF_{25-75\%}$ (small-airway obstruction)

f. **EIA severity** (PEF or FEV_1)
Mild EIA: 15% to 25% decrease
Moderate EIA: 25% to 40% decrease
Severe EIA: 40% or greater decrease

IV. Management

Asthma management should be individualized, addressing the three major airway components: bronchospasm, inflammation, and hyperresponsiveness. Optimal therapy includes patient education, environmental control, pharmacologic therapy, and objective monitoring. Severe cases of asthma require emergency care, which is beyond the scope of this chapter (see the NIH publication in Suggested Readings).

A. **Patient education.** Each athlete and his or her family should be counseled as to the definition and chronicity of asthma, the signs and symptoms of asthma, and the environmental factors that can trigger an attack. They should be instructed on how to use their medication, what the medication is designed to do, what the potential side effects are, how to monitor the medication's effectiveness, and what to do in case of an emergency. The patient and the family should have ample opportunity to ask questions so as to avoid fears and remove misconceptions. Finally, written guidelines should be given to the patient and family.

B. **Environmental control.** Control of exposure to indoor and outdoor allergens is a primary goal of prevention. ***Swimming*** is an excellent exercise recommendation for the person with difficult-to-control asthma owing to the less asthmogenic, warm, humid air at the pool. While avoidance is the first recommendation, allergy immunotherapy may be beneficial if avoidance is impossible and pharmacologic therapy is inadequate. There are several potential outdoor and indoor allergens and irritants. The most common outdoor offenders are pollens, molds, and air pollutants, such as ozone and sulfur dioxide. Practicing indoors or wearing a mask when conditions outside are favorable for asthma provocation can be helpful. Indoor environmental hazards are animal and insect allergens, dust mites, indoor molds, and smoke. Optimally, athletes should not smoke or be exposed to passive smoke. Living in an air conditioned house and having a well-maintained air filtration system can help dramatically.

C. **Pharmacologic therapy.** The pharmacologic management of asthma consists of two components: bronchodilators and antiinflammatory agents. Therapy will be based on the severity of asthma, medication tolerance, and allergen sensitivity.

1. **Bronchodilators**

a. **Beta-adrenergic agonists.** These preparations are first-line therapy for acute bronchoconstriction. These drugs not only relax the bronchial smooth muscle but potently stabilize mast cells. These actions provide preventative as well as acute benefit. Inhaled beta$_2$-agonists are the standard of therapy, since cardiac side effects are minimized. Most (albuterol, bitolterol, metaproterenol, pirbuterol, and terbutaline) are available as metered-dose inhalers (MDIs). Some medications (albuterol, bitolterol, and metaproterenol) can be nebulized. Use of an MDI requires two or three puffs every 4 to 6 hr. If the patient has difficulty using an MDI, either a spacer device can be added or one can try a nebulizer to deliver the medication. Some of the potential side effects are tremor, tachycardia, and paradoxical bronchospasm. Some beta$_2$-agonists (albuterol, metaproterenol, and terbutaline) are available as oral preparations. Oral beta$_2$ agonists have more side effects and are not approved for athletes competing at the level of the National Collegiate Athletic Association (NCAA) or Olympics. A long acting, beta$_2$-agonist recently approved for athletes competing at this level is salmeterol. This drug has a duration of action up to 12 hr but takes approximately 1 hr to deliver therapeutic benefit. Therefore it is not recommended for an acute asthma attack, and it has been linked with fatal asthma if used improperly. In emergent situations where parenteral therapy is required, aqueous epinephrine can be administered. This nonselective beta agonist is a banned substance at the NCAA and Olympic levels.

b. **Methylxanthines.** At one time theophylline and aminophylline were the mainstays of treatment both for acute exacerbations and maintenance. With the advent of beta$_2$-agonists and inhaled steroids, methylxanthines are now used in individuals who are difficult to control with first-line therapies. These medications require careful monitoring owing to their narrow therapeutic windows and increased risk for toxicity. Two oral forms are available, rapid-release and sustained-release preparations. Numerous drug interactions are a problem with either preparation.

c. **Anticholinergies.** Ipratropium bromide is an atropine-like agent that has been used as an adjunct asthma therapy in individuals who have adverse reactions or inadequate responses to beta-agonist drugs. The duration of action is 3 to 4 hr. Peak bronchodilation occurs in 30 to 90 min. While this drug is not specified for refractory asthma, one approved use for it has been as a bronchodilator for chronic obstructive pulmonary disease.

2. **Antiinflammatories**

a. **Glucocorticoids.** In patients with moderate or severe asthma, inhaled glucocorticoids (e.g. beclomethasone, triamcinolone, flunisolide, and dexamethasone) have become the medication of choice to reduce airway inflammation. Dosages range from two puffs q.i.d. to four puffs b.i.d. Proper instruction in usage is necessary to avoid common side effects such as oral candidiasis and dysphonia. Systemic side effects are dose-dependent and unusual with the dosages listed. Dosages for children may need to be adjusted. These medications can be used by athletes in Olympic or international competition provided that a medical letter of need is submitted to the appropriate sport governing body. Systemic (intravenous or oral) glucocorticoids may be required for acute exacerbations of asthma. They are first-line therapy for patients requiring hospital admission. Intravenous or oral preparations are banned for use in athletes in Olympic or international competition.

b. **Khellin derivatives.** Two preparations (cromolyn and nedocromil) that act by stabilizing mast cells to prevent release of inflammatory mediators are available for preventive use. They can be combined with inhaled steroids in select patients with refractory asthma. Cromolyn (two puffs q.i.d.) has no significant side effects but is less clinically predictable than inhaled steroids. It may take 3 to 4 weeks for clinical benefit. Nedocromil is a relatively new agent available for maintenance and/or prevention of asthma. Clinical benefit can be achieved in as little as 3 to 4 days. Like cromolyn, it is not indicated for acute attacks. It is only approved in patients over 12 years of age and dosed at two puffs q.i.d. Side effects include headache, cough, and bitter taste. It may have added benefit over cromolyn in patients with grass-pollen allergies by reducing histamine airway responsiveness.

c. **Leukotriene antagonists.** Leukotrienes are inflammatory mediators formerly known as slow-reacting substances of anaphylaxis. Their bronchoconstricting properties are several times more potent than histamine. Recently, leukotriene antagonists have received approval in the U.S. for the prophylaxis and chronic treatment of asthma in individuals older than 12 yrs. Zafirlukast (Accolate) is the only available leukotriene antagonist in the U.S. and this oral agent has no immediate bronchodilator effect. Therefore, it has no significant value in an acute, evolving asthma attack. For patients with chronic asthma, Accolate shows promise in reducing the need for symptomatic relief and steroids. Clinical benefit usually takes about three days. The recommended dosage is 20 mg twice a day. Food reduces the bioavailability and therefore, doses should be taken at least 1 hr before or 2 hrs after meals. Side effects include inhibition of the cytochrome p450 system and reversible hepatic dysfunction. This medication is approved for use in all athletes.

D. **Objective monitoring.** Twice-daily peak flow monitoring is advantageous to optimize asthma control. It is important for athletes with abnormal resting airway function to monitor peak flows with medication to check for efficacy. Patients need prompt assessment by a physician if their peak flows do not improve above 70% of baseline values after medication.

E. **Athletic participation.** Acute exacerbations of asthma are not compatible with physical activity. Once the acute episode has been brought under control and return of greater than 85% to 90% of baseline pulmonary function is documented, the athlete can return to activity. The asthmatic athlete should be discouraged from scuba diving, as this poses a risk of life-threatening barotrauma due to air trapping (see Chapter 14).

V. Prevention of EIA.

For unrestricted athletic participation, prevention of EIA is highly desirable. Pharmacologic management is superior to nonpharmacologic management in terms of prevention.

A. **Pharmacologic**

1. **The athlete with normal resting airway function.**

a. ***Beta$_2$***-agonists (e.g., albuterol) are up to 95% effective in preventing EIA when used as an aerosol (two puffs with an MDI or nebulizer). They should be used 10 to 15 min prior to competition. **Albuterol** works well for up to 1 to 2 hr. ***Metaproterenol*** is effective for only 30 min. Children can take the medication orally 30 to 60 min prior to exercise, but the medication is not as effective in preventing EIA. Oral beta$_2$-agonists are banned by both the NCAA and the IOC. Written documentation is required by the U.S. Olympic Committee (USOC) for an athlete using an inhaled beta$_2$ agonist. ***Salmeterol*** (Serevent) may provide prevention of EIA for up to 12 hr. This medication should be inhaled 1 hr before exercise (two puffs with an MDI). ***Rapid acting beta$_2$***-agonists should be the only treatment for an acute attack.

b. **Khellin derivatives** (cromolyn and nedocromil), taken (two puffs) 15 to 45 min before exercise, are 70% to 85% effective in preventing EIA for up to 2 hr. They can be used in synergy with beta$_2$ agonists in hard-to-control EIA, and particularly effective for athletes who experience late-phase bronchospasm.

c. **Rapid-release theophylline** is a third-line medication because of its possible side effects. The oral dose is 5 mg/kg 1 hr prior to exercise.

2. **Athletes with abnormal resting airway function.** These athletes typically require a combination of beta$_2$-agonists and inhaled steroids and/or khellin derivatives. The timing of their medications to prevent

EIA is as described previously. ***Inhaled corticosteroids*** have no isolated effect on the early EIA response. However, they may be useful in inhibiting the late-phase response.

3. **Other drugs**
   a. **Anticholinergics.** Ipratropium bromide has not been conclusively shown to prevent EIA but can modulate the symptoms. It can be used in persons who cannot tolerate $beta_2$-agonists.
   b. **Antihistamines** do not prevent EIA but can decrease nasal congested in athletes with allergic rhinitis. Long-acting antihistamines should be taken one hour before activity.
   c. **Calcium antagonists** are believed to inhibit mast cell release and possibly relax bronchial smooth muscle in select patients. They have not been well studied for EIA prevention.
   d. **Leukotriene antagonists.** The data is limited on the effect of these drugs on EIA, but for those patients who do not get sufficient prophylaxis with inhaled $beta_2$-antagonists, and khellin derivatives, and/or inhaled steroids, a trial of zafirlukast administered 2 hours before activity may provide incremental benefit. There is some evidence of the development of drug tolerance with chronic therapy. Therefore, low doses (10–20 mg) may be ineffective over time for EIA prophylaxis.

B. **Nonpharmacologic** (see also section IV.B above, this chapter). Approximately 50% of individuals with EIA are believed to be able to induce a ***refractory period*** following exercise. EIA may be decreased or prevented by performing either high-intensity exercise for 3 to 4 min or a low-intensity warm-up about 1 hr prior to the event. There is no easy way to predict who can or cannot induce a refractory period. Aerobic training may have some preventative benefit by improving cardiorespiratory fitness allowing more efficient work.

Pneumathorax

A pneumothorax is a collection of air within the pleural space, usually resulting from injury to the lung parenchyma with a subsequent air leak. In some cases, a hole in the chest wall may allow air to enter the pleural space because of the negative intrathoracic pressure. A pneumothorax can be an on-the-field medical emergency. Prompt recognition and treatment are critical.

I. Etiology

A. **Traumatic** pneumothorax is usually due to high-energy, blunt trauma, either penetrating or nonpenetrating, and, in athletes, found more commonly than spontaneous pneumothorax. It is most common in collision sports such as football, ice hockey, karate, or boxing. It has been reported in scuba diving, baseball, and softball. Some 3% of clavicular fractures are associated with apical pneumothorax. In athletes, rib fractures rarely result in pneumothorax.

B. **Spontaneous** pneumothorax can occur without evidence of trauma. This has been most associated with running but has also been reported in weight training. One mechanism is rupture of alveolar blebs or bullae, which are often unsuspected, due to increased intrathoracic pressure with physical activity. Individuals with underlying pulmonary disease—cystic fibrosis, chronic obstructive pulmonary disease (CODD), asthma, Marfan's Syndrome) or drug use (cocaine)—may be at higher risk for spontaneous pneumothorax than healthy individuals.

C. **Tension** pneumothorax is a life-threatening emergency. It results from accumulation of air in the pleural space with inspiration that cannot escape with expiration. Compression of the heart restricting venous return and compression of the contralateral lung can occur, producing cardiac arrest.

II. Diagnosis

A. **Clinical presentation.** Localized, pleuritic chest pain, dyspnea, and tachypnea are frequently reported. The chest pain may radiate to the neck, abdomen, or low back. Some individuals with small (up to 25%) pneumothoraces are asymptomatic. Traumatic pneumothoraces usually present with evidence of chest trauma. An athlete with a tension pneumothorax will present acutely ill and may deteriorate rapidly. On physical examination, tachycardia and tachypnea are common. Hyperexpansion of the affected hemithorax with absent or decreased breath sounds is found. Hyperresonance to percusssion, crepitation, and subcutaneous emphysema may be detected. Cyanosis usually indicates a tension pneumothorax and can be seen with contralateral tracheal deviation, neck vein distention, and laterally displaced cardiac impulse.

B. **Chest radiographs** most effectively demonstrate the pneumothorax. Usually, an anteroposterior view is sufficient to confirm the diagnosis, but additional views may be required.

III. Treatment.

Occasionally, if the pneumothorax is small and asymptomatic, the athlete can be followed until resolution is documented. However, surgical intervention with needle aspiration or chest tube placement may be required. On the field, treatment prior to prompt hospital transport should consist of airway maintenance and oxygen administration. Vital signs should be monitored closely for signs of deterioration. If a tension pneumothorax is suspected, emergency management may be necessary prior to transport. A large-bore intravenous catheter should be inserted into the chest over the top of the third or fourth rib in the midclavicular line. A "hissing" sound due to air escaping through the needle is proof of a tension pneumothorax. The needle should be removed, leaving the catheter open to the air. Positive-pressure ventilation via bag and mask or endotracheal tube or spontaneous ventilation should reexpand the lung adequately for transport to the hospital.

IV. Return to activity.

Usually the chest tube can be removed in 24 to 72 hr. There should be no radiographic evidence of pneumothorax before return to activity is permitted. Return to conditioning activities can occur in 3 to 4 weeks, and return to competition should be based on adequate conditioning.

Cystic Fibrosis

Cystic fibrosis (CF) is the most common genetic disorder affecting whites, with an incidence of 1 in 2000. The genetic defect adversely affects epithelial cell chloride permeability. Inheritance is autosomal recessive and multiple organ systems are variably affected. Persons with mild forms of the disease may be participants in competitive or recreational sports. Systems primarily affected are the pulmonary, gastrointestinal, reproductive, and skeletal systems and the sweat glands. Chronic pulmonary disease accounts for the majority of the morbidity, with thick mucus altering pulmonary function and serving as a nidus for infection. Respiratory manifestations include cough, hemoptysis, dyspnea, wheezing, and purulent sputum.

I. Diagnosis.

An abnormal sweat chloride test is diagnostic of cystic fibrosis. Chest radiographs may reveal interstitial disease and bronchiectasis. Sputum culture during exacerbations demonstrates multiple organisms including *Pseudomonas, Staphylococcus aureus,* and *Haemophilus influenza.* Pulmonary function tests show an obstructive pattern similar to that of the asthmatic but with a decreased forced vital capacity.

II. Management.

Therapy must be individualized depending on the extent of organ system involvement. Since this is a progressive disease, an aggressive management plan to decrease the number of respiratory infections is appropriate in all except the mildest cases. Chest physiotherapy, antibiotics, and bronchodilators are the mainstays of treatment. Other treatments include oxygen therapy, glucocorticosteroids, recombinant deoxyribonuclease I, and, in severe cases, lung transplantation.

III. Exercise.

Whether exercise improves life expectancy is debatable, but the quality of life for the patient with CF can be improved with an exercise program. There is a wide range of fitness levels in patients with CF. Athletes with mild CF should be permitted to compete without restriction as their pulmonary function allows. Moderate levels (30 min, three times per week) of aerobic exercise such as swimming, cycling, and running, can improve cardiorespiratory fitness and ventilatory muscle endurance for the recreational athlete. Exercise increases the production of mucus and is an effective pulmonary toilet in concert with chest physiotherapy. Athletes with CF need to be counseled concerning exercise in the heat, since they lose more sodium and chloride in their sweat than do their healthy counterparts. Individuals whose CF causes oxygen desaturation need exercise testing with oximetry monitoring to determine a safe level of exercise.

Chronic Obstructive Pulmonary Disease

It is estimated that 20 million Americans suffer from chronic obstructive pulmonary disease (COPD). Primarily comprising emphysema and chronic bronchitis, this progressive condition of expiratory airflow obstruction generally leads to the development of disabling dyspnea and a subsequent loss of exercise capacity. As a result, the sports medicine physician is likely to encounter it among recreational athletes rather than higher-level performers. The most common etiology for COPD is chronic tobacco use, but genetic factors, including alpha$_1$-antitrypsin deficiency and other medical conditions, may play a role. The natural history of the disease is that of slowly deteriorating pulmonary function, but optimal medical management coupled with a comprehensive exercise program may be of substantial benefit.

I. Pathophysiology.

The pathophysiology of COPD is multifactorial. ***Airways obstruction*** may arise from excessive intrinsic airway reactivity or increased production of respiratory secretions in response to chronic inflammation. Chronic air trapping and hyperinflation cause ***respiratory muscle dysfunction.*** Skeletal muscles may also be weakened by a poor nutritional status and chronic corticosteroid use, both common in COPD patients. The end result is ***generalized deconditioning*** as muscles work less efficiently, lead to lower thresholds of fatigue, and place greater demands on a weakened pulmonary reserve. Progressive ***destruction of alveolar-capillary membranes,*** as in emphysema, causes altered gas exchange, hypoxemia, and poor tissue oxygenation. Pulmonary vascular remodeling, ***pulmonary hypertension (cor pulmonale),*** and right ventricular failure may result from altered hemodynamics in response to chronic hypoxemia. ***Fear and anxiety*** aroused by breathlessness may severely limit the functional status of patients with COPD. Together these factors combine to cause a characteristic obstructive pulmonary pattern, evidenced by a reduction in forced expiratory volume in 1 sec (FEV$_1$) and increased work of breathing. The FEV$_1$ is the standard means by which to assess the clinical course and prognosis. When the FEV$_1$ falls to less than 1 L, 5-year survival is only 50%.

II. Evaluation.

Prior to exercise prescription, patients should undergo a thorough physical assessment to target the major factors contributing to their pulmonary dysfunction.

A. **Physical exam** should assess respiratory rate and breathing pattern, presence of compensatory tachycardia, efficiency of diaphragmatic excursion, posture, and skeletal muscular strength.

B. **Pulmonary function tests** should be used to quantitate the degree of airway obstruction and to predict the maximal sustainable ventilation during exercise (35 times the FEV_1). Ventilatory muscle effort as measured by maximum inspiratory pressure should be evaluated at rest and with activity.

C. **Blood gas analysis** will determine baseline oxygenation, degree of hypercapnia, and acid-base status.

D. **ECG, hematocrit, and thyroid function tests** should be considered as clinically warranted.

E. **Exercise testing** is recommended for all patients. Many protocols exist, most of which are based on a timed walking test (12-min walk) or walking endurance time on a treadmill, providing direct assessment of a patient's exercise performance. Heart rate, blood pressure, ventilation, oxygen saturation, and oxygen consumption can be measured while subjective ratings of breathlessness and perceived exertion are obtained.

III. Management.

The management of the active COPD patient is directed toward the maintenance or improvement of functional capacity and the elimination of any performance-impairing symptoms. Once an exercise evaluation of performance is complete, specific treatments are prescribed to correct those factors which most limit pulmonary function and exercise capacity.

A. **Pharmacologic.**

1. Athletic COPD patients should receive aggressive ***bronchodilator therapy,*** including $beta_2$-adrenergic agonists and inhaled corticosteroids, to improve airway obstruction and increase the FEV_1.
2. **Anticholinergic agents** such as inhaled ipratropium bromide are now recommended in the routine management of virtually all COPD cases, regardless of functional level.
3. **Oral theophylline** may provide some therapeutic benefit in more severe COPD although it remains controversial. ***Oral corticosteroids*** should be reserved for refractory cases with documented steroid responsiveness.
4. **Influenza and polyvalent pneumococcal vaccines** should be administered to all COPD patients because of their increased susceptibility to these pulmonary infections.

B. **Mechanical** Athletic patients with more significant pulmonary disease may benefit from several mechanical interventions. Those with chronic bronchitis can receive vigorous ***bronchopulmonary toilet*** to limit the resultant airway obstruction. COPD athletes who breath inefficiently with high respiratory rates and shallow breaths should practice ***pursed-lips breathing*** to retard exhalation and lead to slower, deeper, more efficient breaths.

C. **Exercise** in chronic pulmonary disease has been shown to improve exercise endurance, anaerobic threshold, and achievable workloads; to decrease the ventilatory requirement and perception of dyspnea and fatigue; and to improve ventilatory efficiency through a slowed respiratory rate. Patients also experience an improvement in sense of well-being and confidence, sleep, and appetite. Athletically active patients with COPD likely exercise for intrinsic physical and psychological reasons. Nevertheless, the beneficial effects of this activity on their pulmonary status should be emphasized. Special care should be taken when patients are exercising on cold, windy days in the winter or hot, humid days in the summer as airway reactivity will be increased. In the setting of an acute exacerbation, regular exercise activities should be halted until airway reactivity decreases and adequate oxygenation with exertion is maintained.

Respiratory Infections

Respiratory infections, particularly of the upper respiratory tract, are among the most common encountered in the care of athletes and their effects on training and performance may be substantial. Proper evaluation and management of these conditions is essential for the athlete's safe return to play.

I. Exercise and Immunity.

A number of studies now support the concept that there is a "J curve" relationship between exercise and the development of an upper respiratory infection. Moderate exercise seems to confer relative resistance to infection while the extremes of a sedentary lifestyle or intense exercise may exert a detrimental effect on the immune status. The exact mechanisms of this effect are not well understood, and further study is clearly indicated.

II. Prevention.

To minimize the risk of infection, avoidance of overtraining, chronic fatigue, inadequate sleep, poor nutrition, and psychological stress is recommended. Athletes who train in large groups or who travel extensively need to be aware of their increased risk for communicable diseases as well.

III. Respiratory infections.

The majority of respiratory infections in athletes and nonathletes alike are viral upper respiratory processes. Other pathogens and other locations in the respiratory tree are less common; nevertheless, these disorders may present with a broad spectrum of clinical manifestations, and a definitive diagnosis is often difficult.

A. **Viral upper respiratory infections** are caused by a number of viral strains including echoviruses, rhinoviruses, coronaviruses, and coxsackie strains. Most cause common cold symptoms (nasal discharge and obstruction, sneezing, sore throat, cough, and hoarseness) without constitutional involvement. The course is self-limited over several days and generally causes little athletic disability. A postviral fatigue syndrome consisting of persistent malaise, fatigue, lassitude, and aching muscles is being increasingly reported. Symptoms may persist for months or years, and no specific treatment is presently available.

B. **Flu-like syndromes** are typically caused by influenza strains, parainfluenza, respiratory syncytial virus, and adenovirus. The clinical picture is one of abrupt onset of intense malaise, myalgias, headache, fever—up to 41°C (106°F)—and nonproductive cough. Substantial morbidity may last 1 to 2 weeks and influenza may occur in pandemics. The course may be complicated by the development of significant airway hyperreactivity, myositis, and influenza pneumonia.

C. **Bronchitis,** an inflammatory condition of the tracheobronchial tree, results from infection with common cold viruses, influenza, adenovirus, *Mycoplasma pneumoniae, Chlamydia pneumoniae,* and *Moraxella catarrhalis.* Patients generally have cough with mild to moderate sputum production and a paucity of systemic signs of infection. Pulmonary function with exercise, however, may be affected, particularly in patients with asthma or reactive airway disease. The course is generally self-limited.

D. **Pneumonia** develops less frequently in the athletic population. Common etiologies are bacterial, most frequently *S. pneumoniae, M. catarrhalis,* and *H. influenzae.* Primary viral etiologies are rare. Clinical manifestations are variable, ranging from indolent to fulminant, but most patients experience shaking chills, fever, pleuritic chest pain, cough with purulent sputum, and dyspnea. Treated patients generally show resolution in 5 to 10 days, but the severity of the acute illness warrants restriction from sports participation.

E. **Atypical pneumonias** comprise the majority of pneumonias in patients under age 40. *Mycoplasma pneumoniae* is the most common etiology. Patients classically present with a flu-like illness with fever, headache, prominent myalgias and malaise. Nonproductive hacking cough with substernal chest pain is prominent. In severe cases, dyspnea may develop. Many patients, however, may have mild symptoms and only a minimal degree of morbidity or dysfunction. Among other etiologies, the presence of diarrhea, renal failure, or central nervous system (CNS) dysfunction should suggest *Legionella* infection.

IV. Management goals are to assess the nature and severity of the illness, initiate appropriate therapy, minimize complications, and plan for a safe return to full sport participation. Athletes should greatly decrease the volume and intensity of their training, obtain adequate rest, and maintain adequate hydration, especially if fever is present. Except for very mild cases, athletes should generally seek a medical evaluation to ensure that appropriate measures are being taken and regardless of other clinical features; athletes with fever should not participate in strenuous physical activities.

A. **Viral upper respiratory infections.** The athlete who has symptoms of the common cold without constitutional involvement may resume regular training after the resolution of clinical illness. It is important to note, however, that mild exercise during sickness with the common cold does not appear to be contraindicated and may thus allow some degree of training to continue. Primary therapy is with decongestants (all sympathomimetics are banned in athletes competing in Olympic/international competition), antitussives, and analgesics. Maintenance of adequate hydration with the use of sympathomimetics is particularly important.

B. **Influenza.** Care is primarily supportive and symptomatic. Initiation of ***amantadine or rimantadine*** therapy (100 mg p.o. b.i.d.) for the treatment of influenza A may be considered within 48 hr of the onset of symptoms in high-risk patients (those with multiple contacts or serious co-morbidities). Therapy should be continued until the patient is asymptomatic for 48 hr. Resumption of training may be allowed after resolution of fever, significant myalgias, and respiratory compromise. A yearly ***influenza vaccination*** should be recommended to all athletes and highly recommended to athletes who compete in the late fall or winter seasons.

C. **Bronchitis.** Care is symptomatic. Marked sputum production or associated signs of infection may prompt antibiotic therapy. In the uncomplicated case, participation is not limited. Those patients with airway reactivity may need additional recuperative time prior to full activities and benefit from short-term inhaled bronchodilator therapy (eg. albuterol MDI, 2 puffs every 4 to 6 hr).

D. **Pneumonia.** Community-acquired pneumonias may cause sufficient morbidity to warrant intravenous antibiotics and hospitalization. Following the resolution of fever, cough, purulent sputum production, and dyspnea and the completion of antibiotic therapy, slow return to activity is permitted.

E. **Atypical pneumonias** are more variable in their clinical presentation. Moderately to severely ill patients require antibiotic therapy (erythromycin, tetracycline, azithromycin, or clarithromycin) and may need hospitalization. Evaluation for return to play is the same as for pneumonia. Those patients with mild clinical symptoms may return to athletic activity prior to the completion of therapy if fever has resolved and respiratory status is stable with exertion. Both of these processes require close follow-up to assess for relapse (seen in 10% of *M. pneumoniae* cases), or late complications.

Suggested Reading

Cooper CB. Determining the role of exercise in patients with chronic pulmonary disease. *Med Sci Sports Exerc* 1995;27:147–157.

Hough DO, Dec KL. Exercise-induced asthma and anaphylaxis. *Sports Med* 1994; 18:162–172.

National Asthma Education and Prevention Program. *Guidelines for the diagnosis and management of asthma. NIH Publication 91-3042.* Washington, DC: U.S. Government Printing Office, 1997:97–4051.

Nieman DC. Exercise, upper respiratory tract infection, and the immune system. *Med Sci Sports Exerc* 1994;26:128–139.

Orenstein DM. Exercise tolerance and exercise conditioning in children with chronic lung Disease. *J Pediatr* 1988;112:1043–1047.

Volk CP, Mc Farland EG, Horsman G. Pneumothorax: on-field management. *Phys Sportsmed* 1996;23:43–46.

28. HEMATOLOGY

E. Randy Eichner

Common hematological issues in sports medicine involve (1) defining the normal hematocrit or hemoglobin (Hb) level for an athlete; (2) understanding the nature of "sports anemia"; (3) deciding if athletes - especially female athletes - are uniquely prone to developing iron deficiency; (4) determining the sites and causes of blood or iron loss in athletes; (5) recognizing the early-warning symptoms of anemia; (6) informing athletes on how to get enough iron from their diet; (7) resolving the debate on whether a low serum ferritin level, in the absence of anemia, can cause fatigue or impair athletic performance; (8) mitigating footstrike or exertional hemolysis; and (9) understanding the sports implications of sickle cell trait. These issues are covered below.

I. Anemia

Anemia, or at least the finding of a low Hb concentration, is a common problem among certain athletes, especially endurance athletes, women more than men. Anemia is defined as a decrease in the circulating red blood cell (RBC) mass; a common criterion is an Hb concentration under 14 g/dL in men or under 13 g/dL in women.

The habit of defining anemia by level of hematocrit should be dropped, because by modern laboratory methods—electronic blood counters—hematocrit is a calculated value and thus more subject to error than is Hb concentration, which is measured directly.

Anemia is not a diagnosis but just a sign of disease, and the potential causes of anemia are many. So the finding of a low Hb concentration calls for thoughtful analysis to pinpoint the cause of the anemia before the proper treatment can be given.

Although any athlete can in theory have any type of anemia—can be born with thalassemia minor or hereditary spherocytosis, for example—the three most common contributors to a low Hb level in an athlete are "sports anemia," iron-deficiency anemia, and "footstrike" hemolysis. Probably the most common, at least in endurance athletes, is sports anemia.

II. Sports Anemia

Athletes, especially endurance athletes (assuming they are training at sea level) tend to have lower Hb levels than do their nonathletic counterparts. In other words, endurance athletes tend to be judged as slightly "anemic" as compared with norms from the general population. This has been called sports anemia.

A. **Mechanism.** The term *sports anemia,* however, poses two problems. First, it is imprecise: there is no one anemia tied to sports. Second, it is a misnomer, because the most common cause of a low Hb concentration in an endurance athlete is not a true anemia. Rather, it is a false anemia, due to regular aerobic exercise, which expands the baseline plasma volume and thus dilutes the RBC and Hb concentration. In other words, the naturally lower Hb level of an endurance athlete is a *dilutional pseudoanemia.*

Dilutional pseudoanemia is most likely an adaptation to the acute loss of plasma volume, or hemoconcentration, that occurs early in each workout. Vigorous exercise acutely reduces plasma volume by (1) increasing mean arterial blood pressure and muscular compression of venules, both of which boost capillary hydrostatic pressure; (2) generating lactic acid and other metabolites in the working muscles, thus increasing tissue osmotic pressure; and (3) producing sweat.

Presumably in adaptation to this repeated hemoconcentration, the body releases renin, aldosterone, and vasopressin to conserve water and salt. Also, albumin is added to the blood. As a result, the baseline plasma volume expands. The increase in baseline plasma volume—and the accompanying dilutional decrease in Hb concentration—range from about 5% in recreational joggers to about 20% in elite marathoners.

B. **Diagnosis.** The diagnosis of dilutional pseudoanemia is enabled by knowing its likely setting (aerobic training) and by excluding other types of anemia, especially iron-deficiency anemia.

C. **Natural history.** The baseline plasma volume waxes and wanes quickly in response to level of physical activity. Plasma volume can expand by 10% within 1 day after a single hard exercise bout or by up to 500 mL after 1 week of intense daily cycling workouts. When daily workouts are stopped, however, the plasma volume shrinks as fast as it once expanded. The rise in baseline plasma volume correlates with the amount and intensity of habitual exercise, so the athletes who train the most and the hardest tend to have the lowest Hb levels.

Athletic pseudoanemia is a cardinal part of aerobic fitness. The rise in plasma volume increases the cardiac stroke volume. This increase more than offsets the fall in Hb concentration per unit of blood, so that more oxygen is delivered to muscles. As a benefit, dilutional pseudoanemia is to be desired, not prevented or treated.

III. Iron-Deficiency Anemia

The most common "true" anemia in athletes, as in the general population, is iron-deficiency anemia. Iron-deficiency anemia is rare in male athletes unless they have bled from the gastrointestinal tract but common in female athletes, who have physiologic depletions of iron. Probably at any one time about 20% of athletic women are iron-deficient and about 5% have iron-deficiency anemia.

A. **Etiology.** The older sports medicine literature suggests that athletic women are especially likely to develop iron-deficiency anemia. This conclusion, however, is unwarranted, because many published studies lack proper nonexercising controls and/or fail to consider the probable presence of dilutional pseudoanemia. In fact, more recent, better-controlled studies suggest little or no difference in iron balance between athletic women and nonathletic controls.

Athletes generally lose trivial amounts of iron in sweat, and hematuria is neither common nor a noteworthy drain of iron; therefore the principal cause of iron deficiency in athletic women, as in nonathletic women, is insufficient iron in their diet to meet their physiologic needs. Women who lose more than 60 mL of blood per menses are more likely to develop iron-deficiency anemia. Pregnancy is another key physiologic depletor of iron stores.

The recommended dietary allowance (RDA) for iron for women is at least 15 mg per day. Many competitive female athletes, however, especially the "low-weight" athletes (e.g., ballet dancers, gymnasts, ice skaters, divers, distance runners) consume no more than 2,000 kilocalories per day, which translates to only 12 mg of iron a day. In other words, they consume too little iron for their needs.

Another factor is the increasing trend among female athletes toward eating vegetarian or vegetarian-like diets. The iron in grains and vegetables is not highly bioavailable, and several studies suggest that female athletes who avoid red meat are prone to iron deficiency. Finally, when evaluating any athlete for presumed iron deficiency, the possibility of gastrointestinal bleeding must be considered. Such bleeding in athletes is covered in Chapter 30.

B. **History and physical exam.** Unlike dilutional pseudoanemia, which causes no symptoms, iron-deficiency anemia causes fatigue that impairs athletic performance. Unlike most other common causes of fatigue, that from mild or moderate anemia occurs only during exertion, not at rest. Often, the first sign of mild anemia is a fall-off in maximal performance. For example, the athlete begins to lose races he or she used to win.

Presenting symtoms of anemia during all-out exertion include (1) undue dyspnea; (2) early and heavy sweating; and (3) heavy, "burning" limbs, nausea, and even retching from the rapid accumulation of lactic acid. As the anemia worsens, the athlete may notice cold intolerance at rest.

One should ask about medications, drug use (including alcohol), change in bowel habits or stool appearance, and any other possible routes of blood loss, including blood donation. Ice-craving or chewing (pagophagia)—and/or the constant eating of raw, crunchy vegetables—can suggest iron-deficiency anemia but is not an indicator of mild anemia. One should look for hemorrhoids or anal fissures and test the stool for occult blood.

C. **Diagnosis.** In the presence of anemia, the *diagnostic triad* for iron deficiency anemia is (1) low RBC mean cell volume (MCV); (2) microcytic, hypochromic RBCs in the peripheral blood smear; and (3) low serum ferritin level (i.e., below 12 ng/dL).

D. **Treatment.** It is crucial to find and correct any source of blood loss. The best treatment for iron-deficiency anemia is ferrous sulfate, 325 mg three times a day with meals. If the athlete cannot tolerate (because of gastrointestinal symptoms) that dose of iron, a smaller dose will do: settle for one tablet a day, with dinner. Ideally, after a delay of about a week, the Hb should rise about 1 g/dL per week. After the Hb is again normal, the athlete should continue to take iron for several months to replenish body stores.

E. **Prevention.** Practical tips for prevention include the following: (1) eat more lean red meat and dark meat of chicken (in contrast to the iron in vegetarian diets, iron in meat is highly bioavailable); (2) to enhance iron absorption from bread and cereal (these staples are iron-fortified), avoid coffee or tea (which contain iron-chelating substances) with meals and consume instead a source of vitamin C, such as orange juice; (3) cook scrambled eggs and acidic foods (e.g., tomato sauce, applesauce, vegetable soup) in cast-iron skillets and pots to leach iron into the food; (4) eat white poultry or seafood (which contain little iron) with dried beans, peas, or other legumes because the animal protein increases the absorption of iron from the legumes.

When an athlete (usually a female athlete) repeatedly develops iron-deficiency anemia despite dietary advice, consider giving ferrous sulfate, 325 mg three times a week, for prevention. If they are otherwise indicated, oral contraceptives can regulate menses and thereby minimize menstrual blood loss.

F. **Low serum ferritin.** The older sports medicine literature suggests that low ferritin alone ("nonanemic low ferritin") is a cause of fatigue. However, the best evidence belies this claim. For example, when mild iron-deficiency anemia was induced by venesection of healthy male runners and the anemia—but not the iron deficiency—was obviated by transfusion, the men's exercise capacity was unchanged from baseline. Also, recent studies agree that when nonanemic female athletes with low ferritin are treated with iron, they experience an increase in ferritin level but not in Hb or exercise capacity. In short, a low serum ferritin level reflects low iron stores but does not impair athletic performance.

The clinical problem is that one cannot always distinguish dilutional pseudoanemia, which does no harm, from very mild iron-deficiency anemia, which impairs athletic performance. If in doubt, a 2-month trial of empiric iron therapy is prudent. An increase in Hb of at least 1 g/dL is the empiric "gold standard" for diagnosing iron-deficiency anemia.

IV. Footstrike Hemolysis

In theory, "footstrike" hemolysis, an *intravascular* hemolysis, the bursting of RBCs in the bloodstream as the foot strikes the ground, has the potential to drain iron stores and contribute to anemia in certain athletes. With intravascular hemolysis, free hemoglobin spills into the plasma, where it binds to haptoglobin, which delivers it to the liver for salvage. The plasma content of haptoglobin, however, can drop to zero if enough red cells—about 20 mL—are hemolyzed. When this happens, some hemoglobin and its iron are lost in the urine.

Fortunately, the footstrikes of most athletes are not forceful enough to exhaust haptoglobin, even during marathons or triathlons. Even if a distance runner were to exhaust haptoglobin in a long race, only tiny amounts of iron would be lost, because haptoglobin is regenerated quickly. The regimens of even elite marathoners thus seem likely only to lower haptoglobin, not to exhaust it. Consequently, footstrike hemolysis is a negligible drain of iron stores and does not cause noteworthy anemia in endurance athletes.

Actually, footstrike hemolysis, initially attributed to impact, is better termed "exertional" hemolysis, because it is seen, for example, in distance swimmers, whose sport involves no impact. It has also been seen in rowers, aerobic dancers, and even weight lifters.

A. **Mechanism.** Probably some exertional hemolysis in athletes is from impact and some from other physical forces, possibly turbulent blood flow in the microvasculature of working muscles, along with the exposure of RBCs traversing such muscles owing to the rigors of dehydration, acidosis, and elevated temperatures.

B. **Diagnosis.** The *diagnostic triad* is (1) high MCV, (2) elevated reticulocyte count, and (3) low serum haptoglobin concentration. All three abnormalities are mild. The blood smear is usually normal, although a rare crenated RBC may be seen. The MCV is slightly elevated (but rarely more than 105 fl) because older (and consequently smaller) RBCs are preferentially destroyed and replaced by younger (and larger) reticulocytes. Visible hemoglobinuria is rare because, as mentioned above, haptoglobin is rarely exhausted.

C. **Treatment.** In general, exertional hemolysis among recreational athletes needs no treatment. It is usually so mild that it causes no anemia; the bone marrow of the iron-replete athlete can easily increase RBC production enough to offset mild hemolysis (i.e., mild reticulocytosis prevents anemia).

   Among elite aerobic athletes, however, even mild hemolysis that causes no anemia can in theory limit the adaptive increase in RBC mass that is part of the key to winning at the world-class level. In this case, treatment involves the following measures to lessen impact: (1) wearing better-cushioned shoes; (2) losing weight; (3) avoiding a "stomping" gait and learning to run "light on the feet;" and (4) running on soft surfaces such as dirt roads or grass.

V. Sickle Cell Trait

Sickle cell trait (SCT), present in about 8% of American blacks and in about one in 10,000 American whites, is generally benign. As a rule, athletes with SCT have no anemia, no blood smear abnormalities, and few or no clinical consequences. Isosthenuria (inability to concentrate urine) does tend to develop with age, which may predispose athletes to dehydration. There is also a small risk for gross hematuria and for splenic infarction at moderate altitude.

In general, SCT does not impair top athletic performance. In laboratory tests of exercise capacity, for example, subjects with SCT perform as well as control subjects. Also, in top-level sports—the National Football League, for example—there are the expected number of players with SCT, suggesting that SCT is compatible with championship performance.

Very rarely, however, especially in harsh environments—as when new to altitude or to a hot, humid climate—SCT athletes who charge recklessly into strenuous workouts are at risk of sickling, collapse, and death.

A. **History and physical examination.** The exercise-induced collapse in SCT has been mistaken for hyperventilation, syncope, heat stroke, or cardiac arrest. But the pattern of collapse in SCT is unique.

   In most cases, the SCT athlete is a football or basketball player new to altitude or summer heat. Collapses have also occurred in runners in distance races. Typically, on the first or second day of team practice, during a bout of intense exercise (e.g., a timed shuttle or track run), the athlete develops excruciating cramping pain in the legs, buttocks, and lower back. This soon leads to collapse on the field, with impaired consciousness, hyperventilation, tachycardia, and hypotension.

B. **Mechanism.** This SCT collapse is caused by (1) sickling of RBCs in working limbs (legs); (2) fulminant rhabdomyolysis from continued exertion in the face of ischemia from sickling; (3) severe lactic acidosis from extreme anaerobic metabolism in ischemic muscles; and (4) shock.

   Unless diagnosis and proper therapy are immediate, the sequence that soon follows is (1) acute renal failure (from released myoglobin, uric acid, and other muscle metabolites); (2) hyperkalemia; (3) ventricular fibrillation; and (4) death.

C. **Diagnosis.** Diagnosis of the exercise collapse in SCT hinges on knowing the unique setting and clinical features described above. Diagnosis of SCT itself is by (1) screening with a simple, fast, blood-drop solubility test (e.g., Sickledex) and (2) confirmation by cellulose acetate hemoglobin electrophoresis.

D. **Treatment.** Prompt recognition, proper diagnosis, and emergent care to prevent acute renal failure and hyperkalemia are critical. Collapsed patients must have full support of vital signs and be given fluids intravenously as they are rushed to the hospital.

E. **Prevention.** All athletes, with SCT or not, should be taught to train wisely, stay hydrated, rest when sick, heed environmental stress and early warning symptoms (e.g., excruciating muscle cramps), and never charge recklessly into maximal exertion.

   Sports medicine physicians can help to educate coaches about this rare but grave syndrome. Coaches should enforce preseason conditioning to the climate that will be encountered and should not schedule all-out runs for the early days of training camp. Probably all young athletes, black or white, should be given the opportunity for informed screening for SCT.

F. **Return to play.** If an SCT athlete survives one collapse, return to the same sport, climate, conditions, and workout is probably inadvisable. Such decisions, of course, must be individualized, but they should be approached with great caution.

Suggested Reading

Eichner ER. Anemia in female athletes. *Patient Fitness* 1989;3:3–11.

Eichner ER. Gastrointestinal bleeding in athletes. *Phys Sportsmed* 1989;17:128–140.

Eichner ER. Sickle cell trait, heroic exercise, and fatal collapse. *Phys Sportsmed* 1993;21:51–64.

Harris SS. Helping active women avoid anemia. *Phys Sportsmed* 1995;23:35–48.

Selby GB, Eichner ER. Hematocrit and performance: effect of endurance training on blood volume. *Semin Hematol* 1994;31:122–127.

29. DERMATOLOGY

Wilma F. Bergfeld and Thomas N. Helm

I. Introduction

Skin disorders are commonly encountered in athletes. Prompt diagnosis and rapid treatment can often prevent time lost from competition or training. Every effort should be made to arrive at a precise diagnosis in infectious dermatoses so that other athletes are not put at risk.

II. Mechanical Problems

A. **Corns** are localized, painful conical thickenings of skin and keratin most commonly found on the dorsa and sides of toes. Calluses are similar but larger and appear primarily on the plantar aspect of feel or hands. Both appear at areas of friction or bony abnormalities. Attention to properly fitted and padded footwear will greatly diminish the likelihood of corns. Pads containing salicylic acid, applied topically, will also cause chemical keratolysis and diminish corns. We favor gentle debridement with a pumice stone after a shower or bath. When the skin has been moistened, the hyperkeratosis can be controlled easily and painlessly, minimizing discomfort. Lotions that contain lactic acid, urea, or propylene glycol are also helpful.

B. **Blisters** are commonly encountered after prolonged shearing forces impact upon the skin. Intraepidermal blister formation is most common. Excessive moisture in footwear from perspiration or from inclement weather increases frictional forces, just as it is more difficult to pull a wet piece of paper across a tabletop than a dry one. If footwear is too loose, excessive movement will exacerbate the condition. Wearing dry shoes with absorbent socks is most important. Foot powder can be helpful and some athletes benefit from the use of emollient lotion.

When blisters occur, they should be left intact whenever possible. The moist and sterile environment within the blister enhances reepithelization. If the blister is in an awkward location, drainage may be achieved by preparing the skin with an alcohol pledgel, inserting an 18-gauge needle, and withdrawing the blister fluid. Removing the blister roof is usually unnecessary and may actually increase discomfort. A thin coating of antibiotic ointment (bacitracin, polymyxin, or mupirocin) will prevent secondary infection. Hydrocolloid dressings can also be used, they enhance healing but may not be worth the additional expense.

C. **Purpura** occur when there is hemorrhage in the skin. At times intracorneal hemorrhage may occur, this is referred to as *talon noir*. Athletes may note the dark discoloration in the skin and fear that they have an atypical pigmented lesion such as a melanoma. In this circumstance, the skin may be gently pared and the pigment will be removed in a painless manner because the hemorrhage is housed in the stratum corneum. Sports with rapid starts and stops such as tennis, racquetball, and basketball are most likely to cause this kind of change.

D. **Abrasion.** Abrasions are commonly encountered in contact sports such as wrestling and football. Gentle cleansing of the affected area with dilute hydrogen peroxide can be followed by the application of a thin coating of antibiotic ointment (polymyxin, bacitracin, or mupirocin). Hydrocolloid dressings can also be used but are usually not necessary. Thick crusts should not be allowed to form, because this may impede healing and lead to a thickened scar. Moistening of wounds and application of an occlusive dressing enhances the rate of reepithelialization.

III. Physical and Climatic Problems

A. **Sunburn.** Sunburn is commonly encountered in fair-skinned athletes, especially those training between the hours of 10 a.m. and 2 p.m. Not only can a rapid exposure to prolonged sun lead to severe burns, but long-term exposure to ultraviolet radiation may predispose to the development of cataracts as well as cutaneous malignancies and, most importantly, melanoma. Use of sunscreens is very helpful. Many athletes may object to heavy creamy or oily products that may leave the skin feeling greasy and can impede sweating. Gel, lotion, and spray products usually circumvent this problem, as they contain an alcohol base and evaporate rapidly. Athletes should be instructed to apply sunscreens approximately 20 min before going out so as to allow adequate time for binding to the stratum corneum. A broad-spectrum sunscreen with a sun protection factor (SPF) of 15 or more that protects against both ultraviolet A and ultraviolet B light is preferred. Even though many sunscreen products are advertised as waterproof, vigorous exertion and sweating may lessen their effect and require reapplication. Should a sunburn develop, soothing compresses, tepid baths, and colloidal oatmeal powder or milk added to the bath all can be soothing. Nonsteroidal anti-inflammatory medications may also lessen pain, and topical emollients will lessen peeling and irritation. Over-the-counter cortisone ointments are helpful for moderate to severe burns.

B. **Pernio.** Pernio occurs from prolonged exposure to cold and is often seen in athletes. Properly insulated shoes, warm socks, and preventing the buildup of moisture within footwear will all help to prevent pernio. When pernio develops, it is characterized by erythematous tender papules and nodules that occur on acral sites. The feet and toes are most commonly involved.

C. **Frostbite.** See Chapter 12.

IV. Infectious Disorders

A. **Onychomycosis.** Onychomycosis is most often due to *Trichophyton rubrum.* Distal subungual onychomycosis is most common; usually the distal nail edge will show yellow discoloration and thickening. Firmly establishing the diagnosis by performing a culture or potassium hydroxide examination is crucial to ensure proper treatment. Oral griseofulvin therapy can be administered but may have to be continued for up to a year or a year and a half, because this is the time it takes for the average individual to grow a new toenail. Itraconazole given at 100 mg twice a day has now been approved for treatment of onychomycosis and is extremely effective when given for 3 months. Other antifungals such as ketoconazole are also very effective but may require closer monitoring because of the greater risk of liver toxicity.

B. **Tinea versicolor.** Tinea versicolor is not due to a true dermatophyte but rather a yeast known *Pityrosporum orbiculare.* Potassium hydroxide examination establishes the diagnosis by revealing short hyphae and small spores. In dark-skinned individuals, tinea versicolor may present as hypopigmented macules. A Wood's light examination of tinea versicolor, unlike vitiligo, would reveal hypopigmentation but not complete depigmentation. The discoloration is due to azelaic acid, which the *Pityrosporum* organism produces and which interferes with normal melanin production. Therapy can usually be performed successfully by applying a selenium sulfite 2 1/2% solution for 10 min to the affected area each night for a week. Alternative treatments include oral ketoconazole therapy of 400 mg administered an hour before exercise. Topical imidazole creams such as econazole nitrate (Spectazole), applied once daily, are also effective and helpful for localized disease.

C. **Fungal infections** are very common in athletes. Sweating and heat predispose to the growth of dermatophytes on the feet and in intertriginous areas. "Athlete's foot" may take a variety of clinical forms. Tense blisters and vesiculopustules may be seen on the plantar surfaces; there may be maceration between the toes; or yellow discoloration and thickening can be seen in the nails. If groin folds are involved, tinea may take on a serpiginous pattern with an erythematous, raised, advancing border. Dermatophyte infections of the skin are frequently classified as tinea pedis, tinea cruris, tinea corporis, tinea capitis, tinea gladiatorum.

1. **Tinea of the foot.** Tinea pedis is the most common type of dermatophyte infection encountered. It is seen most often in westernized countries where the use of shoes is universal. The moisture and heat within footwear allows fungal organisms to grow. Communal locker rooms provide an ideal conditions for the spread of infection. Clinical manifestations may differ. Toe-web infection, known as interdigital tinea pedis, may be identified because of the soggy fissured and scaling appearance between the toes. Itching is often exacerbated when shoes and socks are removed. Dermatophyte fungi are causative, but bacteria such as *Staphylococcus aureus,* gram-negative bacteria, and micrococci add to the problem. Treatment with topical imidazole creams is highly effective, and newer antifungal agents such as terbinafine (an alkylamine) are highly effective. Usual treatment is for 3 or 4 weeks. Some agents such as econazole nitrate (Spectazole) have antibacterial efficacy as well.
2. **Tinea of the groin.** Tinea cruris, also known as jock itch, is encountered most frequently in the warm summer months. Scaling plaques involve the groin folds but spare the scrotum. If scrotal involvement is noted, *Candida* is the more likely culprit. Topical steroid creams may have been applied, and this can lead to a situation known as tinea incognito, where the advancing border is not clearly identified. A potassium hydroxide examination, however, will reveal numerous hyphae. Intertrigo may mimic tinea corporis and is seen more commonly in obese individuals. In intertrigo, the area of erythema and maceration is limited by the body folds.
3. **Tinea of the body.** The clinical appearance of tinea corporis can differ; most commonly an annular appearance (ringworm) is noted, but pustular lesions may be seen, as well as granulomatous lesions. Some zoophilic fungi such as *Trichophyton verrucosum* produce a intensely inflammatory response.

   Topical treatment with a topical imidazole cream for 2 weeks is usually effective. When granulomatous or follicular variants are encountered, oral therapy with either griseofulvin or an antifungal agent such as itraconazole may be considered.
4. **Tinea of the scalp.** Tinea capitis, due to *Trichophyton tonsurans,* is most frequently seen in young children. The dermatophytes that presently cause tinea capitis in the United States do not fluoresce with a Wood's light. Taking a hair sample for culture or performing a potassium hydroxide examination will allow for diagnosis. A selenium sulfate shampoo will prevent spread of spores, but oral therapy is advisable, as topical therapy will not lead to a reliable cure. Oral griseofulvin is helpful, as are itraconazole, ketoconazole, and terbinafine.
5. **Tinea in wrestlers.** *Tinea gladiatorum* is the name given to widespread tinea infection in wrestlers. The close contact and abrasions that result in the skin predispose to infection. Tinea gladiatorum is treated in the same manner as any other cutaneous dermatophyte infection.

D. **Bacteria**

1. Staphylococci and streptococci may cause impetigo, which is characterized by honey-colored crusts occurring in injured skin. The head and neck area is most commonly involved. Sports with close physical contact, such as wrestling, may lead to the spread of impetigo. Bullous impetigo is most commonly caused by staphylococci of phage group II. The staphylococci produce a toxin that causes blistering in the epidermis. Nonbullous impetigo is usually due to group A beta-hemolytic strep. Oral therapy with agents such as erythromycin or dicloxacillin are usu-

ally curative, and topical therapy with aluminum acetate compresses (Burow's solution) at a dilution of 1:40 three times daily can be helpful when combined with topical mupirocin ointment.

2. **Erythrasma.** Erythrasma presents as dull red plaques occurring in axillary or inguinal folds. A Wood's lamp examination will often reveals a coral-red fluorescence because of porphyrin by-products produced by *Corynebacterium.* Soap and water cleansing with antibacterial soap will often eradicate the problem or topical erythromycin cream or gel (Aknemycin or ATS gel) can be used. Oral therapy with erythromycin (250 mg four times daily for 2 weeks) is also very helpful but seldom required.
3. **Pitted keratolysis.** Pitted keratolysis is a disorder occurring most commonly in temperate climates, in which bacteria such as micrococci cause small pits and depressions in the stratum corneum. Biopsy will reveal numerous organisms in the affected areas. Usually athletes affected with this problem have marked hyperhidrosis. The application of topical antibiotic preparations can be of benefit, and products designed to control hyperhidrosis such as topical aluminum chloride (Drysol) are also helpful.

E. **Viruses**

1. **Common warts** are frequently encountered in athletes. Plantar warts can be most vexing, as they can be widespread before they are recognized. Unlike callouses, warts will cause a disruption of the normal dermatoglyphics. Treatment with topical salicylic acid plasters at bedtime, which is painless, can be helpful, but they require diligent and prolonged use. Alternatively, the areas may be pared, and chemical destruction with salicylic acid, nitric acid, or chloroacetic acid may be performed. Other options include the application of liquid nitrogen or cantharone, which may be painful. As a last resort, laser therapy or hyperthermia therapy may be considered.
2. **Herpes simplex virus.** Herpes simplex virus (HSV) is characterized by grouped vesicles and pustules on an erythematous base. Herpes is most commonly encountered on the lips and may be triggered by injury or sunburn. Herpes labialis used to be caused primarily by HSV type I and genital herpes by HSV II, but with changing sexual practices, it is not uncommon to encounter HSV II on the lips. HSV II recurs more frequently than HSV I.

   Herpes gladiatorum. Herpes gladiatorum is a primary herpetic infection of the skin seen in wrestlers. Skin abrasions or lacerations become inoculated with the virus. Systemic symptoms of headache, myalgias, and fever are common.

   Some athletes, such as skiers, who develop recurrent herpes labialis, may benefit from medication with oral acyclovir given in a dosage of 200 mg five times daily for 5 days or acyclovir 400 mg three times daily for 5 days. Valacyclovir (Valtrex) at a dosage of 400 mg three times daily for 5 days and famciclovir (Famvir) at a dosage of 125 mg three times daily are helpful as well, but not yet by the Food and Drug Administration (FDA) approved for herpes labialis. Wrestlers with active herpes lesions should be disqualified from practice, as spread among competitors may result in herpes gladiatorum. If an individual with compromised immunity such as atopic dermatitis or human immunodeficiency virus (HIV) infection develops herpes, widespread herpetic lesions may develop.
3. **Molluscum contagiosum.** Molluscum contagiosum is an asymptomatic to mildly pruritic viral infection induced by the poxvirus. Well established lesions are characterized by an umbilicated pattern. Molluscum lesions may be removed by gentle curettage, light, liquid nitrogen cryotherapy or by Cantharidin. Molluscum lesions are contagious and may be spread among athletes, especially those on swim teams. It is important that all affected individuals be treated.

V. Infestations

A. **Scabies.** Scabies infestation is due to the mite *Sarcoptes scabiei.* In well-established cases, linear burrows may be identified; they are most commonly seen around the wrists or on the ankles or genitalia. In other cases widespread excoriations may be seen with little active dermatitis. Complaints of itching may be disproportionate to objective findings. A skin scraping examined under mineral oil may reveal the mites or its body parts. Treatment with topical lindane or permethrin cream (Elimite) is curative so long as all areas from the neck down are treated, including intertriginous areas, the umbilicus, and the areas underneath the fingernails. All family members in a household should be treated as well, even if they are asymptomatic, because otherwise the infestation may recur. Sexual partners should be treated as well.

B. **Pediculosis.** Pediculosis is an infestation with lice. Pubic lice are usually acquired through sexual contact, but body lice and scalp lice may be encountered through intimate contact. Shaving of the affected body areas is usually not required. Effective treatment includes applying a pediculicide such as permethrin 1% cream rinse (Nix) for 10 min, rinsing the hair, and then reapplying the product in 1 week. Bedding and clothing must be washed. By using a lindane shampoo, organisms may be eradicated, and formic acid rinse will enable removal of nits from affected hairs.

C. **Cutaneous larva migrans.** Cutaneous larvae migrans is a type of infestation encountered in temperate climates in areas such as the Caribbean. An athlete running barefoot on a beach may enable the infecting organism to enter the skin, where it cannot complete its life cycle. The annular or serpiginous track of the worm in the skin will allow for clinical identification. Topical thiabendazole (Mintezol) will lead to eradication of the problem. Alternatively, liquid nitrogen cryotherapy may be directed at the advancing border and lead to death of the organism.

VI. Bites and Stings

A. **Hymenoptera** (bees, wasps, and hornets) bites may be encountered in athletes and usually present as localized pain and swelling in the affected area. Generalized reactions may, however, occur, and even sudden death. Athletes with a history of angioedema, widespread urticarial lesions, or other symptoms of anaphylaxis after being stung by an insect may benefit from having an emergency anaphylactic kit (e.g., Epi-Pen) available. Permethrin-based insect repellents (e.g., Permanone) may also be helpful.

VII. Miscellaneous Disorders

A. **Acne.** Acne vulgaris is prevalent in the population and may be exacerbated by sports. Sports in which helmets and pads are worn may worsen acne by causing follicular occlusion. Acne can be graded into grade I acne, characterized by open and closed comedones; grade II acne, characterized by erythematous papules; grade III acne, characterized by pustules; and grade IV acne, in which deep cysts and nodules occur. Treatment of type I acne usually hinges upon the use of a topical benzoyl peroxide gel (desquam E, benzac, persagel) and a keratolytic agent such as tretinoin cream or gel (Retin-A). If grade II acne is present, introduction of a topical antibiotic such as erythromycin (ATS, erygel) clindamycin (cleocin), or sulfacetamide (Novacet, Sulfacet-R) may be of benefit. If pustular lesions are present, as in grade III acne, oral antibiotic therapy with erythromycin or tetracycline may be considered; if deep cystic lesions are noted, minocycline hydrochloride (Dynacin, Minocin) doxycycline (Monodox), or isotretinoin (Accutane) therapy may be considered. Isotretinoin is a potent teratogen and should be used with great caution in women of childbearing potential. Using alcohol pads to clean helmets and the use of astringents can also be helpful in areas where pads and athletic equipment cause exacerbation.

B. **Contact dermatitis.** Contact dermatitis may result from outdoor sports in which exposure to common allergens such as pentadecyl-catechol the active allergen within poison ivy, poison oak and poison sumac, is encountered. Knowing which allergens are likely to be encountered is important in preventing this problem. When contact dermatitis occurs, cool compresses, application of potent cortisone creams, and occasional use of systemic corticosteroids all may hasten resolution. In other situations, allergies to adhesives within footwear may occur, or to dyes used in equipment such as hockey gloves. In these cases, identifying the offending allergen is most important, and this may be facilitated by patch testing.

C. **Atopic dermatitis.** Individuals with sensitive skin, as from atopic dermatitis, may also note exacerbation with exercise. Sweating may cause an itching sensation in the skin, which promotes a cycle of scratching, itching, and further dermatitis. The use of antihistamines such as hydroxyzine, loratadine, or citrizene may be helpful as well as the judicious use of mild corticosteroids. In many instances selecting appropriate quantity of cream is most important. One requires approximately 9 g of cream to treat 9% of the body area (one upper limb) for a day with t.i.d. application; therefore, if an entire area such as the chest is to be treated for a 10-day period, as much as 180 g of cream will be required. For this reason, it is often worthwhile to prescribe a larger amount of a milder product as well as a more potent agent to be used on the most resistant areas.

D. **Psoriasis.** Psoriasis is a common condition characterized by erythematous and scaling plaques distributed symmetrically, especially over extensor surfaces such as the elbows and knees. Topical corticosteroids may help control psoriasis. Other agents such as topical calcipotriol (synthetic vitamin D) may also be of great benefit and are an exciting addition to the topical armamentarium against psoriasis.

E. **Urticaria.** Urticaria, also known as hives, may occur at any age. This condition has a variety of physical triggers, including pressure, cold, or exposure to the sun. Exercise-induced urticaria may be seen as well. There are also many allergic causes of urticaria, including the ingestion, of fish, shellfish, nuts, eggs, chocolate, strawberries, cow's milk, wheat, yeast, and cheeses.

If urticaria has been present for less than 6 weeks, it is defined as acute urticaria. Symptomatic treatment with antihistamines and soothing topical lotions is usually all that is required. If urticaria persists longer than 6 weeks, further investigation is indicated. Physical uriticaria can often be excluded by history. Dermographism is the most common type of physical urticaria and can last for many months. When the skin is stroked, wheals develop, whereas normally such an exaggerated response would not be seen. Solar urticaria often comes on minutes after exposure to the sun and lasts for a few minutes to 1 or 2 hr. Cold urticaria may be due to familial condition in which a change in skin temperature causes a reaction in from 30 min to 1 or 2 hr. Arthralgias, fever, and tremor may be seen in this rare type of urticaria. Essential acquired cold urticaria is much more common and occurs just a few minutes after cold contact, lasting for 1 or 2 hr. Wheezing may occur. Applying ice in a plastic bag to the arm or immersing the arm in cold water will allow for diagnosis. A first-generation H1-receptor antagonist such as chlorpheniramine maleate, hydroxyzine hydrochloride (Atarax), or diphenhydramine hydrochloride (Benadryl) may be helpful. Second-generation agents may also be used; these include loratadine (Claritin) and citrizene (Zyrtec). It is also very important to avoid the precipitant. The nonsedating antihistamines are most popular among athletes as they cause minimal side effects and are generally safe. It is important to remember that terfenadine (Seldane) can interact with erythromycin as well as some of the oral antifungal agents, potentially causing fatal ventricular arrhythmias.

VIII. Conclusion

Skin problems are commonly encountered in athletes; if recognized promptly, they can be treated in such a way as to minimize morbidity and time lost from training and competition.

Suggested reading

Bergfeld WF, Elston D. Skin problems of athletes. *Sports injuries.* Baltimore: Williams & Wilkins, In: Fu FH, Stone D, eds. 1994:781–795.

Bergfeld WF, Helm TN. Skin disorders in athletes. In: Grana, Kalena, eds. *Clinical sports medicine.* Philadelphia: WB Saunders, 1991:110–118.

Bergfeld WF, Helm TN. The skin. In: Strouss RH, ed. *Sports medicine,* 2d ed. Toronto: WB Saunders, 1991:117–131.

Bergfeld WF, Taylor, JS. Trauma, Sports, and the Skin. *Am J Industr Med* 1985;8:403–413.

Levine N Dermatologic aspects of sports medicine *J Am Acad Dermatol* 1980;3:415–424.

Sedar JI. Treatment of blisters in the running athlete. *Arch Podiatr* Med *Foot Surgery Sports Med* 1978;29–34.

30. GASTROINTESTINAL DISORDERS

Peter Bruno

Gastrointestinal problems are common in the general population and among athletes. There is a paucity of information regarding the gastrointestinal system in relation to exercise; however, more information has come to light owing to heightened awareness of the beneficial effects of exercise. The most common gastrointestinal complaints include belching, bloating, heartburn, nausea, vomiting, chest pain, abdominal pain, diarrhea, and bleeding. With clinical presentation and treatment for the various problems, one must keep in mind that problems vary widely according to the specific sport, level of exertion, condition of the athlete, degree of anxiety, and probably the gender of the athlete. As many as 60% of competitive athletes complain of gastrointestinal symptoms. Of these, 30% admit to similar symptoms when they are nervous about something else; therefore, one must ascertain that such symptoms are not psychogenic in origin; that is, anxiety concerning performance and competition is well recognized as a factor in provoking or exacerbating gastrointestinal symptoms.

I. Nausea and Vomiting

It is well known among athletes that nausea and vomiting are more frequent in those who are poorly trained or who exceed their exertional capacity. This is also true for athletes who have eaten or drunk too much before exercise or attempt to replenish fluid, electrolyte, and carbohydrate late in an endurance event, when gastric emptying is delayed and splanchnic circulation is decreased. Treatment consists of rest and oral rehydration. Patients who are severely dehydrated may require intravenous hydration. In female athletes, pregnancy must be ruled out. Antiemetics, though seldom required, are sometimes used. Examples are Compazine, Tigan, and Thorazine.

II. Gastroesophageal Reflux

Chest pain, belching, regurgitation, and heartburn are common in the general population. Belching and regurgitation are particularly common. Although some studies point out that substernal chest pain is more likely to originate from the esophagus due to reflux or motor dysfunction, a cardiac etiology should be considered before concentrating on the esophagus, especially in patients with known risk factors for coronary artery disease. Gastroesophageal reflux disease (GERD) has been studied extensively in the recent years. Symptoms of GERD may be secondary to the eating of certain foods (e.g., fatty foods, caffeine, mint, citrus fruits or beverages, carbonated drinks). Studies have shown that vigorous exercise can induce GERD in normal subjects. There are studies showing that reflux is more common in the upright position than when subjects are supine. This has been linked to lower esophageal sphincter relaxation. The problem is most likely to occur if food is eaten prior to exercise and with certain types of exercise. Running and swimming are prime offenders. Aerobic exercise with less body agitation, such as bicycling, produces the least reflux.

A. **Management**

1. Treatment of gastroesophageal reflux related to exercise as opposed to eating is empiric. There are no well-accepted studies on the treatment of GERD related to exercise; it is based on clinical judgment. Young people with such symptoms can be treated without further diagnostic workup. However, in individuals who have persistent symptoms or other abnormalities, such as dysphagia or weight loss, endoscopic evaluation should be done to evaluate for abnormalities such as esophagitis or neoplasia. Esophageal manometry or ambulatory 24-hr pH monitoring can serve as diagnostic studies. Patients should be counseled not to eat several hours

prior to exercise. They should avoid foods that delay gastric emptying time and should also be told not to drink too quickly, as this might increase the incidence of aerophagia.

a. Antacids may be used, with care not to use magnesium-containing compounds in athletes prone to diarrhea. As magnesium may cause diarrhea, aluminum-containing antacids and foaming alginate-based antacids such as Gaviscon or calcium carbonate (TUMS or Rolaids) are preferred. For female athletes predisposed to osteoporosis, calcium-containing antacids have the additional benefit of providing a good source of calcium.
b. If the above measures are not successful and symptoms are troublesome, then an H_2-receptor antagonist such as cimetidine, ranitidine, famotidine, or nizatidine might be taken 1 hr prior to exercise. This treatment is seldom necessary unless the athlete already has a history of peptic ulcer disease or dyspepsia.
c. Refractory symptoms of GERD are best treated with proton pump inhibitors, i.e. omeprazole, and lansoprazole.
d. If still necessary, a prokinetic agent such as cisapride taken 1 hr before a meal or exercise might help to increase motility or lower esophageal sphincter tone.
e. In circumstances where all above fails, laparoscopic fundoplication in expert hands is definitive treatment.

III. Abdominal Pain

Abdominal pain occuring during strenuous physical activity, especially running, is referred to as a "stitch." It is well recognized by athletes and coaches and characterized as a transient, sharp, subcostal pain that may occur on either side; it is exacerbated by breathing and decreased by rest. Its etiology is speculative and includes ischemia, muscular spasm, or trapped intestinal gas. The frequency diminishes with training endurance. Abdominal pain that is chronic or persists after rest warrants further medical investigation, a there are rare reports of cecal volvulus, ischemic bowel, hernias, colon cancer, ulcerative colitis, or Crohn's disease presenting as abdominal pain during exercise.

IV. Trauma

Contact sports can lead to traumatic injury of the abdominal wall and visceral organs. Such injuries include abrasions, contusions, muscle sprain, strains, and tears, often resulting in hematomas of the muscle. In most cases ice packs for 48 hr or analgesics are the treatments of choice. Trauma can result in rupture of the diaphragm, with resultant herniation of abdominal viscera into the chest. The hollow visceral organs can also suffer contusion, hematoma, laceration, and rupture. The most serious injuries include laceration or rupture of the spleen, laceration of the liver, and contusion of the pancreas. Typically, these patients develop signs and symptoms of an acute abdomen, possibly with vascular collapse. When such a situation arises, the patient needs immediate resuscitation and surgical evaluation. Further considerations, especially in runners, include cecal slap syndrome thought to be due to excessive motion of the cecum and repetitive jarring.

V. Diarrhea

Watery bowel movements, cramps, fecal urgency, and incontinence are the most common and troubling gastrointestinal symptoms among endurance athletes such as distance runners or triathletes. Surveys reveal that approximately one-third of distance runners have experienced the urge or need to defecate while running and that 20% to 25% suffer from troublesome cramps or diarrhea during or after competitive running. Interestingly, in a survey of triathletes, these symptoms were reduced during the swimming and cycling portion as compared with the running portion. This observation might correlate with the theory that running causes a jiggling effect. Although there is no proof of increasing intestinal transit while an athlete is running, it is believed that the jarring caused by repetitive footfalls during running may stimulate mass movements in the colon.

Runners may also experience the more troublesome form of runner's diarrhea, with lower abdominal cramps, rectal spasm, diarrhea, or fecal incontinence during or immediately following high intensity exertion.

Athletes are not immune to gastrointestinal infections, inflammatory bowel disease, malabsorption, or cancer. It is therefore prudent to rule out other etiologies of these symptoms before blaming them on exercise or running.

A. **Management.** The management of runner's diarrhea is empiric because there are no studies addressing the subject specifically. One should encourage bowel movement prior to exercise. If this is not possible, a light meal might stimulate the gastrocolic reflex and bowel movement. Elimination diets might be worth trying, such as eliminating milk or milk products as well as high-osmolar sugar substitutes such as sorbitol in sugar-free candies or fructose in ice creams or popsicles. If the above measures are ineffective and the physician is sure that there are no non-exercise-related causes, then the occasional use of a prophylactic antidiarrheal might be considered. The preferred drug is loperamide (Imodium) 1 hr prior to competition.

   Athletes who travel to foreign countries to compete are always at risk for contracting **"traveler's diarrhea."** This syndrome is predominantly a result of exposure to different strains of *Escherichia coli* present in foreign areas. Routine precautions such as avoiding tap water, uncooked fruits, vegetables, and ice cubes and eating in better, clean-looking establishments might sometimes not be enough. If diarrhea develops, the athlete must make sure that hydration is maintained. This can be done orally. Bismuth subsalicylate (Pepto-Bismol) 30 to 60 mL every 30 min for eight doses might be effective, but one must be warned that stool will turn black and sometimes the tongue as well, temporarily. Trimetophrim-sulfamethoxazole (Bactrim or Septra one twice a day) as well as ciprofloxacin (Cipro 250 mg or 500 mg twice a day) have been recommended. Loperamide has also been used, but since diarrhea is also the body's mechanism for eliminating an offending agent, such medicine might prolong recovery.

   Pseudomembranous colitis must be considered in anyone who has taken antibiotics in the past several months. Treatment is oral metronidazole or oral vancomycin.

VI. Gastrointestinal Bleeding

Gastrointestinal bleeding is uncommon among athletes with the exception of long-distance runners. Reportedly, up to 20% of marathon runners have occult blood in their stools after competition when tested by the guaiac reagent. The incidence may be higher if more sensitive tests are used. This symptom is likely due to colonic ischemia from reduced blood flow to the bowel during maximal exercise. Use of nonsteroidal antiinflammatory drugs (NSAIDs) has been implicated as a cause. NSAIDs are well known to cause gastrointestinal damage. The exact mechanism(s) remain speculative but likely involve changes in the quality and quantity of mucus, bicarbonate secretion, and mucosal blood flow. NSAIDs are in widespread use among athletes, especially owing to their availability over the counter. However, this does not appear to be a major factor. Although the relationship between NSAIDs, gastritis, and ulcers has been extensively studied, there are no studies to date on NSAIDs and bloody diarrhrea in runners or other athletes. There are, however, published reports of NSAID-associated colitis, which is becoming increasingly recognized as the pathophysiologic mechanism. It is unclear why some athletes develop this while others do not. A death while jogging has been attributed to hemorrhagic gastritis. Gastrointestinal bleeding appears to be related to the runner's level of fitness, the intensity of training, and the intensity of exertion. There are two major theories. The first proposes gastrointestinal ischemia as splanchnic blood flow decreases linearly in relation to $\dot{V}_{O_2max}$ in an effort to increase blood flow to the most active muscle. This decrease in blood flow might be as high as 60% to 80% and—coupled with fluid loss—may provoke a low-flow ischemia to the vulnerable areas of the bowel. The second theory suggests that gastrointestinal bleeding results from trauma of repetitive jarring during running.

Although most cases of G.I. are self-limited and probably related to running, it may be due to a pathological condition. Athletes with gastrointestinal bleeding, just like any other person, require attention and further medical evaluation. Endoscopy is the procedure of choice in the athlete who vomits blood, as source must be identified as soon as possible and therapeutic action taken to prevent untoward results. Lower gastrointestinal bleeding must be evaluated with endoscopy early, as the lesions causing this might be evanescent. Treatment depends on the specific pathology. Usually, bowel rest, rehydration, cautious and judicious use of analgesics, and perhaps sulfasalazine or other products such as mesalamine or osalazine will help to resolve symptoms/condition.

VII. Peptic Ulcer

It is known that many hormones will be increased with exercise. Exercise also increases fasting gastrin concentrations. There is a relationship between the rise in serum gastrin and plasma adrenalin. Acid output in patients with duodenal ulcer, in contrast with normal individuals, increases after exercise. There are some studies showing a decreased incidence of peptic ulcer disease in patients engaged in regular exercise or active individuals as opposed to those who are more sedentary. In light of new data showing a causal relationship between *Helicobacter pylori* and peptic ulcer disease, this factor must be considered. Treatment includes H2 blockers and, in the case of *H. pylori* infection, a proton pump inhibitor plus antibiotics.

VIII. Irritable Bowel Syndrome

Irritable bowel syndrome (IBS) is common in the general population. It is a motor disorder defined clinically by altered bowel habits, abdominal pain, and the absence of detectable organic pathology.

A. **Diagnosis.** Four symptoms that help distinguish IBS from organic disease are (1) visible abdominal distention, (2) relief of abdominal pain by bowel movement, (3) more frequent bowel movements with onset of pain, and (4) looser stools with onset of pain. It generally affects young people and women more than men. The pathophysiology remains unknown, and IBS is therefore usually a diagnosis of exclusion. Treatment includes dietary restrictions, fiber supplementation, antispasmodic agents, and psychological counseling.

IX. Inflammatory Bowel Disease

There is lack of data regarding the influence of exercise on inflammatory bowel disease (IBD). Patients with inactive IBD have little or no problem participating in most sports. However with the effects of exercise on motility and the emotional tension of competition, there might be an increase in symptoms that may or may not be related to the disease. In presence of active disease, however, participation might be hampered by the severity of exacerbation.

The question of possible exacerbations with exercise arises in patients with ileostomy or colostomy as in patients with resections for severe inflammatory bowel disease or other such conditions. With the advent of newer appliances, this type of surgery should cause no limitations in physical activity. However, these athletes should be advised against contact sports, as they pose a risk of trauma. Some of these athletes have continued to participate in sports and sporting events while their associates remained unaware of their medical problem. Medications used for inflammatory bowel disease include sulfasalazine, olsalazine, and mesalamine. Immunomodulators have also been used, including 6 mercaptopurine, azathioprine, and cyclosporine.

X. Constipation

A great deal of myth surrounds the effect of exercise on bowel movement. Constipation is common in bedridden and hospitalized patients and disappears once normal activity is resumed. At present, there is no proof that exercise can be used to treat constipation or that it can cause fecal retention.

XI. Liver Disease

Strenuous exercise has not been shown to aggravate chronic liver disease or cirrhosis. It is wise, however, for patients with prolonged clotting time, enlarged liver or spleen, low platelet count, or esophageal varices to refrain from sports in which they might be subjected to trauma.

A. **Abnormal liver function tests.** Occasionally, the physician is confronted with a well-trained, otherwise healthy athlete with abnormal liver function tests, including elevations in transaminase, bilirubin, and alkaline phosphatase. Mild elevations of liver chemistries are commonly detected incidentally during routine examination with the use of multi-channel analyzers and automated chemistry profiles. The most common pattern involves isolated elevations of aspartate transaminase/ alanine aminotransferase (AST/ALT) in an asymptomatic person. These abnormalities are particularly common in long-distance runners but can occur in other athletes as well. The history should focus on any prior liver disease, episodes of hepatitis, prior abnormal blood tests, rejection as a blood donor, hemolytic disorders, blood transfusion, intravenous substance abuse, alcohol intake and medication use, including NSAIDs, herbal medications, dietary supplements, some vitamins, and anabolic steroids.

B. **Physical examination** should look for icterus, stigmata of chronic liver disease, and hepatosplenomegaly. The most common etiologies for mild elevations of AST and ALT are obesity, alcohol use, and NSAIDs. Suspected medications should be discontinued and blood chemistries repeated in 3 to 4 weeks. Liver disease can be excluded if the serum gamma-glutamyl transpeptidase (GGTP) is normal as well as the glutamic-pyruvate transaminase and albumin. If these are abnormal, further investigations are called for.

C. **Hepatitis A** (see also Chapter 24). Hepatitis serologies should be checked, as athletes in close contact could transmit hepatitis A to each other via the fecal-oral route. Therefore, close personal contacts with infected individuals or ingestion of contaminated water or food can lead to illness. An outbreak was reported in 1970 among members of a football team when they drank contaminated water. Medical management of the athlete is no different from that of other individuals. A more usual circumstance is when one or more members of a team develops acute hepatitis A, especially in teams that travel to endemic areas. In this instance, one must care for the affected individual(s) and for the potentially exposed team members. Hepatitis A has an incubation period of approxmately 4 weeks. The virus is present in the liver, bile, stools and blood during the late incubation period and acute preicteric phase of the illness. Despite persistence of virus in the liver, viral shedding in feces, viremia, and infectivity diminishes rapidly once jaundice becomes apparent. Hepatitis A vaccine has recently become available and has been advised to be given at least 15 days prior to travel to endemic areas. Immune globulin has been advised in the past for travelers and especially for those in close contact with individuals having the disease, but lately there has been a worldwide shortage of the drug. There is also associated risk of other serum-transmitted disease such as hepatits B or C or HIV. Passive immunization is unnecessary unless all team members are in close personal contact with the infected individual. However, in most instances, when a case of hepatitis A is recognized, close contacts have already been exposed, rendering passive immunization irrelevant. Viral concentration in stool is highest during the asymptomatic incubation period and begins to fall with the onset of jaundice. Since there is no specific treatment, care is supportive and should include a balanced diet and observation for increasing jaundice, encephalopathy, prolongation of the prothrombin time, and hypoglycemia, all signs of hepatic failure. If the patient cannot eat or if hepatic failure or bleeding episodes arise, then hospitalization is necessary. There is no evidence that bed rest enhances healing; if the patient is able, moderate exercise has been recommended, though this is still controversial. Most hepatitis A infections are subclinical, and it is recommended that each member of the team have liver enzymes measured to determine who is already affected.

D. **Hepatitis serology.** The presence of IgM antibody to hepatitis confirms acute infection. The presence of IgG antibody without IgM antibody indicates past infection with immunity, hepatitis B and C, as well as other causes. Cytomegalovirus and Epstein-Barr virus should also be considered.

E. **Hepatitis B.** Hepatitis B is primarily transmitted by direct inoculation of infected blood or blood products into a susceptible host. In athletes, this is most likely to occur in contact sports that commonly give rise to open wounds. Onset is often insidious, and incubation period ranges from a mean of 60 to 90 days. The treatment of acute hepatitis B is the same as that for hepatitis A. However, unlike hepatitis A, hepatitis B may occasionally become chronic and lead to cirrhosis. Although there is abundant evidence suggesting that feces are not infectious, body fluids such as saliva and semen have been shown to be infectious, albeit less so than serum. There is no effective treatment for chronic hepatitis B, but interferon has been used with some success. A few infected individuals may become chronic carriers of hepatitis B without evidence of active liver disease. Therefore those with acute hepatitis B should be followed medically until liver function is normal and hepatitis B surface antigen (Hbs Ag) disappears from the serum, documenting full recovery. Further evidence of complete recovery is the demonstration of the antibody to HbsAg in the serum of those previously infected. It is estimated that there are 200 million carriers in the world. Whether to allow chronic carriers of hepatitis B to participate in sports, where they might transmit infection to others, remains an ethical problem. Hepatitis B vaccine was available long before hepatitis A vaccine and is advised for every high-risk individual.

F. **Hepatitis C.** Chronic hepatitis C tends to be an indolent disease, but it is increasingly being diagnosed with the new serologic test available. The mode of acquisition (though there are some data to suggest a higher percentage in individuals with history of blood transfusion) of hepatitis C is unknown in 80% to 90% of patients. A significant number of affected patients will progress to chronic liver disease and cirrhosis. Patients with symptoms, progressing abnormalities, or chronic hepatitis should be referred for evaluation.

G. **Anabolic androgenic steroid intake** to increase strength, muscle growth, and endurance can cause a reversible cholestasis similar to that due to estrogens and is another potential cause of serious abnormal liver function in athletes. It has been associated with peliosis hepatis, hepatocellular carcinoma, and hepatic adenomas. The use of these agents is to be discouraged, and they are banned in many competitive sports.

XI. Other G.I. Conditions

Hemorrhoids are not a problem peculiar to athletes but may present difficulty in the course of practice or competition. They should be considered in the differential diagnosis when an athlete complains of rectal pain or bleeding.

Recent epidemiologic studies have supported the idea that physical activity may be protective against colon cancer, but the mechanism remains uncertain.

Superior mesenteric artery syndrome has been reported in a wrestler. Symptoms consists of postprandial bloating, abdominal pain, and vomiting. This syndrome is attributed to duodenal obstruction as the superior mesenteric artery falls across the duodenum at about the third lumbar vertebra. Rapid, severe weight loss is a recognized contributing factor.

Anorexia nervosa and bulimia have also been reported in athletes and nonathletes. It is imperative that coaches and physicians recognize these disorders and address them in their early stages (see Chapter 21).

IX. NEUROLOGICAL PROBLEMS

31. HEAD INJURIES

Robert C. Cantu

Recognition of Head Injury

The head and spine are unique in that their contents are incapable of regeneration. The brain and spinal cord cannot regrow lost cells, as can the other organs of the body; thus injury to these structures takes on a singular importance. Recognition of a head injury is easy if the athlete has a loss of consciousness. It is the far more frequent mild head injury, in which there is no loss of consciousness but rather only a transient loss of alertness, that is much more difficult to recognize. More than 90% of all cerebral concussions fall into this mildest category, where there has not been a loss of consciousness but rather only a brief period of posttraumatic amnesia or loss of mental alertness. Because the dreaded second-impact syndrome can occur after a grade 1 concussion, just as it can after more serious head injuries, it becomes very important to recognize all grades of concussion.

Mechanism of Injury

Three distinct types of stresses can be generated by an acceleration force to the head: the first is a compressive; the second is tensile, the opposite of compressive and sometimes called negative pressure; and the third is shearing, a force applied parallel to a surface. Uniform compressive and tensile forces are relatively well tolerated by neural tissue, but shearing forces are very poorly tolerated.

The cerebrospinal fluid (CSF) that surrounds the brain acts as a protective shock absorber, converting focally applied external stress to compressive stress, because the fluid follows the contours of the sulci and gyri of the brain and distributes the force in a uniform fashion. The CSF, however, does not totally prevent shearing forces from being imparted to the brain, especially when rotational forces are applied to the head. These shearing forces are maximal where rotational gliding is hindered within the brain, as at the dura mater–brain attachments and the rough, irregular surfaces between the brain and the skull especially prominent at the base of the frontal and middle fossa.

In understanding how acceleration forces are applied to the brain, it is important to keep in mind Newton's law that force equals mass times acceleration, or, stated another way, force divided by mass equals acceleration. Therefore, an athlete's head can sustain far greater forces without injury if the neck muscles are tensed, as when the athlete sees the collision coming. In this state, the mass of the head is essentially the mass of the body. In a relaxed state, however, the mass of the head is essentially only its own weight and therefore the same degree of force can impart far greater acceleration.

Assessment of Injury

In assessing a head injury, if the athlete is unconscious, it must be assumed that he or she has suffered a neck fracture and the neck must be immobilized. In assessing a conscious athlete, the level of consciousness or alertness is the most sensitive criterion both for establishing the nature of the head injury and subsequently following the athlete. Orientation to person, place, and time should be ascertained. The presence or absence of posttraumatic amnesia and the ability to retain new information—such as the ability to repeat the names of four objects 2 min after having been given them or the ability to repeat one's assignments with certain plays—should be determined. It is also important to ascertain the presence, absence, and severity of neurologic symptoms such as headache, light-headedness, difficulty with balance, coordination, and sensory or motor function. Whereas a complete but brief neurologic examination involving cranial nerve, motor, sensory, and reflex testing is appropriate, it is the mental exam and especially of level of consciousness that should be stressed.

The Glasgow Coma Scale
When time permits the Glasgow Coma Scale (Table 31-1) can be very useful not only in predicting the chances for recovery but also in assessing whether the head-injured athlete is improving or deteriorating. An initial score above 11 is associated with more than a 90% chance of an essentially complete recovery, whereas an initial score below 5 is associated with more than an 80% chance of death or a persistent vegetative state.

Differential Diagnosis

The differential diagnosis with a head injury includes a cerebral concussion (see Table 31-2 for severity of concussion), the second-impact or malignant brain edema syndrome, the postconcussion syndrome, and intracranial hemorrhage.

Concussion
In a grade 1 concussion—which is the most common type of cerebral concussion, accounting for 90%— there is no loss of consciousness and the period of posttraumatic amnesia is brief. It is often difficult for the physician on the sidelines to recognize that the player has sustained a concussion. The word "ding" is commonly applied to this injury. With a grade 2 or 3 concussion, there are periods of unconsciousness and the injury is obvious to medical personnel. Occasionally an athlete's injury is said to be a grade 2 or 3 concussion because he or she has experienced extended periods of posttraumatic amnesia but has not actually been unconscious. By definition, periods of posttraumatic amnesia lasting more than 30 min but less than 24 hr, even in the absence of unconsciousness, would equate with a grade 2 concussion, whereas a period of posttraumatic amnesia greater than 24 hr would equate with a grade 3 concussion.

Second-Impact Syndrome
The second-impact syndrome occurs when an athlete is still symptomatic from an initial head injury and sustains a second head injury. Typically the athlete is stunned for 30 to 60 sec and then rapidly deteriorates, with fixed, dilated pupils, cessation of respiration, and decerebrate or decorticate posturing. In no other condition does the athlete deteriorate from a conscious to a decerebrate state so rapidly.

Table 31-1. Glasgow Coma Scale[a]

Eye opening (E)	
Spontaneous	4
To speech	3
To pain	2
No response	1
Motor response (M)	
Obeys commands	6
Localizes pain	5
Withdraws from pain	4
Decorticate posturing	3
Decerebrate posturing	2
No response	1
Verbal Response (V)	
Orientated	5
Confused conversation	4
Inappropriate words	3
Incomprehensible sounds	2
No response	1

[a] The patient's score is the sum of the ratings on E, M, and V.

Table 31-2. Severity of concussion

Grade	Feature	Duration of feature
Grade 1 (mild)	PTA	<30 min
	LOC	None
Grade 2 (moderate)	PTA	>30 min, <24 hr
	LOC	<5 min
Grade 3 (severe)	PTA	>24 hr
	LOC	>5 min

PTA, posttraumatic amnesia; LOC, loss of consciousness.

Intracranial Hematoma

In the case of an intracranial hematoma, there is usually a loss of consciousness. With the *epidural hematoma,* consciousness may be regained shortly thereafter. This lesion typically occurs with a skull fracture from a blow received in the temporal area. There is usually no associated brain injury and death usually results from the mass of the rapidy expanding blood, which causes brain herniation. Typically this athlete will experience headache and then deteriorating levels of consciousness within 15 to 30 min after the initial injury.

On the other hand, *the subdural hematoma,* which is the most common cause of death due to athletic head injury, and continues to carry a 30% to 40% percent mortality rate even at the finest neurosurgery centers, is usually associated with loss of consciousness and the failure to regain consciousness. It is the severe associated brain injury that causes death in a significant percentage of cases.

The *intracerebral hematoma* usually occurs deep within the the brain and is associated with an extremely severe acceleration injury to the head. Typically consciousness is not regained unless this lesion is extremely small.

The *subarachnoid hemorrhage* may be seen from a ruptured congenital vascular lesion such as an aneurysm or arteriovenous malformation. This condition also can result from a severe contusion or bruise of the brain.

Types of Injury

Diffuse Axonal Injury

This condition results when severe shearing forces are imparted to the brain and axonal connections are literally severed in the absence of intra- cranial hematoma. The patient is usually deeply comatose with a low score on the Glasgow Coma Scale and negative head computed tomography. Immediate neurosurgical triage for treatment of increased intracranial pressure is indicated.

Treatment

Immediate Treatment

With a head injury, the ABCs (airway, breathing, and circulation) of first aid must be followed. Before a neurologic exam is undertaken, the treating physician must determine the airway is adequate, breathing is adequate, and circulation is being maintained. Thereafter the physician may direct his or her attention to the neurologic exam, as discussed under Assessment of Injury above.

Definitive Treatment

Definitive treatment of grades 2 and 3 concussions as well as the second-impact syndrome and intracranial hematoma should take place at a medical facility with neurosurgical and neuroradiologic capabilities. In the case of intracranial hematoma, definitive surgical evacuation is indicated, in the case of the closed head injuries and more severe degrees of concussion, observation with careful neurologic monitoring is appropriate.

What Tests to Order and When to Order

After a grade 1 concussion, observation alone may be all that is indicated. In instances of grade 2 and 3 concussion, however, computed tomography (CT) or magnetic resonance imaging (MRI) of the brain is recommended. These athletes should be removed from the play and sent to a definitive neurologic facility where such imaging can take place. In the case of the second-impact syndrome and intracranial hemorrhage, emergent scanning with either CT or MRI is also appropriate.

When to Refer

All head injuries other than the grade 1 concussion should be referred for neurologic or neurosurgical evaluation following the athlete's removal from play.

When to Operate

Closed head injuries such as concussions and diffuse axonal injury of the brain do not require surgery. However, significant intracranial blood accumulations—whether epidural, subdural, or intracerebral—may require prompt surgical evacuation. A congenital vascular anomaly such as an aneurysm or arteriovenous malformation may require planned, deliberate surgical intervention.

Appropriate Time Course for Resolution

Table 31-3 provides guidelines for return to competition after a cerebral concussion, whether of grade 1, 2, or 3, and whether this was the first, second, or third concussion sustained in a given season. An athlete who has experienced the second-impact syndrome and who is in the small minority who survive without significant morbidity would not be allowed to return to a contact or collision sport. Also, an athlete who has undergone surgery for an intracranial hemorrhage would be ill advised to return to contact or collision sports, since both the surgery and the underlying hemorrhage have altered CSF dynamics and the ability of the CSF to protect the brain from subsequent head injury. It should be noted that the guidelines presented are those used by the author. Other guidelines for return to play have been proposed and may be found elsewhere.

Table 31-3. Guidelines for return after concussion

	First concussion	Second concussion	Third concussion
Grade 1 (mild)	May return to play if asymptomatic[a] for 1 week	May return to play in 2 weeks if asymptomatic at that time for 1 week	Terminate season; may return to play next season if asymptomatic
Grade 2 (moderate)	May return to play if asymptomatic for 1 week	Must be asymptomatic for a minimum of 1 month; may then return to play if asymptomatic for 1 week; consider terminating season	Terminate season; may return to play next season if asymptomatic
Grade 3 (severe)	Must be asymptomatic for a minimum of 1 month; may then return to play if asymptomatic for 1 week	Terminate season; may return to play next season if asymptomatic	

[a] "Asymptomatic" means no headache, dizziness, or impaired orientation, concentration, or memory during rest or exertion.

Principles of Rehabilitation and Return-to-Play Criteria

Neural tissue itself is incapable of being rehabilitated. Where there has been significant neurologic impairment, the athlete would not be allowed to return to competition. When there has been complete neurologic recovery, the athlete would be allowed to return to competition according to the guidelines in Table 3, but only when and if his or her general physical condition and conditioning, especially of the neck muscles, had returned to its preinjury status.

Other conditions that would preclude return to contact/collision sports include spontaneous subarachnoid hemorrhage, permanent neurologic sequelae from head injury, and a posttraumatic seizure disorder.

Suggested Reading

Cantu RC. Criteria for return to competition after head or cervical spine injury. In Cantu RC, Micheli LJ, eds. *American college of sports medicine: guidelines for the team physician.* Philadelphia: Lea & Febiger, 1991.

Cantu RC. Criteria for return to competition following a closed head injury. In: Torg JS, ed. *Athletic injuries to the head, neck, and face,* 2nd ed. Chicago: Year Book, 1991.

Cantu RC. Guidelines for return to contact sports after a cerebral concussion. *Phys Sportsmed* 1986;14:75–83.

Cantu RC. Head and neck injuries in the young athlete. In: Micheli LJ, ed. *Sports Injuries in the young athlete.* Philadelphia: WB Saunders, 1988.

Cantu RC. Head injury in sports. In: Grana WA, Lombardo JA, eds. *Advances in sports medicine and fitness.* Chicago: Year Book, 1988.

Cantu RC. Minor head injuries in sports. In: Dyment PG, ed. *Adolescent medicine: state of the art reviews,* Philadelphia: Hanley & Belfus, 1991.

Cantu RC. Second impact syndrome: immediate management. *Phys Sports Med* 1992;20:55–66.

32. INJURIES OF THE CERVICAL SPINE

Joseph S. Torg and James J. Guerra

I. Epidemiology.

Injury to the cervical spine as a result of participation in competitive or recreational sports is not uncommon. A broad clinical spectrum of injuries to the cervical spine and associated structures can occur. Fortunately, catastrophic injuries to the cervical spine and spinal cord are rare. Although relatively uncommon, these injuries represent a sobering proportion of athletic injuries that can produce permanent, irrevocable disability. Accordingly, health care professionals engaged in treating athletes should have an appreciation of the prevention, recognition, and early management, of these injuries, the basic principles of their treatment, and the advisability of return to play.

II. Prevention

A. **Mechanism of injury.** Axial loading is the predominant force in athletic injuries of the cervical spine. In contact sports, the cervical spine is repeatedly exposed to potential injurious forces. These forces are usually dissipated by controlled cervical motion, with the paravertebral muscles and intervertebral discs absorbing the energy. However, when the head is lowered to ram an opponent (i.e., ***spearing***) the cervical spine straightens, assuming the characteristics of a segmented column. When the spine assumes this position, axial forces can no longer be dispersed by controlled cervical motion. At the moment of collision, the head stops and the fragile cervical spine is compressed between the head and oncoming trunk. If the compressive force, estimated at merely 750–1,000 lb, exceeds the ability of the intervertebral discs and vertebral bodies to resist it, fractures and dislocations can occur.

B. **National Collegiate Athletic Association (NCAA) Football Rules Committee, 1976.** In the early 1970s, improvements in helmet design had encouraged the use of the head as the primary point of contact in blocking, tackling, and head butting, resulting in increased injuries of the cervical spine. In 1976, ***the NCAA Football Rules Committee banned "spearing"*** and using the head as the initial point of contact. As a direct result of this rule change, there has been a precipitious decline in these injuries. Players employing head-first tackling techniques should be strongly counseled regarding the perils of head-first impact and coached in proper and safe tackling techniques.

III. Emergency Management

A. **Who is at risk?** The clinical manifestations of cervical spine injuries are extremely variable, and the clinical picture may not always be representative of the seriousness of the injury. All unconscious players should be managed as though they had a significant neck injury until proven otherwise. Since most athletes tend to minimize symptoms and underreport injuries, any athlete who complains of neck pain, even without a neurologic deficit, should be suspected of having a potential cervical spine injury.

B. **Preparation.** Since severe injuries to the cervical spine are infrequent, the on-site medical team typically has little if any prior experience. The emergency management protocol should be familiar to the entire medical staff beforehand, so as to avoid confusion in the true emergency situation. The team physician or trainer should be the designated "captain," supervising the on-the-field management. Necessary emergency equipment should include, at a minimum:

1. A spine board and stretcher
2. Equipment necessary for the initiation and maintenance of cardiopulmonary resuscitation (CPR)
3. Bolt cutters or a sharp knife for removal of face mask
4. Ambulance on site for football and on call for other sports
5. Telephone access for communicating with hospital emergency department

C. **Assessment.** The single most important objective in the acute assessment of the athlete with a suspected cervical spine injury is the prevention of further injury. This necessitates an examination that does not disturb the longitudinal alignment of the spine. The first step is to immobilize the head and neck by supporting them in a stable position while applying gentle cervical traction. Next, a standard cardiopulmonary evaluation is performed. The ABCs (airway, breathing, and circulation) are checked, followed by an evaluation of the level of consciousness. If the cardiopulmonary status is stable, the mouthpiece is removed and the airway simply maintained until transportation is available. No attempt to move the athlete, even if he or she is unconscious, is made except to transport the patient or to initiate CPR.

D. **Management of the athlete who stops breathing.** Establishing the airway is paramount. If in the prone position, the athlete must be turned to a face-up position while avoiding independent movement of the head and neck. This is accomplished by log-rolling the athlete into the face-up position, preferably onto a spine board for later transportation. In order to initiate rescue breathing, ***the face mask and the helmet are removed.*** The type of face mask that is attached to the helmet determines the method of removal. Older single- and double-bar masks require the use of a bolt cutter for removal, whereas newer masks are attached by plastic loops that can be cut with a sharp knife or scalpel. Once the face mask has been removed, an airway must be established by either of two techniques:

1. **Jaw-thrust maneuver.** The rescuer grasps the angles of the victim's mandible and displaces the jaw anteriorly.
2. **Head tilt–jaw lift technique.** The rescuer places one hand under the athlete's lower jaw on the bony part near the chin and lifts the chin forward while the other hand gently presses on the victim's forehead tilting the head back. Care must be exercised not to overextend the neck. Rescue breathing and CPR are then initiated according the current standards of the American Heart Association.

E. **Transportation.** Lifting and carrying the athlete on the spine board requires five people—four to lift and the leader to maintain immobilization of the cervical spine. It is extremely important that the leader remain in control, and the ambulance crew should be receptive to taking orders. ***At no time should the helmet or chin strap be removed during the transportation process.*** The shoulder pads create a relative anterior translation of the thorax which is balanced by the elevation created by the helmet. Removing the helmet with the shoulder pads intact places the neck in extreme hyperextension. The helmet should be removed only when the patient reaches the emergency room, where it can be removed in a controlled manner.

F. **Medical treatment for spinal cord injury.** The role of steroid treatment for spinal cord injury remains somewhat controversial. Methylprednisolone has been shown to be effective in improving motor and sensory deficits after spinal cord injury if the drug is administered within 8 hr of injury. Therefore, acute management should include parenteral steroids. The recommended treatment protocol is an initial ***30mg/kg bolus of methylprednisolone followed by a 5.4 mg/kg/hr infusion for the next 23 hr.***

IV. Specific cervical spine considerations in the athlete

A. **Acute cervical sprain syndrome.** The most common athletic injury to the cervical spine is the acute cervical sprain syndrome. It is a collision injury seen in contact sports.

1. **Clinical presentation.** The athlete complains of having "jammed" the neck, with subsequent pain localized to the cervical area. Characteristically, the athlete presents with limited motion of the cervical spine but without radiation of pain or paresthesias. Neurologically, the patient is intact without focal signs.
2. **Radiographs.** Radiographs are normal. After acute symptoms subside, if the athlete continues to demonstrate limited cervical motion, lateral flexion and extension radiographs are indicated to rule out occult fractures or instability. Clinical instability has been defined by White and Panjabi as greater than ***3.5 mm*** of translation or more than ***11 degrees*** of increased angulation as compared with either adjacent vertebra. If flexion and extension radiographs are negative, marked limitation of cervical motion, persistent pain, or radicular symptoms should be further evaluated with magnetic resonance imaging (MRI) to rule out an intervertebral disc injury.
3. **Treatment.** Treatment of athletes with cervical sprains should be tailored to the degree of severity. The majority of sprains can be managed effectively with conservative modalities, including soft cervical collar immobilization, antiinflammatory agents, and analgesics. Physical therapy is also effective in obtaining full, spasm-free range of motion.
4. **Return to Play.** The athlete with less than a full, pain-free range of cervical motion, persistent paresthesia, or weakness should be protected and excluded from activity. Return to contact activity may occur when the athlete demonstrates full, pain-free motion and is neurologically intact with a stable cervical spine.

B. **Transient quadriplegia.** Transient quadriplegia is a temporary, totally reversible phenomenon due to neurapraxia of the cervical spinal cord from a deformation of the spinal cord without fracture or dislocation. It has been clearly associated with developmental narrowing or stenosis of the cervical spine.

1. **Clinical presentation.** The syndrome is characterized by transient motor and sensory abnormalities and is most commonly seen in football players. The sensory changes can include burning pain, numbness, tingling, and loss of sensation, while motor changes range from paresis to complete paralysis in both upper and/or both lower extremities. The fact that ***both*** sides of the body are involved is important in differentiating this entity from the more commonly occurring "burner" or "stinger," which is usually due to a brachial plexus neurapraxia. Transient quadriplegia typically last 10 to 15 min and complete neurologic recovery is the rule, although in some cases gradual resolution may occur over a 24- to 48-hr period. Except for the burning paresthesia, neck pain is usually not present at the time of injury.
2. **Incidence.** The reported occurrence rate of transient quadriplegia is 1.3 per 10,000, indicating that the problem is more prevalent than expected.
3. **Etlology.** Transient quadriplegia is thought to occur from a "pincer mechanism." According to this theory, the developmentally narrow spinal canal is further compromised by extreme flexion or extension, creating a pincer between the vertebral body and the subjacent spinous process and causing transient compression of the cord.
4. **Radiographs.** Routine radiographs of the cervical spine in athletes who have had an episode of transient quadriplegia are negative for fracture, subluxation, and dislocation. However, evidence of cervical stenosis is invariably present. It may be present as either an isolated finding or in association with congenital fusions, ligamentous instability, or intervertebral disc disease. The routine lateral radiograph of the cervical spine should be evaluated for stenosis using the ***Pavlov ratio*** method. The ratio method for determining the diameter of the sagittal spinal canal compares the anteroposterior width of the spinal canal with the antero-

posterior width of the corresponding vertebral body at its midpoint. This method for determining narrowing of the cervical spinal canal is independent of magnification factors caused by varying radiographic techniques, since the spinal canal and vertebral body are in the same anatomical plane and are, thus, similarly affected by magnification. A spinal canal–vertebral body ratio of less than 0.80 is indicative of significant cervical stenosis and has been present with very few exceptions, at one or more levels in all athletes who have experienced an episode of cervical cord neuropraxia. The sensitivity of the ratio, or the probability of radiographic stenosis in a symptomatic individual, is nearly 100%. However, 12% of the general population and 33% of football players without a history of transient quadriplegia have a ratio of less than 0.80 at one or more cervical levels as well. Therefore, the ratio method has a low positive predictive value and ***preparticipation screening radiographs in asymptomatic players are not recommended.*** Such exams do not contribute to safety, are not cost effective, and only confound the issue.

5. **Prognosis.** The concern is whether athletes who have experienced an episode of cord neurapraxia are prone to future clinical episodes but, importantly, are not predisposed to further permanent neurologic injury. A recent study using computed tomography (CT) analysis of the cross-sectional area of the spinal canal has clearly demonstrated a strong correlation between the tightness of the canal and future episodes of transient quadriplegia. Although previously symptomatic athletes with more stenotic canals are more prone to future occurrences, transient quadriplegia is not a risk factor for permanent neurologic sequelae. Of the 117 known quadriplegics in the National Football Head and Neck Injuries Registry, none had experienced prior episodes of cord neuropraxia. Moreover, of the 45 athletes in the transient quadriplegia cohort within the registry, none have gone on to develop permanent quadriplegia. This is believed to be due to the difference in the mechanism of injury. The pincer mechanism, as in transient quadriplegia, is in direct contrast to the axial loading mechanism seen with fractures and dislocations of the cervical spine that result in permanent neurologic loss. Therefore, on an epidemiologic and pathophysiologic basis, an episode of **cord neurapraxia in the presence of uncomplicated cervical stenosis in a stable spine does not appear to be either a harbinger of or to predispose to permanent neurological injury.**
6. **Return to play.** With respect to the advisability of return to play, the incidental finding in an asymptomatic patient of a canal–vertebral body ratio of less than 0.8 represents no contraindication to participation in contact sports. In those individuals with a ratio of 0.8 or less who have experienced an episode of cervical cord neuropraxia, there is a relative contraindication to continued participation. These cases must be determined on an individual basis, depending on the understanding of the player and parents and their willingness to accept any presumed theoretical risk. Contact sports are absolutely contraindicated in those individuals who experience a documented episode of cervical cord neuropraxia in the presence of any of the following:
   a. Ligamentous instability
   b. Acute intervertebral disc hemiation
   c. MRI evidence of cord defects or swelling
   d. More than one recurrence

C. **"Spear tackler's spine."** This is a recently described condition that occurs in football players who habitually employ spearing techniques using the head as the initial point of contact. It is important to recognize this condition, since it represents an absolute contraindication to continued participation in contact sports.

1. **Clinical presentation.** Athletes typically present because of complaints, referable to the cervical spine or brachial plexus, resulting from football injuries. The diagnosis is made through the pathognomonic radiographic findings. Early recognition of this entity is imperative because the athlete is at high risk for permanent neurologic injury.
2. **Radiographs.** The entity consist of the following triad:
   a. Loss of the normal cervical lordosis
   b. Cervical stenosis
   c. Posttraumatic radiographic changes

   The key to the diagnosis is loss of the normal cervical lordosis. This is best visualized on an erect lateral radiograph in neutral alignment. The straightened cervical spine assumes the characteristics of a segmented column, which predisposes the spine to permanent neurologic injury with axial loading. The combination of a spear-tackler's spine and head-first tackling téchniques creates an extremely dangerous situation with potentially catastrophic sequelae.
3. **Etiology.** The triad of radiographic changes is thought to be due to repetitive microtrauma to the spinal structures caused by habitual use of spear tackling techniques.
4. **Return to play.** The spear tackle's spine represents an absolute contraindication to further participation in contact sports. The straightened cervical spine may be a reversible or a fixed deformity. In those instances in which the loss of cervical lordosis is of a reversible nature, a return to actvitity may be considered when the normal lordotic curve returns.

D. **Axial load "teardrop" fracture.** A complete discusssion of all acute cervical spine fractures is beyond the scope of this manual. However, the reader should be aware of the *axial load teardrop fracture* and its implications for the athlete. It is important to differentiate this fracture pattern from the more benign *isolated teardrop fracture,* which portends a much better prognosis.

1. **Clinical presentation.** Athletes who sustain axial load teardrop fractures typically present after attempting a tackle with significant neural element compression, ranging from nerve root compression to complete spinal cord paralysis.
2. **Radiographs.** Radiographically, the axial load teardrop fracture consists of a three-part, two-plane fracture in which there is a sagittal vertebral body fracture as well as fractures of the posterior neural arch. Although the name of the fracture focuses attention on the fracture of the anteroinferior vertebral body, it is the unstable fracture pattern that is responsible for encroachment on the spinal cord, resulting in the paralysis that frequently accompanies this injury. This fracture pattern should be differentiated from the *isolated teardrop fracture* of the anteroinferior corner of the vertebra, which is usually not associated with permanent neurologic sequelae.
3. **Etiology.** Axial loading of the cervical spine has been clearly identified as the mechanism of injury.
4. **Return to play.** The axial-load teardrop fracture constitutes an absolute contraindication to continued participation in contact sports.

V. Guidelines for return to play.

With respect to the advisability of return to play for athletes who have sustained an injury to the cervical spine, the easiest and perhaps most prudent advice was traditionally to prohibit further contact sports. This approach had been employed historically owing to limited objective data pertaining to postinjury risk factors as well as the potential for severe permanent disability should things go awry. Recently, criteria for return to contact activities for specific bony, ligamentous, and congenital anomalies have been established. These guidelines have been based largely upon epidemiologic information compiled from over 1,200 cervical spine injuries documented by the National Football Head and

Neck Injury Registry as well as from "educated" conjecture based upon recognized injury mechanisms.

A. **Absolute prerequistes.** It should be emphasized that in order to be considered for return to contact activities, the athlete must absolutely meet *all* of the following prerequisites:
   1. The athlete must have a normal neurologic examination.
   2. The athlete must demonstrate a full range of cervical motion.
   3. The athlete must be pain-free.
   4. The athlete must have a stable cervical spine.

B. **Classification.** General guidelines to assisit the clinician, as well as the patient and parents, in the decision-making process have been established.

Table 32-1. Guidelines for the Advisability of Return to play[a]

	No contraindication	Relative contraindication	Absolute contraindication
Congenital conditions			
Odontoid anomalies			X
Spina bifida occulta	X		
Atlantooccipital fusion			X
Klippel-Feil syndrome			
Mass fusions			X
Fusion ≤2 interspaces			
Upper cervical spine			X
C3 or below	X		
Developmental conditions			
Transient quadriplegia		X	
Spear tackler's spine			X
Traumatic conditions—upper cervical spine			
Atlantoaxial instability			X
Atlas (C1) fractures			
Healed nondisplaced		X	
Healed displaced			X
Odontoid fractures			
Healed nondisplaced		X	
Healed displaced			X
Surgical fusion, C1-C2			X
Fibrous union			X
Traumatic conditions—Lower Cervical Spine			
Healed compression fractures	X		
Healed burst fractures			X
Healed teardrop fracture dislocation			X
Cervical instability			
White and Panjabi criteria[b]			X
Healed 1–2 level fusion		X	
Healed >2 level fusion			X

[a] Return to play is predicated upon the athlete meeting all of the following conditions: (1) The athlete must have a normal neurologic exam. (2) The athlete must demonstrate a full range of cervical motion. (3) The athlete must be pain-free. (4) The athlete must have a stable cervical spine. The reader is advised to see the Suggested Readings for a more extensive discussion of the criteria for the return to play.

[b] White and Panjabi have defined clinical instability as greater than 3.5 mm of translation or more than 11 degrees of increased angulation as compared with either adjacent vertebra (*Spine* 1984;9:512).

Each injury or condition has been divided into categories that represent either:

1. No contraindication
2. Relative contraindication
3. Absolute contraindication

C. **Return-to-play criteria for specific injuries or conditions.** It must be understood that these recommendations are meant only as general guidelines and not as absolute directives. Each case must be individualized with respect to specific injury pattern, the specific sport in question, and the age and activity level of the athlete. Guidelines regarding the relative safety of return to contact activity following cervical spine injury or the identification of congenital anomalies are outlined in Table 32-1. The reader is advised to see Suggested Reading, below, for a more extensive discusssion.

D. **Return-to-play criteria following cervical spine fusion.** A stable one-level anterior or posterior fusion that does not involve the atlas (C1) in a patient who is asymptomatic, neurologically intact, pain-free, and has a normal range of cervical motion presents no contraindication to continued participation in contact activities. A two- or three-level fusion presents a relative contraindication, and a fusion of more than three levels constitutes an absolute contraindication.

Suggested Reading

Guerra JJ, Torg JS. Evaluation and rehabilitation of the cervical spine in the athlete. *Sports physical therapy section home study course.* 1996;1–16.

Torg JS, Gennarelli TA. Head and cervical spine injuries. In: DeLee JC, Drez D, eds. *Orthopaedic sports medicine,* vol 1. Philadelphia: W.B. Saunders, 1994;417–462.

Torg J, Glasgow S. Criteria for return to contact activities following cervical spine injury. *Clin Sports Med* 1991;1:12–26.

Torg JS, Pavlov H, Genuario SE, et al. Neuropraxia of the cervical spinal cord with transient quadriplegia. *J Bone Joint Surg* 1988;68A:1354–1370.

Torg JS. *Athletic injuries to the head, neck and face.* St. Louis; Mosby–Year Book, 1991.

Torg JS, Vegso JJ, Sennett BJ. The national football head and neck injury registry: 14-year report on cervical quadriplegia, 1971 through 1984. *JAMA* 1985;254: 3439–3443.

Torg JS, Vegso JJ, O'Neill J. The epidemiologic, pathologic, biomechanical, and cinematographic analysis of football-induced spine trauma. *Am J Sports Med* 1990;18:50–57.

33. PERIPHERAL NERVE INJURIES OF THE SHOULDER GIRDLE

Robert D. Leffert

I. OVERVIEW

Injuries to the peripheral nerves are not the most common injuries in sports. This makes their diagnosis more difficult or unlikely than that of some of the more common entities that are encountered. Consequently, their management may be less familiar to those who render care to injured athletes. For these reasons, a systematic approach to examination must include evaluation of the peripheral nervous system to eliminate the possibility that a nerve injury may be responsible for loss of function. Even when there is an obvious musculoskeletal lesion, it may not be the entire cause of the problem.

In the United States, the majority of sports-related peripheral nerve injuries are associated with contact sports, and those about the shoulder girdle are the most common.

II. Diagnosis of Nerve Injury

A. **History.** The history may appear obvious if an athlete is injured in a contact sport. The episode may be witnessed by other players, trainers, or team physicians. In some cases, however, the mechanism may not be obvious, so that it may be necessary also to interview others besides the patient to determine the course of events. In a professional sporting event, there may be videotape that can be helpful. It is also important to obtain a past history of any prior nerve injuries or underlying neurological conditions, although the latter would be unlikely in a competitive athlete. If there is a fracture or dislocation and the patient is not seen immediately, it is important to determine when the loss of neurological function occurred, whether immediately, after immobilization or reduction or gradually thereafter. When emergency treatment has been rendered on the playing field or at another facility, written notes from the person rendering the treatment can be extremely helpful in management and should be sought.

Not all peripheral nerve problems affecting athletes can be directly related to an easily identifiable traumatic event. In some cases there may be a nerve entrapment that has a subtle presentation. These cases require that the caregiver have a working knowledge of the kinesiological requirements of the athletic activity. In addition, the duration and frequency of participation may be important in formulating of the diagnosis. As with any medical history, questions regarding general condition, underlying generalized disorders that could predispose to neuropathies, and the possibility of both prescribed or self-administered drugs should not be overlooked.

B. **Physical examination.** In cases of trauma incurred in a contact sport, a brief screening examination of the peripheral nervous system is conducted in parallel with that of the musculoskeletal system. There is really no excuse for not performing it, since it can be accomplished in less than 2 min and without sophisticated equipment. Once it has been determined whether or not there are fractures, dislocations, or serious muscle injury, the neurological examination can be performed and modified as necessary to take these into account. For example, a patient whose shoulder has been dislocated will be in severe pain. Nevertheless, prior to reduction, in addition to radiographs, the integrity of the axillary nerve can be accurately assessed by asking the patient to contract the deltoid muscle isometrically and by testing light touch in the autonomous zone of the axillary nerve. It is possible to manually muscle-test the injured athlete accurately under these circumstances, and all four limbs should be rapidly assessed. The testing of sensibility need not be complex or time-consuming, since only light touch and appreciation of pinprick need be tested in most cases.

C. **Radiographic examination.** As in any type of musculoskeletal injury, appropriate three-plane radiographs of the injured area of the limb are necessary. When there is a nerve injury accompanying a closed fracture, the level of the bone lesion may be assumed to be the level of the nerve injury. This is particularly true of transverse fractures, although spiral fractures may involve longer lengths of nerve by traction. Those with severe displacement or sharp bone fragments can be expected to result in more severe nerve injuries, varying from traction to actual laceration of the nerve.

D. **Electrodiagnostic testing.** Electrodiagnostic testing of muscles thought to be denervated by nerve injury should ordinarily be delayed until 3 weeks postinjury in order to ensure that the electrical changes have time to develop. Unless there is reason to believe that a nerve injury preexisted the one under consideration, the only reason to study an acute injury is to define an innocent lesion, neurapraxia, by means of nerve conduction velocity determination, since normal conduction can be found distal to an area of compression or nerve contusion that will block normal impulses and function. The combination of nerve conduction velocity determination and needle electromyographic (EMG) examination can objectively confirm the location and degree of severity of the nerve lesion in most cases.

III. Types of Nerve Injury.

A clinically useful classification of peripheral nerve injury is that of Seddon, who defined three types of nerve injury as follows:

A. **Neurapraxia.** A physiological interruption of nerve conduction that does not involve disruption of the anatomic components of the nerve. It results in loss of motor power and sensory function within the cutaneous distribution of the nerve, although the latter may be less impaired than the former. Most neurapraxias are due to nerve compression, although sometimes mild traction may be responsible. They can result from external compression on the limb as well as internal compression or traction due to fractures or dislocations. The duration of neurological loss can range from minutes to approximately 4 to 6 weeks, during which time the EMG shows no evidence of denervation. Nerve conduction in the areas of the nerve not directly affected will often be normal, with a local delay in conduction delineating the involved area. The prognosis for complete recovery is excellent, although the limb may still require splints to avoid development of contractures.

B. **Axonotmesis.** This lesion results from more severe compression or traction and produces loss of motor and sensory function in the distribution of the nerve. Unlike neurapraxia, this does represent an anatomic lesion that may be observed at the microscopic level. The axon is transected but the supporting elements of the nerve are preserved, so they can serve as a conduit for nerve regeneration when it occurs. These lesions may occur acutely as a result of crush injuries, fractures, blows to the musculature of the limb, or hemorrhage within closed fascial spaces. All have in common the production of elevated pressure within the compartment, which ultimately impairs the circulation to the muscles and nerves. Such lesions may also be seen in muscle groups subjected to unaccustomed, prolonged exercise, such as long runs or hikes. The limb becomes swollen and painful, and the nerves and muscles are compressed and lose function. Diagnosis is clinical, confirmed by measurements of compartment pressure. Failure to recognize the problem and to decompress the fascial compartment surgically will result in permanent loss of function and possibly even the limb itself.

IV. Special Injuries

Injuries to the following are considered: the spinal accessory nerve, brachial plexus, thoracic outlet syndrome, long thoracic nerve, suprascapular nerve, and axillary nerve. Electromyography is instrumental in the diagnosis of these injuries. Further, the EMG can be used to follow the course of the patient to determine if nerve recovery is occurring (see above).

A. **The spinal accessory nerve** is a cranial nerve rather than a peripheral nerve, and injuries to it are unusual in athletics. It innervates the major suspensory muscle of the scapula, the trapezius. Weakness of this muscle can significantly impair the athlete and even affect ordinary activities of daily living. Most of these injuries are the result of traction on the shoulder girdle and may result from violent blows to the shoulder, which stretch the nerve. They may accompany acromioclavicular or sternoclavicular subluxations or dislocations.
   1. **History.** Most athletes complain of severe pain—even with activities of daily living—weakness, and deformity. They note difficulty elevating and abducting the arm. They may complain of a dull ache or heavy feeling about the arm.
   2. **Physical Examination** is best performed from behind the patient. There may be atrophy (or asymmetry) of the trapezius/neckline, drooping of the shoulder, and—on attempting to elevate the arm—scapular winging, as the scapula falls laterally and forward due to the weight of the arm. There is also weakness of abduction and forward elevation, especially above the horizontal.
   3. **Treatment.** Initially range of motion to prevent stiffness, modalities, heat and cold, transcutaneous electrical nerve stimulation (TENS) and resistance exercises may help eliminate the pain and to improve the drooping of the shoulder as well as the winging and weakness. A cloth harness (Biomet hemi-hook harness) may help relieve the pull on the shoulder. If there is no evidence of recovery by examination or EMG by 3 months, the nerve should be explored surgically.

B. **Burners and stingers** are relatively common in athletics, particularly among football players, where up to 50% of players may have the symptoms in a 4-year collegiate career. The most common mechanism for the production of the symptoms is that of traction on the upper trunk of the plexus when either the head and shoulder are forced apart by a blow or the shoulder pad is forced into the neck and causes a contusion. Local stretch can range from mild elongation of the nerves with almost instantaneous recovery to serious structural neural damage accompanied by local hemorrhage. The C5-C6 nerve segments and/or upper trunk tend to be most commonly affected.
   1. **History.** The symptoms come on acutely with a blow to the shoulder girdle or a fall during a tackle and are usually those of an intense burning or stinging sensation extending from the lateral aspect of the neck into the shoulder girdle, arm, and often also the thumb and index finger. Most of these injuries are of very short duration and are unaccompanied by persisting neural deficits. In fact, many will have resolved by the time an athlete reaches the sidelines for evaluation. Up to 10%, however, may involve persistent pain, numbness, and weakness lasting several hours or days.
   2. **Physical examination** may include varying amounts of numbness and weakness depending on the nerves involved and the severity of injury. Those athletes with the more severe stretch injury and structural damage to the nerve may have persisting pain, numbness, and weakness of the muscles innervated by the injured nerves. The more common muscles with weakness are the deltoid, supraspinatus, and biceps.
   3. **Differential diagnosis** includes cervical intervertebral disc herniation and infraclavicular brachial plexus injury associated with shoulder dislocation. In cases where an injured player has severe neck and interscapular pain that is increased by tilting the head toward the affected side or where there is a sudden feeling of electric shock through the body when the neck is flexed, there is a likelihood of a herniated cervical disc. For such a player to continue playing would risk permanent neurological damage, possibly quadriplegia. In a very rare instance, a player may sustain actual neurotmesis of the brachial plexus during a football

game or rugby match. This may prove to be either a root avulsion from the spinal cord or a rupture further distally in the plexus. These lesions are caused by a very great amount of trauma and have a very poor prognosis.

4. **Treatment.** It is important to attempt to define the extent of injury so that proper treatment can be given. Players whose symptoms subside very quickly may return to the game. Those with any neurologic residua should be benched, with follow-up neurological evaluation. They may return to sports when all the symptoms are resolved and neurological examination is normal. Patients who have recurrent stingers do run an increased risk of permanent neurological injury.

C. **Thoracic outlet syndrome and effort-induced thrombosis.** Paresthesias, numbness, and weakness of the upper limb that is felt with overhead activities and weight lifting may be due to compression of the neurovascular structures within the thoracic outlet. This may occur in the absence of cervical ribs and may rest on a muscular or postural basis. In those athletes who do repetitive overhead exercise and are symptomatic, there is a danger of acute thrombosis of the subclavian vein.

1. **History.** Clinical presentation depends on which neurovascular structures are most affected. The patient may complain of pain in the neck or shoulder or numbness and tingling involving either the entire upper limb or the forearm and hand. Most often paresthesias involve the ulnar nerve distribution (C8-T1). Patients may complain of arm weakness or fatigue. Symptoms are usually reproduced by specific athletic activities. Tennis players may report that they experience weakness in the arm and hand with their backhand swing. Rarely, a hyperdeveloped weight lifter may experience similar symptoms. Athletes with effort-induced thrombosis present with acute pain (within 24 hr of the activity), swelling, and numbness of the limb.
2. **Physical examination.** This will vary based on the which neurovascular structures are most involved and to what extent. Occasionally there will be coolness and pallor with arterial involvement and edema, venous engorgement, and cyanosis with venous obstruction of the involved extremity. Adson's test, Wright's test, and the overhead stress test are provocative maneuvers to aid in the diagnosis.
3. **Special tests.** Electrodiagnostic tests are helpful if positive but do not rule out the diagnosis if negative (normal). Venography showing occlusion of the axillary or subclavian vein is indicated to diagnose effort-induced thrombosis.
4. **Treatment.** Whereas the other varieties of thoracic outlet compression can usually be managed by postural corrective exercises, the patient with effort thrombosis must be treated acutely with intravenous thrombolytic agents followed by anticoagulation. In addition to postural corrective exercises, a regimen of rest, non-steroidal anti-inflammatory drugs, and TENS followed by muscle strengthening of the shoulder girdle often is effective. For those patients who cannot achieve relief of symptoms by conservative management and are incapacitated by them, surgical decompression of the thoracic outlet is occasionally indicated as a last resort.

D. **Palsy of the long thoracic nerve** results in winging of the scapula. Acute scapular winging may occur as a spontaneous phenomenon with no obvious cause for the loss of function of the nerve to the serratus anterior muscle, in which case it is labeled "idiopathic." Other common causes of injury to the long thoracic nerve include acute trauma such as forceful shoulder depression and contralateral bending of the cervical spine. Serratus palsy may also be found in high-level volleyball players because of repeated irritation of the long thoracic nerve. Although this is usually an axonotmesis, it has a good prognosis for recovery in most cases.

1. **History.** The athlete will complain of pain in the shoulder or periscapular region after an acute injury or repetitive activity, often also noting loss of power in the shoulder and difficulty in raising the arm above horizontal. There may also be discomfort as the scapula hits the back of a chair.
2. **Physical examination.** The patient should be examined from behind for winging of the scapula with wall push-ups or active arm-forward elevation.
3. **Treatment.** Winging is best treated with rest until the muscle recovers. The time for recovery may be as long as 18 months, during which the function of the shoulder girdle will be severely compromised. It is important to maintain shoulder range of motion during this time.

E. **The suprascapular nerve** is most often entrapped at the level of the suprascapular notch, before it innervates the supraspinatus and then the infraspinatus muscles. In some cases, where only the infraspinatus is affected, the entrapment may either relate to the spinoglenoid ligament or the presence of a ganglion coming from the posterior aspect of the shoulder joint. Here again, players engaging in repetitive overhead motions, such as volleyball players and throwers, develop an injury to this nerve. Direct trauma may also be a cause of suprascapular nerve injury.

1. **History.** Athletes complain of a vague ache in the posterior or superior aspect of the shoulder, which may be accompanied by weakness about the shoulder. When the injury is atraumatic in origin, the onset is gradual and insidious and, without treatment, progressive. Patients may note that pain is exacerbated by exercise and/or arm elevation.
2. **Physical examination.** Both arm abduction and lateral rotation will be weak. The extent of actual atrophy and weakness of the supraspinatus and/or infraspinatus muscles is determined by the extent of involvement and duration of nerve injury. Tenderness may exist in the infraspinatus fossa and/or suprascapular notch.
3. **Special tests.** MRI and ultrasound can demonstrate ganglia if they are present. Confirmation of the diagnosis is by electrodiagnostic testing including EMG and nerve conduction velocity determination.
4. **Treatment.** If there is significant atrophy of the rotator cuff muscles, the nerve should be surgically decompressed. If there is no atrophy, a trial of rest and physical therapy is indicated. If an EMG confirms the diagnosis and the symptoms do not resolve after 3 to 4 months of conservative treatment, surgical decompression is indicated.

F. **Axillary nerve**

The axillary nerve is at risk in dislocations and fracture-dislocations of the glenohumeral joint because the nerve is directly stretched by the humeral head and neck. Therefore, prior to reduction, the function of the nerve should be assessed as advised above. In those cases in which there is no evidence of recovery by three months post-injury, the nerve should be surgically explored.

There is another mechanism for injury to the axillary nerve of players in heavy contact sports. These injuries occur in the absence of dislocations, but rather are the result of direct crush injuries to the nerve with hemorrhage as it runs its course in the subfascial plane of the muscle. The prognosis for these injuries is poor.

The question of whether total lack of the function of the deltoid is compatible with high-level athletic performance depends on the sporting activity and the requirements of the individual player. Obviously, a throwing athlete would be incapacitated by such an injury. A player who did not have to throw might still be able to compete, and we have seen several of them who continue in professional football even with paralysis of the deltoid. If the rotator cuff is intact, they can still elevate the arm, although obviously, they lack strength.

Suggested Reading

Clancy WG. Brachial plexus and upper extremity peripheral nerve injuries. In:Torg JS, ed. *Athletic injuries to the head, neck and face.* Philadelphia: Lea & Feiberger, 1982;215–222.

Ferretti A, Cerullo G, Russo G. Suprascapular neuropathy in volleyball players. *J Bone Joint Surg* 1987;69A:260–263.

Leffert RD. Neurological problems. In:Rockwood CA Jr, Matsen FA III, eds. *The shoulder.* Philadelphia: WB Saunders, 1990;750–790.

Perlmutter GS, Leffert RD, Zarins B. Direct injury to the axillary nerve in athletes playing contact sports. *Am J Sports Med* 1997;25:65–68.

Schulte KR, Warner JJP. Uncommon causes of shoulder pain in the athlete. *Orthop Clin North Am* 1995;26:505–528.

Vastimaki M, Kauppila LI. Etiologic factors in isolated paralysis of the serratus anterior muscle: a report of 197 cases. *J Shoulder Elbow Surg* 1993;2:240–243.

34. EXERCISE-RELATED HEADACHES

John M. Henderson

I. Background

A. **Epidemiology**

1. Headache is one of the most common presenting complaints to the primary care specialist's office/clinic.
2. Nontraumatic headache triggered by exertion is also common and can be a confounding experience for the physician as well as the patient.
3. Post-traumatic, exertion-induced headache is anecdotally common but poorly documented and not well understood.
4. The single most important factor in the diagnosis of headache is that the presence of ominous disease is not overlooked, especially intracranial malignancies, vascular diseases, indolent infections, occult trauma, inflammatory and suppurative processes.

B. **Incidence/frequency**

1. The true incidence of exercise-related headache in the general population is not known because of self-treatment and lack of reporting.
2. The incidence of these headache in sports is also not known because the true incidence of its common causes, such as minor head trauma, is not known and because the complaint is often trivialized (particularly in football, rugby, soccer, and boxing).
3. Over half the athletes sustaining a minor head trauma/concussion still complain of a headache at rest 1 week later. Many of these athletes complain of an exertional headache several weeks to months later.
4. The common exertion-induced headache may not be preceded by a traumatic event. These complaints can have an insidious onset over days to weeks or may develop suddenly. These headaches are more common in the groups of athletes whose sports involve short, explosive anaerobic bursts and who are characteristically self-critical and introspective (dance, wrestling, gymnastics, diving, fencing, and marksmanship events like archery, riflery, modern pentathlon).
5. Nearly everyone who lives below 1,000 ft above sea level and recreates or competes in a sport above 5,280 ft above sea level experiences an exertional headache for the 48 to 72 hr during which acclimatization occurs.
6. Headaches induced by resistance training/weight lifting and accompanied by nausea and vomiting, with crescendos of deep boring pain and an inability to find a comfortable position, could signal an intracranial hemorrhage. Systolic blood pressure increases to the range of 300 to 400 torr during some weight-training activities and can contribute to intracranial etiologies.
7. Headache can herald an illness caused by *Mycoplasma pneumoniae.*
8. Headache can be the hallmark of withdrawal from certain drugs, such as alcohol, codeine, and clonidine.
9. Headache associated with personality changes and inappropriate behavior can be due to insidious etiologies such as chronic subdural hematoma, meningioma, second-impact syndrome, heavy metal poisoning, and illicit drug use. Headache and eye pain can signal glaucoma or corneal abrasion or uveitis/iritis. Headache and throat pain can signal streptococcosis.

II. Etiologies of Exercise-Induced Headaches

A. **Intracranial etiologies**

1. Postconcussion syndrome
2. Dural rent

3. Increased Intracranial pressure
    a. Cerebral contusion
    b. Second-impact syndrome
    c. Cerebritis with viral syndrome
    d. Aseptic meningitis
4. Decreased Intracranial pressure
    a. After spinal surgery
    b. After spinal anesthesia
    c. Volume contraction

B. **Muscle traction / tension (MTT)**
1. MTT & temporal mandibular joint (TMJ) problems
    a. From excessive chewing (gum, tobacco, sunflower seeds, etc.)
    b. bruxism
2. Cervical spine DJD
    a. Osteoarthrosis
    b. Spondylosis
    c. From repetitive falling, flexion-extension activities (wrestling, swimming)
3. Facet syndrome
    a. Basilar-atlas facet syndrome
    b. Atlas-axis facet syndromes
    c. From head and neck posture (cycling, gymnastics, wrestling, tennis)
4. Occipital neuralgia
    a. From overtight head gear (batting helmet, football helmet)
5. Levator syndrome
    a. From prolonged neck extension (cycling with extension bars)
6. Rhomboid syndrome
    a. From rapid arm motions (racquetball, tennis, golf)
7. Thoracic somatic dysfunction
    a. From incorrect posture (bobsledding, marksmanship)

C. **Problems related to sensory end organs**
1. Eye
    a. Increased intraocular pressure (barotrauma, scuba, inversion)
    b. Corneal abrasion with orbicularis muscle spasm
    c. Occult fracture (racket and club sports)
2. Ear
    a. Middle-ear effusion (barotrauma)
    b. Vestibulitis (dance, gymnastics, skating)
3. Nose
    a. Sinusitis
    b. Blunt trauma (rugby, soccer, wrestling)
4. Mouth
    a. Periodontitis
    b. Dental abscess

D. **Problems related to metabolic derangements**
1. Ketosis headache from fasting/dieting (wrestling, dance, gymnastics, skating)
2. Hypoglycemia headache from relatively excessive insulin during/after exercise
3. Lower oxygen tension (acute mountain sickness)
4. Oxygen desaturation (exercise-induced bronchospasm)
5. Hyponatremia from volume contraction
6. Chronic iron-loss anemia
7. Overtraining
8. Hypokalemia

E. **Neurologic disorders**
1. Partial complex seizures with complex symptomatology
2. Status migrainosus
3. Multiple sclerosis

F. **Vascular disorders**
   1. Temporal arteritis
   2. Migraine headache
   3. Vascular permeability/histamine headache

G. **Nonorganic/psychologic headaches**
   1. Pleasure paradox (enjoyable activity becoming unpleasant work)
   2. Depression
   3. Adjustment reaction
   4. Secondary gain

H. **Medication problems**
   1. Adverse reaction to any medication
   2. Rebound headache from any analgesic
   3. Drug withdrawal headache

III. Treatment Strategies.

Due to the nature of this problem, nondrug and drug-oriented treatment plans must be individually tailored.

A. **Nonpharmacologic treatment**
   1. Relaxation techniques—myofascial release techniques for the posterior cervical, scalp, and facial muscles
   2. Ceremonial practice—practicing the competitive event in small tolerable parts up to the headache threshold
   3. Anticipation training—using imagery techniques to lessen performance anxiety
   4. Cervical spine training—range of motion exercises to enhance facet motion and suppleness of the cervical soft tissues
   5. Physical therapy—accupressure therapy: progressive blunt pressure over trigger point areas of tenderness; physical modalities; cryotherapy and electrical stimulation over tense areas of the upper back and posterior neck muscle groups

B. **Do not overlook or trivialize**
   1. Diet—the following items should be limited, since they can have a triggering effect on headaches:
      a. Refined sugar—candy, icings, glazed toppings
      b. Salt—prepared, processed, frozen foods
      c. Spices—nutmeg, monosodium glutamate
      d. Herbs—ginseng, cocoa
      e. Mild cholinergic poisoning from insecticides on unwashed fruits and vegetables
   2. Equipment—sports gear should be checked to assess their contribution to the headache trigger:
      a. Headgear—helmet, ear pads, chin straps, inner shock absorbing liner
      b. Chest-wall protector—shoulder and arm straps
   3. Mechanics—the motion involved in the sport can be assessed to search for contributions to the headache trigger:
      a. Spine, particularly neck; posture
      b. Trunk posture
      c. Upper arm position
   4. General fitness
      a. Aerobic power—the ability to sustain low-level work by large muscle groups over long periods of time is part of the foundation of treatment. This includes walking, running, cycling, nordic skiing.
      b. Flexibility—posterior shoulder, cervical, and low lumbar passive and active ranges of motion usually need improvement to enhance competitive performance.

C. **Drug treatment strategies.** Remember that all these medications have unwanted side effects and may decrease the patient's athletic performance. Many of these substances are banned by the major international and national governing bodies of various sports. Additionally, medication compliance drastically decreases when the medication dosage schedule requires more than once-a-day dosing.

1. Acute abortive treatment of the exertional headache
   a. Empiric diagnostic and therapeutic trial of sumatriptan (Imitrex), a selective agonist for vascular 5-HT1D. This can be used as a diagnostic as well as therapeutic trial. It is contraindicated in gravid athletes or those who have coronary artery disease.
      i. Imitrex-sumatriptan available as 1. autoinjector 6 mg, 2. oral tablets 25 and 50 mg, 3. inhaled spray 20 mg. Zomig-zolmitriptan available as oral tablet 2.5 and 5 mg.
   b. Analgesic cocktails
      i. Combination parenteral analgesic agents: dihydroergotamine (DHE-45) 1 to 2mg i.m., metoclopramide (Reglan) 5 to 10 mg i.m., and hydroxyzine (Vistaril) 25 to 100 mg i.m. **or** meperidine (Demerol) 25 to 75 mg i.m., promethazine (Phenergan) 12.5 to 25 mg i.m., and chlorpromazine (Thorazine) 6 to 12 mg i.m.
      ii. Single parenteral analgesic agent: ketorolac (Toradol) 30 to 60 mg i.m.
      iii. Inhaled agents: intranasal butorphanol (Stadol) 1 mg (one puff)—agonist at opioid receptors k and u, and dihydroergotamine (Migranol) (DHE-45) one puff
2. Break the "exertion-headache cycle"
   a. Empiric use of a nonnarcotic analgesic around the clock
      i. Acetaminophen (Tylenol) 650 mg q8h
      ii. Acetaminophen plus butalbitol (Axocet) q8h
      iii. Acetaminophen plus butalbitol plus caffeine (Fiorinal) q12h
      iv. Propoxyphene (Darvon) 65 mg q8h
   b. Around-the-clock nonsteroidal antiinflammatory drugs (NSAIDs)
      i. Aspirin 650 mg q.i.d. (cheapest but associated with dyspepsia and ulcers)
      ii. Ibuprofen (Motrin) 200 to 800 mg t.i.d. (cheap but can also cause dyspepsia)
      iii. The newest NSAIDs are more expensive but have fewer gastrointestinal, neurobehavioral, and renal complications:
         - Oxaprozin (Daypro) 600 mg b.i.d.
         - Nabumetone (Relafen) 750 mg b.i.d.
         - Etodolac (Lodine) 400 mg t.i.d.
   c. Empiric use of a beta blocker to reduce vascular reactivity
      i. Propanolol (Inderal) 10 mg b.i.d.-t.i.d.
      ii. Nadolol (Corgard) 20 to 80 mg q.d.
      iii. Metoprolol (Lopressor) 50 to 100 mg q.d.
      iv. Atenolol (Tenormin) 25 to 50 mg q.d.
   d. Empiric use of a tricyclic antidepressant having anticholinergic effects to reduce norepinephrine reuptake:
      i. Amitryptiline (Elavil) 25 mg h.s.
      ii. Doxepin (Sinequan) 10 to 50 mg h.s.
      iii. Imipramine (Tofranil) 10 to 50 mg h.s.
   e. Empiric use of a preexertional/preevent analgesic as for abortive treatment
      i. See III.C.1.a or III.C.1.b
   f. Empiric use of herbal teas
      i. Chamomile, rose hips, dandelion, jasmine
3. Modify the associated complaints without causing a decrement in the athlete's physical abilities by sedation, decreased cardiac output, or dampening of the neuromuscular unit's excitability.
   a. Mild, short-onset/limited-action hypnotic to affect the sleep pattern
      i. Zolpidem (Ambien) 5 mg h.s.
   b. Hormone replacement to influence the perimenstrual and menopausal dysphoria and depression

i. Medroxyprogesterone (Provera) 2.5 mg for days 19 through 25 of the cycle
ii. Estrogen/progestin combination agent (Prempro) 1 q.d.
iii. Trial of low-dose oral birth-control pills containing levonorgestrael 50 to 125 μg plus ethinyl estradiol 30 to 40 μg (Triphasil or Tri-Levlen)
iv. Esterified estrogens plus methyltestosterone (EstraTest) 1.25/2.5 mg q.d.
v. Estradiol (Estrace) 1 to 2 mg q.d.

c. Serotonin manipulation to influence neurotransmitters
   i. Selective serotonin inhibitor (serotonin antagonist): ondansetron (Zofran) 4 to 8 mg h.s. or cyproheptadine (Periactin) 4–8 mg h.s.
   ii. Selective serotonin reuptake inhibitors for underlying dysphoric affective disorder (serotonin agonists)
      - Paroxetine (Paxil) 20 to 40 mg q.d.
      - Sertraline (Zoloft) 50 to 100 mg b.i.d.
      - Bupropion (Wellbutrin) 75 to 150 mg b.i.d.
      - Nefazodone (Serzone) 100 mg b.i.d.
      - Fluvoxamine (Luvox) 50 to 100 mg h.s.

d. Nonsedating antihistamine for its central effect as well as for its upper-airway decompression
   i. Loratadine (Claritin) 10 mg q.d.
   ii. Astemizole (Tavist) 1.34 to 2.68 mg b.i.d.

e. Calcium channel blocker to minimize vasospasm
   i. Nifedipine (Procardia) 10 to 30 mg b.i.d.–t.i.d.
   ii. Isradipine (Dynacirc) 2.5 mg q.d.
   iii. Amlodipine (Norvasc) 2.5 to 5 mg q.d.

f. Alpha-adrenergic manipulation.
   i. alpha antagonists/blockers prazosin (Minipres) 1 to 5 mg b.i.d. or terazosin (Hytrin) 1 to 5 mg q.d.
   ii. alpha agonists/stimulants: clonidine (Catapres) 0.2 to 2.0 mg b.i.d. or guanfacine (Tenex) 1 to 2 mg h.s.

IV. Suggested Workup

A. Remember the biopsychosocial basis of this complaint

B. Refrain from the temptation to order serum and imaging studies to assess every etiology listed above. No currently available imaging study contributes to the evaluation and treatment of most of the etiologies listed above. A thorough history is more important than studies of cerebrospinal fluid.

C. Based on a provisional diagnosis, trials of the least noxious medications could be useful if the athlete's response is monitored closely.

D. Correction of the underlying or associated problems should be the focus of treatment. Make sure there is not a treatable underlying endocrine, vascular, infectious, neurologic, cardiac, or psychiatric condition.

V. Treatment Goals

A. Short-term goal is to keep the athlete functional
   1. Reassure the athlete of the ongoing pursuit of a somatic etiology while recognizing the probable psychologic/emotional contribution to this problem. Try not to alter the athlete's schedule to cater to the headaches.
   2. Keep work and recreational schedules as normal as possible.
   3. Reassess the "fun component" of the sport. Is there a pleasure paradox?
   4. "Manage" the head pain without trying to "ablate" it.

B. Long-term goal is to manage the discomfort.
   1. Daily suppression therapy (preventive therapy)
   2. Episodic crisis intervention (abortive therapy)
   3. Patient education to minimize effects on lifestyle and competition

C. Reassess the headaches and the complaints periodically, especially if there are dramatic changes in the severity or pattern of symptoms as well as associated dysfunctional symptoms such as loss of balance, visual disturbances, or clumsiness. These should signal the need to reconsider further evaluation with imaging or neurophysiologic studies.

VI. Immediate Treatment for Exercise-Induced Headaches

A. Check for trauma
   1. Cervical spine trauma
   2. Head trauma
   3. Maxillofacial trauma
   4. Ear-nose-throat and dental trauma

B. Recheck equipment

C. Check vital signs

D. Ice massage over painful area and at the nuchal ridge

E. Passive soft tissue manipulation
   1. Accupressure over trigger point of tenderness
   2. Massage, efflurage and frappage for trapezius, rhomboids, levator, splenius
   3. Myofascial release techniques for deep cervical extensors

F. Active exercises
   1. Shoulder shrugs, shoulder range of motion (ROM) exercises
   2. Cervical spine ROM and progressive resistance exercises
   3. Scalp and facial exercises: frontalis, orbicularis

G. Before using any headache medication, ask
   1. Is this substance banned by the sport's governing body or agency?
   2. Will the substance alter the athlete's cognitive abilities or eye-hand reaction time?
   3. Will the substance stigmatize the athlete?
   4. Can the athlete's response be monitored?

H. Apply reasonable "return to play" criteria

I. Make arrangements to reassess this athlete in a controlled office setting

Suggested Reading

Headache Classification Committee of the International Headache Society. Classification and diagnostic criteria for headache disorders, cranial neuralgias, and facial pain. *Cephalalgia* 1988;8(suppl 7):5–30.

Henderson J. The impact of head injuries on the return of athletes to sports participation. *Sports Med Arthrosc Rev* 1995;3:308–313.

Sandler M. *Migraine: a spectrum of ideas.* Oxford, England: Oxford University Press, 1990.

35. THE ATHLETE WITH EPILEPSY

Gregory L. Landry and David T. Bernhardt

I. General.

Without scientific studies to guide them, physicians are reluctant to allow young people with epilepsy to participate in sports. There is always concern that participation will either provoke seizures or that seizures during participation will increase the risk of injury. As in the case of other medical conditions, practitioners focus on the risk of participation rather than benefits of physical activity. This often leads them to advise the athlete with epilepsy to refrain from participation. Fortunately, an increasing number of physicians are urging participation of athletes with epilepsy in most sports. Despite statements in the 1960s stressing the risks of sports participation, the American Medical Association and the American Academy of Pediatrics have since issued statements discussing the benefits of exercise.

II. Definition and Epidemiology.

Simply stated, epilepsy is a disorder characterized by recurring seizures. Caused by abnormal electrical discharges within the brain, seizures are characterized by sudden, brief, repetitive and stereotypical alterations of behavior. A person must have more than one seizure to be diagnosed with epilepsy. About 10% of the population will have a seizure at some time during their lives, but only 1% to 3% will develop epilepsy. Head injury is the leading cause of epilepsy, with other potential etiologies including toxic/metabolic problems, neoplasms, infections, degenerative disorders, and developmental abnormalities.

III. The Classification

system for epilepsy used most frequently is the one proposed by the International League Against Epilepsy. Seizures are divided into three main types: partial, generalized, and unclassified. Partial seizures (formerly called temporal lobe or psychomotor seizures) are classified as either simple or complex depending on level of consciousness. Consciousness is preserved in simple partial seizures whereas complex partial seizures are associated with impairment of consciousness. Partial seizures are characterized by loss of awareness of the environment and often associated with semipurposeful movements such as lip smacking, picking at clothing, or walking aimlessly. Partial or complex seizures may progress into a grand mal, generalized tonic-clonic convulsions. Generalized seizures are convulsive or nonconvulsive. The classic grand mal seizure begins with a tonic phase for 15 to 30 sec followed by up to 5 min of generalized clonic movements with tongue biting and urinary and/or fecal incontinence. Nonconvulsive generalized seizures include absence seizures (petit mal), which tend to occur in otherwise healthy children, and atonic seizures, which tend to occur in severely impaired children.

IV. Treatment.

Most childhood epilepsies respond favorably to anticonvulsant medications. Approximately 60% of individuals with epilepsy can achieve good control of seizures with one or more medications. Some 80% of patients with generalized seizure disorders may achieve good control. Epilepsy is not always a lifelong disorder. More than half of children are seizure-free after 2 to 4 years on medications; if slowly withdrawn from anticonvulsant medication, they will not experience a recurrence. Prognostic factors include severity of electroencephalographic (EEG) abnormalities, age of onset, and rapidity of withdrawal of the medications.

V. Mortality.
It has been estimated that the death rate among patients with epilepsy is about 1 per 100,000, which is about double the rate for age-matched controls. Deaths during or soon after a seizure account for 10% to 15% of the mortality rate. It has been reported that bathtub drownings are the most common cause of seizure-related deaths. One study reported that the risk of drowning during recreational swimming is four times greater for epileptic children than for their nonepileptic peers. The risks of these activities are not well studied and remain controversial. Suicide accounts for 7.2% of deaths among epileptics—five times the suicide rate of the general U.S. population.

VI. Benefits of Participation in Sports
for the individual with epilepsy are both physical and psychological. Few studies have been performed to document these benefits. Based on the paucity of reports of exercise-related seizures in the literature, exercise appears to pose little risk for the epileptic children. There is increasing evidence that exercise-induced seizures are rare in adults. It is not clear why a few patients will trigger a seizure with exercise while the majority enjoy a protective effect from activity. Exercise does not appear to alter anticonvulsant metabolism significantly. There is no direct relationship between the metabolic changes that occur during exercise and altered brain electrophysiology.

VII. Risk Factors for Participation in Sports
include many variables such as degree of seizure control, a history of exercise-induced seizures, the potential for injury to the athlete should a convulsion occur during the activity, physical skills or handicaps, the athlete's motivation, side effects of anticonvulsant medication, and environmental factors that might increase the likelihood of seizures.

Probably the most important factor is the degree of control of the epilepsy—i.e., the frequency of seizures. For example, a compliant athlete who has had no seizures in the last year might be allowed to participate in almost all sports. An athlete who has very poor control of seizures (e.g., who has had more than ten seizures in the past year) probably should participate only in low-risk sports.

Because many sports involve trauma to the head and body, there is concern about the risk of blunt head trauma to the epileptic athlete as opposed to the nonepileptic athlete. There is minimal evidence that head trauma increases the risk of seizures in athletes with epilepsy. It remains unclear whether there is any increased risk with repeated head trauma, as occurs in American football or with frequent heading of the soccer ball.

VII. Classification of Sports.
Sporting activities have been grouped by risk to the patient with epilepsy in Table 35-1. In general, aquatic sports, and sports involving altitude carry the highest risk; operating machinery is also risky. These groupings are meant to serve as a guideline for the practitioner when advising the athlete regarding risk of participation. All eligibility decisions must be considered on an individual basis, taking all the factors listed above into consideration.

VIII. Long-term Management.
Eligibility decisions depend to a great degree on the documentation of seizure frequency, and since the athlete may not remember seizure activity, it is important to gather information from the families of athletes with epilepsy. With children, school authorities may be helpful. As with most chronic conditions, close follow-up by the athlete's primary care physician is important until 1 to 2 years of excellent control are documented. Anti-convulsant serum levels should be monitored to document compliance with medication regimens and to make sure that the dose prescribed produces therapeutic levels in the athlete.

Table 35-1. Categories of sporting activities by approximate risk for the athlete with epilepsy or others around the athlete

High risk
Diving
Scuba diving
Parachuting
Rock climbing
Hang gliding
Aviation
Downhill skiing
Motor racing
Boxing
Ski jumping
Rodeo
Cycling
Moderate risk
Waterskiing
Swimming
Canoeing
Crew (rowing)
Fishing
Wind surfing
Surfing
Sailing
Archery
Wrestling
Low risk
Skating
Table tennis
Badminton
Ballet
Billiards
Curling
Cross-country skiing
Golf
Fencing
Bowling
Handball
Squash
Baseball
Softball

If a breakthrough seizure occurs, serum anticonvulsant levels should be obtained. If these are shown to be subtherapeutic, adjustments in medication dose should be made before the athlete returns to sport participation.

IX. Team Physician's Role.

The team physician covering an athletic event must be fully familiar with first-aid measures for seizures.

A. **Generalized tonic-clonic seizures** produce the most anxiety in all concerned. As with any emergency situation, it important for the physician to stay calm and to protect the athlete from injury during the seizure. Be sure that the head, arms, and legs cannot strike anything, causing injury. The athlete should be turned on one side with the head down to prevent aspiration of saliva or vomitus. *Nothing* should be forced into the mouth during a convulsion. More importantly, it is dangerous to place one's fingers into the patient's mouth during a seizure; fingers have been lost in this way. In the postictal period, it is important to monitor the airway. Most generalized seizures last less than 5 min. If the seizure lasts more than 5 min or this is the athlete's first convulsion, emergency medical services should be summoned for transport. Any athlete suffering a seizure during a collision sport should be transported, since the seizure may be related to brain injury. When covering an athletic event, the physician's first responsibilities are first aid and attention to the ABCs (airway, breathing, and circulation)—not stopping the seizure with medication.

B. **Partial seizures** are not as much of a problem unless they become generalized. Athletes with partial seizures, like those with generalized seizures, may be very tired during the postictal period and should be allowed to rest.

X. Summary.

Athletes with epilepsy can play most sports without significantly increasing their risk of seizures or increasing the risk of injury. Close monitoring of the frequency of seizures in athletes with epilepsy and compliance with anticonvulsant medication regimens helps to reduce the risk of participation. Since many factors are involved in assessing the risk of sports participation, eligibility must be determined on a case-by-case basis.

Suggested Reading

Bennett DR. Epilepsy. In: Goldberg B, ed. *Sports and exercise in children with chronic health conditions.* Champaign, IL. Human Kinetics Publishers, 1995.

Gates JR, Spiegel RH. Epilepsy, sports and exercise. *Sports Med* 1993;15(1):1–5.

X. MUSCULOSKELETAL INJURIES

36. IMAGING

Leanne L. Seeger and Lawrence Yao

Although a thorough history and physical examination by a skilled practitioner are the backbone of diagnosis and therapeutic planning for the injured athlete, diagnostic imaging can often enhance the clinical evaluation of both acute and overuse injuries. The effective use of diagnostic imaging is a four-step process; determining the need for imaging, selection of an appropriate imaging modality, case-specific image acquisition, and image interpretation.

When the indication for imaging has been established and the appropriate modality chosen, the imaging study must be tailored to best answer the relevant clinical question. Hence, effective diagnostic imaging is facilitated by open communication between referring clinicians and radiologists. The appropriate, well-tailored imaging examination performed with state-of-the-art equipment may fail if it is interpreted by an inexperienced reader. Finally, an accurate imaging interpretation must be integrated into the overall clinical context before treatment can be planned. Not every imaging abnormality (e.g., meniscal tear in the knee, rotator cuff tear, disc herniation in the spine) is symptomatic, and careful clinical assessment is the ultimate arbiter for the relevance of any "abnormality" on imaging tests.

A guide to the appropriate selection and application of different imaging modalities follows.

I. Plain Radiography

Conventional radiography is often the initial imaging examination undertaken for the individual with musculoskeletal injury or pain. Plain films can cost-effectively exclude nontraumatic causes of pain, such as arthritis or tumor, and they are sufficient to diagnose most traumatic fractures.

Examination of a joint for a traumatic injury generally requires at least three views; anteroposterior (AP) or posteroanterior (PA), lateral, and oblique. Subtle pathology such as a nondisplaced fracture may be seen on only a single projection. Two views will usually suffice for following fracture healing or surgical fixation.

The imaging requisition should indicate the desired examination, pertinent clinical history, and the specific location of the complaint. Whenever possible, the examination should be focused on the area of concern. For example, it is not appropriate to request "radiographs of the forearm to include the wrist and elbow." Abnormalities of the proximal and distal joints will easily be overlooked due to x-ray beam divergence at the edges of the film and distortion of osseous structures. If the proximal and distal joints are of clinical concern, separate examinations of each joint are required.

Most imaging centers have radiographic protocols for each body part. Specific clinical concerns may, however, demand special views. Some of these special projections are discussed below.

A. **Shoulder.** In the setting of acute trauma or suspected degenerative or overuse conditions, the routine series includes AP views with internal and external rotation of the humerus and a view perpendicular to the bony glenoid, such as the axillary view. The axillary view should not be attempted after reduction of an acute glenohumeral dislocation because positioning for this view may redislocate the shoulder. In this setting, a transscapular or transthoracic view will provide necessary information regarding glenohumeral alignment. The West Point view (prone axillary) projects the anteroinferior glenoid rim in profile and is useful in detecting nondisplaced or minimally displaced Bankart fractures. Hill-Sacks fractures will best be detected on a standard AP internal rotation view where the posterolateral humeral head is seen in profile. The supraspinatus outlet view (transscapular with 15 degrees caudal tube tilt) may be useful in suspected impingement syndrome by depicting acromial morphology and anterior acromial spurs (Fig. 36-1). This view may mask soft tissue calcifications, and calcific tendinitis is best evaluated with the standard AP internal/external rotation and axillary examination. While osteoarthritis of the glenohumeral joint is usually adequately assessed on standard AP views, the Grashey view (perpendicular to the glenohumeral joint rather that to the shoulder girdle) better depicts early narrowing of the glenohumeral joint space. Acromioclavicular joint arthritis is adequately evaluated on standard AP views. Acromioclavicular joint laxity can be demonstrated with an AP view that includes both joints on one image, both with and without weights.

B. **Elbow.** In acute trauma, radiographic evaluation of the elbow should include a minimum of three views; AP, lateral, and lateral oblique. Some centers include the medial oblique view in the trauma series. The lateral film should be obtained with the elbow in 90 degrees of flexion to allow evaluation of the fat pads anterior and posterior to the joint. The anterior fat pad should normally be concave or straight and the posterior should not be visible. A convex anterior fat pad and/or visualization of the posterior fat pad indicates distension of the joint from either synovitis (inflammation) or fluid (effusion). In the setting of acute trauma, this usually indicates the presence of an intraarticular fracture. An angled radial head view may assist in identification of a nondisplaced fracture of the radial head or neck. Olecranon bursitis is evident radiographically as fullness of the soft tissues over the olecranon process on the lateral film; this may be infectious or traumatic.

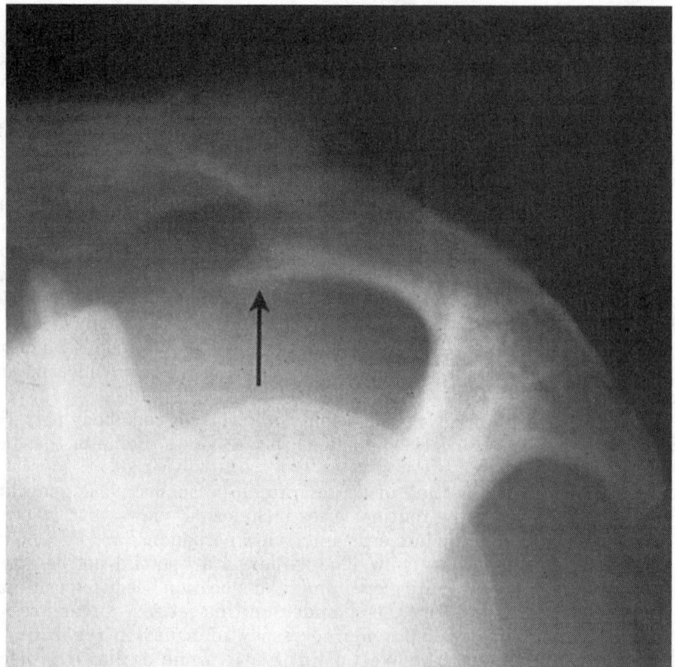

Fig. 36-1. Outlet view radiograph of the shoulder. This projection allows evaluation of acromial morphology. In this patient with impingement syndrome, the anterior acromion lies low with respect to the distal clavicle, and a spur is present at the insertion of the coracoacromial ligament on the anterior acromion (*arrow*).

C. **Hand and wrist.** The routine hand series consists of posteroanterior (PA), fan lateral (to separate the fingers), and PA 45 degree oblique views. These views are sufficient to diagnose most metacarpal fractures and abnormalities of the phalanges or carpals. If a specific digit or the wrist is the site of pain, a dedicated series of the area of concern is preferable.

The routine radiographs for evaluation of the wrist are AP, lateral, oblique, and coned navicular projections. Radial and ulnar deviation views may demonstrate widening of the scapholunate or lunotriquetral space secondary to a tear of the intercarpal ligament. Because intercarpal laxity varies between individuals, comparison films of the opposite wrist add specificity.

D. **Pelvis.** The standard plain film evaluation of the pelvis is the AP projection. Bilateral 45 degree oblique projections (Judet views) assist in identification and classification of acetabular fractures. Inlet and outlet views improve detection of sacral and pubic rami fractures. On pelvic radiographs, the sacral arcades, ilioischial line (posterior acetabular column), and iliopubic line (anterior acetabular column) should be evaluated for continuity. The sacroiliac joints and symphysis must be examined for diastasis. If there is a clinical question of inflammatory sacroiliitis, the radiographs should include a PA view of the sacrum and bilateral PA oblique views of the sacroiliac joints to better display these joints in profile.

E. **Hip.** The hips are typically evaluated on the AP and frog-leg lateral views. These provide nearly perpendicular views of the proximal femur but only one projection of the acetabulum. The frog-leg lateral view requires abduction and external rotation of the hip. The axiolateral (groin lateral) view provides a nearly orthogonal view of the joint without moving the affected hip. For this projection, the film cassette is placed along the lateral aspect of the hip. The contralateral hip is flexed, and the angled, cross-table x-ray beam travels beneath the flexed femur. This produces a roughly medial-to-lateral view of the acetabulum and proximal femur.

F. **Knee.** If an acute fracture is suspected, radiographs should be obtained with the patient supine. AP, lateral, and axial patellar (sunrise) views comprise the initial evaluation. The lateral radiograph should be taken with a horizontal x-ray beam in order to detect a lipohemarthrosis (layering of suprapatellar fluid and fat). This finding is indicative of an intraarticular fracture, with liberation of marrow fat. If a lipohemarthrosis is present and a fracture is not detected on routine radiographs, additional views (bilateral oblique, tunnel view) or cross-sectional imaging is indicated. The tunnel view better depicts the intercondylar notch and the posterior weight-bearing articular surface of the femoral condyles and affords an additional view of the tibial plateau.

In the patient with chronic knee pain, weight-bearing radiographs should be obtained to permit accurate evaluation of medial and lateral joint space loss and femorotibial alignment. A weight-bearing PA radiograph with the knee in 45 degrees of flexion may be more sensitive for early joint-space narrowing but is more difficult to perform. In addition, this view distorts alignment of the joint and obscures the femur proximal to the condyles. The Merchant view is an angled-beam, axial view of the patella with the knees in 45 degrees of flexion. This view assesses patellofemoral alignment and the congruence angle but can only be done reproducibly with the aid of a special positioning device and film holder.

G. **Foot and ankle.** Radiographic evaluation of the foot or ankle requires three separate views of each part; AP, lateral, and oblique. When the injury involves the forefoot or midfoot, foot films should be obtained. If the injury involves the hindfoot or the ankle joint, the ankle series is indicated. Evaluation of malalignment of the foot (including subtle Lisfranc injuries) require weight-bearing radiographs, but these should be avoided if a fracture is suspected. Stress views of the ankle (eversion, inversion, anterior drawer) may gauge insufficiency of the angle ligaments. Since the normal range of ligamentous laxity is broad, the asymptomatic ankle should be imaged for comparison.

H. **Long bones.** The long bones are usually adequately imaged in two orthogonal projections; AP (or PA) and lateral. Oblique views rarely provide additional information. The examination should concentrate on the area of the bone of concern, and the request should indicate if the clinical complaint relates to only one part of the bone (proximal, distal). In cases of a focal complaint, skin markers may be used to assure that the x-ray beam is properly centered.

I. **Cervical spine.** Plain radiography of the cervical spine is usually obtained for traumatic injury or suspected degenerative disease (degenerative disc disease and/or osteoarthritis of the facet or uncovertebral joints). A full routine evaluation consists of five views; AP, lateral, bilateral oblique, and odontoid (open-mouth) views. All views should be evaluated for bony alignment. The AP view depicts alignment of the facets and uncovertebral joints. Shift of the cervical airway may suggest soft tissue edema. The lateral film should include the upper body of T1; if this is obscured, a swimmer's view is necessary. Vertebral body fractures, subluxation, and disc-space narrowing are best identified on the lateral projection, and prevertebral soft-tissue swelling may be a clue to occult bony or ligamentous injury. Narrowing of the AP diameter of the spinal canal (normal ≥12 mm) may indicate congenital or acquired spinal stenosis. The oblique projections depict the patency of the intervertebral foramina. The odontoid view is essential for evaluation of the dens, the C1 lateral masses, and alignment of the C1-C2 articulation. The pillar view (AP, 30-degree caudal beam angulation) provides supplemental information about the lower facets and lamina and may be indicated by suspicious findings on routine views or a hyperextension mechanism of injury.

In the setting of suspected ligamentous injury and normal standard routine radiographs, lateral flexion and extension views may document instability. These views should be taken only on a conscious, cooperative patient. Magnetic resonance imaging (MRI) is a safer and more sensitive means of diagnosing ligamentous injury of the spine.

J. **Thoracic spine.** Plain radiographic evaluation of the thoracic spine consists of the AP and lateral projections. Oblique views are difficult to obtain and rarely provide additional information. The upper thoracic spine is usually not well seen on the lateral view owing to overlap of bony and soft tissue structures of the shoulder girdle. Evaluation of the AP view should include assessment of the paraspinal stripe, which may be displaced by hematoma or soft tissue mass.

K. **Lumbar spine.** Radiography of the lumbar spine is indicated for acute trauma, radicular symptoms, or pain refractory to conservative measures. Standard projections include AP, lateral, bilateral oblique, and a lateral view coned to the L5-S1 disc space. Vertebral alignment and disc-space height are best assessed on the lateral projection. Pars interarticularis defects are usually detectable on the lateral radiograph; however, oblique views are helpful for confirmation of a defect and determination of laterality. The oblique films also best display osteoarthritis or laxity of the facet joints. Lateral flexion and extension and AP side-bending views assist in demonstrating instability. Assessment of scoliosis should only be done on upright films. AP side-bending films may help determine the major curvature and the flexibility of the curves.

II. Magnetic Resonance Imaging

MRI has become a powerful and versatile tool for evaluating the musculoskeletal system. It depicts soft tissue anatomy with clarity and detail unmatched by other modalities and is the most sensitive and specific means to detect radiographically occult bony injury. Diagnostic applications of MRI usually demand high image spatial resolution. This typically requires high field strength (1 to

1.5 tesla) and specialized, local receiver coils. High-quality studies can be acquired at lower field strengths but will generally entail significantly longer study times. The design of some low-field-strength units (open architecture) may be better tolerated by the claustrophobic patient.

A multiplicity of MRI scan options and pulse sequences exist that may be variously used to advantage for different clinical indications. Perhaps more than any other modality, MRI should be tailored to the clinical indication in order to optimize diagnostic efficacy. Most MRI scans are acquired with spin-echo or fast spin-echo pulse sequences. The highest resolution is obtained with three-dimensional acquisition techniques that are currently available only for gradient-echo pulse sequences. The bone marrow space is generally best evaluated on Tl-weighted spin-echo images, which display fatty marrow as white or on fat-suppressed spin echo or STIR (short tau inversion recovery) images, on which marrow fat is dark. STIR pulse sequences depict edema and fluid with exceptional sensitivity.

A. **Shoulder.** MRI may be indicated for evaluation of the rotator cuff or the labrocapsular mechanism of the shoulder. A rotator cuff tear is evident as well-defined fluid intensity within a cuff tendon on high-quality images. Anterior or posterior labral tears are best detected on high-resolution axial images. Coronal oblique images may demonstrate SLAP (superior labrum, anterior and posterior) lesions. Labral tears may be difficult to distinguish from advanced labral degeneration on MRI. After an acute glenohumeral dislocation, hemarthrosis may help define the location and extent of a Bankart lesion. MRI arthrography (see below) is preferred for evaluation of the patient with atraumatic, multidirectional instability.
B. **Wrist.** The role of MRI in the evaluation of traumatic disorders of the wrist is evolving. Effective evaluation of intercarpal ligament and triangular fibrocartilage tears requires high-resolution three-dimensional image-acquisition techniques and local coils that are not universally available. MRI effectively detects radiographically occult scaphoid fractures and may also determine the viability of bone marrow after nonunion of a scaphoid fracture.
C. **Knee.** MRI is the imaging method of choice for evaluation of internal derangement of the knee. Meniscal and cruciate ligament pathology is accurately detected on routine high-field-strength, thin-section images. In addition to detecting meniscal tears, MRI also provides information about the size and orientation of the tear, and may detect displaced fragments from a flap or bucket-handle tear (Fig. 36-2). MRI may thus assist in preoperative decision making and predicting meniscal repairability. While most collateral ligament injuries are treated conservatively, MRI can detect and gauge acute collateral ligament injuries while excluding additional pathology that would require surgical intervention.
D. **Ankle and foot.** Most injuries of the ankle and foot can be adequately managed based on careful physical examination and plain radiography. MRI sensitively detects ligamentous and tendinous injury, and may help plan surgical intervention. All extrinsic foot tendons are easily imaged, and the location and extent of tears can be determined. In the case of the Achilles tendon, MRI may gauge the severity of partial ruptures and thereby influence patient management.
E. **Spine.** MRI is the preferred imaging modality for diagnosis of disc herniation and/or degeneration. In the setting of long track or radicular signs, MRI may also be indicated to assess the adequacy of the spinal canal and the intervertebral foramina. In the setting of acute trauma, MRI can detect radiographically occult fractures and ligamentous or muscle injuries. MRI more sensitively and safely detects acute ligamentous injury of the spine than flexion and extension radiographs.
F. **Fracture.** MRI is the most sensitive means to diagnose radiographically occult fractures, and it also defines the presence of trabecular injury. To confidently exclude a clinically suspected traumatic or fatigue fracture, a normal plain film evaluation should be followed by MRI. Fractures will be

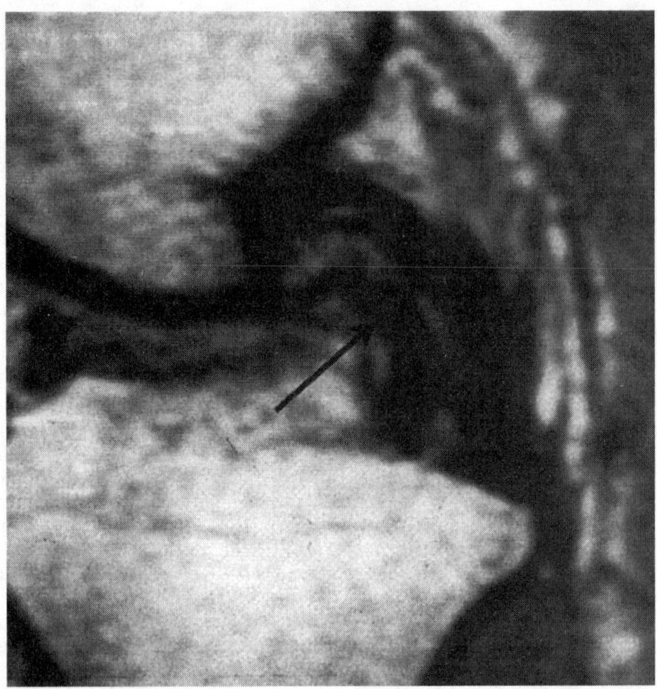

Fig. 36-2. Bucket-handle meniscal tear. Sagittal MRI shows a centrally displaced meniscal fragment (*arrow*) in the intercondylar notch, anterior to the posterior cruciate ligament.

manifest by marrow, periosteal, and/or soft-tissue edema on MRI; occasionally the actual fracture line will be evident (Fig. 36-3).

G. **Osteochondritis dissecans.** MRI is useful for the detection of radiographically occult osteochondritis dissecans and can determine the stability of an osteochondral fragment (Fig. 36-4). MRI can also differentiate between nondisplaced osteochondral fractures and purely trabecular injury. High-resolution images can also detect radiographically occult, purely chondral lesions or defects along the joint surface.

III. Radionuclide Bone Scan

Radionuclide bone scanning (typically with ^{99m}TcMDP) has been largely supplanted by MRI for the evaluation of bone trauma in many settings. The bone scan is, however, a highly sensitive technique and has the advantage of being able to survey large areas of the body. Disadvantages of bone scanning include its nonspecificity (traumatic, degenerative inflammatory, and neoplastic conditions will all demonstrate increased tracer uptake), radiation exposure, and the long duration of the examination (2 to 4 hr from injection to image acquisition).

Conventional static images will detect most bony injuries. When a fracture of a small bone is suspected (carpal navicular, hallux sesamoid), pinhole images may be necessary to achieve adequate spatial resolution and anatomic detail. Soft-tissue injury may be indirectly depicted as focal increased tracer uptake at sites of tendinous, ligamentous, or capsular insertions.

Single photon emission computed tomography (SPECT) bone scanning acquires projectional data that can be reconstructed into cross-sectional images

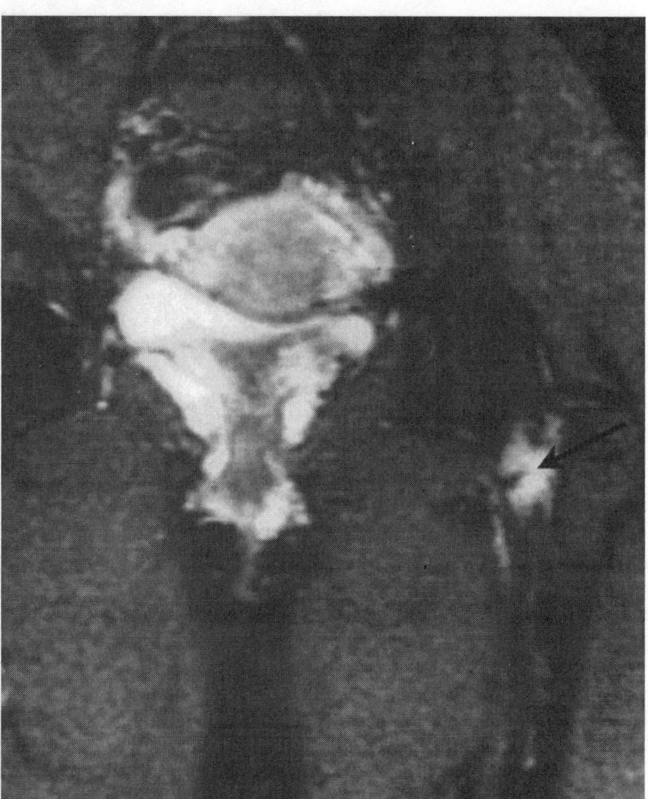

Fig. 36-3. Stress fracture of the proximal femur. This runner complained of left hip pain. Plain radiographs were normal. Coronal MRI reveals high signal intensity marrow edema in the medical femoral neck (*arrow*). The fracture is evident as a low signal intensity line.

in arbitrary planes (axial, coronal, sagittal, oblique). This method is preferred for regions of complex bony anatomy such as the spine. Triple-phase scanning is generally reserved for suspected inflammatory processes and plays little or no role in the evaluation of sports injuries.

A. **Bony trauma.** Radiographs should always be the first study obtained for suspected fracture. If the clinical suspicion for an occult or fatigue fracture is high, the bone scan may be indicated by its high sensitivity for these lesions. Fractures are identified as focal areas of increased tracer accumulation that reflect increased blood flow and osteoblastic activity. The pattern and intensity of increased tracer localization may gauge the degree of bony injury in fatigue states. Stress reaction appears as a broad, diffuse, mild increased uptake, and stress fractures show focal, intense cortical uptake. Shin splints show findings that may be scintigraphically indistinguishable from stress reaction, appearing as broad-based, periosteal tracer accumulation.

B. **Spondylolysis.** Spondylolysis (pars interarticularis fractures) may be symptomatic or asymptomatic. Increased scintigraphic activity on bone scan is suggestive of a more acute spondylolysis or abnormal motion, either of which could explain low back pain (Fig. 36-5). Increased scintigraphic activ-

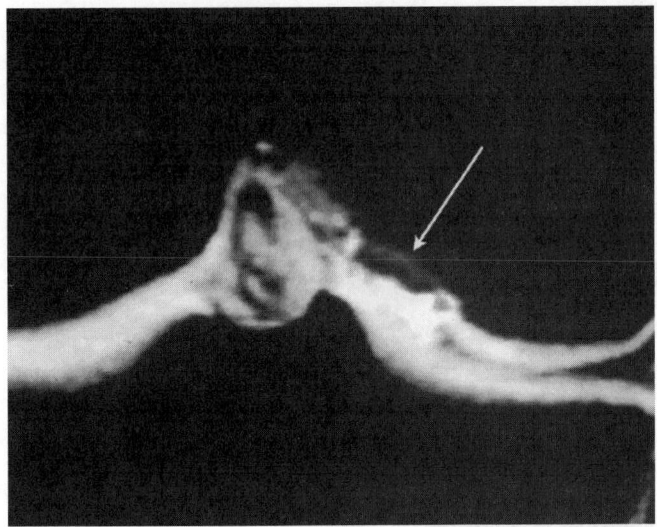

Fig. 36-4. Osteochondritis dissecans of the medial femoral condyle. The coronal MRI reveals that the osteochondral fragment (*arrow*) is surrounded by high signal intensity. This indicates instability.

ity may also indicate that a pars defect has the potential to heal (most go on to become nonunions or fibrous unions), and this finding may influence management.

C. **Hallux sesamoid fracture.** When plain radiographs are normal or show a bipartite hallux sesamoid, radionuclide bone scans can be useful for determining the presence of a stress fracture of the sesamoid or sesamoiditis.

IV. Computed Tomography (CT)

CT is less frequently indicated for primary fracture diagnosis than for aiding fracture management. Intravenous contrast is not necessary for the CT evaluation of most sports conditions. Newer CT scanners can acquire images in a helical mode, which reduces scan times and produces a three-dimensional image data set. Axial images from a helical acquisition can be reconstructed at arbitrarily close, overlapping intervals, which greatly improves multiplanar image reformations. Reformatted images in appropriate oblique imaging planes can aid in the depiction of complex anatomic surfaces and compensate for the inability of CT to directly image in nonaxial planes. Whenever possible, however, it is better to image anatomy directly in the optimal imaging plane by positioning the body part of interest (properly.) CT is well tolerated and can often speed diagnosis more than radiographic evaluation.

A. **Sternoclavicular and inferior radioulnar dislocations.** These injuries can be difficult to detect clinically and radiographically. A limited CT scan can quickly make the diagnosis. In the case of the inferior radioulnar joint, both wrists should be scanned in both supination and pronation. Only a few selected images through the joints of interest are necessary for diagnosis.

B. **Tarsal coalition.** Tarsal coalitions can easily be diagnosed on thin-section axial CT images. Direct coronal images are of added benefit. These are obtained with the knees flexed and the foot resting flat on the table.

C. **Carpal navicular fracture.** Initial fracture diagnosis can be made on radiographs or MRI, but direct sagittal CT can be especially useful to assess fracture healing or nonunion. These images can be obtained with the patient

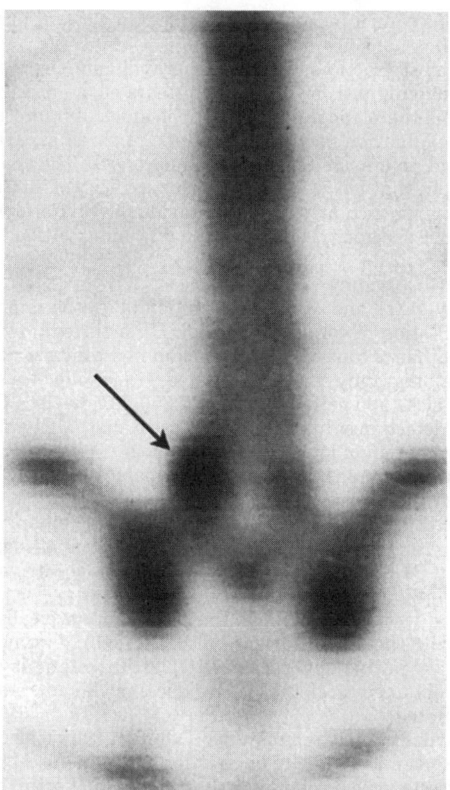

Fig. 36-5. Pars interarticularis defect. Plain radiographs revealed bilateral pars defects, but the patient was experiencing pain only on the right. The coronal SPECT image from a ^{99m}TcMDP bone scan reveals intense tracer activity confined to the symptomatic side (*arrow*). This suggests persistent motion or increased osteoblastic activity.

prone, arm overhead, with the wrist in radial deviation to place the long axis of the navicular parallel to the x-ray beam.

D. **Spondylolysis.** Fatigue fractures of the pars interarticularis predominate at L5 and are usually detectable on routine radiographs. Subtle cases can easily be confirmed on thin-section axial CT images. A pars fracture can be misinterpreted on standard 10-mm axial CT images as volume averaging of the adjacent facet joint. Fracture healing, in those rare cases when it occurs, can be much better assessed on CT than on plain radiography.

V. Arthrography

MRI has supplanted arthrography in many practice settings. At present, arthrography is still more reliable than MRI in evaluating internal derangement of the wrist, although MRI technology continues to improve image resolution. Arthrography is still less expensive and better tolerated by the claustrophobic patient than MRI and carries negligible risk.

A. **Shoulder.** The shoulder arthrogram is a simple and accurate way to diagnosis a full-thickness rotator cuff tear. The size and extent of a cuff tear cannot usually be accurately determined by arthrography alone. Labrocapsular lesions cannot be adequately evaluated without further evaluation by CT or MRI.

B. **Wrist.** In most practices, wrist arthrography remains the most reliable and accurate imaging test for diagnosis of tears of the triangular fibrocartilage complex and the scapholunate and lunotriquetral interosseous ligaments. A complete evaluation requires injections of three separate compartments (radiocarpal, inferior radioulnar, and midcarpal). The clinical utility of wrist arthrography may be limited by the nonspecificity of intercompartment communications, particularly in older individuals. Bilateral wrist arthrography may improve specificity, but is more costly and invasive.

VI. MRI and CT Arthrography

The sensitivity of CT and MRI studies of joints can be improved by the intra-articular instillation of contrast material. CT arthrography can be performed with dilute iodinated contrast alone or iodinated contrast and air (double contrast). MRI arthrography can be performed with saline or a dilute solution of a gadolinium chelate and saline (typically 1:250, Magnevist). CT arthrography is preferable for detection of intraarticular loose bodies. MRI arthrography is superior for the evaluation of joint surface pathology. As in other applications, MRI has the advantage of multiplanar imaging capability, while CT is faster and better tolerated by the claustrophobic patient.

A. **Shoulder.** Either CT or MRI arthrography is helpful in detecting labrocapsular pathology and Bankart lesions. MRI arthrography is probably better than CT arthrography for the evaluation of intrinsic labral tears and SLAP lesions.

B. **Hip.** Labral lesions can occur in the hip and are typically located anterosuperiorly. With the proper surface coils, MRI arthrography is preferable to CT arthrography in this application. If CT arthrography is used, thin sections should be obtained (preferably in a helical mode) and multiplanar reformations evaluated.

C. **Knee.** The detection of remnant tears after partial meniscectomy is problematic with conventional MRI. The question of new meniscal pathology after partial meniscectomy is a potential indication for MRI arthrography of the knee.

D. **Osteochondritis dissecans.** In cases of osteochondritis dissecans that warrant further imaging evaluation after radiographic detection, stability and coverage of chronic osteochondral lesions are probably best evaluated with a high-resolution MRI arthrogram.

VI. Ultrasonography

Ultrasound (US) is a portable, noninvasive, and highly operator-dependent imaging technique. Attractive features of US imaging are the lack of ionizing radiation, lower cost, and real-time (dynamic) imaging capability. It may be especially helpful for the evaluation of patients who are too large or claustrophobic to undergo MRI. US is an accurate technique for the evaluation of tendon integrity. Tendon tears typically appear as focal, hypoechoic alterations in the normally regular, intermediate echo texture of the normal tendon; the echogenicity of tendons, however, is dependent on the angle of sonification. Tendon sheath effusions are readily detected.

A. **Rotator cuff.** In the hands of an experienced user, US is nearly as accurate as MRI for diagnosing full thickness rotator cuff tears. US may detect a large percentage of partial-thickness tears as well. Examiners will routinely evaluate both shoulders to assess for asymmetry in cuff thickness and echo texture.

B. **Achilles tendon.** US can accurately detect ruptures of the Achilles tendon. Rupture severity is probably better gauged by MRI.

C. **Extensor hood injuries of the hand.** High-resolution US may be useful in the often difficult evaluation of the extensor hood and may help localize ruptures of the sagittal band—an injury that may occur in boxing and the martial arts.

Suggested Reading

Berquist T H, ed. *MRI of the musculoskeletal system.* New York: Raven Press, 1990.

Greenspan A. *Orthopaedic radiology: a practical approach.* New York: Gower Medical Publishing, 1992.

Seeger LL, ed. *Diagnostic imaging of the shoulder.* Baltimore: Williams & Wilkins, 1992.

Stoller DW. *Magnetic resonance imaging in orthopaedics and sports medicine.* Philadelphia: Lippincott, 1987.

37. FRACTURES

Peter J. Fowler and Bruce C. Twaddle

Fractures

A ***fracture*** is defined as a cortical infraction of bone with the disruption of at least one cortex. ***Stress fractures*** occur when a specific bone is ***repeatedly loaded*** beyond the threshold it is capable of withstanding.

Almost all fractures can reliably be made to heal. Of greater concern in the long term are the associated joint and soft tissue injuries, which may result in ongoing morbidity. Awareness and active management of these related problems is essential, particularly in the competitive athlete.

I. Terminology

Fractures are described by their specific characteristics, often referred to as **"the personality of the fracture."** Such a classification serves to direct investigation of associated injuries and to identify treatment options (Table 37-1).

A. **Bone or bones** involved.

B. **Closed or compound.** Compound fractures are those that have at some point communicated with the external environment. If there is a skin laceration through which a fractured end of the involved bone may have exited, the fracture must be assumed to be compound.

C. **Section of bone involved.** The position of a fracture within a bone is identified by its relation to the growth plates:

Intraarticular	The fracture extends into the joint
Epiphyseal	The fracture involves the area between the joint and its adjacent growth plate
Metaphyseal	The fracture involves the area adjacent to the growth plate but removed from the adjacent joint
Diaphyseal	The fracture involves the zone between the two growth plates

D. **Deformity.** A deformity is described with reference to the relative position of the more distal segment of a fractured bone to the more proximal segment and can be varus, valgus, anterior, posterior, or rotational.

E. **Fracture orientation.** This can be transverse, oblique, spiral, or segmental (more than one fracture in the same bone).

II. Etiology

Forces that exceed a bone's capacity to withstand them are the commonest cause of fractures. Most bones are designed to resist axial forces. Excessive loads, such as rotational or bending, applied in other directions are more likely to result in fractures.

III. History

The history is usually diagnostic or at minimum generates a high index of suspicion.

A. A ***significant force*** or ***load*** is applied in an ***abnormal manner.*** This is ***painful*** and usually ***easily recalled.*** A ***pop or crack*** may be heard or felt. Nausea may be experienced.

B. **Deformity** of the limb may be present. This can be dramatic.

C. There is ***immediate inability*** to continue with the activity. **Pain is** ***instantaneous*** and ***constant*** and is not alleviated by either the application or release of any load. The individual requires assistance to leave the area.

D. The affected limb becomes ***functionless*** except for the most trivial tasks.

E. **Swelling** occurs rapidly and noticeably.

Table 37- 1. Fracture Types

Fracture type	Description
Avulsion	Involves a tendon or ligament and its insertion or origin with a piece of bone
Impaction	Compression of the cortex or joint surface
Simple linear	There is one fracture line dividing the bone into two parts
Comminuted	There is more than one fracture line dividing the bone into three or more parts

IV. Physical Examination

Confirms the diagnosis.

A. **Deformity** of the area may be present. ***Comparison*** to the opposite side is often helpful.
B. **Swelling** at the site of injury is usually evident.
C. **Palpation** directly over the bone is painful, often exquisitely so. The pain is usually well localized and ***percussion*** along the affected bone confirms the injury site.
D. **Movement** of the affected part both actively by the patient and passively by the examiner is painful. ***Crepitus*** at the fracture site may be audible or palpable.
E. **Function** of the affected part is usually dramatically impaired.

V. Diagnostic Tests

(Table 37-2). Confirmation of a cortical infraction on imaging studies is diagnostic.

VI. Special Tests

A. **Stress films.** On occasion the use of stress films to demonstrate instability of a joint injury without an associated fracture may be useful e.g., ankle sprains, thumb metacarpo-phalanged (MCP) joint injuries. Injecting local anesthetic into the region prior to the film may increase its effectiveness. These are also useful in children in demonstrating growth-plate injuries, which may be unstable, particularly about the knee.
B. **Arthrography.** On occasion the injection of air or dye into a joint prior to plain x-rays or CT scanning may increase the detection of articular surface and/or associated soft tissue injury.

VII. Natural History

With appropriate immobilization, virtually all fractures will eventually heal. In the athlete, it is important to be mindful of the implications of time away from training and competition. In all patients, it is important to recognize the types of fractures that require intervention in order to reduce long-term disability. These include vascular or neurological complications, articular surface displacement, angular or rotational deformity, and associated soft tissue injury and instability.

VIII. Prevention

It is important that coaches and athletes understand the safety features incorporated into the rules of sports as well as the necessary equipment and technical aspects that minimize the likelihood of injury.

IX. Treatment Options

Factors in selecting the appropriate treatment:
The “personality” of the fracture.
The temporal relationship of the fracture to the athlete’s particular “season.”
Whether the individual is playing or practicing.
The demands of a particular sport or position.
The aspirations of the individual athlete.

Table 37-2. Diagnostic tests

Test	Description
Plain radiographs	Cortical disruption evident on at least two views Special views may be required to demonstrate subtle injuries
Plain tomography	Demonstrates true configuration and extent of fractures, particularly those involving joint surface displacement or disruption
Scintigraphy	Appropriate for:
Bone scan (technetium labeled)	Situations where there is a high index of suspicion but not a clearly identifiable fracture on plain films Situations where interpretation of films is difficult due to previous injury or other disease Stress fractures Situations where failure to identify a fracture may have significant consequences, (e.g., scaphoid, femoral neck, talus, spine)
CT scan	Particularly effective in imaging cortical bone Accurately identifies Fracture Degree of comminution Direction of each component Extent of joint involvement in intraarticular fractures
MRI	Beneficial in determining the extent of any associated soft tissue injury Occult fractures not seen on radiographs

CT, computed tomography; MRI, magnetic resonance imaging.

X. Immediate Treatment

A. **Rule out or manage hemodynamic or respiratory shock and neurological compromise.**

B. **In compound fractures,** attempt to reduce any exposed or protruding bone unless there is gross contamination. Note the state and contamination of the wound for future reference. Cover the laceration and control any bleeding.

C. **Realign and splint** the affected limb.

D. **Apply traction** and return the limb to ***normal alignment*** to allow initial splintage.

E. **Temporary splintage** can be achieved with semirigid immobilization by ***padding*** the area and adding some form of rigid support. Choices are wooden or metal splints, plaster or synthetic casting, premade canvas and aircasts or improvisational materials such as rolled-up newspapers or magazines.

Padding that circumferentially constrains the affected area will cause constriction with subsequent swelling and should be prepared and applied so that this is avoided. Ideally, the joints above and below diaphyseal fractures are immobilized to maximize patient comfort.

F. **Continued observation** of the patient and the neurovascular status of the limb is essential throughout treatment and particularly after any change in treatment.

XI. The most appropriate treatment depends on the injury, the individual patient, and the treating physician. Options include:

A. **"Watchful neglect,"** e.g., the use of splints or padding during activity.

B. **Supportive padding and splinting** for most metatarsal, metacarpal, and some humeral fractures.

C. **Application of casts** for undisplaced ankle and wrist fractures.
D. Open reduction and internal fixation, e.g. in midshaft forearm fractures and displaced intraarticular fractures.

The application of splints and casts may cause stiffness, or "cast disease," to occur when the device is removed. The recognition and treatment of the soft tissue component of all injuries is as important as the management of the fracture. Any treatment that achieves adequate stability but allows motion is advantageous. When caring for the athlete, it is important to remember that the first responsibility of the treatment provider is to prescribe what is best for the patient and the injury. Personal aspirations and the inconvenience to the team or sport are important to recognize but should remain secondary considerations. Time to return to sport varies with each injury and requires a balance between minimizing risk of reinjury and achieving the required level of function. Initially, it is advisable to return to practice only. These issues have been dealt with in greater detail in other chapters.

Stress fractures

Stress fractures are mechanical failures of bone caused by repetitive mechanical loading beyond the tolerance of a specific bone. They may be precipitated by a single event, but the failure has occurred over time.

I. Etiology

Most stress fractures occur following a change in the training or performance schedule which increases the mechanical load on a particular bone. Physiological conditions such as amenorrhea and osteoporosis may also be contributing factors. An increase in the mechanical stresses on bone results in microinjuries that trigger the normal cascade of responses to bone injury. Unfortunately, with the repeated application of load, a disordered response with accelerated resorption of bone occurs. This eventually results in a weakening of the affected region and subsequent mechanical failure or fracture.

II. Incidence

The incidence of stress fractures is uncertain, but particular fractures are more common in specific sports (Table 37-3).

III. History

Since radiological changes may be subtle, a diagnosis of stress fracture often depends on a high index of suspicion aroused by the vulnerablity of athletes in particular sports as well as changes in exercise intensity. Following are typical components of the history:

A. A specific event may be recalled, but often the patient has experienced ***pain*** in the area for some time. This is associated with an increase in the intensity of exercise. The background discomfort is often interrupted by a more intensely painful and acute event.
B. The body ***habitus*** of the patient may not be that traditionally associated with the sport involved.
C. Firm bony ***swelling*** over the area and occasionally a ***deformity*** of a gradual or more acute onset may be noticeable to the patient.
D. **Pain** is of varying intensity, localized to the area involved and aggravated by activity; it occurs with both loading and unloading of the affected part.
E. In women, it is important to determine the presence of ***amenorhea*** or any other condition that may be predispose the individual to local or generalized osteopenia and subsequent stress fracture.
F. A history of a ***previous stress fracture*** may be significant.

IV. Physical Examination

Clinical features are similar to those of acute fractures but may be less dramatic.

Table 37-3. Stress Fractures Associated with Particular Sports

Area of stress fracture	Sport/activity	Area of stress fracture	Sport/activity
Pelvis	Running Walking	Patella	Basketball Baseball (catching)
Femur	Running Basketball Jumping	Metacarpal	Tennis Handball
Tibia	Running Soccer Swimming Ballet Basketball Aerobics	Ulna	Javelin Tennis Curling
Fibula	Running Skating Aerobics	Humerus	Baseball (pitching) Cricket
Metatarsal	Running Walking Marching Swimming Soccer Ballet	Rib	Tennis Baseball (batting) Rowing Golf
Os calcis	Basketball Volleyball	Spine (pars intraarticularis)	Gymnastics Cricket (bowling) Waterskiing Football (lineman)

A. **Deformity** may be present and may be of gradual onset.
B. **Swelling** may accompany an acute exacerbation. ***Bony swelling*** may occur with a history of sufficient duration.
C. There is localized ***bony tenderness,*** the hallmark of a fracture.
D. **Pain** with ***movement*** of the affected part is characteristic. Stressing the bone involved may increase the intensity of the pain.
E. **Function** is limited by pain for a longer period of time than could be expected with sprain or strain.

V. Diagnostic tests

Evidence of cortical disruption is diagnostic but may be more subtle than in fractures (Table 37-4).

VI. Prevention

Prevention of stress fractures depends on recognition of those patients at risk. Patients who rapidly increase their training or competitive demands, who are amenorrheic or skeletally immature (bones are relatively osteoporotic), and who develop overuse syndromes are among those "at risk." Clear counseling of athletes, trainers, coaches, and often parents regarding potential hazards of improper training programs is an important part of prevention. Prescribing oral contraceptives for amenorrheic women athletes is a recognized method of lowering the risk of stress fractures in this group.

VII. Treatment options

Many stress fractures are ***errors in training*** by an athlete at a particular time in his or her development. Recognition and correction of these by athletes,

Table 37-4. Stress Fracture Diagnostic Tests

Test	Description
Plain radiographs	Cortical disruption Evidence of preexisting bony reaction or attempted healing
Scintigraphy	Diagnostic when history and physical exam indicate stress fracture but there are minimal changes on plain film
CT Scan	May be diagnostic when pain is present and plain radiographs are normal
MRI	Useful when there is pain, no definitive physical findings, and no apparent abnormalities on plain radiographs

coaches, and parents are fundamental in the management of these potentially recurring injuries. Treatment options are similar to those in an acute injury.

A. **Relative rest** and appropriate ***splintage*** until symptoms have resolved and radiological healing has occurred.
B. **Cast application** may be necessary, depending on the fracture and its location. This often effectively ensures complete rest from activity.
C. **Internal fixation** may be required, particularly in stress fractures that have a high incidence of delayed or nonunion—e.g., fifth metatarsal (Jones) and femoral neck fractures. Internal fixation may allow earlier return to training or sport but should not be chosen for this reason alone. There are recognized complications associated with internal fixation, which, in the long term, may have a significant effect on performance. The primary rule in treating athletes is *first, do no harm.*

The fundamental purpose of the health care provider is to give advice that will result in the maximum likelihood of recovery from a specific ailment. In treating athletes, particularly those predisposed to stress fractures, altering treatment and shortening lay-off periods to appease the individual are decisions that will compromise outcome. Education of all involved parties in the prevention of stress fractures and adjusting training programs once stress fractures have been successfully managed are essential components of treatment.

Suggested reading

Adams JC, Hamblen DL. *Outline of fractures: including joint injuries.* Edinburgh: Churchill Livingstone, 1992.

Browner BD, Jupiter JB. *Skeletal trauma.* Philadelphia: WB Saunders, 1991.

Reid DC, Bone: a specialized connective tissue. In: *Sports Injury Assessment and Rehabilitation.* New York: Churchill Livingstone, 1992:103–128.

Rockwood C.A., Green D.P. *Fractures.* Philadelphia: JB Lippincott, 1991.

38. SOFT TISSUE AND OVERUSE INJURIES

Wayne B. Leadbetter

As the most frequent disability associated with athletic competition and recreational athletics, injuries to the dense connective tissue of ligament, tendon, and associated muscle are sometimes as difficult to qualify as to quantify. While many of these "injuries" create symptoms of inflammation, they may also be degenerative tissue responses. These difficulties have significant implications for efficacy, timing, and overall choice of treatment. The goal of sports medicine therapy is to minimize the adverse effect of traumatic inflammatory response while promoting tissue repair, thereby expediting a safe return to performance. To do so, the sports medicine clinician must become familiar with the biological capabilities of human tissue and its limitations and appreciate basic differences between acute and chronic (overuse) forms of soft tissue sports trauma.

I. Spectrum of Soft Tissue Sports Injury

Sports-induced soft tissue injuries are characterized by a spectrum of interrelated cell-matrix responses associated with failed cell-matrix adaptation and the processes of inflammation, repair, and degeneration. It is helpful to define these terms in order to more fully understand the observed clinical problems.

A. **Trauma** implies an injury from a mechanical force that is applied external to the involved tissue, causing structural stress or strain that results in a cellular or tissue response.

B. **Load and use** are normal, basic physiologic requirements for tissue maintenance or renewal.
   1. **Load** is a measure of external mechanical force; it is described by the terms *strain* and *stress.*
   2. **Use** implies the accumulation of load over time—i.e., a rate in addition to movement. Such repetition is seen in endurance sports in the form of cyclic loading.

C. **Strain and stress**
   1. **Strain** is the deformation of a structure in response to external load. It is a complex physical signal for tissue adaptation, with the final tissue response resulting from the interrelation of several factors, including strain mode (i.e., tension, compression, or shear), direction, rate, frequency, duration, distribution, and volume.
   2. **Load-induced tissue strain** is a powerful cell-matrix stimulus causing changes in cell proliferation, differentiation, matrix organization, altered deoxyribonucleic acid DNA synthesis, and altered tissue mechanical properties. Both sports and rehabilitative exercise cause load-induced tissue strain.

D. **Sports injury** is the loss of cells or extracellular matrix resulting from sports-induced trauma. Like other wounds, an athletic wound is a disruption of normal anatomic structure and function. All wounds result from pathologic processes, beginning inside or outside the involved part. Although there is much overlap, wounds are generally characterized by their mode of onset, mechanism of injury, and—most importantly—progression of healing.
   1. **Acute injury** is characterized by rapid onset, a macrotraumatic mechanism, and an orderly and timely reparative process that results in the sustained restoration of anatomic and functional integrity.
   2. **Chronic injury** is of more subtle onset, often the result of a microtraumatic mechanism; it fails to proceed through an orderly and timely process to produce anatomic and functional tissue integrity, or it may have proceeded through the repair process without establishing a sustained anatomic and functional result.

E. **Sports-induced inflammation** is a localized tissue response initiated by injury or destruction of vascularized tissues exposed to excessive mechanical load or use. It is a time-dependent, evolving process characterized by vascular, chemical, and cellular events leading to tissue repair, regeneration, or scar formation. Clinically, sports-induced soft tissue inflammation may spontaneously resolve; or it may evolve into a chronic inflammatory response (Fig. 38-1).

1. **Five cardinal signs of inflammation:**
    a. **Heat.** *Calor*—metabolic radiant energy.
    b. **Redness.** *Rubor*—increased vascularity (angiogenesis) and blood flow.
    c. **Swelling.** *Tumor*—extracellular edema and matrix changes.
    d. **Pain.** *Dolor*—stimulation of afferent nerve endings by noxious mediators.
    e. **Loss of function.** *Functio laesa*—decrease performance caused by direct damage, inhibiting pain, edema, contracture, or atrophy.

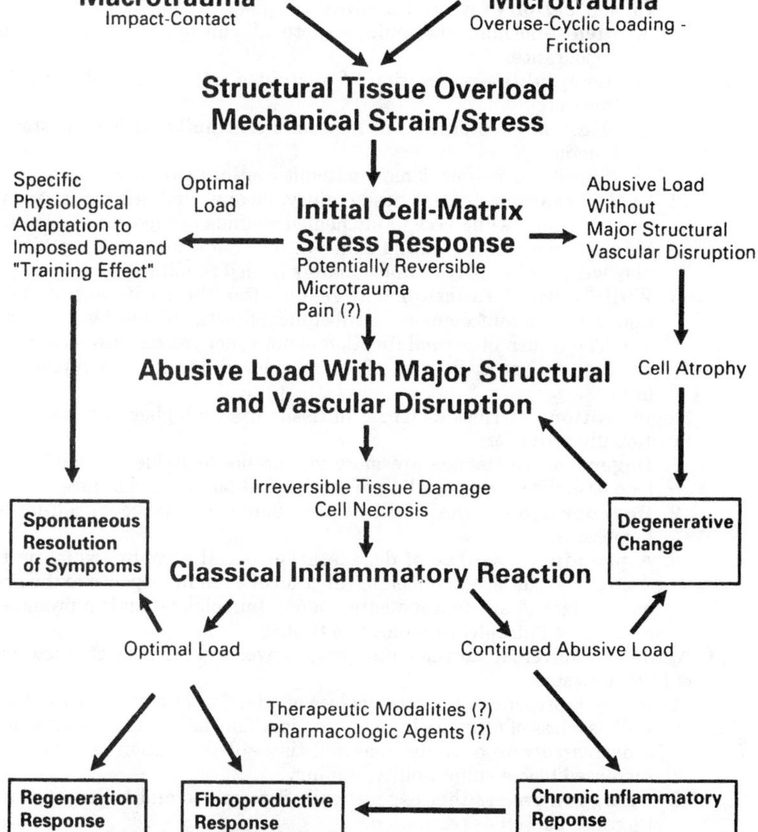

Fig. 38-1. Schema of the theoretical pathways of sports-induced inflammatory response. (From Leadbetter WB: An introduction to sports-induced inflammation. In: Leadbetter WB. Buckwalter JB. Gordon SL, eds. *Sports-induced inflammation: clinical and basic science concepts.* Park Ridge, IL. American Academy of Orthopaedic Surgeons, 1990:2, with permission.)

2. **Not all sports injuries** produce a classic inflammatory pattern or response after injury—e.g., articular cartilage, chronic tendon injury.

F. **Necrosis** is that structural change occurring in cells subsequent to their death in a living organism.
   1. **Necrosis** always stimulates inflammation if there is an adequate tissue vascular supply.
   2. **The severity of sports injury** depends upon the extent of cell necrosis.

G. **Repair** of soft tissue injury is defined as the replacement of damaged or lost cells and extracellular matrices with new cells and matrices.
   1. **Regeneration** is a form of repair that produces new tissue that is structurally, biochemically, biomechanically, and functionally **identical** to normal tissue. Muscle tissue has some limited capability for regeneration.
   2. **Acutely injured tissue,** such as tendon or ligament is repaired by scar deposition, and never exactly replicates the histologic or biomechanical properties of the original structures. Such deficiencies are partly compensated for by the increased volume of scar.

H. **Healing** is a complex dynamic process that results in the restoration of anatomic continuity due to an orderly, logical repair process.
   1. **Classification of wound healing** adequacy.
      a. **Ideal**—normal anatomic structural continuity, function, and appearance.
      b. **Acceptable**—restoration of sustained anatomic continuity and function.
      c. **Minimal**—restoration of anatomic continuity without sustained function.
      d. **Failed**—no restoration of anatomic continuity or function.
   2. **In the treatment** of soft tissue injury, ideal wound healing is rarely if ever obtained, while acceptably healed wounds are more common. It is the challenge of the treating clinician to avoid returning the athlete to play with a minimally or inadequately healed condition.
   3. **While normal function** may result after the treatment of sports injury, it is not uncommon for subclinical functional deficiencies to persist. The return of normal function is not synonymous with ideal tissue healing—i.e., good function often is achieved despite scar repair after injury.

I. **Degeneration** describes a change in tissue from a higher to a lower, less functionally active form.
   1. **Degenerative tissues** are more vulnerable to sudden dynamic overload or cyclic overuse leading to mechanical fatigue and failure.
   2. **Degeneration** is the result of a profound imbalance in cell-matrix homeostasis.
   3. **A prominent source** of degeneration is cell atrophy, which is the decrease in the size, number, or function of a cell in response to the presence or lack of an environmental signal. Immobilization is a prominent cause of cell atrophy in connective tissues.

J. **Aging** is a universal, decremental, progressive, and intrinsic characteristic of human tissues.
   1. **Aging** represents a progressive loss of adaptive or training capacity as well as a loss of ultimate level of function. This failure is associated with a decreased rate of tissue renewal, tissue degeneration, and eventual increased tissue vulnerability to injury.
   2. **Aging** is a process that is genetically determined and multifactorial in its cause as well as regulation.
   3. **Aging** is a contributing cause of tissue degeneration occurring after sports injury. However, while one tissue may be losing functional capacity rapidly, other tissues may be quite young functionally and never, depending on longevity, get an opportunity to age.
   4. **Aging** does not occur at the same rate in all species or in all individuals of the same species in exactly the same way.

II. Tissue Response to Load or Use

A. **Homeostasis** is a process by which connective tissues renew their cell populations and their matrix contents.
   1. The process involves cell signaling by mechanical stimuli—mainly strain deformation in tension, compression, or shear, thereby altering cell behavior.
   2. **Load and use** are basic requirements of tissue maintenance.

B. **Adaptation** is a process by which advantageous change is achieved in the function or the constitution of an organ or tissue to meet new conditions.
   1. A **maladaptation** is a disadvantageous change in an organ or tissue.
   2. In sports, different modes of training result in different tissue responses. This has been characterized as the principle of **specific adaptation to imposed demand (SAID)**.

C. **Overload versus overuse** are terms that are interrelated and yet not synonymous. Generally, sports injury risk increases as load increases or as use increases.
   1. **Overload**—excessive, rapid increase in resistance implying the potential for sudden tissue injury.
   2. **Overuse**—repetitive motion without necessarily increasing resistance, implying the potential for fatigue.

D. **Overuse injury** occurs when a structure is exposed to repetitive force beyond the abilities of that specific structure to withstand such a force. Overuse injury is manifested at the tissue and clinical level.
   1. **Tissue overuse injury** is that point at which loss of tissue homeostasis and degeneration results in loss of cell matrix integrity. This may be either asymptomatic or symptomatic.
   2. **Clinical sports overuse injury** occurs at the point where the damage of cells or matrix resulting from overuse or abusive exercise pattern becomes symptomatic to the athlete or produces loss of function.

E. **Loading of injured connective tissues** may be either tolerant or intolerant.
   1. Tolerant loading promotes soft tissue healing by the following mechanisms:
      a. Improving efficiency of tissue repair
      b. Better organization of extracellular matrix
      c. Realignment of collagen fibers along lines of stress
      d. Increased mass of tissue
      e. Increased rate of collagen synthesis
      f. Increased tissue strength and resistance to deformation
   2. **Intolerant** loading disrupts soft tissue healing and recovery by:
      a. Excessive deformation of extracellular matrix and collagen fibers
      b. Tissue disruption
      c. Increased tissue laxity
      d. Increased inflammation
      e. Increased fibrosis and fibroarthrosis

F. **The therapeutic role of rest** has long been clinically recognized to aid recovery, especially after chronic injury. However, it is never a singular solution. In the modern therapy of sports injury, rest must be balanced with rehabilitative activity.
   1. Rest may allow tissues to heal but, because of atrophic side effects, may also be detrimental. Rest will not predictably increase tissue tolerance to load.
   2. Rest allows cellular repair to theoretically "catch up" after injury.
   3. The frequency and duration of the rest cycle is important and will vary with each individual injury, type of tissue, and genetic endowment. The clinical observation of "quick healers" and "slow healers" remains poorly understood.
   4. Forms of rest include:
      a. Total
      b. Protected dynamic activity (e.g., brace, orthotic, taping, etc.)

c. Altered activity (i.e., change in frequency, intensity, or duration of exercise)

III. Seven Basic Mechanisms of Sports Injury

There are only seven basic mechanisms by which an athlete may sustain injury: (1) *contact* and (2) *dynamic overload* are of sudden onset; (3) *cyclic impact* and *overuse* are chronic and revealed primarily by the taking of an accurate history; (4) *structural vulnerability,* (5) *inflexibility,* (6) *muscle imbalance,* and (7) *rapid growth* are the focus of the physical examination. These mechanisms may occur singularly, as in acute tissue damage resulting from contact or collision; more commonly, however, these mechanisms are seen to occur in combinations, especially in the endurance athlete. In total, these seven mechanisms form the foundation for the clinical diagnosis of all sports injury. The following is a checklist of what to look for during the clinical history and examination:

A. **Contact** is the most obvious source of acute macrotraumatic injury. It generally results in a classic inflammatory wound-repair reaction initiated by the onset of bleeding, hematoma, and clot formation. Direct muscle contusions and severe ligamentous sprains with possible traumatic joint dislocations are typical examples of soft tissue contact injury. **Impact** is a related corollary of contact. This often underrecognized mechanism of injury is exemplified by the cumulative microtrauma experienced by tissues exposed to repetitive load. For example, the ground-reactive force at midstance in running is 250% to 300% of body weight. A 70-kg runner at 1,175 steps per mile absorbs at least 220 tons of force per mile! While contact may produce more notorious injuries, it is the cumulative damage of impact that produces the more common spectrum of overuse injuries.

B. **Dynamic overload** describes that tissue failure resulting from sudden intolerable strain deformation. An acute tendon rupture or muscle strain is often the result of dynamic overloading during jumping, sprinting, or kicking. Tendons are particularly at risk during the eccentric loading that may occur when an athlete is landing or throwing.

C. **Overuse or overload** represents a failed cumulative cell-matrix adaptive response as the result of a summation of repetitive unresolved strains or stresses of a tissue. It is often seen in the context of cyclic loading or overtraining. Some 30% to 50% of all sports injuries are related to overuse. Of these, 70% are caused by training errors. In the presence of other mechanisms, overuse is often the "lighted fuse" prior to the occurrence of an injury crisis.

D. **Structural vulnerability** may contribute to fatigue and eventual tissue failure secondary to focal overload and excessive strain or stress. Hyperpronation of the foot during running, pathologic laxity of the ligamentous support of a joint, or malalignment of the lower extremity—as seen with excessive persistent femoral anteversion or genu varum—are examples of structural vulnerability capable of contributing to the onset of injury during sports play.

E. **Inflexibility** describes a loss of range of motion of a joint involving both periarticular tissue and ligament as well as the subtended muscle tendon units. Joint inflexibility may lead to biases in articular contact, thereby initiating a cycle of articular degeneration. A shortened, preloaded muscle is more vulnerable to strain.

F. **Muscular imbalance** is a mechanism interrelated with that of inflexibility resulting primarily from improper muscle conditioning and usage. Repetitive abusive patterns of muscle overuse during athletic activity promote muscular imbalances secondary to muscular fatigue microtear, scarring, and functional maladaptations. A fatigued muscle is more vulnerable to strain.

G. **Rapid growth** is a mechanism seen in the growing or child athlete. The terms "overgrowth syndrome," along with "growing pains" emphasize the muscular imbalances and flexibilities coincident with changing skeletal proportions during maturation; these create potential dynamic overload of soft tissue structures. Acquired inflexibilities and muscular imbalances during periods of growth may often persist for inordinate periods of time, even into adulthood, in the absence of appropriate rehabilitation and conditioning.

IV. The Principle of Transition

as originally defined by Leadbetter states that "*sports injury is most likely to occur when the athlete experiences any rapid change in use of the involved part.*"

1. **Transitional injury** is rate-dependent. Sudden ill-timed changes in activity are more injurious.
2. **Abrupt changes** in training volume (i.e., intensity, duration, or frequency) have been shown to be the most prominent cause of overuse injuries in endurance sports. It is a common error in overtraining injury.
3. **Examples of transitional risks** include any attempt to increase performance level; any change in the athlete's playing positions; improper training; changes in equipment; environmental changes such as a new surface or a different training altitude; abrupt alterations in frequency, intensity, or duration of training; attempts to master new techniques; return to sport too soon after injury; and even body growth itself.

V. Pathophysiology of Soft Tissue Injury

A. **Acute macrotraumatic tissue response** may result from a sudden compression, laceration, extreme tensile load, or shear. The moment of injury is defined by the onset of vascular disruption and initiation of the clotting mechanism with platelet activation (Fig. 38-2). A cascade of overlapping processes characterizes "classic inflammation and repair": inflammation, cell replication, angiogenesis, matrix deposition, collagen protein formation, contraction, connective tissue remodeling, and—in the case of exposed wounds—epithelialization. These highly ordered and interdependent events are summarized in phases that display great disparity in their duration (Fig. 38-3). While phase I subsides in a few days, phase III may last indefinitely and in most tissues up to at least a year. Severe muscle strain, spontaneous tendon ruptures, ligamentous tears and sprains, or surgical wounds typically generate

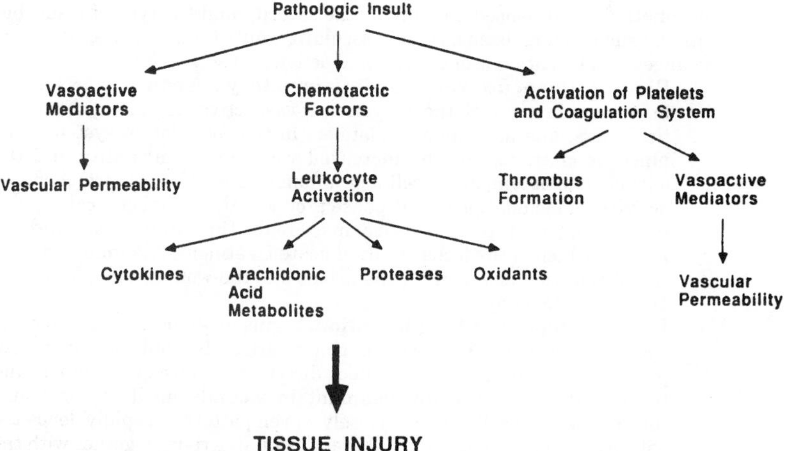

Fig. 38-2. Mediators of the inflammatory response. (From Fantone JC. Basic concepts in inflammation. In: Leadbetter WB, Buckwalter JB, Gordon SL, eds. *Sports-induced inflammation: clinical and basic science concepts.* Park Ridge, IL: American Academy of Orthopaedic Surgeons, 1990, with permission.)

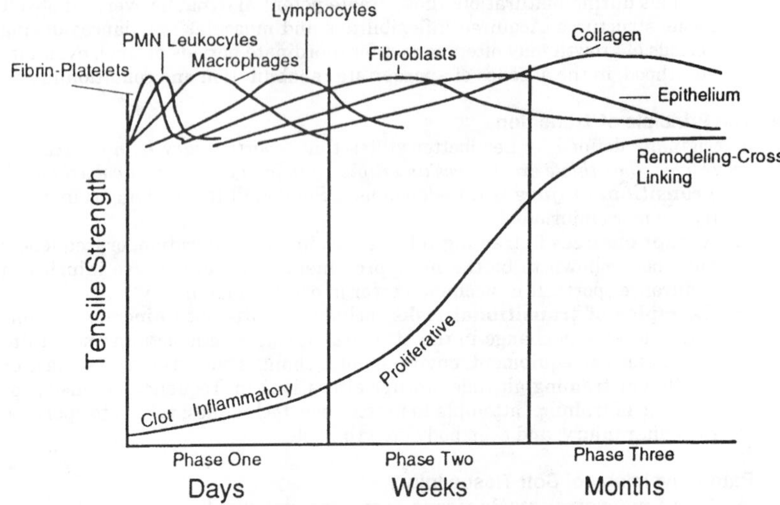

Fig. 38-3. Ideal wound healing model. Originally derived from the study of skin lacerations, a variety of factors may distort the actual healing sequence in tendon. Although this diagram is an accurate portrayal of cell matrix wound healing events, note that the temporal relationship of the various phases is such that the duration of phase one is measured in hours or a few days, but phase three may extend indefinitely. Normal tendon is not regenerated, however, PMN = polymorphonuclear cell. (Adapted from-Gamble JG. The musculoskeletal system: physiological basics. In: Hunter-Griffin L, ed. *Athletic training and* sports medicine. 2nd ed. New York, Raven Press, 1988:105, with permission.)

this type of response. In the athlete, this represents an optimum sequence of events that is influenced not only by the severity and the type of insult but also by such factors as age, tissue vascularity, nutrition, genetics, hormonal changes, local treatment measures, and activity level (Fig. 38-4).

1. **Phase I, the acute vascular inflammatory response,** starts at the moment of injury with the activation of vasoactive mediators, chemotactic factors, and activation of platelets in the coagulation system. This phase is characterized by increased vascular permeability and the edema that accompanies cellular inflammation. The intense chemical activity and exudation of this phase produces the initial clinical signs of injury and, with increasing edema, create the **zone of secondary injury,** which is the focus of initial acute treatment. Assuming no coincident infection or repetitive disturbance to the wound, this phase usually lasts 3 to 5 days.
2. **Phase II, repair and regeneration,** begins in 48 hr and lasts on average 6 to 8 weeks. This phase is characterized by multipotent macrophages that appear to be the major directors of subsequent repair and fibroblasts which remain dominant in wounds until repair stops. Initially type III collagen in a loosely woven pattern is rapidly deposited within a fibrin matrix. This exuberant cellular activity together with the vascular proliferation and in ingrowth is known as **granulation tissue.**
3. **Phase III, the remodeling maturation phase,** is characterized by a trend toward decreased cellularity and an accompanying decrease in synthetic activity, increased organization of extracellular matrix, and a more normal biochemical profile. Collagen maturation with a shift to

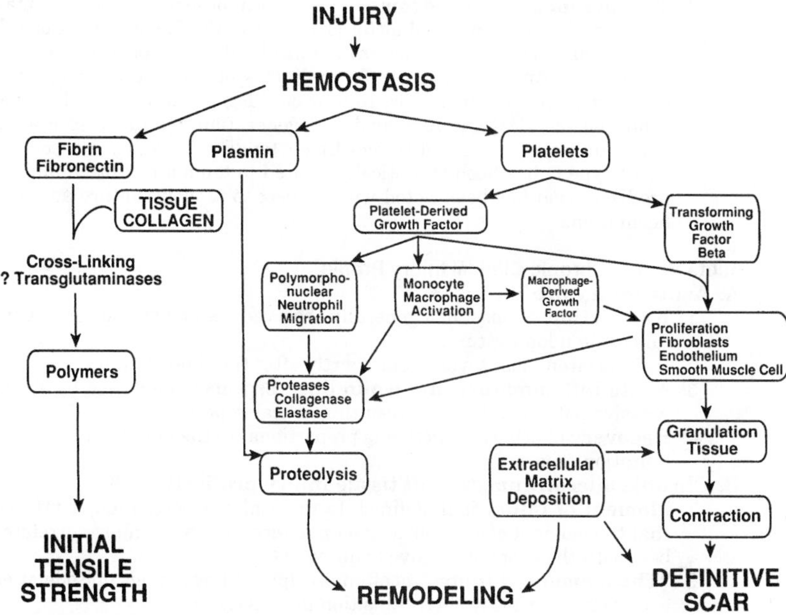

Fig. 38-4. Summary of events in macrotraumatic wound response. (From Martinez-Hernandez A. Basic concepts in wound healing. In: Leadbetter WB, Buckwalter JB, Gordon SL, eds. *Sports-induced inflammation: clinical and Basic Science Concepts.* Park Ridge, IL: American Academy of Orthopaedic Surgeons, 1990:78, with permission.)

type I collagen and a functional linear realignment of collagen fibrils is usually seen by 2 months after injury in ligament and tendon. However, final biomechanical properties can be reduced by as much as 30% despite this remodeling effort. The exact end point at which remodeling ceases in the soft tissue injury response has not been determined. Normal histology is often replaced by scar, the material properties of which never equal those of the original intact tissue.

B. **Chronic microtraumatic injury response,** typically the result of overuse or overload and abusive exercise, this injury response may be inflammatory-dominant or structural degenerative–dominant.

1. **Inflammatory-dominant** is typically a response of irritated synovial tissue due to direct trauma, friction, intrabursal bleeding (hemobursa), intraarticular bleeding (hemarthrosis), or associated arthritis. Clinically, the cardinal signs of inflammation may be prominent.
2. **Structural degenerative–dominant** is a pattern of connective tissue injury response resulting from failed adaptation to increased exercise demand, most often in combination with some form of failed healing and repair. There is characteristically diminished or no organized inflammation. Progressive degeneration often leads to tissue rupture. Tendons most frequently display this type of response. Joint menisci and articular cartilage are other examples. The propensity for this type of response in ligament is less well understood but is suspected to occur. It has been suggested that these changes result from hypoxic injury as a result of the diminished blood supply frequently seen in tendon. The exact pathoetiology remains controversial.

3. **The mesenchymal syndrome** is the clinical observation of what may be a genetically determined factor or factors in the failed healing of soft tissue injury. Tendinosis appears in multiple sites in approximately 15% of patients. An association with tendinosis of the lateral epicondyle extensor carpi radialis brevis, rotator cuff degeneration, carpal tunnel syndrome, cervical and lumbar disc degeneration, plantar fasciosis, de Quervain's syndrome, and trigger-finger tendinosis has been observed. Blood type O has been statistically related to tendon rupture. Familial predisposition has been noted with respect to tendon rupture and disc herniation.

IV. Acute Versus Chronic Clinical Injury Profile

A. **Acute injury profile** (Fig. 38-5)

1. **Known time** of onset of a generally observed trauma episode or a spontaneous tendon rupture.
2. **Pain** is often most severe at or shortly after the time of injury.
3. **Acute inflammatory and wounding response** is followed by a progressive pattern of healing, resulting in scar repair.
4. **Recovery** of athletic function is proportional to the quality of the rehabilitation program.

B. **Chronic microtraumatic soft tissue injury profile** (Fig. 38-6)

1. **Moment of injury** is ill defined. In the athlete's perception, it may be that the moment of most obvious pain in terms of tissue injury correlates best with the onset of abusive training.
2. **"The moment of injury"** is often precipitated by a crisis episode after overexertion or too rapid a transition in activity.
3. **The examiner's ability** to ferret out abusive training patterns is critical to the diagnosis.
4. **The accumulation of hypertrophic scar,** adhesions, chronic granulation tissue, degenerative change, and adverse tissue effects of microtrauma imply that recovery will be slower.

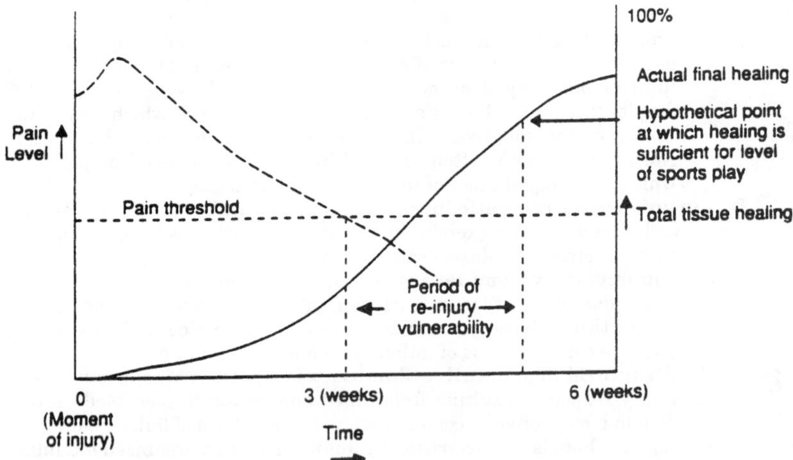

FIG. 38-5. Hypothetical profile of acute macrotraumatic tissue injury. This profile is typical of an acute partial tendon strain or the pattern of healing in other acutely injured connective tissues such as a lateral-collateral ligament sprain in the ankle. Curved dashed line = pain; curved solid line = tissue healing. (From Leadbetter WB. Cell-matrix response in tendon injury. *Clin Sports Med* 1992:11553–557, with permission.)

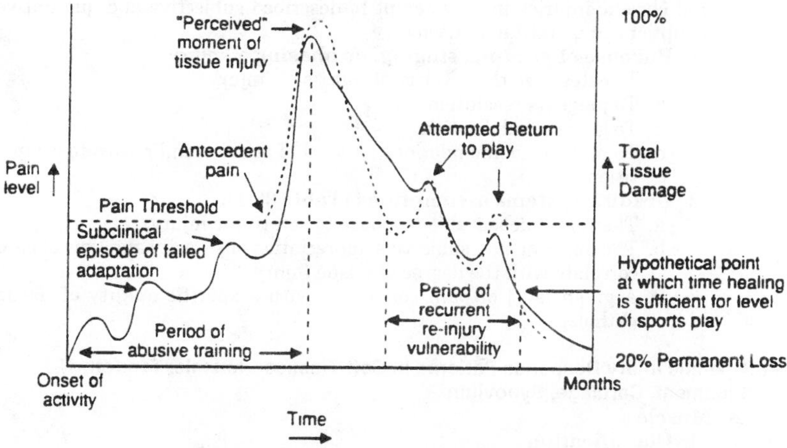

Fig. 38-6. Profile of chronic microtraumatic soft tissue injury. This profile is typical of overuse tendon injury. Solid line = percentage of tissue damage. (From Leadbetter WB. Cell matrix response in tendon injury. *Clin Sports Med* 1992:11 533–557, with permission.)

C. **Clinical significance of the injury profile**
   1. **Acute injury treatment** traditionally centers on the suppression of the acute inflammatory phase and reduction of pain. A period of reinjury vulnerability develops as pain falls below the athlete's threshold of perception, which typically precedes the full and final healing phase of the injured soft tissue. Paradoxically, the more comfortable the athlete is made to feel, the more likely it is that activity will be resumed prior to adequate healing. The period of vulnerability is lengthened by the adverse effects of inappropriate immobilization but would be shortened by functional rehabilitation or protective bracing, which would either expedite fibrogenesis or avoid placing a load on an injured part.
   2. **Chronic injury** treatment must be taken into account in the history for proper recommendation and adjustment of activity. The athlete must be counseled that the period of vulnerability to recurrent or new injury is likely to be far longer, as the subclinical tissue microtrauma is often well established when the patient first perceives the injury. It is more likely that there will be resulting degenerative change or permanent loss of tissue integrity. The athlete's expectations, therefore, must be realistic, and moderate return to activity advocated. Surgery may be required to stimulate repair.

V. Sources of Pain in Soft Tissue Injury

are multifactorial and include both inflammatory and biomechanical sources.

A. **Chemical sources of pain** include the following:
   1. **Synovium**
   2. **Fibroblasts**
   3. **Tendon or ligament elongation** beyond elastic limits
   4. **Retinacular pain** in the knee
   5. **Substance P**, a peptide nociceptor stimulating substance

B. **Pain may be due to inflammation as opposed to degeneration.**

C. **Pain grading** is a concept used throughout sports medicine. Grading, staging, or phasing concepts for sports trauma have been applied to both acute and chronic injuries in an attempt to described subjective and qualitative symptoms in quantitative terms.

1. **Purpose of grading, staging, or phasing** of injury
   a. To categorize the severity of soft tissue injury
   b. To judge its resolution
   c. To guide rehabilitation
   d. To make recommendations on level of activity and return to competition
2. **Grading systems assumptions (Table 38-1):**
   a. There is a measurable response to soft tissue injury.
   b. The duration and subjective appreciation of severity and type of pain correlate with the degree of tissue injury.
   c. A given level of pain correlates with a specific quality of tissue pathology.

VI. Specific Injury Response Patterns in Soft Tissues—Muscle, Tendon, Ligament, Cartilage, Synovium

A. **Muscle**

1. **Classification**
   a. Acute strains and avulsions
   b. Contusions
   c. Delayed-onset muscle soreness (DOMS) syndrome and exercise-induced injury
   d. Contracture
2. **Contributing factors** to strain injury include:
   a. Passive overstretching or preloading
   b. Sudden voluntary or concentric contracture
   c. Fatigue
3. **The pathophysiology** of muscle injury is characterized by both acute-phase inflammatory responses in strain injury and a variety of metabolic disturbances of muscle homeostasis with overexertion. While regeneration of muscle fibers and incomplete muscle tears is theoretically possible, most completely disrupted muscles heal by a combination of regeneration and scar. This may result in restrictive adhesions, reduced contractile force, and restricted adjacent joint function.
4. **Muscle injury** is characterized similarly to ligament injury:
   a. First-degree or mild strains are defined by minimal structural damage, minimal hemorrhage, and early resolution.
   b. Second-degree or moderate muscle strains are defined as partial tears most often at the myotendinous junction, accompanied by pain, inflammation, and functional loss.
   c. Third-degree or severe strains are accompanied by obvious hemorrhage, swelling, and often complete or palpable muscle tissue disruption.
5. **A muscle contusion** results from an external force sufficient to cause muscle damage.
   a. Severity may be graded by measuring the restriction in range of motion of the subtended joint. A mild contusion causes loss of less than one-third of the normal range of motion of the adjacent joint, whereas a severe contusion limits the joint motion to less than one-third of normal excursion.
   b. Two types of injury occur:
      1. Intermuscular hematoma—a hemorrhage occurring along intermuscular septal or fascial sheaths.
      2. Intramuscular hematoma—a hemorrhage occurring within muscle substance. It is thought that intramuscular hematomas are more difficult to resolve and are associated with scar contracture, myositis ossificans, and acute compartment syndrome secondary to hemorrhage.

Table 38-1. Clinical grading of sports-induced soft tissue inflammations

Grade	Subjective pain pattern	Physical signs	Tissue damage	Healing potential	Relevant therapeutic measures	
I	Pain alter activity only. Duration of symptoms less than two weeks. Spontaneous relief within 24 hr.	Nonlocalized pain.	Microinjury	Potential spontaneous resolution	Proper warmup and conditioning. Avoidance of abrupt transition in activity level.	Training coaching and self-help measures often effective.
II	Pain during and after activity, but no significant functional disability. Duration of symptoms greater than two weeks, less than 6 weeks.	Localized pain. Minimal or no other signs of inflammation.	Microinjury	Potential spontaneous resolution	Analysis of technique and efficiency. Decrease transitional abuse and improve training.	Training coaching and self-help measures often effective.
III	Pain during and after sport lasting for several days despite rest with rapid return upon activity. Significant functional disability. Duration of pain greater than 6 weeks. Night pain may occur.	Intense point tenderness with prominent inflammation (edema, effusion, erythema, crepitus, etc.).	Macroinjury	Permanent scar and residual tissue damage more likely	Medical assessment of structural vulnerability (e.g., flat feet, inflexibility, muscle weakness, etc.). Protected activity (e.g., bracing). Modification or substitution of different sports exercise to avoid excessive load on injured part.	Medical diagnosis and opinion valuable.
IV	Continuous pain with sport and daily activity. Total inability to train or complete. Night pain common.	Grade III symptoms plus tissue breakdown, atrophy, etc. Impending or actual tissue failure.	Macroinjury	Permanent scar and residual tissue damage more likely	Surgical treatment often indicated to stimulate fibrous scar and repair or create structural alteration such as releases or decompression, potential permanent withdrawal from activity (e.g., degenerative joint disease, tendon rupture).	Medical diagnosis and opinion valuable.

Adapted from Leadbetter WB, Buckwalter JA, Gordon SL, eds. *Sports-induced inflammation: Clinical and basic science concepts.* Park Ridge, IL: American Academy of Orthopaedic Surgeons, 1990.

6. **Myositis ossificans traumatica** is a condition of heterotopic ossification response, usually confined to a single muscle or muscle group occurring after a prior episode of trauma, either single or repetitive.
   a. Clinically, myositis ossificans can be a source of considerable and lengthy disability to the athlete due to inflammatory pain and contracture.
   b. The most common clinical findings are soft tissue mass with restriction of joint motion.
   c. Historically, these lesions have been confused with osteosarcoma, with dire treatment consequences. Distinguishing features include the decreasing pain and size of the myositis mass as the lesion matures, and the intramuscular location of the myositis lesion. In questionable cases, the patient needs careful follow up and often repeat x-ray or MRI.
   d. Common sites include quadriceps femoris, hamstrings, and biceps brachii.
   e. In one study, approximately 70% of athletes afflicted by moderate or severe muscle contusions developed heterotopic ossification. Reinjury of a contused quadriceps was associated with 100% development of myositis ossificans.
   f. A presentation of pain, palpable mass, and associated flexion contracture after muscle injury strongly suggests the possibility of early myositis ossificans. The most important differential diagnosis of myositis ossificans is malignancy. The advent of magnetic resonance imaging (MRI) has made this less difficult to distinguish.
   g. The condition is generally self-limiting; surgical biopsy is discouraged to avoid confusing the benign pseudomalignant histology of bony callus with a true malignancy. In rare cases, the surgical removal of a symptomatic lesion is indicated for persistent pain, usually no sooner than a year or more after onset.
7. **Delayed onset muscle soreness (DOMS)** appears 12 to 48 hr after exercise sessions and represents a distinct clinical syndrome associated with the exertional muscle injury.
   a. DOMS is characterized by tenderness on muscle palpation, increased muscle stiffness, and restriction of range of motion. It is often seen as part of the "getting in shape" experience.
   b. While the exact mechanism remains unresolved, there is considerable evidence for both inflammatory and metabolic dysfunction secondary to ultramicroscopic muscle damage.
   c. Acute compartment syndromes may result from excessive exercise-induced muscle damage.
   d. The rapid use of muscles and discoordination of normal agonist–antagonist protective dampening reflexes contributes to the onset of DOMS.
   e. **Myoglobinuria** is seen to some degree with all intense exercise. However in rare cases, exertional rhabdomyolysis has occurred secondary to derangements in intracellular calcium and the stimulation of muscle proteolysis resulting in myoglobin-induced kidney failure as well as multiple organ failure. There is some evidence that such a severe inflammatory myopathy may be potentiated by viral infection.

B. **Tendon Injury**
   1. **Classification** (Table 38-2)
      a. Acute and chronic peritenonitis
      b. Degenerative tendinopathy, tendinosis, or cystic degeneration.
      c. Spontaneous rupture
   2. **Enthesopathy** is an injury in which tendon fibers are either microtorn or inflamed at their bony insertion.
   3. **The tendinosis lesion** is a site of failed adaptation and failed healing that may be initially asymptomatic or lead to progressive tendon degeneration, pain, nodularity, or rupture (Fig. 38-7).

Table 38-2. Terminology of tendon injury

New	Old	Definition	Histologic findings	Clinical signs and symptoms
Paratenonitis	Tenosynovitis Tenovaginitis Peritendinitis	An inflammation of only the paratenon, either lined by synovium or not.	Inflammatory cells in paratenon or peritendinous areolar tissue.	Cardinal inflammatory signs: swelling,pain, crepitation, local tenderness, warmth, dysfunction.
Paratenonitis with tendinosis	Tendinitis	Paratenon inflammation associated with intratendinosis degeneration.	Same as I, with loss of tendon collagen fiber disorientation, scattered vascular ingrowth but no prominent intratendinous inflammation.	Same as I, with often alpable tendon nodule, swelling, and inflammatory signs.
Tendinosis	Tendinitis	Intratendinous degeneration due to atrophy (aging, microtrauma, vascular compromise, etc.).	Noninflammatory intratendinous collagen degeneration with fiber disorientation, hypocellularity, scattered vascular ingrowth, occasional local necrosis or calcification.	Often palpable tendon nodule that can be *asymptomatic,* but may also be point tender. Swelling of tendon sheath is absent.
Tendinitis	Tendon strain or tear A. Acute (less than 2 weeks) B. Subacute (4–6 weeks) C. Chronic (over 6 weeks)	Symptomatic degeneration of the tendon with vascular disruption and inflammatory repair response.	Three recognized subgroups: each displays variable histology from purely inflammation with acute hemorrhage and tear, to nflammation superimposed upon preexisting degeneration, to calcification and tendinosis changes in chronic conditions. In chronic stage there may be: 1. Interstitial microinjury 2. Cystic tendon degeneration 3. Frank partial rupture 4. Acute complete rupture	Symptoms are inflammatory and proportional to ascular disruption, hematoma, or atrophy-related cell necrosis. Symptom duration defines each subgroup.

Data from Clancy WG. Tendon trauma and overuse injuries. In: Leadbetter WB, Buckwalter JA, Gordon SL, eds. *Sports-induced inflammation.* Park Ridge, IL: American Academy of Orthopaedic Surgeons, 1990; and Puddu G, Ippolito E, Postacchini P. A classification of Achilles tendon disease. *Am J Sports Med* 1976; 4:145–150.

4. **Current classifications** of tendon injury emphasize the distinction between peritenon or synovial inflammation versus direct involvement of the tendon substance (i.e. a structural dominant complaint).
5. **The pathohistology** of acute peritendinitis reveals inflammatory cell reaction, edema extravasation of plasma proteins, and accumulation of fibrin in the subperitenon space. Crepitation is caused by the presence of fibrin. Chronic peritenonitis is caused by the fibroblastic proliferation, the presence of myofibroblasts, thickening of the peritenon, degenerative changes in the peritenon tissues and adhesions.
6. **Spontaneous tendon rupture** is highly associated with tendon degeneration.
7. **Dystrophic calcium pyrophosphate** salts precipitate in degenerative tendon tissue as a result of mitochondrial injury. In such calcification,

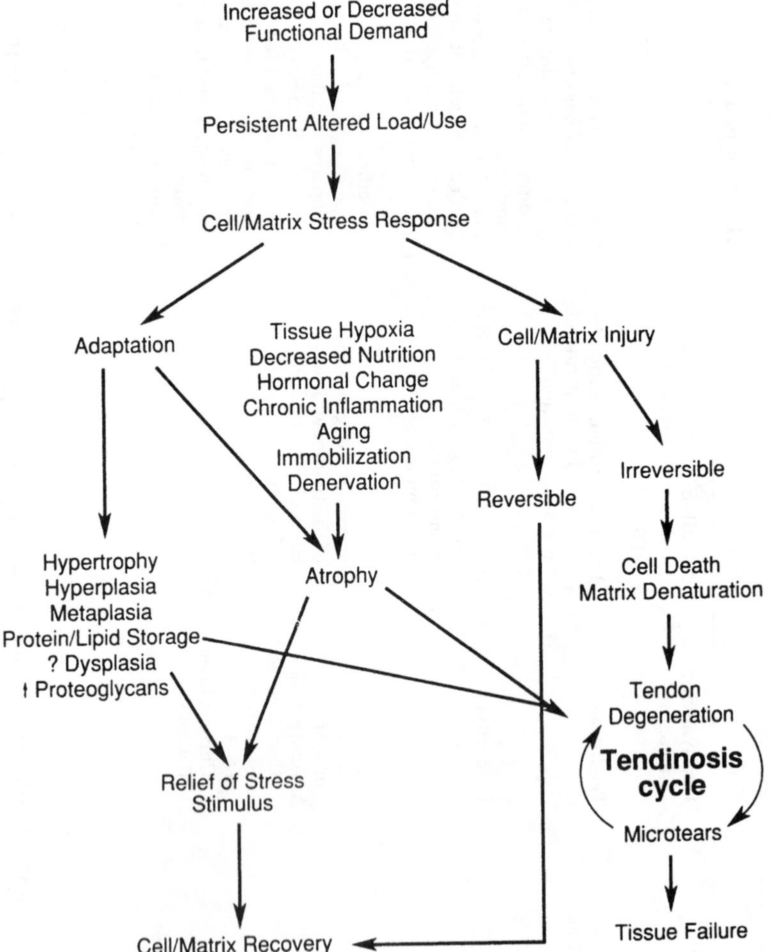

Fig. 38-7. Cell matrix response to change in functional level. In this model, tendinosis results from a failed cell matrix adaptation to excessive changes in load use. Such failure is modified by both intrinsic and extrinsic factors.

calcium deposited in the damaged collagen matrix appears as chalky hydroxy apatite crystals. Visible on x-ray, these deposits are the "tombstones" of tendon injury.

C. **Ligament injury**
   1. **Classification** (Table 38-3)
   2. **A sprain** is an acute injury to a ligament. With some notable exceptions, healing of sprained ligamentous tissue is analogous to healing in other vascularized tissues. Intraarticular ligaments such as the anterior cruciate ligament heal poorly. The reason for this disparity is multifactorial and not well understood.
   3. **Ligaments** display viscoelastic behavior—i.e., nonlinear deformation with respect to load. Therefore the more rapidly a ligament is loaded, the more strain resistance develops. This observation underlines the importance of slow static stretching of both tendon and ligament. The disability of ligament injury is joint instability and the loss of subtle proprioceptive feedback to both joint and muscle function.

D. **Cartilage and synovium**
   1. **Classification of chondral injury**
      a. Partial thickness injury—laceration, flap tear, chondromalacia
      b. Complete chondral separation
      c. Osteochondral fracture
   2. **Stages of articular degeneration**
      a. Stage I—softening and deformation
      b. Stage II—articular fissures, early fragmentation, and chondromalacia
      c. Stage III—prominent articular degeneration, chondromalacia, and early separation
      d. Stage IV—complete dissolution of articular surface and articular fragmentation with subchondral bone exposed (eburnation)
   3. **Contributing factors to articulate cartilage degeneration**
      a. Joint surface overload
      b. Excessive body weight
      c. Limb malalignment
      d. Acute trauma or articular fracture

Table 38-3. Schemes for assessing ligament injury

Grade	Severity	Degree	Structural involvement	Exam	Performance deficit
1	Mild	1	Negligible	No visible injury Locally tender, only joint stable	Minimal to a few days
2[a]	Moderate	2	Partial	Visible swelling, Marked tenderness +/- stability	Up to 6 weeks (may be modified by protective bracing)
3	Severe	3	Complete	Gross swelling, Marked tenderness, Antalgic posture Unstable Joint	Indefinite, minimum of 6–8 weeks

[a]In present schemes for clinical classification of soft tissue injury, it is the intermediate qualities of trauma that form a "gray zone" in clinical decision making.

e. Genetic predispostion
f. Chronic joint instability
g. Chronic inflammatory synovitis
h. Loss of normal functional protection (e.g., anterior cruciate ligament deficiency or meniscectomy of the knee)

4. **The pathophysiology** of articular cartilage injury and degeneration is characterized by a lack of the classic wound healing response. Because of an absence of blood vessels, lymphatics, and nerves, partial-thickness cartilage injuries do not repair themselves. In cartilage lesions, an inflammatory response is generally possible only when subchondral bone is also injured, because this type of injury allows inflammatory and reparative cells to enter the wounded area from the marrow. Healing of full-thickness osteochondral lesions takes place by fibrocartilaginous replacement. When normal cartilage is exposed to excessive pressure or shear, isolated chondrocyte necrosis can occur, resulting in loss of matrix and the softening of the articular surface known as chondromalacia. Inflammatory symptoms associated with cartilage injury may be caused by shedding of matrix breakdown products and secondary stimulation of the synovium leading to further degeneration and continued softening, with eventual total loss of the articular covering exposing the underlying subchondral bone in advanced arthritis.
5. **Osteochondritis dissecans** is a unique osteochondral lesion often seen in childhood involving separation of a fragment of bone and cartilage from the articular surface (see Chapter 51).
6. **Osteochondral contusion** describes a lesion now recognized by MRI to be associated with episodes of joint instability or overload, as typically demonstrated in the pivot shift with anterior cruciate ligament deficiency of the knee. There is evidence that this osseous subchondral microfracture may involve chondrocyte necrosis of the overlying articular cartilage is surface. The clinical significance of these findings remains controversial but is concerning.

E. **Synovial injury**

1. **Classification**
   a. Joint synovitis
   b. Peritenonitis
   c. Bursitis
2. **The pathophysiology** of the synovial membrane is inflammatory-dominant. Various cytokines may be released from the synovium, promoting articular damage. The majority of synovial lining cells (type B cell) express fibroblast characteristics allowing complications of fibroarthrosis and capsular fibroplasia to arise, so-called adhesive capsulitis.
3. **Intrasynovial bleeding** due to direct trauma (i.e., hemobursa or hemarthrosis) rapidly triggers an inflammatory process.
4. **Synovitis** resulting in chronic joint effusion markedly inhibits subadjacent muscle function and contractile strength. The pain of physical joint distention and pathologic chemical events further disables the injured athlete. Aspiration can be therapeutically beneficial in decompressing joint distention as well as aiding in further diagnosis of the underlying condition. Synovial flow analysis and appearance may distinguish acute trauma from chronic inflammation or even sepsis.

VII. Summary of the Pathologic Basis for Clinical Treatment of Sports Injury

A. **The clinical assessment** of athletic injury must take into account the following:

1. There are basic differences in the patterns of acute traumatic and chronic overuse tissue response.
2. The clinical predictability of soft tissue healing in sports-induced trauma is frustrated by a number of variables, especially with respect to the definition of the severity of injury and its exact onset.

3. Sports trauma tissue response is a time-dependent cellular process with unique limitations defined by the variable biological behavior of the tissues involved and the unique demands of the activity. Transition plays an important role in the determination of this process.
4. Degeneration is a common result of extensive tissue overload or overuse; as such, it must be distinguished from inflammation as well as aging.
5. Posttraumatic pain has multiple potential etiologies, only one of which is inflammatory. The failure to distinguish inflammation from degenerative pain can lead to ineffective therapy.

B. **The role of therapeutic prescription** must be continually redefined and reassessed in face of the known pathophysiology of athletic injury.
   1. Pharmocologic modifiers such as nonsteroidal antiinflammatory drugs (aspirin, NSAIDs, corticosteroids) are best suited for treating inflammatory processes, notably synovitis. However, in the total treatment of the injured athlete, they are primarily adjunctive and rarely the only solution. Without attention to a comprehensive therapeutic program, antiinflammatory therapy generally fails to restore sustained function.
   2. Physical modalities—such as ice, heat, electric stimulation, and ultrasound—can be useful adjuncts in the reduction of pain and the secondary effects of injury. However, their ability to significantly promote healing remains controversial and poorly understood as to timing, dosage, and duration.
   3. Exercise rehabilitation remains a singularly important solution to sports-induced injury. However, claims that rehabilitation will promote healing assume that tissue necrosis and degeneration are not excessive. When tissues retain their ability to heal after injury, regulation of connected tissue biology and repair by the controlled application of rehabilitative load or use has a proven empiric benefit. Explanations to this observed therapeutic response include:
      a. Training effect upon remaining uninjured tissues
      b. Improvement of the kinetic linkage function with decreased force at the injury site
      c. Induced cellular reparative response at the site of the injury
      d. Avoidance of secondary functional loss due to atrophy or contracture

C. **Rest**
   1. Rest alone does not predictably restore sustained function. Retraining and reconditioning are generally required after injury to counter the effects of disuse.
   2. The concept of protected activity during recovery after injury holds that for any given problem there is some range of acceptable load and use that will provide greater stimulation than damage at the injury site. The application of such a concept is generally based upon both clinical experience and trial and error.

D. **Healing versus functional recovery**
   1. Healing is a tissue effect resulting from repair. As such, it is not synonymous with functional recovery.
   2. Functional recovery is a multifactorial regaining of the use of the injured part. Injury is never an isolated event and should always be seen as a part of a kinetic link rehabilitation. It is possible to have significant sustained functional recovery in the face of incomplete healing when injuries are not too extensive. The choice to allow an attempt at sports play in the face of incomplete healing is dependent on several variables including the skill of the athlete, the position played, the inherent nature of the injury and the importance of the competition. Such decisions are among the most difficult to make in the care of the athlete and inherently require a complete discussion of the risks and benefits by all parties (Fig. 38-8).
   3. **In the injured athlete** the normal tissue homeostatic balance must be restored from its disrupted state. The relative balance of this restora-

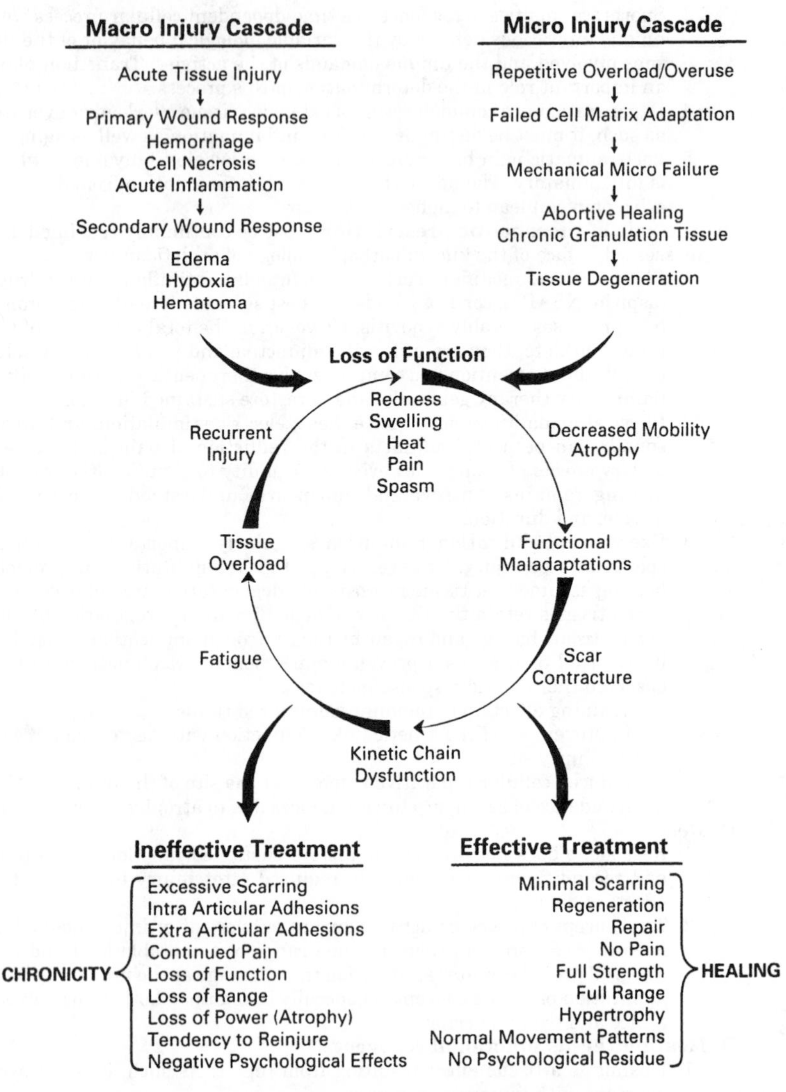

Fig. 38-8. Injury-pain cycle. The promotion of healing and performance depends upon accurate diagnosis of excessive inflammatory response and adequate rehabilitation.

tion versus disruption lies at the crux of differentiating the healthy noninjured or "normal" from the injured, diseased, or "pathologic" condition.

E. **Aging** is characterized by a reduced ability to adapt to environmental stress and loss of tissue homeostasis. The maintenance of tissue homeostasis or continued connective tissue renewal under conditions of physiologic stress depends upon retaining adaptive ability. Aging is a mutable process, the effects of which can be retarded or reversed by therapeutic exercise.

Suggested Reading

Leadbetter WB. Soft tissue athletic injury. In: Fu FH, Stone DA, eds. *Sports injuries: mechanisms, prevention, treatment.* Baltimore: Williams & Wilkins, 1994:733–780.

Leadbetter WB. Anti-inflammatory therapy in sports injury: the role of nonsteroidal drugs and corticosteroid injection. *Clin Sports Med* 1995; 14:353–410.

Leadbetter WB. Aging effects upon the repair and healing of athletic injury. In: Gordon SL, Gonzalez-Mestre X, Garrett WE Jr, eds. *Sports and exercise in midlife.* Park Ridge, IL: American Academy of Orthopaedic Surgeons, 1993:177–233.

Leadbetter WB, Buckwalter JA, Gordon SL. *Sports-induced inflammation: clinical and basic science concepts.* Park Ridge, IL: American Academy of Orthopaedic Surgeons, 1990.

Reid DC. *Sports injury: assessment and rehabilitation.* New York: Churchill Livingstone, 1992.

39. THE SHOULDER—MUSCULOTENDINOUS INJURIES

Russell F. Warren

I. Anatomy and Kinesiology.

The musculotendinous unit of the shoulder may be divided into intrinsic (rotator cuff) and extrinsic musculature. The rotator cuff may be considered a primary mover, which provide motion, as well as an active stabilizer, centering the humeral head on the glenoid. The rotator cuff includes the following four musculotendinous structures: the subscapularis anteriorly, the supraspinatus superiorly, and the infraspinatus and teres minor posteriorly. The extrinsic muscles move the humerus in coordination with the rotator cuff. This action has been termed a *force couple.* The extrinsic muscles include the deltoid, pectoralis major, latissimus dorsi, and teres major. The biceps functions both as intrinsic and extrinsic muscles to help stabilize the glenohumeral joint as well as to flex the humerus and elbow. It is active in throwing activities.

The glenohumeral joint is also dependent on the scapular musculature, which, through movement on the chest wall, positions the arm for athletic activities. Dysfunction in these muscles, such as the trapezius and serratus anterior, result in a loss of scapular control and thus winging of the scapula. Such winging is usually secondary to nerve dysfunction but may occur primarily as a result of muscle weakness.

The rotator cuff acts via the subscapularis as an internal rotator. It should be noted that the latissimus dorsi and teres major and pectoralis major are also strong internal rotators. The infraspinatus and teres minor are external rotators, while the supraspinatus is particularly active in elevation. The cuff muscles are active in concert to center the humeral head during elevation and rotation. In sports, the level of activity of the cuff will vary with the phase of throwing and the quality of the athlete. Thus, throwing activities, which have been divided in four basic phases, will see activity increase from the windup to the cocking phase. While the cuff activity will decrease during the acceleration phase, posterior cuff and biceps activity will increase during the deceleration phase.

II. Muscle Tendon Injury—Pathophysiology

Strain injury may present in differing ways in the shoulder, depending on the athlete's age, the presence or absence of cuff degeneration, and type of athletic activity. In addition, shoulder instability can lead to rotator cuff injury. In throwing sports, the shoulder is subjected to repetitive activities during which high forces are generated that will stress the cuff and labrum. Speeds of up to 7,000 degrees per second are seen during the acceleration phase, with high forces at the end of the cocking and deceleration phases. Swimming can also generate high forces dependent on the stroke and phase involved. In addition, certain sports that involve contact or heavy lifting may impose sudden high loads that cause acute disruption of the muscle tendon unit. These failures of the muscle tendon unit may occur gradually from fatigue, repetitive activity, and/or acute injury.

A. ***Fatigue*** will prevent the humeral head from being centered during elevation, thus stressing the associated tendons, labrum, and biceps. With fatigue, the humeral head will migrate superiorly, which will result in increased cuff compression.

B. ***Repetitive activity*** is dependent on a muscle unit that is capable of endurance activity as well as generating high forces for short periods. In this setting, the cuff is also dependent on its environment for satisfactory function, thus it must be able to glide easily through the subacromial space without excessive contact on the acromion or acromioclavicular (AC) joint.

III. The Impingement Syndrome

The *impingement syndrome* is a sequence of cuff failures that occur over time, particularly in older patients. Three phases are described: (1) cuff edema without tearing, (2) cuff degeneration, and (3) full-thickness cuff tears. It was felt that the anterior third of the acromion was specifically related to cuff failure, as it was thickened and had a spur forming in the coracoacromial ligament. This pathogenesis of cuff disease in patients in their fifties is fairly typical, but in contrast, there is often some degree of instability or increased translation present in the young athlete, which leads to the presence of high forces in the tendon and ultimate failure with or without associated acromial changes. In addition, contractures are common in throwing athletes, leading to altered kinematics and tendon strain. Most throwers will have increased external rotation at 90 degrees of elevation with losses of internal rotation at 0 and 90 degrees. This resultant posterior contracture has been noted to result in increases of anterior translation and possible compression.

Impingement syndrome may result from extrinsic compression or internal injury. ***Extrinsic compression*** may result from (1) ***fatigue,*** leading to increased superior migration; (2) ***hooked acromion,*** either congenital, which is rare, or secondary to increased compression, which is more common; (3) ***a thickened AC joint,*** (4) ***lateral sloping of the acromion***; (5) ***coracoid impingement*** and/or; (6) ***enlargement of the greater tuberosity,*** either congenital, degenerative, or fracture malunion.

Internal impingement may occur with or without associated instability. Increased anterior translation may cause or be associated with internal impingement. In essence, during throwing activities with the shoulder at 90 degrees abduction and with 90 degrees of external rotation (or more), the deep surface of the supraspinatus is placed in contact with the posterior superior labrum and glenoid. At this site, the high forces that are generated may result in cuff failure or damage to the labrum. Normally, with external rotation at 90 degrees, the humeral head will translate posteriorly, relieving cuff strain. With mild capsular failure, the posterior translation will be lost, resulting in cuff failure at the articular side of the supraspinatus and mild instability, which will be difficult to note on examination.

Finally, a sudden, violent acute injury may occur resulting in failure of the cuff or extrinsic muscles. The failure will depend to some degree on arm position and the forces applied. Thus, with the arm at 90 degrees of elevation, if the arm is driven higher, forcing the greater tuberosity into the superior glenoid, the supraspinatus will impact and be injured, possibly resulting in a full-thickness tear. In older patients, this will be more likely. In addition, as the tuberosity impacts the labrum, a superior labral injury will occur. This has been called a SLAP (superior labrum, anterior and posterior) lesion, with four stages described. With the shoulder at 90 degrees and working with weights, a sudden force or overload may rupture the pectoralis major.

The magnitude and site of each of these injuries will vary depending on arm position, forces applied, and the presence or absence of prior tendon degeneration and muscle fatigue. An understanding of these components of injury may allow us to prevent injury better and create improved treatment regimens.

In its classic sense, the impingement syndrome is generally seen in older (above age 45) athletes, realizing that cuff failure may also occur in young athletes, but then it is often associated with instability . In addition, acute injury to the cuff or tendons can occur, resulting in ruptures or simply a contusion to the muscle tendon unit that will mimic a full-thickness tear clinically but will usually improve with time. The presence of prior degeneration in older athletes will make rupture more likely.

A. Chronic Stage I and Stage II Impingement

1. **History.** These patients typically are in their forties or early fifties and present with shoulder pain often related to a specific activity. They complain of pain at the deltoid patch, difficulty in lying on the shoulder because of pain, pain with overhead activity, weakness (especially diminished strength at 90 degrees above elevation), and occasionally

mild crepitation. Patients with mild or moderate cuff disease will have pain with specific activities as well as night pain.

2. **Physical Examination** will reveal ***tenderness*** over the anterior humeral head and subacromial regions; there may also be tenderness at the AC joint. Range-of-motion testing will reveal a ***decrease of internal rotation*** and mild losses of elevation, especially active elevation. There should be a smooth scapular thoracic rhythm, and no shoulder shrug should be noted. Inspection will reveal minimal or no atrophy of the supraspinatus or infraspinatus regions. Strength should be intact with ***painful eccentric loading at 90 degrees*** of forward elevation. Stability should be assessed and is usually normal, though one may see mild anterior translation. The neurovascular examination is unremarkable. Special tests include a positive ***impingement sign,*** a positive ***abduction sign,*** and positive ***impingement test*** (see Appendix 6). The adduction test and O'Brien maneuver are negative.

   Recognition is dependent on noting the painful arc at 90 degrees aggravated with internal rotation and the impingement sign of painful forced elevation at 170 to 180 degrees. Instability must be assessed carefully. Usually there is an internal rotation contracture with losses of internal rotation at 0 and 90 degrees. The impingement test performed by relieving painful elevation with a subacromial injection of lidocaine may be used to confirm the impression.

3. **Further Studies.** ***Radiographs*** may well be helpful in evaluating shoulder pain if the condition is chronic or if high forces are applied. As a standard series, we will obtain in patients above 40 years of age a true anteroposterior (AP) view, a West Point view, and Stryker Notch view. In older patients, we will use a true AP view in internal and external rotation, an axillary view, an outlet view, and a weighted AP view at 45 degrees of elevation. With these projections, one can note, in the chronic cases, acromial spurs, an acromial angle, AC joint arthritis, and enlargement of the greater tuberosity. In addition, we look for glenohumeral arthritis, bone lesions (benign or malignant), and signs of instability.

   In young patients, the x-ray will often be negative; in the chronic state, acromial changes with thickened dense bone, acromial spurs, and a change from a convex to concave will be noted.

4. **Treatment.** The treatment of chronic cuff injury includes paying attention to the mechanism of injury so as to avoid further injury and ***decreasing load*** to the cuff. ***Antiinflammatory medications,*** such as oral nonsteroidal antiinflammatory drugs (NSAIDs) early and injectable corticosteroids with late or chronic cases, are very useful. Formal or home therapy to ***increase flexibility*** and then gradually ***increase strength and endurance*** are mainstays of treatment. Then a gradual resumption of high loads is permitted.

   In the athlete one often finds a contracture and a lack of sufficient strength for the given activity. Thus a program of lowered stress on the shoulder (i.e., decreased yardage in swimming, missing of a period of throwing) combined with improved flexibility and strength will gradually allow a return to full activity. It may require 8 to 10 weeks to significantly improve strength in a graduated fashion.

   Initially, NSAIDs (avoiding injections) are begun, combined with a stretching program to decrease the previously noted contractures at 0/90 degrees. Strength work must include the rotator cuff, extrinsic muscles, and scapulothoracic muscles. Concentric and eccentric work is important, progressing initially from a 0 degree position to a 90 degree position for overhead sports. The activity itself often will have to be decreased but not entirely eliminated in the early stage. In a later stage, a period off from the activity while building flexibility and endurance could be important.

   Upon resumption of the activity, careful observation by an experienced coach will be of value to avoid repeating poor habits that may lead to reinjury. Thus a thrower who "opens" too soon or over strides must have his or her technique adjusted accordingly.

5. **Failure of Conservative Treatment.** If the patient is not improving by 3 to 4 months, a ***cortisone injection*** will be considered. This again can be combined with lidocaine to note pain relief, initially helping to confirm the diagnosis. In patients with cuff disease secondary to instability, pain relief with the injection may occur; however, as their symptoms are not due to subacromial impingement, decompression would not be of benefit.

   If ***surgery*** is being considered in the younger athlete, magnetic resonance imaging (MRI) may be of value to note the presence or absence of cuff disease and labral injury. In patients in their forties and fifties who are active in tennis, it is often not necessary but will aid in preoperative planning, as the presence of a full-thickness cuff tear will significantly alter the postoperative program.

   Surgical options will vary on the type of pathology that resulted in cuff failure. Arthroscopy will generally be helpful to fully evaluate the rotator cuff and the degree of degeneration in the joint as well as to perform decompression as needed. During the exam under anesthesia, particular attention is important to avoid missing instability.

   Standard arthroscopic evaluation of the joint and subacromial space is performed. The surgeon will look for cuff degeneration and signs of instability. If there is degeneration of the cuff and the acromion is abnormal, with spurring and fraying of the coracoacromial ligament, debridement followed by subacromial decompression is performed. The AC joint is resected if painful or only debrided inferiorly if it is enlarged by spurs and playing a role in impingement. If it is prominent, the greater tuberosity is abraded. If identified, a full-thickness cuff tear is repaired either with a miniarthrotomy or an arthroscopic repair. If instability is present and there is no evidence for impingement, this is addressed at this time or later, after a second course of physical therapy.

   Thus, rotator cuff degeneration is treated with cuff debridement, acromioplasty, possible AC joint resection, possible tuberosity debridement, and cuff repair if necessary. If instability is the main problem, then rehabilitation is attempted, followed by surgical stabilization if necessary.

6. **Return to Sports.** With nonoperative treatment, this is based on the type of sport. Return is based on when the athlete is pain-free, which may be as early as 4 to 6 weeks. Surgical treatment usually takes 3 to 6 months before the athlete is able to return to full, unrestricted pain-free activity.

B. **Impingement Stage III—Full-Thickness Cuff Tears—Chronic**

1. **History.** These patients will frequently present in a manner similar to those described earlier with cuff degeneration. Typically they are older (average age, 58) but can be seen specifically in those sports where repeated activity such as throwing leads to earlier cuff degeneration and full-thickness tears. More commonly, in patients below age 35, one will see acute injury resulting in either a cuff contusion or a full-thickness tear. Thus, a direct or indirect load on an already degenerated cuff in skiers below 45 years of age will result in a full-thickness tear, while a 25-year-old skier may only have a contusion. These patients complain of pain that is increased with activity and/or stress, pain that is increased at 90 degrees, night pain, pain when lying on the shoulder, and, often, crepitation.

2. **Physical Examination.** Reveals tenderness over the proximal humeral head and subacromial region. Range of motion (ROM) usually reveals mild to major loss of elevation, though young patients may have normal active ROM. Frequently, especially with larger tears, the shrug sign is present, as is altered scapulothoracic rhythm. Young patients may note increased translation on stability testing, while there may be a true dislocation in older (above age 40) patient.

3. **Ancillary Studies.** See discussion of impingement syndromes, above, for radiographic changes. Depending on the degree of suspicion and the patients need for full function, an early MRI may be of value in deciding on appropriate management both for younger and older patients. The

MRI will help to define the size of the tear, note the degree of degeneration and cuff atrophy, and indicate the outlook for a satisfactory repair. It should be noted that cuff contusion can occur and confuse the issue and that some cuff tears in older patients will be so chronic and degenerative, with large losses of tissue, that a repair may not be warranted or feasible.

4. **Treatment.** Older patients (above age 70), good function may best be restored through rehabilitation with progressive strengthening exercises combined with NSAIDs. Young patients, especially those with high demands or poor function and a positive MRI, are best treated with early surgery to maintain strength and power.

   In patients making heavy demands on shoulder function, such as certain athletes, an early surgical approach to cuff repair is indicated. In older patients, whose demands are probably less, a period of rehabilitation may suffice. However, if there is a marked shrug sign and weakness in external rotation, a large tear is probably pres-ent. Generally in patients in their fifties and sixties, such a tear, if acute, is superimposed on chronic degeneration of the tendon. Thus the urgency of repair is not apparent and one can delay to see the effects of rehabilitation. In contrast, in younger patients, a cuff tear is often more acute, the tendon is not particularly degenerated, and future high performance will commonly require a repair before the tendon becomes fixed and retracted.

C. **Impingement III—Full-Thickness Cuff Tears—Acute**

In contrast to older patients, where cuff degeneration is already present, full-thickness rotator cuff tears in the young athlete are relatively uncommon. Cuff tears may occur acutely in association with a dislocation. This is more common in patients past the age of 40, where the supraspinatus tendon may fail, or in patients over 50, where the subscapularis may rupture. However, it may occur in young athletes as well, thus creating a posterior mechanism for anterior instability. We have seen this particularly in football, where an acute first-time dislocation occurs and the supraspinatus fails, causing instability without labral injury. The reduction may be easy or difficult; but during the recovery phase, the patient will continue to complain of pain and subsequent weakness. In this setting, an MRI should be obtained. If a significant (full-thickness) tear seen, in a young, active athlete, an early repair is suggested.

In contrast, in older patients, an acute tear usually has a component of degeneration with and there is a history of prior symptoms. Therefore management would tend to be similar to that of a chronic tear. The exception would be based on the degree of sudden weakness and loss of motion, particularly external rotation, suggesting a large or massive tear. In this situation, an early repair would be advised in an active patient.

1. **Return to Sports:** Following rotator cuff repair, return to sports is variable and may take up to a year or more following surgery. However, many high-level throwing athletes cannot return to the same level of sports activity.

IV. Coracoid Impingement

This uncommon entity produces symptoms resembling biceps tendinitis and instability. It is often iatrogenic from prior surgical procedures but can be a primary condition.

A. **History.** Typically the patient is middle-aged and presents with painful adduction and pain while lying on his or her shoulder. The dull pain is in the front of the shoulder, though it may radiate.

B. **Physical Examination.** Shoulder motion may be limited, particularly adduction and internal rotation. Pain may be elicited by forward elevation and internal rotation, adduction, or internal rotation.

C. **Studies.** Radiographs may reveal a long coracoid, calcification in the subscapularis or a space-occupying lesion posterior to the coracoid may be present. A subcoracoid injection of lidocaine that eliminates the pain will confirm the diagnosis. Computed tomography (CT) with the arm in adduction reveals that with coracoid impingement, the humeral-to-coracoid distance is reduced.

D. **Treatment.** A local injection with lidocaine and corticosteroid, posterior to coracoid, is the first step. Then the internal rotation test at 90 degrees of forward elevation is repeated. Failure to recover with just the injection should be treated with resection of the tip of the coracoid to shorten it by 1 cm. Care must be taken to reattach conjoined tendons.

V. Cuff Contusion

We have become more aware that a cuff contusion may occur and mimic the dysfunction of a full-thickness cuff tear.

A. **History.** These lesions have tended to occur in contact sports—such as football, rugby, or skiing—where a direct blow to the shoulder results in marked pain and limitation of motion. The patient will present with inability to elevate the arm beyond 50 to 60 degrees initially, with slow improvement generally over 2 to 3 months.

B. **Physical Examination.** Often patients will have a shrug sign and altered scapulothoracic motion. Their pain is proximal on the humeral head. Passive elevation will be to 150 degrees in some patients. Pain with passive abduction to 90 degrees and a positive impingement sign may be noted. On occasion there is significant swelling over the humeral head.

C. **Radiographic Studies.** Radiographs should be carefully evaluated for a small crack in the greater tuberosity, but often none is seen. An MRI will frequently show a bone bruise and/or crack in the tuberosity combined with an increased signal in the supraspinatus but no full-thickness tear.

D. **Treatment.** It should be explained to the patient that a cuff contusion may require 8 to 12 weeks to clear completely and that, on occasion, surgery is required to improve motion by removing scar tissue from the subacromial space. Subacromial decompression of soft tissue only may have a dramatic effect in improving active motion and relieving pain.

E. **Return to Sports.** This may require up to 2 to 3 months in cases treated nonoperatively. Surgical intervention may provide dramatic results with 6 weeks of postoperative rehabilitation, depending on the sport and the position played.

VI. Subscapularis Rupture

Rupture of the subscapularis tendon has become increasingly apparent with the more frequent use of the MRI. It has been identified as a cause of dislocation in patients over age 50.

A. **History.** Subscapularis rupture can occur when a high load is applied to the arm when it is at 90 degrees of elevation and 90 degrees of external rotation. Subsequently the patient may note pain and clicking particularly at the 90/90-degree position. If the disruption is complete, the biceps tendon will subluxate medially with a painful click. This may occur with external rotation at 90 degrees or on internal rotation of the arm. Partial loss of the subscapularis also occurs in association with supraspinatus failure and will add to the dysfunction.

B. **Physical Examination.** There may be ecchymosis anteriorly if the condition is acute. Weakness on resisted internal rotation and increased passive external rotation may be seen, as well as a positive lift-off test.

C. **X-rays.** These will generally be negative except in adolescents, where an avulsion of the lesser tuberosity may occur. In some patients this will calcify over time, leaving a long bony projection on the proximal humerus. MRI is diagnostic for tendon injury to the subscapularis.

D. **Treatment.** Surgery is generally the rule, particularly if the biceps tendon is subluxated medially (into the joint).

E. **Return to Sports.** This can be expected after 4 to 6 months.

VII. Biceps Tendon Injuries

There are four main categories of biceps injuries: (1) SLAP (superior labral anterior and posterior) injuries: (2) proximal biceps ruptures; (3) proximal biceps tendinitis; and (4) midhumeral muscle ruptures.

A. **SLAP Lesions**

These are lesions of the superior labrum that occur from the 10- to the 2-o'clock position on a right shoulder. They may involve the biceps anchor.

The labrum in this position is subject to considerable anatomic variability, making the classification difficult at times. The labrum at 12 o'clock may be meniscal or simply flat at its attachment site; the attachment may be recessed or on the edge of the glenoid. Additionally, there is a perforation anteriorly under the labrum at 2 o'clock in about 20% of shoulders. If a superior tear extends into this perforation, stability may be further compromised. SLAP lesions have been classified into four types: (1) labrum frayed at 10 to 2 o'clock; (2) labrum detached superiorly, including biceps anchor, (3) bucket-handle tear of labrum, biceps anchor intact; and (4) labrum and partial biceps displaced into the joint, and partially still attached anchor.

Patients with SLAP lesions may present acutely or with a chronic pain pattern, which is particularly seen in throwers. The injury may occur as a result of a direct blow with the arm at 90/90 degrees, resulting in compression and disruption of the labrum from 10 o'clock to 1 o'clock. In addition, repetitive throwing activities with internal rotation and the deceleration of the follow-through phase may lead to biceps avulsion and/or labral injury at 10 o'clock to 2 o'clock. Conversely, with the arm at 90 degrees of elevation and external rotation, internal impingement may occur, creating a similar injury in the posterior superior labrum and on the articular side of the supraspinatus.

1. **History.** The patient will complain of pain with activity. Often there is no complaint at rest. There may be a sense of repeated clicking associated with pain, particularly on elevation and internal rotation. Weakness overhead is frequently present. Looseness of the shoulder may be noted, but with no episodes of subluxation or dislocation.
2. **Physical Examination.** Often there is tenderness along the biceps proximally while there is full active and passive ROM. Stability testing may reveal a mild increase of anterior translation, though there is no apprehension. The adduction maneuver often produces pain deep in the joint, while the O'Brien maneuver is positive with internal rotation (pronation) of the arm. Speeds test (resisted elevation of arm with elbow at 0 degrees) may cause pain due to biceps irritability.
3. **Other Studies.** X-rays are usually negative. MRI may be useful, though it is not always diagnostic. If the MRI is well done, using proper software and selected views, the biceps anchor can readily be seen. This can be diagnostic of a SLAP lesion.
4. **Treatment.** Initially this consists of a period of observation combined with strengthening and stretching, which may be of value. Typically, however, pain will persist. A thrower will note loss of velocity and control, pain being associated particularly with the follow-through phase. ***Operative treatment*** consists of arthroscopic evaluation and treatment. Type I lesions may be debrided if necessary but are rarely symptomatic. Labral reattachment for type II, labral debridement for type III, and labral debridement and biceps reattachment for type IV are currently recommended. Reattachment procedures may be performed with a suture or implant technique.
5. **Return to Activity.** This will vary with the degree and type of SLAP lesion; it generally ranges 3 to 6 months.

B. **Biceps Tendinitis**

Lesions of the proximal biceps were felt to be quite common during the 1960s and 1970s. However, it was gradually realized that isolated lesions were uncommon but were frequently found in association with cuff disease as a component of the impingement syndrome.

1. **History.** Patients may note pain with activity, particularly with forward elevation of the arm and elbow flexion. Patients will also note pain at night and while stressing the biceps. They note that the pain is proximal along the bicipital groove.

2. **Physical Examination.** The impingement sign will generally be positive, but it is negative in an isolated lesion. Isolated biceps tendinitis may occur if there is an injury to the bicipital groove or a fracture of the lesser tuberosity. More commonly, biceps degeneration is seen with compression from the anterior acromion. There is tenderness along the bicipital groove, and, as noted above, the impingement sign may be present or absent. Speed's test—resisted elevation of the arm in adduction—is often positive, although it has low sensitivity. Yergason's sign—resisted elbow supination and flexion with the arm in adduction—may produce pain at the shoulder: however, its value is questionable.
3. **Treatment.** Local injection of lidocaine in the bicipital groove is of value for diagnostic purposes. Adding corticosteroids to the injection may also be of value in the management of this problem. NSAIDs and other measures as outlined for impingement syndrome are of benefit when the two entities coexist. ***Surgical intervention*** includes acromioplasty for combined processes, while isolated biceps tendinitis is treated with biceps tenodesis.
4. **Return to Sports.** This occurs when the athlete is pain-free, usually 4 to 6 weeks when there is no surgery and 3 to 6 months when there is surgical intervention.

C. **Biceps Instability**

Again, as noted earlier, biceps instability is most commonly associated with injury to the subscapularis tendon. It is not seen as an isolated injury. At times subscapularis injury is only partial, allowing the tendon to slip over the proximal aspect of the lesser tuberosity. It may also be seen with supraspinatus tears to the rotator interval if the subscapularis fails either partially or completely.

1. **History.** These patients note pain with passive external rotation or active internal rotation.
2. **Physical Examination.** This reveals weakness on internal rotation; the lift-off test is positive. Yergason's test will result in a snap of the proximal tendon with resisted elbow flexion, pronation, and shoulder external rotation.
3. **Studies.** Plain radiographs are of no benefit in diagnosing this problem, though MRI will reveal subscapularis tear or injury as well as showing the biceps position medial to the lesser tuberosity.
4. **Treatment.** In most patients, repair of the subscapularis with repositioning of the biceps is required. Often repair of the rotator interval and transverse ligament is also needed.

D. **Biceps Muscle Rupture**

This relatively rare injury has been described in the military, where an individual has parachuted out of a plane.

1. **History.** There is usually a history of direct injury or trauma, often as the biceps muscle is contracted—for example, when the straps to the parachute strike the midarm as the chute deploys, causing a complete or partial rupture of the muscle belly in one or both arms.
2. **Physical Examination.** This reveals marked swelling with pain and limited elbow flexion, especially weakness and limitation of resisted elbow flexion and increased pain with passive elbow extension.
3. **Treatment.** This includes aspiration of the hematoma, resting of the arm and elbow in a sling, and gradual resumption of activities over 6 weeks. Surgery has not routinely been required in these patients.
4. **Return to Sports.** This usually occurs by 6 weeks.

VIII. Pectoralis Major Injury

The pectoralis major is a major internal rotator and flexor of the humerus. It is highly active while heavy loads are applied to the shoulder, particularly in forward flexion and overhead positions. There are two heads to the muscle, sternal and clavicular; they insert on the humerus anterior to the biceps groove. Injury may occur at the bony insertion or along the muscle tendon junction or, rarely, it is restricted to the muscle belly itself.

A. **History.** Usually the patient is a young, muscular individual who felt a sharp pain or snap in the chest with forceful activity, such as weight lifting (bench press). The presenting complaints are usually weakness, pain, and/or deformity.

B. **Physical Examination.** Acute, marked swelling and tenderness along the site of injury are usual. Rupture of the inferior sternal component is easy to miss, and swelling may make the rupture less obvious, accounting for frequently missed diagnoses. There is often a defect that is accentuated by having the patient push both palms together at chest level—loss of the axillary fullness. There also is tenderness over the site of injury during isometric testing. In the chronic state, the defect is more obvious. There is a mild decrease in internal rotation strength, with more weakness noted on bench pressing. Acute injury will often result in ecchymosis in the axilla and anterior chest.

C. **Treatment.** The issue of the need to repair this large chest wall muscle will be dependent on the strength requirements and subjective impressions of the patient. Athletes who require heavy bench-press activities to maintain bulk and power for their sport are best managed operatively. Body builders will generally require repair for cosmetic and weight-lifting issues. Throwing athletes are also best served by an early repair. Some athletes may elect to avoid surgery if power is less of an issue.

On occasion, discomfort in the muscle belly may be a chronic complaint. If so, a late reconstruction can be performed. We have performed late repairs up to 5 years after injury.

Injuries restricted to the muscle belly may be treated nonoperatively, but a late reconstruction once scar tissue has formed might be considered subsequently.

IX. Miscellaneous

A. **Return to Sports.** Highly demanding activities, such as unlimited weight lifting, should be avoided for 6 months.

Other muscle tendon strains particularly to the latissimus dorsi, may occur about the shoulder in athletes. Injuries of these tendons should be carefully evaluated as to the degree of injury. If a complete disruption is suspected, an MRI is of value to note the site and ease of repair. Musculotendinous injuries about the shoulder require a careful evaluation based on sound anatomic principles and a through understanding of the forces applied in a particular sport. Early surgery, when indicated, is important, as is protection with a good rehabilitation program for lesser degrees of injury.

Suggested Reading

Blevins FT, Warren, RF, Cavo D, et al. Arthroscopic assisted rotator cuff repair: results using a mini-open deltoid splitting approach. *Arthroscopy* 12(1):50–59, 1996.

Blevins FT, Hayes WM, Warren RF. Rotator cuff in contact athletes. *Am J Sports Med* 24:263–267, 1996.

Pagnani MJ, Speer KP, Altchek DW, et al. Arthroscopic fixation of superior labral lesions using a biodegradable implant: a preliminary report. *Arthroscopy* 2:194–198, 1995.

Snyder SJ, Karzel RP, Del Pizzo W, et al. SLAP lesions of the shoulder. *Arthroscopy* 6:274–279, 1990.

Walch G, Boileau P, Noel E, et al. Impingement of the deep surface of the supraspinatus tendon on the posterosuperior glenoid rim: an arthroscopic study. *J Shoulder Elbow Surg* 1: 238–245, 1992.

Neer CN II. Impingement lesions. *Clin Orthop* 173:70–77, 1983.

40. THE SHOULDER—INSTABILITY AND MISCELLANEOUS

Jon J. P. Warner and Ronald A. Navarro

I. Instability

A. **Definitions.** Glenohumeral ***instability*** represents a spectrum of disorders from shoulder ***subluxation,*** which is the symptomatic translation of the humeral head relative to the glenoid articular surface, to shoulder ***dislocation,*** which is complete displacement out of the glenoid. As the shoulder joint is normally lax, clinical subluxation or dislocation requires excessive translation of the humeral head relative to the glenoid in association with symptoms. We classify shoulder instability based on its frequency, etiology, direction, and degree. Such a classification allows treatment to be tailored to the natural history in each case.

Instability can result from ***macrotrauma*** such as a unidirectional ***anterior*** dislocation occurring after a football player is tackled. Repetitive ***microtrauma*** from overhead activities—such as swimming, tennis, or throwing—can result in subtle degrees of subluxation, either *anterior* or ***posterior*** in direction. ***Atraumatic*** instability occurs without any known injury. Many of these individuals are preadolescents with ***voluntary*** instability. These individuals can be further classified into two subgroups. The first includes those who have voluntary instability that is *position-dependent.* Instability occurs in a posterior direction when the patient places the arm in a position of flexion, adduction, and internal rotation. These patients often respond to rehabilitation. The second group of patients have *muscle-dependent* voluntary instability, which results from *selectively contracting* muscles to create a dislocation or subluxation. Some of these individuals have an underlying psychiatric disturbances and tend to use their instability for secondary gain. They are best managed by psychiatric counseling and a therapy program. Many patients with ***involuntary*** posterior instability can demonstrate a positional type of instability as well.

B. **Anterior Instability**

1. **Anatomy.** A relative surface-area mismatch of the larger humeral head in the smaller glenoid predisposes this joint to instability. Stability is largely provided by static and dynamic soft tissue structures including the labrum, capsule (glenohumeral ligaments), and rotator cuff. Clinical conditions such as *glenoid fractures, glenoid dysplasia, and labral detachment* can lead to instability. The ***glenohumeral ligaments*** represent discrete thickenings in the capsule. There is a significant variation among individuals in the size of these ligaments, though in all individuals they elongate toward end ranges of rotation to prevent excessive rotation or translation. The capsule (and ligaments) are normally lax structures. In addition, the capsular injury to these structures that occurs with a shoulder dislocation can occur at their attachment site (Bankart lesion), along their length (rupture), or in combination. The ***glenoid labrum*** is the fibrocartilaginous thickening along the glenoid rim, which contributes to stability of the joint by functionally deepening the glenoid cavity and acting as an anchoring point for the glenohumeral ligaments and capsule. ***A Bankart lesion*** represents detachment of the anterior labrum from the glenoid due to subluxation or dislocation. This lesion has been implicated as the primary injury occurring with a traumatic dislocation. An associated impression fracture of the posterolateral margin of the humeral head (***Hill-Sachs lesion***) may be created when the head dislocates over the anterior glenoid rim.
2. **Types. Subcoracoid** dislocation is the most common form of dislocation. Medial dislocations are sometimes called ***subclavicular*** disloca-

tions and imply greater degrees of injury to the capsuloligamentous structures with an associated increased risk of brachial plexus injury. ***Intrathoracic*** dislocations fortunately are rare, and ***subglenoid*** and ***subacromial*** dislocations are described below.

Others have described two different categories of anterior instability: **t**raumatic **u**nilateral dislocation with a **B**ankart lesion which usually requires **s**urgery (**TUBS**) and **a**traumatic **m**ultidirectional **i**nstability that is **b**ilateral and responds to **r**ehabilitation, rarely requiring an **i**nferior capsular shift (**AMBRI**). Although this distinction may be helpful, in practice there is usually a degree of overlap between labral injury *and* capsular injury, which are associated with instability.

3. **Etiology.** Traumatic anterior instability is most commonly associated with forceful trauma to an abducted and externally rotated arm (macrotrauma). Anterior instability due to atraumatic etiologies is rare, though congenital and neuromuscular causes have been reported. Atraumatic instability is usually multidirectional.
4. **Incidence.** Traditionally, 95% of all instability is anterior in direction and is the result of a single trauma. More recently, experience has suggested combination with inferior instability to be common also.
5. **History.** Age and chief complaint are important factors. Instability is more common in younger individuals and younger age is associated with a higher recurrence rate. Furthermore, young patients who have recurrent subluxation may complain only of pain and have no sense of instability. A frequent complaint is that the arm "goes dead" when the patient is trying to throw a ball or place the arm overhead.
6. **Physical examination.** With dislocation, an anterior and axillary fullness is present with a prominent acromion posteriorly. Atrophy may indicate nerve injury (i.e., axillary) or concomitant rotator cuff tear. The sensory and motor exam should document function of the axillary nerve. Rotator cuff tears present with limitation of active range of motion but preservation of passive range. A positive apprehension test and a positive relocation test increase the sensitivity of the examination, although these are not specific tests (see Appendix 6). Generalized ligamentous laxity should be documented if present. Impingement signs should alert the examiner to possible concomitant rotator cuff pathology. Glenohumeral translation testing provides information about laxity but not necessarily instability of the joint (see Appendix 6). This is best performed under anesthesia with the arm in varying degrees of abduction. The amount of translation is graded on the basis of final position of humeral head with respect to the glenoid. The term *trace translation* refers to a small amount of humeral head translation. Grade I translation is seen when the humeral head rides up the glenoid slope but not over the rim. Grade II describes a humeral head that rides up and over the glenoid rim but reduces when stress removed. Grade III translation occurs when the humeral head rides up and over the glenoid rim and remains dislocated on removal of stress. In general, anterior translation of grade III is consistent with instability.
7. **Diagnostic tests.** ***Standard radiographs*** help locate the humeral head with respect to the glenoid in orthogonal planes.
   a. **True anteroposterior (AP) view of the glenohumeral joint.** Obtained by angling the x-ray beam 45 degrees lateral to the plane of the thorax. This allows the glenohumeral joint to be seen in true profile, without any overlap of the humeral head on the glenoid. If the arm is also in internal rotation, a Hill-Sachs lesion may be detected.
   b. **Axillary lateral.** This view will determine if there is any static subluxation of the head out of the glenoid and will allow detection of a bony Bankart lesion (glenoid fracture). If the arm cannot be abducted, one can obtain a Velpeau axillary view.

c. **Transscapular Y view.** This view is a true lateral of the scapula. If an axillary view cannot be obtained, this will permit assessment of the humeral head position.

8. **Special tests**
   a. **Radiographs**
      i. **West Point view.** A modified lateral view to evaluate the anteroinferior glenoid rim for the presence of a fracture or bony Bankart lesion.
      ii. **Stryker notch view.** This makes it easier to assess for the presence of a Hill-Sachs lesion.
   b. **Magnetic Resonance Imaging (MRI).** Recent advances have improved the diagnostic sensitivity and specificity of this test. It allows for detection of Bankart lesions and can help to suggest capsular injury. Arthrography in association with MRI may add more information.
   c. **Computed tomography (CT) arthrogram.** CT after an arthrogram allows for detection of a Bankart lesion (labral avulsion). Arm internal and external rotation followed by cuts that reveal the continued presence of dye where the capsule should be tight indicates capsular laxity.
   d. **Subacromial injection.** As with all shoulder pathology, examination findings of impingement should be addressed. If a subacromial injection of 1% lidocaine relieves symptoms, concomitant impingement syndrome may be present. This can have effects on the treatment plan chosen.
9. **Natural history.** The single most important factor for predicting the likelihood of recurrence is the age of the individual at the time of the initial dislocation. The recurrence rate may be higher than 80% in athletes under the age of 20 and decreases significantly in those sustaining a dislocation in their fourth or fifth decade of life. The reason for this high recurrence rate in younger individuals is the propensity for the development of a Bankart lesion with a traumatic anterior dislocation. The incidence of this lesion approaches 70% to 80% and is associated with a high failure rate of conservative management. Older persons (thirties to fifties) appear to develop a stiff shoulder if immobilized and also appear to have adequate spontaneous healing of injured capsuloligamentous structures, which results in a much lower recurrence rate.
10. **Prevention.** Avoidance of the offending position is the best preventive measure. Avoidance of traumatic mechanisms also helps to prevent anterior instability. Rotator cuff strengthening also may be utilized in the patient who may be at higher risk for instability (ligamentous laxity, higher-risk sporting events).
11. **Treatment options**
    a. **Initial treatment.** Early treatment includes reduction of the dislocation, usually with some variation of the traction-countertraction technique. An acute dislocation can often be reduced on the playing field. Most successful reductions take place in a controlled environment, with adequate sedation. Results of postreduction radiographs and neurovascular examination should be carefully documented. In older patients, it is important to evaluate the rotator cuff to make sure that it is not torn.
    b. **Nonoperative treatment.** A conservative approach is most appropriate after a first episode of traumatic anterior dislocation. Most surgeons favor a 2- to 6-week period of immobilization, depending on the patient's age (longer for younger patients). This is followed by a period of intense rehabilitation including rotator cuff and scapular stabilizer, strengthening, emphasizing the internal rotators.
    c. **Surgical treatment.** In most cases this approach is reserved for individuals with recurrent instability despite a conservative pro-

gram. This begins with an ***examination under anesthesia*** to confirm both the degree and direction of a patient's instability as compared with contralateral shoulder translation on drawer testing. Then ***diagnostic arthroscopy*** is performed to define pathology, including a Bankart lesion, capsular tear, Hill-Sachs lesion, SLAP lesion, rotator cuff tear, and articular injury. Appreciation of these individual components of pathology help to decide on the form of operative repair best suited to each individual case. The current treatment options are arthroscopic Bankart repair or open capsulorrhaphy.

i. **Arthroscopic treatment.** The most common repair techniques use either suture fixation or absorbable tac fixation to repair the Bankart lesion. The advantages of these techniques are less surgical morbidity, less operative time, less postoperative pain, and less loss of motion. Unfortunately, growing experience with these approaches continues to achieve a success rate inferior to that with open repairs. Currently the overall recurrence rate is about twice that seen with open repairs.

ii. **Open bankart repair plus/minus capsular shift.** This procedure remains the standard against which all arthroscopic procedures compared. These approaches all repair a Bankart lesion through drill holes or suture anchors. They also permit capsular tightening to treat associated capsular laxity or injury. Overall, the failure rate in the treatment of traumatic anterior instability is less than 5%.

12. **Return to play**

a. **After closed reduction.** After immobilization, a rehabilitation program is begun that consists of active assisted range-of-motion exercises and strengthening of the rotator cuff as well as periscapular muscles (serratus anterior, rhomboids and trapezius). At 3 months, isokinetic strengthening is begun. When full motion is obtained as well as strength equivalent to the uninjured side, a sports-specific activity rehabilitation program is begun. Return to forceful overhead motions is permitted at 5 to 6 months. Occasionally, a commercially available brace may be used to restrict abduction and external rotation in athletes engaged in contact sports.

b. **After surgery.** The arm is maintained in a sling and swath for 1 to 4 weeks. Therapy is begun after the sling is removed. Usually at 4 months, the patient is permitted to swim and begin tossing a ball or hitting ground strokes in tennis. At 6 months after surgery, the patient is permitted to begin throwing with more force. Contact sports are usually allowed after 6 to 8 months, depending on progress with physical therapy.

C. **Posterior instability**

1. **Anatomy.** The ***posterior capsule*** is the thinnest portion of the shoulder capsule. ***Bankart lesions*** can be seen in association with posterior instability. The ***reverse Hill-Sachs lesion*** is an impression fracture of the anterolateral margin of the humeral head that is created when the head dislocates over the posterior glenoid rim. In most cases the major pathology is capsular laxity.

2. **Types.** ***Subacromial*** dislocations are those which are posterior and inferior to the acromion.

3. **Etiology.** Most athletes with posterior instability will have posterior and inferior subluxation from repetitive microtrauma to the joint capsule. Sports often associated with this type of instability are those that require repetitive arm motions overhead or in front of the body. These include swimming, football, volleyball, and softball. A greater percentage of posterior instability is attributable to atraumatic causes.

4. **Incidence.** Acute traumatic posterior dislocation is felt to represent only 4% of all shoulder dislocations; however, this is a commonly missed condition in the emergency department setting.
5. **History.** Repetitive overhead activities can lead to microtrauma and eventual posterior instability, often evidenced only as vague complaints of pain. Offensive football linemen develop traumatic posterior subluxation due to blocking maneuvers in which the arm is axially loaded in adduction and internal rotation. The diagnosis is initially missed in 50% to 80% of the cases. Epilepsy or a known electrical shock should create suspicion of a posterior dislocation. Voluntary instability and associated psychological disturbance must always be ruled out in patients with posterior instability.
6. **Physical examination.** The hallmark of chronic, fixed posterior dislocation is a limitation of external rotation as compared with the contralateral extremity. The patient typically holds the arm internally rotated. There is flattening of the anterior aspect of the shoulder, with prominence and rounding of the posterior aspect of the shoulder. There can also be evidence of anterior prominence of the coracoid. Patients with more subtle posterior subluxation will often have posterior glenohumeral joint line tenderness and crepitation. The ***posterior apprehension test*** can help confirm the diagnosis (Appendix 6). ***Fukuda's jerk test*** slowly moves the seated patient's subluxated/dislocated shoulder from forward flexion to extension, while maintaining 90-degree abduction, and reduces it over the posterior glenoid rim with an audible and palpable shifting.
7. **Diagnostic tests**
   a. **Anteroposterior (AP) Shoulder.** When the humeral head is normally superimposed on the glenoid, a smooth, bordered ellipse is made. Distortion of this *elliptical overlap shadow* can indicate the presence of a posterior dislocation. Also with posterior dislocations, the glenoid may appear to be *vacant.* A *positive rim sign* is present if the distance between the humeral head and the anterior glenoid rim is greater than 6 mm. Also, if the head is internally rotated, it has the profile of a light bulb.
   b. **Axillary lateral.** Flexion of the arm may allow for posterior translation to be detected. The center of the humeral head should line up with the true center of the glenoid on this view. If it is posterior on this view, instability is detected.
8. **Special tests.** See above.
9. **Natural history.** Because of the relative rarity of this entity, the true natural history is not clear. Recurrence has been seen to be far less frequent in traumatic posterior dislocation than in traumatic anterior dislocation. An increased recurrence rate has been noted in younger patients, in cases with an atraumatic etiology, and when a large bony defect is noted in either the glenoid or the humeral head.
10. **Prevention.** Modifications in throwing, including emphasizing the lower extremity during follow-through, can be helpful.
11. **Treatment options**
    a. **Initial treatment.** The treatment of acute posterior dislocation begins with attempts at closed reduction. It must be noted that attempts at closed reduction of an acute dislocation with a large reverse Hill-Sachs lesion or a chronic locked dislocation carry a significant risk of humeral head fracture. After suitable sedation, the patient is positioned supine. Lateral traction is applied to the arm and gentle internal rotation is used to unlock any impaction fracture of the humeral head that may exist. Excessive external rotation is to be avoided as it may lead to displacement of a head fragment. Posterior head pressure followed by longitudinal traction on the

adducted arm generally positions the arm to allow for relocation after a final external rotation maneuver. Failure to reduce the joint indicates need for a surgical open reduction with complete muscle paralysis.

b. **Nonoperative treatment.** In cases of subluxation, a conservative approach is employed initially, emphasizing strengthening of the external rotators and posterior deltoid.

c. **Surgical treatment.** Posterior capsular stabilization is indicated in patients who have failed nonoperative management and have recurrent traumatic posterior instability or in individuals with an irreducible dislocation. Recent experience has been good in terms of return to work following surgery. In cases of recurrent posterior subluxation or dislocation, an open capsular shift and Bankart repair are performed. In cases of a locked dislocation, an anterior approach allows reduction and the subscapularis is transferred into the reverse Hill-Sachs lesion.

12. **Return to play.** Postoperative management consists of 6 weeks of immobilization. Active assisted range-of-motion exercise is then begun and strengthening is initiated at 12 weeks. As with anterior procedure, competitive throwing and contact sports are usually delayed from 6 to 9 months.

D. **Inferior and multidirectional instability (MDI).** MDI encompasses a spectrum of atraumatic, microtraumatic, and macrotraumatic types of injuries. The diagnosis of MDI is especially important to make because the traditional approaches to management of instability, *both* by conservative and surgical measures, are likely to fail. The hallmark of this clinical condition is a component of symptomatic inferior instability in addition to anterior and/or posterior instability.

1. **Anatomy.** MDI is characterized by stretching of the static shoulder stabilizers. This may be due to congenital laxity or acquired laxity from repetitive microtrauma. In the atraumatic type, a large inferior capsular pouch exists without anterior labral detachment. In the traumatic type of MDI, a Bankart lesion may exist in addition to a capacious pouch. Recently, the superior structures of the glenohumeral joint (biceps tendon, superior capsule, rotator interval, and supraspinatus muscle) have received attention with regard to etiology in MDI.

2. **Types.** A ***subglenoid*** dislocation is significant in that the degree of displacement implies a significant injury to the glenohumeral ligaments in multiple planes. ***Luxatio erecta*** is a specific type of inferior dislocation that occurs with the arm overhead. In this position, the head slips inferior to the glenoid and can become locked there. MDI instability has been classified into types according to directions of major instability. ***Type I*** patients have global instability with anterior, posterior, and inferior instability. ***Type II*** instability is anterior and inferior, while ***type III*** is posterior and inferior. ***Type IV*** patients have only anterior and posterior instability, with no significant inferior component.

3. **Etiology.** The vast majority of patients fall into groups of atraumatic and microtraumatic etiology. Consideration must be given to Ehler's-Danlos and Marfan's syndromes in patients with hyperextensibility of the joints.

4. **Incidence.** MDI is seen in approximately 1% of all types of instability.

5. **History.** The patients often present with bilateral complaints. Most patients with this diagnosis will not present reporting a sense of instability but rather will have pain whenever they use the arm overhead or especially when carrying heavy loads with the arm at the side. Issues relating to the possible presence of ligamentous laxity should be probed.

6. **Physical examination.** Diagnosis is made by demonstrating excessive laxity, which is symptomatic in at least two planes. Inferior laxity should be present. Inferior laxity is assessed using the ***sulcus sign*** (see

Appendix 6). The degree of inferior laxity is assessed by measuring the distance between the inferior border of the lateral acromion and the superior aspect of the humeral head. Translation of less than 1 cm represents a 1+ sulcus, 1 to 2 cm indicates a 2+ sulcus, and greater than 2 cm represents a 3+ sulcus. A 3 + sulcus sign is diagnostic of inferior instability. Approximately 50% of individuals will have clinical signs of generalized ligamentous laxity, including the ability to oppose the thumb to the forearm, parallelism of dorsiflexed phalanges with the radius and ulna, elbow hyperextension beyond 10 degrees, knee hyperextension beyond 10 degrees and the ability to touch the palms of the hands to the floor with the knees kept straight. Impingement findings can be seen in 20% of patients with MDI and represent secondary irritation of the rotator cuff.

7. **Diagnostic tests and special tests.** As above.
8. **Natural history.** In the absence of intervention, MDI will continue to be symptomatic.
9. **Prevention.** As in other types of instability, the affected patient can avoid the arm position that lead to pain. Individuals who have generalized laxity may undergo preventative strengthening of the shoulder if they are participating in sports that risk overuse.
10. **Treatment.** This begins initially with a prolonged trial (6 months to 1 year) of therapy. In the atraumatic case, up to 70% of these patients may respond to a rehabilitation program of rotator cuff and axioscapular muscle strengthening. However, those individuals with a posttraumatic or microtraumatic etiology of their MDI, especially if they continue to participate in sports requiring repetitive overhead motions, will not be likely to respond to conservative treatment. Rehabilitation focuses on the strengthening and improvement in endurance of the dynamic stabilizers and the periscapular musculature. Isokinetic muscle testing may be useful and proprioception training can also be helpful. ***Surgical*** repair of this problem should be considered only for patients who are disabled by their instability and who have failed an intensive therapy program. Currently, arthroscopic repair techniques are experimental. In cases where surgery is required, the approach is some form of capsular shift that reduces the capsular laxity in an inferior as well as anterior or posterior direction. Postoperative immobilization is much longer (about 6 weeks) than with unidirectional instability procedures because capsular healing must be more extensive to prevent recurrence.
11. **Return to play.** The shoulder is immobilized in a sling and swath for 6 weeks. Following immobilization, active assisted range-of-motion exercise is begun, followed by strengthening. The goal of postoperative treatment is to gradually regain motion while strengthening the shoulder. Recovery of motion often takes 6 months to 1 year in these patients.

II. Uncommon Causes

A. **Snapping scapula.** This term refers to an auditory and palpable phenomenon about the symptomatic scapulothoracic (ST) articulation.

1. **Types.** Two broad categories have been proposed: (1) changes in the congruence of the anterior scapular surface and the underlying chest wall and (2) changes in the interposed soft tissues, muscles, or bursae between the scapula and the chest wall.
2. **Etiology.** This entity can be due to inflammation of the ST bursa or due to a bony incongruity. In rare cases an individual may have a scapular osteochondroma, which “washboards” over the chest wall with shoulder motion.
3. **History.** Some athletes may present with pain and sometimes a “grinding” sensation that may be audible over the ST articulation. They have pain in this region, and onset may or may not be after a specific trauma. Some patients can reproduce this voluntarily.

4. **Physical examination.** There is audible or palpable grinding over the scapula with shoulder motion and periscapular tenderness just medial to the scapular margin.
5. **Diagnostic tests.** A transcapular Y view may reveal an exostosis at the inferior angle or spurring at the superior angle as well as an osteochondroma if present.
6. **Special tests.** Alleviation of the pain with local injection of 1% lidocaine into the ST bursa, can be diagnostic. A CT can also reveal any osseous lesion present.
7. **Treatment.** Avoidance of the motions that increase discomfort coupled with axioscapular muscle strengthening, including shoulder shrugs with weight and push-ups, may alleviate symptoms. Rarely, infiltration with local steroid preparations has been helpful. Occasionally, resection of the ST bursa, with or without resection of a prominent superior medial corner of the scapula, may be indicated.
8. **Return to play.** Maintenance of full elbow, glenohumeral, and ST range of motion should be a part of the early posteporative regimen. Periscapular stabilization exercises should continue. At 6 weeks postoperatively, the athlete can begin gentle tossing. Return to sports participation can then proceed as tolerated.

B. **Effort thrombosis**

1. **Anatomy.** Compression of the axillary vein can occur between the first rib and the clavicle, the subclavian muscles, or the costocoracoid ligament.
2. **Definition.** This condition is called *effort thrombosis* because of its frequent association with repetitive vigorous activity or blunt trauma with direct or indirect injury to the axillary vein.
3. **Etiology.** Compression in the costoclavicular space can occur with hyperextension of the neck or hyperabduction of the arms. Risk factors for development of deep venous thrombosis include stasis, intrinsic mechanical pathology, or a hypercoagulable state (Virchow's triad). Hypercoagulability is most commonly seen in female athletes taking oral contraceptives and in dehydrated athletes, such as wrestlers, who use several different methods to lose water weight before matches. Athletes who use their arms in an overhead position are predisposed to effort thrombosis syndrome. The overhead position stretches the subclavian vein and may result in tears of the intima of the vein.
4. **History.** Symptoms include activity related-fatigue; numbness and heaviness of the involved upper extremity; dull, aching pain; and swelling. Symptom onset is usually within the first 24 hr following the inciting activity. The symptoms that are usually present immediately following activity often subside after a period of rest.
5. **Physical examination.** The superficial veins may be dilated, the arm may appear to be cyanotic, and there may be tenderness to palpation in the axilla or deltopectoral groove.
6. **Diagnostic test.** If the symptoms are suggestive of venous obstruction but physical examination is equivocal, exercise testing may be beneficial at provoking the thrombotic state.
7. **Special tests.** A venogram will show total occlusion of the axillary or subclavian vein and marked venous collateral return.
8. **Treatment options**
   a. **Conservative.** Initial treatment consists of rest, heat, and elevation of the involved arm. Pain and swelling usually revolve in 3 to 4 days although 80% to 85% of conservatively treated patients may experience residual symptoms because of continued occlusion of the vein with inadequate collateral flow.
   b. **Anticoagulation.** Another option is anticoagulation with heparin followed by warfarin in the acute phase to prevent progression of the thrombus. However, 50% of the patents continued to have symptoms with this treatment.

   c. **Thrombolysis.** Recently, thrombolytic agents such as streptokinase, urokinase, and tissue-plasminogen activator (TPA) have been used for lysis of intravenous clots, although they are much more effective with acute clots than chronic clots. TPA has been shown to be more effective and is more specific for clots with less systemic bleeding complications than the other options.
9. **Return to play.** Little has been written regarding return to athletic activity following treatment, and this is not predictable based on the existing literature. Early motion with avoidance of provocative positions is advisable in the first month after therapy has provided an effect. In later months, return to overhead activities can proceed as long as the athlete remains assymptomatic.

C. **Deltoid disruption**

1. **Etiology.** Strains and contusions can occur after a direct blow to the upper arm when it is in a position of abduction or forward elevation. In throwing sports, the anterior deltoid can be injured during acceleration and the posterior deltoid can be injured during deceleration. Acromioclavicular (AC) dislocations can lead to deltoid injury in the setting of a distal clavicle rupture through the deltotrapezius fascia (grade V AC dislocation). Inadequate reattachment of the deltoid following shoulder surgery can lead to this entity as well.
2. **Incidence.** Strains are relatively common. Traumatic disruption is a rare clinical entity. Iatrogenic cases are uncommon after routine procedures.
3. **History.** The athlete will complain of pain, swelling, and weakness in the area of the deltoid. If a true disruption has occurred, he or she may complain of a defect in the normal contour of the deltoid musculature.
4. **Physical examination.** Ecchymosis and local tenderness may be present in the setting of a contusion. Motion is limited and weakness secondary to pain may occur. After a complete rupture, the signs and symptoms noted above will be heightened and loss of normal contour with a palpable defect will often he seen. In the setting of multitrauma, more life-threatening injuries may direct attention away from this diagnosis until late retraction of the tissues had taken place. If iatrogenic detachment has occurred, a palpable defect can be appreciated. This too can be masked by local swelling.
5. **Treatment.** Strains and contusions require early ice and immobilization until less tender. After 6 to 10 days, mobilization, stretching, and strengthening gradually occur. Any true deltoid avulsion from its bony anchor, either from trauma or after surgery, requires surgical repair. Delays in diagnosis create reconstructive difficulties owing to severe scarring and atrophied tissues. Distal retraction of the deltoid can be a difficult problem to reconstruct. Tendon to bone reconstruction is recommended. Midsubstance injuries are often difficult to repair and require protection in an abduction brace.
6. **Return to play.** Contusions and strains usually heal uneventfully with complete return to activities in 2 to 4 weeks depending on the severity of the injury. The prognosis for deltoid disruptions is guarded. If the reconstruction is successful and no defect is seen residually, the athlete's function must be assessed. Often the loss of strength can significantly impair an athlete is performance to the degree that prior levels cannot be met.

D. **Stress fractures.** These are less common in the upper extremity, although numerous case reports have described proximal humeral, coracoid, and acromial infractions after repeated loading. The etiology is the same as for all stress fractures: repetitive microtraumatic overload.

1. **History and physical examination.** The athlete has pain with activity; without treatment and continued use, he or she may have constant pain. Examination reveals point tenderness and occasionally swelling and erythema.

2. **Diagnostic tests.** Plain radiographs are usually unremarkable.
3. **Special tests.** Bone scans can localize the stress fracture and CT or MRI can confirm the diagnosis.
4. **Treatment.** This consists of rest and avoidance of offending activities, with a majority healing in within 6 to 8 weeks. In rare cases of nonhealing, the fracture may require open reduction and internal fixation (ORIF) with bone grafting.
5. **Return to athletic activity.** This should be gradual, with full competition only after the athlete is symptom-free and without any motor weakness.

Suggested Reading

Allen AA, Warner JJP. Shoulder instability in the athlete. *Orthop Clin North Am* 1995; 26:487.

Bigliani LU, Pollock RG, McIlveen SJ, et al. Shift of the posteroinferior aspect of the capsule for recurrent posterior glenohumeral instability. *J Bone Joint Surg* 1995; 77A:1011.

Schulte KR, Warner JJP. Uncommon causes of shoulder pain in the athlete. *Orthop Clin North Am* 1995; 26:505.

Warner JJP, Caborn D N. Overview of shoulder instability. *Crit. Rev Phys Rehab Med* 1992; 4:145–198.

Warner JJP. Shoulder In: In Miller MD, Cooper DE, Warner, JJP, eds. *Review of sports medicine and arthroscopy.* Philadelphia, W.B. Saunders, 1995:113–164.

41. THE CLAVICLE

William N. Levine, Evan L. Flatow, and Louis U. Bigliani

The clavicle is the upper extremity's only bony articulation to the appendicular skeleton. As such, it is important in sports activities, and injuries to the clavicle and its two articulations are commonly seen in athletes. Most injuries are acute traumatic injuries to the clavicle and the acromioclavicular (AC) and sternoclavicular joints, while the AC joint is also susceptible to overuse injury (osteolysis).

I. Fractures of the Clavicle

are very common injuries that affect athletes as well as the general population. Such a fracture may occur following a fall onto an outstretched hand or the tip of the shoulder. However, trauma, such as occurs in contact sports, is a more common cause in adult patients. The incidence of clavicular fractures has been estimated to be 5 % of fractures; however, they are the most common fracture of childhood. They account for nearly half of all injuries to the shoulder girdle. The most common fracture of the clavicle (80%) in adults and children occurs in the middle third of the bone.

Fractures of the distal third of the clavicle account for 12% to 15% of clavicular fractures. These fractures are classified based on the integrity of the coracoclavicular ligaments and the status of the acromioclavicular joint (Fig. 41-1). Type I distal clavicular ('interligamentous') fractures have a portion of the conoid ligament attached to the medial fragment. Since the coracoclavicular ligaments effectively span the fracture, the lesion is stable and heals readily. In type II distal clavicular fractures, the conoid ligament is ruptured (or occasionally avulsed with a fragment of bone) from the medial shaft, which allows the arm and distal fragment to displace inferiorly. In a type III distal clavicular fracture, the fracture involves the articular surface of the distal clavicle, so that posttraumatic osteolysis or arthritis may occur.

Fractures involving the inner third of the clavicle are the least common type, accounting for 5% to 6% of all clavicular fractures. Since the costoclavicular ligaments usually remain intact, there is rarely any significant displacement.

A. **History.** Athletes will complain of pain and deformity at the clavicle or shoulder following a fall on the outstretched hand or direct trauma in contact sports.

B. **Physical examination.** Deformity at the level of the clavicle or AC joint may be noted. Skin tenting may warrant an immediate attempt at closed reduction. The clavicle's close proximity to the subclavian artery, as well as the brachial plexus, make it imperative to rule out injuries to these structures. Careful evaluation of pulses on the affected extremity may reveal discrepancies that could signify a vascular injury. The lungs must be examined for the presence of symmetric breath sounds to rule out pneumothorax.

C. **Diagnostic tests.** Clavicular shaft fractures are best evaluated with a standard anteroposterior (AP) view that often shows the proximal fragment to be displaced upward and the distal fragment downward. The 45-degree cephalic-tilt view more accurately assesses the anteroposterior relationship of the proximal and distal fragments. For distal-third fractures, anterior and posterior 45-degree oblique views should be obtained in addition to a standard AP view.

D. **Special tests.** In rare instances, computed tomography may be necessary to further delineate the extent of the injury and assess intraarticular extension.

E. **Natural history.** Clavicular shaft fractures heal completely with normal return of function in more than 95% of patients. The reported incidence of nonunion is 0.9% to 4.0%. Type II distal clavicular fractures, however, have a reported incidence of nonunion of 30%. Patients should be warned that the

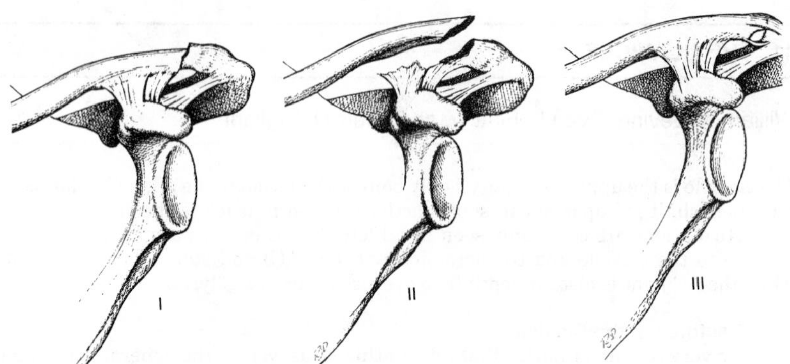

Fig. 41-1. Neer's classification of distal clavicle fractures: Type I—Minimal displacement with intact ligaments. Type II—Displaced with detachment of the ligaments from the medial fragment. Type III–Articular surface fracture.

bump may remain and that clothes may fit imperfectly, since the "width" of the shoulder (from the sternum to the shoulder joint) may be diminished on the affected side. In extremely rare cases, especially when an intercalary fragment is rotated down, compression of the underlying nerves or vessels may occur.

F. **Treatment.** Apply a sling and swathe for acute fractures of the clavicular shaft. Figure of eight splints can also be used but are associated with complications. This is maintained until the athlete is comfortable and has painless range of motion of the extremity. This will usually be in 2 to 4 weeks. It is rare that a fracture of the clavicular shaft requires surgery. Nondisplaced distal clavicular fractures can be treated in the same fashion. Type II distal clavicular fractures with wide displacement and instability are treated with open reduction and internal fixation. If the distal fragment is small or osteoporotic or the fracture involves the acromioclavicular joint, the distal fragment is resected primarily and the coracoacromial ligament is transfered to the medial fragment with supplemental subcoracoid fixation using heavy suture. Proximal-third clavicular fractures are quite rare and usually require only symptomatic treatment with a sling and swathe.

G. **Return to sport.** The athlete should not return to noncontact sports until the fracture has healed, range of motion is painless and full, and strength is near normal. This routinely will take at least 6 weeks from the time of the injury. More conservative treatment is required for athletes involved in contact sports. There is a propensity for refracture at the healed site, therefore 4 to 6 months are usually required before return to collision athletics is allowed.

II. Injuries of the acromioclavicular (AC) joint

account for a high percentage of injuries to the shoulder girdle and AC separations are, after glenohumeral instability, the second most common type of shoulder instability. These injuries are much more common in males and contact athletes. Most injuries of the AC joint result from a fall with an adducted arm, striking the shoulder against the ground. Much less commonly, a fall onto an outstretched hand can cause a less severe injury of the AC joint with preservation of the coracoclavicular ligament.

Classification of these injuries is based on the degree of distal clavicular displacement, the integrity of the acromioclavicular and coracoclavicular ligaments, and the integrity of the fascia overlying the deltoid and trapezial musculature. Six types of injury have been noted by Rockwood (Fig. 41-2). Type

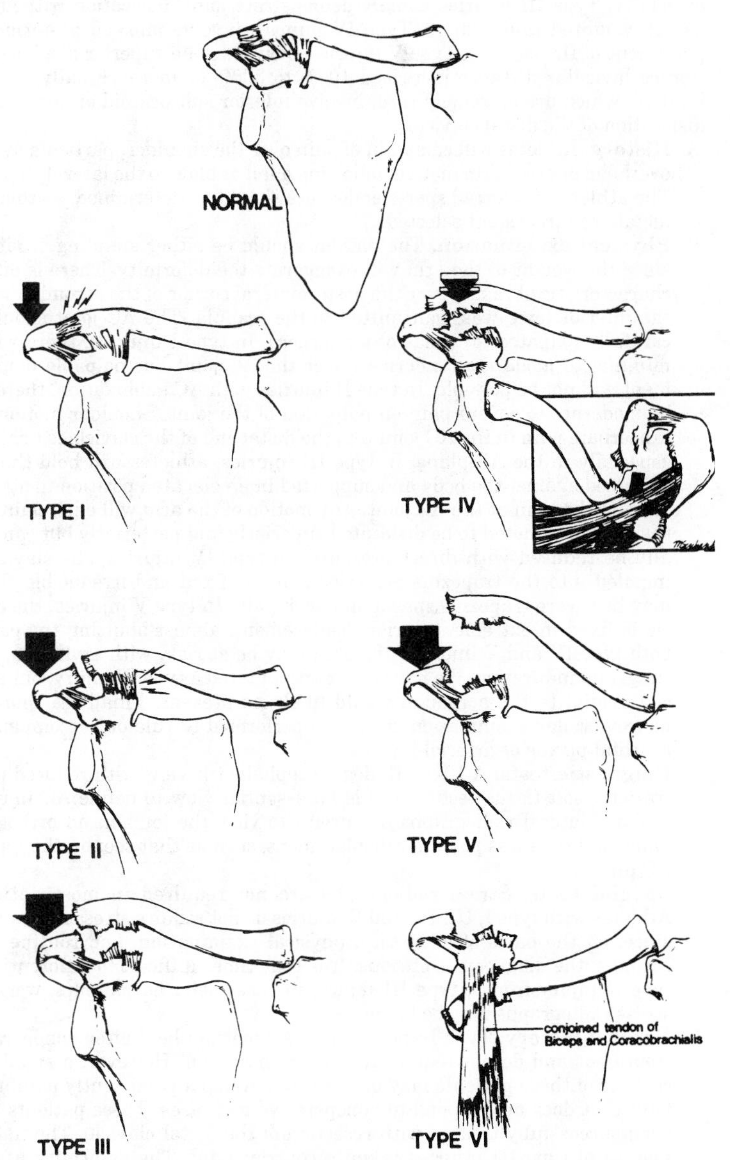

Fig. 41-2. Rockwood classification of AC separation: Type I—Normal radiograph. Type II—AC ligaments disrupted, CC ligaments intact. Type III—AC and CC ligaments disrupted. Type IV—Type III with severe posterior displacement of clavicle. Type V—Type III with deltotrapezial disruption and 100% to 300% superior displacement of the clavicle. Type VI—Type III with subcoracoid displacement of clavicle.

I injuries have normal radiographs despite a tender AC joint. Type II injuries will show widening of the acromioclavicular joint as compared with the opposite extremity. Type III injuries usually demonstrate joint dislocation without the use of weighted radiographs. Type IV injuries involve marked posterior displacement of the clavicle. Type V injuries show extreme superior displacement (coracoclavicular distance increased 100% to 300% or more). Finally, type VI injuries, which are extremely rare, involve inferior subcoracoid or subacromial dislocation of the distal clavicle.

A. **History.** Athletes will complain of pain over the shoulder, particularly with overhead or cross arm motion, following a fall or blow to the lateral shoulder. The athlete's preferred sports endeavors should be determined, as this may dictate the treatment selected.
B. **Physical examination.** The patient should be either standing or sitting, since the weight of the arm will exaggerate the deformity. There is often a characteristic abrasion over the posterolateral corner of the acromion where the inferior force was transmitted to the scapula. The AC joint should be carefully palpated for areas of tenderness. In type I injuries, there will be minimal to moderate tenderness over the AC joint but palpable displacement will not be possible. In type II injuries with AC subluxation, there will be moderate to severe pain on palpation of the joint. Shoulder motion will exacerbate pain in the AC joint and the distal end of the clavicle is unstable, especially in the AP plane. In type III injuries, athletes will hold the arm adducted against the body and supported in an elevated position to attempt relief of the pain at the AC joint. Any motion of the arm will elicit pain, and the clavicle is noted to be dislocated superiorly and posteriorly but can usually be reduced with direct pressure. In type IV injuries, the clavicle is impaled into the trapezius posteriorly and is fixed and irreducible. There may be severe trapezius spasm and neck pain. In type V injuries, the clavicle is fixed in extreme superior displacement, almost abutting the ear. In both type IV and V injuries, the skin may be at risk, with erythema, mottling, and induration. We have never encountered a type VI injury, but a sulcus medial to the acromion would likely be present. Finally, a thorough neurovascular examination should be performed to rule out accompanying brachial plexus or arterial injuries.
C. **Diagnostic tests.** A 10- to 15-degree cephalic tilt view with reduced penetration ("soft tissue technique") is an essential view to define AC injuries. Axillary lateral radiographs are useful to view the joint in an orthogonal plane and to assess posterior displacement, such as that seen in the type IV AC injury.
D. **Special tests.** Stress radiographs are not required in most patients. Athletes with type I, III, IV, and V injuries do not require stress radiographs since, on the basis of of history, physical examination, and routine radiographs, the diagnosis is obvious. It is sometimes difficult to differentiate a type II injury from a type III injury, in these selected patients, weighted stress radiographs may be helpful.
E. **Natural history.** Type I and II injuries generally heal after nonoperative treatment and do not require further intervention. However, a small percentage of these patients may progress to develop a persistently painful AC joint that does not respond to nonoperative measures. These patients have been successfully treated with resection of the distal clavicle. The natural history of type III injuries is quite controversial. The deformity usually remains, but in many patients the pain gradually resolves and a full return of function is achieved. However, some patients, especially overhead athletes and heavy laborers with dominant-arm involvement, develop chronic trapezius ache and spasm, altered scapular tracking, and limiting throwing.
F. **Treatment.** A sling is provided for comfort for the first several days following type I AC joint injuries. Ice in the first 24 hr and immediate range-of-motion exercises are recommended. Type II injuries are treated with ice, rest, and sling support. Range-of-motion exercises may be more painful than

in the type I injuries, so full motion is delayed for several days. Inferior drooping of the arm is the primary deformity, as opposed to superior dislocation of the clavicle, so attention is focused on supporting the arm and keeping it elevated. Lifting and carrying are avoided for 4 to 6 weeks. Operative treatment is recommended for type III injuries in most overhead athletes (e.g., baseball, tennis). Although this remains controversial, we feel that the results following operative treatment are superior to those following nonoperative treatment. Nonoperative management is preferred for contact athletes (e.g., hockey, football, lacrosse), with sling support until the pain recedes. All type IV and V injuries are treated surgically. Operative management of types III, IV, and V injuries includes resection of the distal clavicle, transfer of the coracoacromial ligament to the end of the clavicle, and coracoclavicular fixation with sutures.

G. **Return to sports.** This may occur within several days to a week following a type I AC injury if full, painless motion is present. Type II injuries can take substantially longer to heal. However, typical return to sports is allowed between 2 to 3 weeks from the time of injury if pain is eliminated with shoulder motion. Return to sports is delayed for a minimum of 4 months in patients with type III, IV, or V injuries who undergo surgical reconstruction. Healing of the soft tissues, strengthening of muscles, and recovery of full shoulder motion are necessary prior to return to sports.

III. Osteolysis of the Distal Clavicle

is characterized by resorption of the distal end of the clavicle, which is often insidious in onset and may take many months to complete its course. The etiology of distal clavicular osteolysis remains unclear. A leading theory maintains that it is caused by avascular necrosis of the lateral end of the clavicle. Many patients, however, will have a history of trauma or repetitive microtrauma such as that seen in weight lifters. The incidence is unknown, but the disease is significantly more prevalent in males.

A. **History.** This usually includes either a traumatic event, such as a fall on the shoulder, or repetitive microtrauma, as with weight lifting.

B. **Physical examination.** Tenderness to palpation is a very specific finding. Cross-body adduction and internal rotation may exacerbate the symptoms; however, these maneuvers are not specific.

C. **Diagnostic tests.** Elimination of pain by selective injection of 1% lidocaine into the AC joint confirms the source of pain. Routine radiographs of the AC joint will confirm the diagnosis of distal clavicular osteolysis. Focal cystic erosions, soft tissue calcification, and apparent widening of the acromioclavicular joint space are all characteristic radiographic features.

D. **Special tests.** Bone scans have been used to assist in the diagnosis of distal clavicular osteolysis, but they are rarely indicated.

E. **Natural history.** The condition may resolve if the athlete is willing to give up exacerbating activities (usually an unacceptable option). Continued activity, however, usually results in persistent pain, though the extent of osteolysis does not tend to progress more than 3 cm from the AC joint.

F. **Treatment.** Initial treatment includes elimination of exacerbating events, a trial of nonsteroidal antiinflammatory drugs, and—if the pain is severe—an AC injection. We prefer a combination of 1% lidocaine, 0.25% bupivicaine, and a depot corticosteroid compound. For those failing conservative treatment or those unwilling or unable to alter their activity, surgery with distal clavicular excision is recommended.

G. **Return to sports.** Athletes can continue to compete in sports as pain allows. For those requiring surgery, a sling is required for comfort and support in the immediate postoperative period. This can usually be discarded after the first or second week. Emphasis is placed on regaining full motion during the initial postoperative period, with strengthening added later. The total time of rehabilitation varies, but most athletes can return to their sport by 6 to 8 weeks.

IV. Sternoclavicular separation.

The sternoclavicular (SC) joint is the least commonly injured joint of the shoulder girdle. Most SC dislocations are displaced anteriorly and both types can be the result of direct or indirect trauma. The incidence of sternoclavicular dislocation is less than 1% of all joint dislocations. The incidence of physeal injuries to the medial clavicle is unknown. However, given that the medial epiphysis does not ossify until age 18, most SC "dislocations" in patients 25 years of age and younger are probably physeal separations.

Sternoclavicular joint injuries are classified into three grades. A grade I injury is a mild sprain with no ligamentous damage or instability. A grade II injury is a moderate sprain with a subluxated joint and partial disruption of the surrounding ligaments and capsule. Finally, grade III injuries involve gross disruption of the ligaments and dislocation (either anteriorly or posteriorly).

A. **History.** The mechanism of injury should be sought, especially direct trauma to the medial clavicle, as from a kick to the area or indirect forces, especially a violent compression of the shoulder toward the midline combined with an anterior or posterior force. The patient should be specifically questioned as to any difficulties breathing or swallowing and as to sensations of neck fullness or choking, any of which may suggest a posterior SC dislocation compressing the trachea or other vital structures.

B. **Physical examination.** Grade I injuries will show mild tenderness on palpation without evidence of instability. In grade II injuries, there will be more discomfort on palpation and subluxation will be evident. Manual stressing of the joint will often reveal anteroposterior instability. In anterior grade III injuries, the medial clavicle is visibly and palpably prominent anterior to the sternum. The patient usually holds the affected extremity across the chest and supports it with the opposite arm. Posterior SC dislocations are potentially more dangerous and may be associated with severe symptoms. Venous congestion, breathing difficulties, shortness of breath, pneumothorax, and difficulty swallowing are all possible.

C. **Diagnostic tests.** Routine radiographs often underestimate SC joint injuries. A 40-degree cephalic tilt view of both sternoclavicular joints should be obtained if SC joint pathology is suspected, but it may be difficult to interpret.

D. **Special tests.** Tomograms can be helpful in further evaluating injuries of the SC joint. However, if such an injury is suspected, computed tomography is the imaging modality of choice. This may be particularly helpful in picking up epiphyseal fractures.

E. **Natural history.** Grade I and II injuries heal completely with little to no residual effect. Anterior grade III and asymptomatic posterior injuries also usually heal without sequelae.

F. **Treatment.** All grade I injuries are treated with a sling. The length of treatment is dictated by the patients' symptoms. The sling is usually worn for the first week and activities are encouraged by the fifth day. A sling is also used for grade II injuries and is usually worn for 10 to 14 days. Anterior grade III injuries are usually not reduced due to their inherent instability. Patients are instructed about the instability and the generally benign natural history. Acute posterior grade III SC dislocations are treated with closed reduction in the operating room after other life-threatening injuries are ruled out. A figure of eight bandage is then applied for 4 to 6 weeks. If closed reduction is unsuccessful or the dislocation is chronic and there are symptoms of compression of the trachea or great vessels, open reduction is performed with the assistance of a chest surgeon.

   Finally, we do not routinely reduce either anterior or asymptomatic posterior Salter-Harris fractures of the medial clavicle epiphysis. Remodeling of these injuries is often dramatic and typically results in a painless, stable joint.

G. **Return to Sport.** Athletes with grade I injuries can return to competition within the first week if they are asymptomatic and have regained full, painless motion. Grade II injuries, however, require a longer convalescence, typically 6 weeks, to allow the elongated ligaments time to heal. Athletes with grade III injuries can return after 6 weeks if they are no longer symptomatic and have full range of motion of the affected extremity. However, collision sports and activities that might drive the medial clavicle further back are avoided for 3 months after a grade III posterior SC dislocation regardless of the chosen treatment.

Suggested Reading

Bigliani DU, Flatow EL. History, physical examination, and diagnostic modalities. In: McGinty, JB, Caspari, RB, Jackson, RW, Poehling, GG, eds, *Operative arthroscopy*. New York, Raven Press, 1991:453–464.

Bigliani DU, Nicholson GP, Flatow EL. Arthroscopic resection of the distal clavicle. *Orthop Clin North Am* 1993;24:13–141.

Flatow EL. The biomechanics of the acromioclavicular, sternoclavicular, and scapulothoracic joints. In: Heckman JD ed. *Instructional course lectures.* Rosemont IL: American Academy of Orthopaedic Surgeons, 1993;42:237–246.

Weinstein DM. McCann PD, Fithian DC et al. Surgical treatment of complete acromioclavicular dislocations. *Am J. Sports Med* 1995;23:324–331.

Williams GR Jr, Rockwood CA Jr. Injuries to the acromioclavicular joint, the sternoclavicular joint, clavicle, scapula, coracoid, sternum, and ribs. In: DeLee JC & Drez DJ Jr. eds. *Orthopaedic sports medicine,* vol 1. Philadelphia: W.B. Saunders, 1994: 481–545.

42. THE ELBOW

Champ L. Baker, Jr., and Charles A. Gottlob

The diagnosis and treatment of athletic elbow injuries have improved as our understanding of the functional anatomy and biomechanical demands placed on this complex joint during sports has increased. Conditions can be classified as acute or chronic overuse injuries involving either the bony or soft tissue structures about the joint, or both, and further categorized according to the location of the presenting symptoms.

I. Specific Fractures

Anteroposterior (AP) and lateral x-rays are standard for all suspected fractures. In cases where other x-ray views or additional radiographic studies are helpful, this is noted in the text.

A. **Olecranon fractures** occur either from a direct blow to the elbow or indirectly through a forceful triceps muscle contraction after a fall on the flexed upper extremity. They can be isolated or associated with a dislocation.

1. **Classification.** Olecranon fractures are classified as either undisplaced (displaced less than 2 mm) or displaced (displaced more than 2 mm). To be treated as undisplaced, the fracture must remain stable through 90 degrees of flexion and the patient must be able to actively extend the elbow against gravity.
2. **Physical examination.** To evaluate the integrity of the triceps mechanism, check for the ability to extend the arm actively against gravity. Rule out the presence of an associated neurovascular injury, usually involving the ulnar nerve.
3. **Treatment**
   a. **Undisplaced fractures** can be treated in a long arm cast or splint in 45 to 90 degrees of flexion. Motion from 0 to 90 degrees is allowed at approximately 3 weeks. Full motion and functional rehabilitation are delayed until clinical and radiographic union have occurred (average, 6 to 8 weeks).
   b. **Displaced fractures** are best treated with open reduction and internal fixation (ORIF) and early active motion.
4. **Olecranon stress fractures** have been reported in throwing athletes. Patients present with insidious-onset posterior elbow pain, made worse with activity. If x-rays are negative, a bone scan may be required to make the diagnosis. Initial treatment consists of immobilization, rest, and nonsteroidal antiinflammatory drugs (NSAIDs). Delayed unions can require ORIF or partial excision of the olecranon tip.

B. **Coronoid process fractures** typically occur in conjunction with elbow dislocations. The coronoid process is important for both AP and valgus joint stability.

1. **Classification.** Type I fractures involve only the tip of the coronoid process. Type II fractures involve up to 50% of the process; Type III fractures involve greater than 50% of the process and are therefore unstable.
2. **Physical examination.** The normal triangle formed by the olecranon tip, lateral epicondyle, and radial head is disrupted in an elbow dislocation.
3. **Treatment.** Type I and II fractures are managed with closed reduction, long arm splinting or casting, and early active motion (within 3 weeks). Type III fractures typically require ORIF followed by early protected motion.

C. **Fractures of the distal humerus**

1. **Supracondylar fractures.** These extraarticular fractures are more common in children with open physes. In adults, always suspect intraarticular extension of the fracture (i.e., intercondylar fracture).

a. **Mechanism of injury.** A supracondylar fracture usually results from a fall on the outstretched hand or a direct blow to the posterior aspect of the elbow.
b. **Classification** is based on distal fragment displacement: there are extension (posterior displacement) and flexion (anterior displacement) types.
c. **Physical examination** focuses on the neurovascular status of the limb. Injuries to the brachial artery and all three major nerves (median, ulnar, and radial) have been reported. Rule out the presence of a forearm compartment syndrome.
d. **X-rays.** Supplemental AP and lateral tomograms or computed tomography (CT) scan may be required to rule out intraarticular extension of the fracture.
e. **Treatment.** Treat undisplaced fractures with a long arm splint or cast and begin active motion within 3 weeks. Treat displaced fractures with ORIF and early active motion.

2. **Intercondylar fractures.** These complex T-Y intraarticular fractures occur with high-energy mechanisms of injury and can be accompanied by concomitant soft tissue and neurovascular injuries.
   a. **Classification.** Intercondylar fractures are classified as undisplaced, displaced, displaced and rotated, or comminuted.
   b. **Physical examination.** Examine the skin for evidence of an open fracture. Rule out neurovascular injuries and forearm compartment syndrome.
   c. **X-rays.** AP and lateral tomograms or CT scan with 3D reconstruction may be needed to clarify the fracture pattern.
   d. **Treatment.** Stable ORIF is typically required to allow early active motion.

D. **Fractures of the radial head** fractures are relatively common in the adult athlete. Often, they appear radiographically benign (occult); the diagnosis requires a high index of suspicion.

1. **Mechanism of injury.** Fractures of the radial head usually occur from a fall on the outstretched hand.
2. **Classification.** Type I fractures are undisplaced; type II fractures are displaced marginal fractures involving one-third of the radial head, 30 degrees of angulation, or 3 mm of displacement; type III fractures have comminution of the entire head; and type IV fractures are associated with a dislocation.
3. **Physical examination.** Pain is reproduced with passive supination and pronation, and the radial head is tender to palpation.
4. **X-rays.** Special radial head–capitellum views are helpful. An isolated posterior fat pad sign combined with a consistent mechanism of injury, history, and examination is suggestive of an occult fracture.
5. **Treatment.** Type I fractures are treated with a sling or splint, followed by early active motion within 1 to 2 weeks. The treatment of type II fractures remains controversial; options include splinting and early motion, ORIF, and radial head excision. Type III fractures generally require radial head excision. Type IV fractures are managed with reduction of the dislocation, followed by appropriate treatment for the radial head fracture, according to its type. Occult fractures are treated like type I fractures.
6. **Return to sports.** Criteria include radiographic and clinical union, a functional range of motion, and strength and stamina sufficient to withstand the demands of the athlete's sport and position.

II. Dislocations

The elbow is the most commonly dislocated joint in children, second only to the shoulder in adults. Up to 20% of dislocations are associated with neurovascular injuries of the brachial artery, ulnar nerve, median nerve, radial nerve, or anterior interosseus nerve.

A. **Mechanism of injury.** Posterior dislocations result from a posterolateral force applied to the elbow from a fall on the outstretched hand with the elbow near full extension. Anterior dislocations generally result from a direct blow to the posterior elbow.
B. **Classification** is based on the direction of displacement of the proximal ulna: posterior, posterolateral, posteromedial, medial, lateral, or anterior. Posterior and posterolateral dislocations are the most common types.
C. **Physical examination.** The normal triangular relationship between the olecranon, lateral epicondyle, and radial head is disrupted. Examine carefully for an associated neurovascular injury.
D. **X-rays.** AP and lateral radiographs demonstrate the dislocation. Rule out associated fractures, most often of the radial head, coronoid process, or medial epicondyle.
E. **Treatment.** After initial x-rays, reduce the elbow by gentle closed manipulation, with sedation as needed. Postreduction x-rays verify concentric reduction and rule out interposed soft tissue or bony fragments. Reassess elbow stability after reduction. A long arm splint or bivalved cast is applied at 90 degrees of flexion. For stable reductions, begin early active motion as soon as symptoms permit. For unstable reductions, a fracture brace allows early active motion with an extension block that is gradually decreased after 3 weeks. Reevaluate neurovascular status immediately postreduction and during the 24 to 36 hr following the injury. Nonconcentric reductions should be studied further with tomograms or a CT scan.
F. **Return to sports.** Criteria are similar to those listed in under I. Specific Fractures, above. Full recovery can require 6 to 18 months.

III. Olecranon Bursitis

is an inflammation of the subcutaneous bursa overlying the olecranon process, can be acute or chronic, septic or aseptic. This problem is rare in children because the bursa is not developed before the age of 7 years.

A. **Mechanism of injury.** Acute bursitis usually results from a direct blow to the elbow point, as in an ice hockey collision or a fall on artificial turf. Chronic cases develop from repeated trauma, with gradual fluid accumulation. Septic cases usually involve a hematogenously seeded *Staphylococcus aureus* infection, or, less often, direct inoculation via a laceration or injection.
B. **History** depends on the duration of the problem. In acute cases, the elbow is swollen and painful and lacks full motion. A direct blow to the elbow is often recalled. Chronic cases present as insidious fluid accumulations. Swelling can become quite impressive but is often painless. Septic bursitis is occasionally accompanied by systemic signs and symptoms, such as fever.
C. **Physical examination.** Swelling and tenderness are confined to the posterior elbow. Inspect for abrasions or lacerations. Motion is limited at the extreme of flexion. In septic cases, the bursa is warm and erythematous.
D. **X-rays** are usually not helpful. They can show calcifications in chronic cases.
E. **Treatment.** Treat aseptic bursitis with a compression dressing and pad to prevent subsequent trauma. Aspirate the bursa if motion is significantly limited by swelling. Always aspirate the bursa and send the fluid for gram stain and cultures if there is any suspicion of infection. Treat septic bursitis with incision and drainage, open wound management, and antibiotics. Bursal excision is indicated only rarely for chronic refractory cases.
F. **Return to sports.** The athlete may compete with appropriate protective gear to prevent further insult to the bursa.

IV. Chronic or Overuse Injuries

In general, x-rays are needed to rule out physeal injuries in children and calcifications. Magnetic resonance imaging (MRI) can be helpful in certain cases; these are noted in the text.

A. **Definition.** The term *overuse injury* is used to describe a broad array of injuries that result from repetitive microtrauma. Repeated submaximal loading of the soft tissue and bony elbow structures results in an insidious inflammatory process, which leads to pain and ultimately failure of the overloaded structures. Inadequately conditioned athletes who use poor sport-specific mechanics (e.g., throwing motion) or equipment (e.g., tennis racquet grip size) are vulnerable to these problems. The pattern of injury depends largely on the athlete's age, sport and position, and level of athletic involvement.

B. **Epicondylitis**
   1. **Medial epicondylitis (golfer's elbow)** is a painful tendinitis of the common flexor-pronator origins, adjacent to the medial epicondyle.
      a. **Pathoanatomy.** The origins of the pronator teres and flexor carpi radialis origin are routinely involved. Chronic overload results in inflammation, microtears, and occasionally calcifications.
      b. **Etiology.** Sports often associated with this injury include golf, racquet sports, bowling, baseball, and swimming.
      c. **Incidence.** Medial epicondylitis is approximately one-fifth as frequent as its lateral counterpart.
      d. **History.** Athletes present with insidious, activity-related medial elbow pain and swelling. Question the player about participation in at-risk sports. Provocative activities include the acceleration phase of throwing, the tennis serve, and forehand racquet strokes.
      e. **Physical examination.** Tenderness is well localized 1 to 2 cm distal to the medial epicondyle; there can be associated swelling and palpable calcifications. Resisted wrist flexion and pronation are painful. Rule out associated ulnar neuritis and valgus instability.
   2. **Lateral epicondylitis (tennis elbow)** is a painful tendinitis involving the common extensor origin at the lateral epicondyle. It is one of the most frequent causes of lateral elbow pain in the athlete.
      a. **Pathoanatomy.** The extensor carpi radialis brevis is most often involved. Inflammation leads to microtears, or occasionally frank rupture of the extensor origin.
      b. **Etiology.** Commonly implicated sports include tennis, racquetball, squash, and fencing.
      c. **Incidence.** More than 50% of recreational tennis players suffer from lateral epicondylitis. Peak incidence is in the fourth and fifth decades of life.
      d. **History.** Athletes complain of insidious-onset lateral elbow pain exacerbated by inciting activities. Acute-on-chronic pain is suggestive of a frank rupture of the extensor origin.
      e. **Physical examination.** Tenderness is localized to 2 to 5 cm distal and anterior to the lateral epicondyle. Symptoms are reproduced with resisted wrist extension while the elbow is extended. Rule out signs of compressive neuropathy, radiculopathy, and intraarticular pathology.
      f. **X-rays.** MRI can be helpful in ruling out an acute-on-chronic rupture of the extensor origin.
   3. **Conservative treatment** is successful in most cases of medial and lateral epicondylitis.
      a. **Reduce inflammation** with rest, NSAIDs, ice, and possibly counterforce bracing. Corticosteroid injections may be used judiciously.
      b. **Rehabilitation** involves regaining pain-free range of motion and adequate flexibility, followed by progressive strengthening exercises.
      c. **Return to sports** should be gradual and only after the patient is pain free and the involved extremity's strength nears 80% of that on the contralateral side. Modify sport-specific throwing and stroke mechanics as needed.
   4. **Surgical treatment** is indicated after at least 6 months of failed conservative care.
      a. **Medial epicondylitis.** Surgical options include elliptical excision of diseased tissue, followed by side-to-side closure of the defect, versus

elevation of the flexor-pronator origin, followed by debridement and reapproximation.

b. **Lateral epicondylitis.** The common extensor origin is elevated, the pathologic tissue is debrided, and the tendon is reapproximated.

5. **Prevention.** Proper conditioning emphasizing flexibility, strength, and stamina, in combination with proper sport-specific mechanics and equipment, can reduce the athlete's risk of medial and lateral epicondylitis.

C. **Injury of the ulnar collateral ligament (UCL).** Throwing sports or activities that simulate the throwing motion subject the medial elbow to repetitive valgus stresses, which can result in tension injuries to the ulnar collateral ligament, the flexor-pronator muscle mass, and the ulnar nerve. While often seen in baseball pitchers, similar problems can develop in javelin throwers, quarterbacks, swimmers, volleyball players, and tennis players.

1. **Pathophysiology.** Chronic valgus overload produces a continuum of injuries from flexor-pronator strain and tendinitis to UCL attenuation to complete tearing of the ligament. The body's failed attempts at repair can result in ligament calcifications or an elbow flexion contracture. Less often, the UCL ruptures acutely, usually in the presence of an underlying chronic injury. Tension overload of the medial elbow can also produce ulnar neuritis.
2. **History.** Overhead athletes, particularly throwers, complain of activity-related medial elbow pain during the late cocking and acceleration phases of the throwing motion. These symptoms of insidious onset ultimately result in an inability to throw effectively. Pain also occurs when striking the ball during batting. In acute ruptures, the pain is sudden and can be associated with a "pop," and then the athlete is unable to throw. Symptoms of ulnar nerve irritation can be present.
3. **Physical examination.** Chronic cases reveal a flexion contracture and UCL tenderness. Painful resisted wrist flexion and pronation suggests injury to the flexor-pronator muscle mass. Ecchymosis can be present in acute cases. Valgus stress testing with the elbow at 20 degrees of flexion is positive if the ligament is incompetent (see Appendix 6). Rule out commonly associated problems, such as loose bodies and ulnar neuropathy.
4. **Diagnostic tests.** Plain x-rays can reveal UCL calcifications or avulsions off the medial epicondyle. The gravity stress x-ray is helpful in determining the degree of valgus instability. MRI can demonstrate the extent of injury, and arthrograms are positive in complete tears when performed early.
5. **Natural history.** In addition to medial tension injuries, chronic valgus overload can ultimately result in lateral compartment compression injuries and posterior compartment shearing injuries.
6. **Treatment**
   a. **Nonoperative.** Manage chronic UCL insufficiency with rest and NSAIDs, followed by rehabilitation emphasizing strength, endurance, proper mechanics, and an interval return-to-throwing program. In general, nonoperative measures are less successful for acute ruptures in athletes who wish to continue throwing.
   b. **Operative.** Consider surgical reconstruction of the anterior band of the UCL in overhead athletes who have failed at least 6 months of conservative treatment. Concomitant ulnar nerve transposition is indicated when signs and symptoms of ulnar neuritis are present. Resection of calcifications without reconstruction of the ligament should be undertaken with caution, as this can increase instability. Acute ruptures in athletes who wish to continue throwing are also indications for reconstruction.
7. **Return to sports** after nonoperative treatment is contingent upon the athlete's ability to complete a return-to-throwing program without symptoms, which can require more than 3 to 6 months of rehabilitation. Following UCL reconstruction, athletes may return to throwing no ear-

lier than 6 to 12 months postoperatively after completing a similar return-to-throwing program.

8. **Prevention** requires proper off-season conditioning to maintain flexibility, strength, and sport-specific coordination. Return to throwing should be gradual and supervised.

D. **Posterolateral rotatory instability** of the elbow describes a recurrent pattern of coupled posterolateral proximal ulnar and radial head subluxation or dislocation relative to the distal humerus. The signs and symptoms of this relatively infrequent disorder are typically vague, and the diagnosis is often elusive.

1. **Pathophysiology.** Instability is produced by injury to the lateral collateral ligament complex, most notably the lateral ulnar collateral ligament. The annular ligament is usually intact; therefore, there is no proximal radioulnar dissociation. Instead, both the radiohumeral and ulnohumeral articulations subluxate or dislocate posterolaterally about the distal humerus as the elbow is supinated and extended.
2. **Etiology.** This instability pattern is typically posttraumatic. Common complex mechanisms of injury affecting the lateral ligament include elbow dislocations or excessive tennis elbow releases and radial head excisions. Rarely, sprains of the isolated lateral ligament can occur from varus stresses.
3. **History.** Patients have vague complaints of lateral elbow pain and clicking, clunking, or locking during activities that require combined elbow extension and supination.
4. **Physical examination.** The lateral pivot shift maneuver reproduces the subluxation by combining axial loading, valgus stress, and supination of the elbow at 20 to 30 degrees of flexion. As the elbow is flexed, a "clunk" indicates reduction (see Appendix 6).
5. **Stress lateral x-rays** taken during the lateral pivot shift maneuver can show subtle instability.
6. **Treatment.** A pronation-extension block splint can reduce symptoms in patients with low elbow demands. Definitive surgical treatment involves repair of avulsed ligaments or, more often, reconstruction of the lateral ulnar collateral ligament with a free tendon graft.
7. **Return to sports.** Following surgical reconstruction, the elbow is protected for 6 to 18 weeks. Allow sports no sooner than 6 months postoperatively, after completion of a range-of-motion and strengthening program.

E. **Tendon injuries**

1. **Brachialis muscle and anterior capsular strain** results from repetitive overuse of the flexed and pronated forearm, as in rock climbing, weight lifting, gymnastics, and bowling. Hyperextension injuries or direct blows to the anterior elbow can also produce this injury. Complete brachialis tendon ruptures do occur, most frequently with elbow dislocations.
   a. **Pathophysiology.** Chronic overload results in inflammation and microtears. The body's attempts at repair can lead to a flexion contracture. Bleeding into the tissues can result in heterotopic ossification and further loss of motion.
   b. **History.** Patients complain of activity-related anterior elbow pain, with or without a loss of extension.
   c. **Physical examination** is often nonrevealing. A flexion contracture can be present. Brachialis tendon tenderness and pain reproduction with hyperextension or resisted elbow flexion suggest the diagnosis. Rule out high median nerve compression and distal biceps tendinitis or rupture.
   d. **X-rays** can be helpful if heterotopic ossification is suspected.
   e. **Treatment** is as for other overuse injuries. Begin with rest, ice, and NSAIDs, followed by rehabilitation aimed at restoring motion, strength, and endurance.

f. **Return to sports** is individualized according to the patient's symptoms.

2. **Distal biceps tendon.** Acute and overuse injuries of this structure are potential sources of anterior elbow pain in the athlete.
   a. **Distal biceps tendinitis.** Tendon inflammation results from friction across the bicipital tuberosity during repetitive elbow hyperextension or forceful flexion and supination.
      i. **History.** Insidious-onset anterior elbow pain with activities is characteristic.
      ii. **Physical examination** is often significant only for distal biceps tendon tenderness and pain with resisted supination or elbow flexion.
      iii. **Treatment** is initial rest, ice, NSAIDs, and compression, then rehabilitation to regain motion, strength, and endurance. Therapeutic modalities can be of benefit.
   b. **Rupture of the distal biceps tendon** is usually an acute event, though it can be superimposed on a history of chronic tendinitis.
      i. **Pathophysiology.** Forceful, eccentric biceps muscle contraction against resistance suddenly overloads the tendon, avulsing it from the bicipital tuberosity.
      ii. **History.** Patients recall the exact moment of injury and report a history of sharp anterior elbow pain that diminished quickly, to be replaced by a persistent dull ache. Patients also note a bulge in the biceps muscle mass and elbow weakness.
      iii. **Physical examination.** Ecchymosis is present within 2 to 3 days of the injury. A biceps muscle bulge is usually palpable, and the bicipital tuberosity is tender. Weakness is appreciated more in supination than in flexion.
      iv. **X-rays** rule out an annular ligament rupture with radial head dislocation.
      v. **Treatment.** Complete tendon rupture results in 30% and 40% strength deficits in elbow flexion and supination, respectively. Although these deficits may be acceptable to a sedentary individual, they are usually not so for the athlete. Surgical repair with a double-incision approach is the treatment of choice for active individuals.
      vi. **Return to sports** should occur no earlier than 3 to 6 months postoperatively, after completion of a supervised rehabilitation program.
3. **Triceps tendon**
   a. **Triceps tendinitis** is a relatively uncommon cause of posterior elbow pain. Tendon inflammation results from repetitive forceful elbow extension, as in the tennis serve or the late acceleration and deceleration phases of throwing.
      i. **History.** Typically, throwing athletes complain of insidious-onset, activity-related posterior elbow pain near the end of the throwing motion.
      ii. **Physical examination** is notable only for tenderness at the triceps insertion and pain reproduction with resisted elbow extension. Rarely, tendon calcifications are palpable.
      iii. **Treatment** is usually nonoperative: rest, ice, NSAIDs, and modalities followed by a supervised interval throwing program. Do not inject corticosteroids because of the risk of iatrogenic tendon rupture.
      iv. **Return to sports** is based on patient symptoms.
   b. **Triceps tendon rupture.** The triceps tendon is one of the least common sites of acute tendon rupture. Forceful eccentric triceps loading, as in weight lifting, a fall on the outstretched hand, or a

direct blow produces this injury. Anabolic steroid use or local corticosteroid injections have been implicated in some cases.

i. **History.** Acute posterior elbow pain from an injury as described above favors the diagnosis. There can be a history of triceps tendinitis, anabolic steroid use, or corticosteroid injection.

ii. **Physical examination.** Ecchymosis usually occurs within 2 to 3 days. A palpable tendon defect near the insertion and an active extension lag are generally present.

iii. **X-rays** can reveal a small avulsion fracture of the tip of the olecranon process or tendon calcifications from previous episodes of triceps tendinitis.

iv. **Treatment.** Early exploration and transosseous repair of the tendon yields excellent results and is the treatment of choice for this injury.

F. **Nerve injuries**

1. **Ulnar neuropathy at the elbow (cubital tunnel syndrome).** The superficial location and restrictive local anatomy of the ulnar nerve make it vulnerable to injury during sports. Ulnar nerve entrapment, the second most common compressive neuropathy of the upper extremity after carpal tunnel syndrome, can be an isolated entity or associated with other sources of medial elbow pain, such as UCL insufficiency or medial epicondylitis.

a. **Pathophysiology.** The ulnar nerve can be injured by a direct blow to the medial elbow or indirectly by repetitive compression, traction, or friction. Compression typically occurs at the arcade of Struthers, the medial intermuscular septum, the cubital tunnel, or the flexor carpi ulnaris. Space for the nerve is decreased by space-occupying lesions (e.g., soft tissue calcifications, bone spurs, and flexor muscle hypertrophy) and by elbow flexion. Valgus elbow stresses can produce nerve traction injuries. Rapid, repetitive elbow extension and flexion with subsequent ulnar nerve subluxation can lead to nerve friction injuries. Hence, overhead athletes are at particular risk for ulnar nerve injuries. The throwing motion creates repetitive valgus stresses on the elbow and forceful flexion and extension. Also, medial bone spurs and UCL calcifications, not uncommon in the symptomatic throwing athlete, can result in further nerve compression.

b. **History.** Athletes initially have vague complaints of activity-related medial elbow pain and hand clumsiness or heaviness. Later, pain, paresthesias, and numbness can radiate down the forearm and into the two ulnar digits. Concomitant symptoms of UCL laxity or medial epicondylitis can exist.

c. **Physical examination.** Tenderness and boggy swelling are localized to the cubital tunnel. Overhead athletes can have a flexion contracture. Passive elbow flexion and extension can reveal ulnar nerve subluxation or dislocation. Tinel's sign behind the medial epicondyle and the elbow flexion test (a provocative test like the Phalen test of the wrist—see Appendix 6) are usually positive. Initially, the neurologic examination is normal; later, sensory or motor deficits or both can occur in the ulnar nerve distribution. Rule out UCL laxity and medial epicondylitis.

d. **Diagnostic tests.** Plain x-rays, plus the cubital tunnel view, rule out impinging soft tissue calcifications or bone spurs. Electromyography (EMG) and nerve conduction velocity (NCV) studies are useful in defining the extent of the injury but not critical to the diagnosis. False-negative studies are not uncommon.

e. **Treatment**

i. **Nonoperative.** Direct injuries can be treated with padding and protection of the ulnar nerve. Nonoperative treatment of indirect injuries is often less successful. Initial treatment is rest,

NSAIDs, and elbow splinting in midflexion at night. A 2- to 3-week period of continual splinting can help athletes with recurrent ulnar nerve subluxation. It is critical to refrain from the provocative activities to ensure the success of nonoperative care, but this is often unacceptable to the competitive athlete. Corticosteroid injections have not proved effective. Athletes with valgus overload should modify their throwing techniques.

ii. **Operative.** Failure of conservative treatment, refractory nerve subluxation, fixed neural deficits, and medial elbow surgery for other reasons point to operative intervention. Because competitive players tend to be unwilling to give up sports, surgery is often needed. This includes complete ulnar nerve release from the arcade of Struthers to the flexor carpi ulnaris, with anterior nerve transposition, either subcutaneously or, preferably, submuscularly. Any UCL insufficiency should also be addressed.

f. **Return to sports.** Postoperative flexor-pronator muscle rehabilitation is painstaking, and return to throwing is typically delayed for at least 6 months.

2. **Posterior interosseous nerve (PIN) syndrome.** The radial nerve's terminal motor branch can become entrapped around the lateral elbow, causing pain. PIN syndrome is often confused with lateral epicondylitis and has, therefore, been termed “resistant tennis elbow” by some.
   a. **Pathoanatomy.** Nerve compression commonly occurs at four sites: adjacent to the radial recurrent vessels (leash of Henry) or at the leading edge (arcade of Frohse), the midportion, or the distal edge of the supinator muscle.
   b. **History.** Initially, patients complain of vague, activity-related lateral elbow pain very similar to the pain of tennis elbow. Pain can radiate down the dorsoradial forearm. Late in the course, subjective weakness of the wrist and digital extensors can occur. Because the PIN is a motor nerve, sensory complaints are absent.
   c. **Physical examination** shows tenderness 2 to 5 cm distal to the lateral epicondyle and pain reproduction with resisted supination or passive pronation. Pain with resisted long finger extension is a nonspecific finding. With advanced compression, motor weakness of the PIN-innervated muscles can be present.
   d. **Diagnostic studies.** EMG and NCV studies are helpful when positive, but false-negative studies are not uncommon.
   e. **Treatment.** Nonoperative care includes rest, ice, NSAIDs, and protective equipment as necessary. Failure of at least 6 months of conservative treatment for objective motor weakness or EMG-documented, ongoing PIN injury are reasons for surgical nerve release.
3. **Median nerve compression.** Repetitive use of the elbow in sports can result in median nerve compression at the distal arm or proximal forearm. The pattern of symptoms produced has been collectively termed *pronator syndrome.*
   a. **Pathoanatomy.** The median nerve can be compressed at four anatomic sites: the ligament of Struthers, the lacertus fibrosus, the pronator teres, or the fibrous arch of the flexor digitorum superficialis.
   b. **History.** Complaints are vague, including easy forearm fatigability and activity-related forearm discomfort that radiates proximally into the arm. Later, motor or sensory symptoms of the median nerve distribution can mimic carpal tunnel syndrome.
   c. **Physical examination.** Like the history, physical findings are subtle. The pronator mass can be constricted distal to the medial epicondyle from tightness of the lacertus fibrosus, or it can feel indurated and tense. The pronator region is tender and Tinel's sign is typically positive there. Pain is reproduced by resisted pronation,

long finger flexion, or simultaneous elbow flexion and supination. With prolonged compression, median nerve distribution motor or sensory changes can occur. Isolated anterior interosseous nerve compression is not associated with sensory findings.

d. **Diagnostic studies.** EMG and NCV studies have been unreliable.

e. **Treatment.** Conservative measures include NSAIDs, ice, and avoiding provocative activities. Corticosteroid injections are rarely indicated. Failure of conservative treatment and objective neurologic deficits are indications for surgical release of the median nerve.

G. **Valgus extension overload syndrome** refers to a variety of signs and symptoms related to posterior compartment elbow changes from repetitive valgus stresses. The syndrome is most often described in throwing athletes. Other inciting activities include the tennis serve, the hockey slap shot, and the javelin throw.

1. **Pathophysiology.** Rapid, forceful elbow extension and valgus stresses due to the throwing motion lead to medial shear of the posterior compartment. The olecranon tip's medial aspect impinges against the olecranon fossa's medial aspect, causing chondromalacia, reactive spurring, flexion contracture, and, ultimately, loose body formation. The underlying mechanism for this pattern of injury is chronic valgus overload.
2. **History.** Patients complain of posterior elbow pain during the pitching motion's late acceleration and follow-through phases. The pain can be severe enough to cause early ball release and loss of control. As posterior compartment osteophytes develop, full extension is lost. Loose bodies can cause locking or catching.
3. **Physical examination.** Flexion contractures are common. Posterior pain is reproduced by forced elbow extension combined with valgus stress. Grating with passive range of motion is suggestive of loose bodies. Evaluate UCL integrity.
4. **Diagnostic studies.** Plain x-rays, including an axial view, demonstrate osteophytes at the olecranon tip's medial aspect. CT scans can assist in identifying loose bodies.
5. **Initial treatment** comprises rest, NSAIDs, flexor-pronator strengthening exercises, and a return-to-throwing program that focuses on improving technique. Once significant posterior impingement and osteophytes or loose bodies are present, nonoperative methods are generally not curative. Arthroscopic debridement and removal of loose bodies has been very successful in returning athletes to throwing.
6. **Return to sports.** Following arthroscopic debridement, most patients gradually return to supervised throwing within 3 months. However, because the primary pathology, UCL laxity, typically is not addressed, symptoms can recur. Most authors believe that it takes several years for osteophytes, loose bodies, and significant symptoms to redevelop.

H. **Little Leaguer's elbow.** This term refers to the spectrum of injuries affecting the skeletally immature elbow from repetitive stresses secondary to pitching and other overhead activities. The development of this problem appears more related to the frequency and technique of pitching than to the type of pitches thrown. Demands placed on the developing elbow's vulnerable physes and epiphyses during throwing produce three general patterns of injury: medial tension, lateral compression, and posterior shear or traction. Although described predominantly in adolescent pitchers, these injuries have also been reported in gymnasts and other overhead athletes.

1. **Medial epicondylar osteochondrosis and stress fractures.** Repetitive valgus stresses on the growing elbow from the pull of the UCL and flexor-pronator musculature result in medial epicondylar traction injuries, including traction apophysitis and ultimately an avulsion (stress fracture) of all or part of the medial epicondyle: the most common manifestation of Little Leaguer's elbow.

   a. **Anatomy.** The medial epicondylar apophysis ossifies near the age of 6 years and fuses to the distal humerus by the age of 17 years.

b. **History.** Traction apophysitis is typified by insidious, activity-related medial elbow pain, diminished pitching effectiveness, and decreased pitching distance. Flexion contractures are frequent. Avulsions are often accompanied by more acute discomfort.

c. **Physical examination** is most notable for medial epicondylar point tenderness and a flexion contracture in excess of 15 degrees. The medial epicondyle is often enlarged compared with that on the uninjured side. Valgus stability should be determined. Ecchymosis is common in acute avulsions.

d. **Diagnostic studies.** Plain x-rays confirm the diagnosis and demonstrate a spectrum of abnormalities, including epiphyseal fragmentation and enlargement, physeal widening, and partial or total epiphyseal avulsion. Comparison with the uninvolved side is helpful. In medial epicondylar avulsion, evaluation of valgus stability with gravity stress x-rays is critical in determining appropriate treatment.

e. **Treatment.** Traction apophysitis usually responds to conservative treatment of cessation of throwing for 2 to 3 weeks, ice, and NSAIDs. This is followed by exercises emphasizing range of motion, strength, proper throwing mechanics, and a return-to-throwing program after motion is regained. Treatment of stress fractures or avulsions depends upon the degree of displacement and valgus instability. Nondisplaced, stable injuries are treated as outlined above. Avulsions with more than 5 mm of displacement or 2 to 3 mm of instability on stress x-rays should be treated surgically, with ORIF.

f. **Return to sports.** Regardless of the treatment method, competitive throwing is resumed after pain-free, full range of motion is regained and the athlete has successfully completed an interval throwing program. This usually requires approximately 6 weeks from the time full motion returns.

2. **Capitellar osteochondrosis (Panner's disease) and osteochondritis dissecans (OCD).** Valgus overload subjects the radiocapitellar joint to compression injuries. In the growing elbow, the compression injury manifests as either Panner's disease (ages 7 to 12 years) or OCD (ages 13 to 16 years). Although pathology has been reported in the radial head and neck, it typically involves the capitellum.

   a. **Anatomy.** The capitellum ossifies at approximately 6 months of age and fuses to the distal humerus at the age of 13 years in females and 14.5 to 15 years in males.

   b. **Pathophysiology.** The exact mechanism of injury may be different for the entities. Current thinking is that repetitive compressive trauma jeopardizes the growing capitellar ossification center's precarious blood supply, resulting in aseptic necrosis. Panner's disease tends to involve a larger part of the ossific nucleus in younger persons; loose bodies and late degenerative changes are rare. In older persons, OCD involves more focal changes in subchondral bone and capitellar cartilage changes and it is more often associated with loose bodies and late degenerative changes.

   c. **History.** Children with Panner's disease have acute or subacute activity-related lateral elbow pain and decreased motion. Adolescents with OCD have insidious-onset lateral elbow pain, decreased motion, and catching or locking if loose bodies are present. In both conditions, pitchers ultimately lose the ability to throw effectively.

   d. **Physical examination** for the two entities reveals similar findings: radiocapitellar joint tenderness and a flexion contracture. In OCD, loose bodies can cause mechanical grating.

   e. **Diagnostic studies.** Standard x-rays confirm the diagnosis. In Panner's disease, the ossific nucleus is fragmented, with areas of rarefaction and reossification like those seen in Perthes' disease of the hip. In OCD, a focal sclerotic subchondral lesion is encircled by rarefaction; loose bodies can be present. Supplemental CT scans, CT arthrography, and MRI scans help to define the lesion's size and the presence of loose bodies.

f. **Treatment.** Panner's disease usually runs a benign, self-limited course and is therefore treated symptomatically. Initial treatment includes rest, and sometimes immobilization, until symptoms subside (3 to 4 weeks). This is followed by range-of-motion exercises and finally a supervised return-to-throwing program once full, pain-free motion is achieved and radiographic healing has occurred. OCD treatment depends upon the stage of the disease. Stable lesions with intact overlying articular cartilage can be treated as outlined above. Large, partially detached lesions can be reduced and fixed arthroscopically, with or without bone grafting. Smaller lesions are excised arthroscopically and the bed is curetted. Loose bodies are also best treated with excision and curettage of the base.

g. **Prognosis.** Panner's disease has a favorable prognosis; most athletes return to throwing. The OCD prognosis is more guarded and related to the stage of the disease. Return to throwing after treatment is possible in asymptomatic players who have radiographic healing. Once fragmentation is significant, the risk of late arthritic changes, loose bodies, and ongoing symptoms exceeds 50% in some series. Thus, many surgeons dissuade athletes from returning to highly provocative activities such as pitching and gymnastics.

3. **Olecranon osteochondrosis (traction apophysitis).** Repetitive stresses applied to the developing olecranon apophysis through the pull of the triceps invoke an injury pattern analogous to that of Osgood-Schlatter disease. In addition to throwing athletes, olecranon osteochondrosis has been seen in gymnasts, divers, and hockey players.
   a. **Anatomy.** The olecranon apophysis ossifies around age 8 years in girls and age 10 years in boys and fuses at the ages of 14 and 16 years, respectively.
   b. **Pathophysiology.** Repetitive microtrauma to the vulnerable apophysis leads to progressive fragmentation, irregular ossification, and widening of the physis. Later in adolescence, apophyseal overgrowth can occur, producing a flexion contracture but rarely loose bodies. Finally, incomplete physeal fusion or frank avulsion fracture can occur. Incompletely fused apophyses are at increased risk for fracture in young adulthood.
   c. **History.** Vague posterior elbow pain accompanies activities requiring forceful elbow extension. A flexion contracture can be present.
   d. **Physical examination** reveals swelling of the olecranon tip and as well as tenderness and pain reproduction with passive hyperextension and resisted active extension. Flexion contractures are not uncommon, but loose bodies are rare.
   e. **Diagnostic studies.** Standard x-rays, plus an axial view, demonstrate the pathology. Bone scan can aid in the diagnosis of stress fracture or incomplete physeal fusion.
   f. **Treatment.** Simple traction apophysitis is treated with rest, ice, and NSAIDs, followed by range-of-motion exercises, strengthening, and a return-to-throwing program. Incomplete physeal fusion refractory to symptomatic care is best treated with ORIF and bone grafting. Frank avulsion fractures also require surgical stabilization.
   g. **Prognosis** for return to throwing is generally favorable.

I. **Loose bodies**
1. **Congenital.** Several accessory centers of ossification about the elbow may or may not be the source of symptoms.
   a. **Medial epicondylar accessory ossification**
   b. **Olecranon** (os patella cubitii)
   c. **Olecranon fossa** (os supratrochleare)

2. **Acquired loose bodies** are often the result of the acute and chronic injuries discussed above (e.g., OCD, valgus extension overload syndrome, chronic UCL laxity).
   a. **Osteochondral fractures**
   b. **Degenerative conditions**
   c. **Synovial chondromatosis**
3. **History.** Patients note intermittent joint pain, locking, or grating with activity.
4. **Physical examination.** This reveals loss of motion with palpable crepitation.
5. **Diagnostic studies.** Standard x-rays, supplemented with plain tomography or CT.
6. **Treatment.** Arthroscopic removal is the treatment of choice for symptomatic loose bodies.

Suggested Reading

Andrews JR, Craven WM. Lesions of the posterior compartment of the elbow. *Clin Sports Med* 1991; 10:673–652.

Caldwell, GL Jr, Safran MR. Elbow problems in the athlete. *Orthop Clin North Am* 1995; 26:465–485.

Norkus SA, Meyers MC. Ulnar neuropathy of the elbow. *Sports Med.* 1994; 17:189–199.

O'Driscoll SW, Bell DF, Morrey BF. Posterolateral rotatory instability of the elbow. *J Bone Joint Surg* 1991; 73:440–446.

Thomas DR, Plancher KD, Hawkins, RI. Prevention and rehabilitation of overuse injuries of the elbow. *Clin Sports Med* 1995; 14:459–477.

43. THE WRIST AND HAND—BONE AND LIGAMENT INJURIES

Arthur C. Rettig and Dipak V. Patel

Introduction

Injuries to the wrist and hand in sports comprise approximately 3% to 9% of all athletic injuries. A 10-year survey (from January 1977 to October 1986) of all injuries at the U.S. Olympic Training Center in Colorado Springs showed that 9% of injuries involve the wrist and hand. It is estimated that 14% of injuries occurring in high school football may involve the hand and wrist.

I. Acute Ligamentous Injuries of the Wrist—Carpal Instabilities.

Ligamentous injuries of the wrist may cause a significant disability in an athlete whose sport requires a stable wrist with good mobility. Attempts should be made to make a specific anatomic diagnosis in every case so that a reasonable treatment program may be initiated. A careful history of the injury and a detailed physical examination may be supplemented with stress testing, stress radiographs, bone scan, arthrography, magnetic resonance imaging (MRI), and arthroscopy ***when necessary.*** Standard radiographs are taken to rule out injuries of the bone.

A. **Diagnosis.** A careful history of the mechanism of injury is important. The patient with an acute injury presents with pain, swelling, and restriction of joint motion. History of a "pop" or a tearing sensation in the wrist may be obtained. On physical examination, point tenderness may help in localizing the pathology. Both active and passive range of motion (ROM) should be recorded and compared with that of the opposite normal wrist. Provocative tests, such as the scaphoid shift (Watson's sign) and Reagan's Shuck test (See Appendix 6) may also help make the diagnosis.

B. **Investigations.** Radiographic evaluation of the athlete with suspected ligamentous injury of the wrist includes standard anteroposterior, lateral, and oblique views; lateral and anteroposterior stress views; and a clenched-fist posteroanterior view. We emphasize that comparison radiographs of the opposite normal wrist should be obtained.

A radioisotope bone scan may be indicated in cases where ligamentous injury is suspected but plain radiographs are normal. Arthrography is useful in detecting complete disruption of the intrinsic ligament. This is frequently combined with a cine study to evaluate carpal motion. MRI offers promise as a method of investigation for ligamentous injuries of the wrist. Computed tomography (CT) is of little help in ligamentous injuries but may be needed to evaluate accompanying bony lesions. ***We emphasize that radiological investigations should not be used as a substitute for a good history and physical examination.***

If the initial radiographs are negative but the injury appears to be major, it is important to obtain a specific diagnosis early and a further workup is indicated. A bone scan may be obtained to rule out occult fracture and arthrography may be used to rule out complete scapholunate or triquetrolunate ligament disruption. If these studies are not diagnostic, one may consider obtaining MRI scan or performing arthroscopy.

C. **Management.** If the injury appears to be relatively minor clinically, a splint is applied and the athlete is reexamined in 10 to 14 days. Partial tears of the scapholunate and triquetrolunate without bony injury or with mild injury of the extrinsic ligament may be treated expectantly. Most partial ligamentous tears will respond to 4 to 6 weeks of immobilization. The athlete may then be able to participate in sports using a splint.

II. Carpal Instabilities

A. **Classification.** Wrist instability patterns may be thought of simply as radial, ulnar, and midcarpal. The most common instability pattern is radial. The mechanism of injury is usually a fall on the outstretched hand, which affects the thenar eminence and involves dorsiflexion, ulnar deviation, and intercarpal supination stress. This injury may be associated with fracture of the scaphoid and triquetrum (injury of the greater arc). Ulnar instability or insufficiency of the triquetrolunate ligament may be the result of a reverse Mayfield lesion due to impact on the hypothenar eminence with initial injury of the triquetrolunate ligament. Midcarpal instability (nondissociative) is frequently caused by repetitive activities, and in many instances no history of trauma is given. It is thought to result from insufficiency in the ulnar portion of the capitotriquetral ligament.

B. **Diagnosis.** Wrist instability in a chronic setting may present as aching pain in the wrist and forearm. This type of pain increases with repetitive sports activities and decreases with rest. Point tenderness is most important in attempting to localize pathology. In all cases, range of motion, both active and passive, should be noted and compared with that of the opposite wrist. Provocative tests, such as the scaphoid shift (Watson's sign) for scapholunate dissociation and Reagan's shuck test evaluates the triquetrolunate ligament; are more reliable in assessing chronic instability (see Appendix 6). A "catch-up clunk" test for midcarpal instability has also been described and is the hallmark of this syndrome. Radiographic investigation such as cinearthrography are most important in diagnosing chronic instability.

C. **Management of specific instabilities**

1. **Scapholunate instability.** In cases of grade III scapholunate disruption, open repair of the torn ligaments with pinning is the standard treatment for the acute injury. This procedure may be performed as long as anatomic reduction is possible, particularly in the first 9 months postinjury. In late cases, dorsal capsulodesis in addition to primary repair has been advised. The criteria for the capsulodesis also demand that the carpus be reducible.
2. **Triquetrolunate instability.** Repair of the lunotriquetral ligament in acute cases or lunotriquetral arthrodesis may be indicated in cases of triquetrolunate instability, although results of these procedures are less predictable. Athletes undergoing limited arthrodesis or reconstruction procedures usually do not obtain maximum strength and range of motion for 6 to 12 months, but limited sports participation with protective splinting may be possible at 3 to 4 months. In all cases, a complete discussion with the athlete of the expected residual wrist range of motion following reconstruction and the possible limitation this may impose regarding return to sport is mandatory.

D. **Dislocations of the carpus.** Most carpal dislocations occur secondary to dorsiflexion, ulnar deviation, and intercarpal supination and represent stage 4 of Mayfield's progressive perilunar instability scheme. This injury pattern results in either dorsal perilunate dislocation or volar lunate dislocation—severe injuries that require urgent attention. Diagnosis is best made on a true lateral radiograph of the wrist. The injury represents disruption of the scapholunate and triquetrolunate ligaments, the volar radioscapholunate ligament, and, usually, the dorsal extrinsic ligaments. Goal of treatment is attainment of anatomic reduction as rapidly as possible. Successful closed reductions in acute perilunate dislocations have been documented in professional football players. In many cases, open reduction, ligament repair, and pin fixation is required. In dislocation of the carpus or significant injuries with open reduction and repairs performed, return to sport is not recommended for 3 to 6 months.

III. Fractures

A. **Fracture of the distal radius.** Distal radial fractures comprise 8% to 15% of all bone injuries and are commonly seen in athletes. The mechanism of injury is a fall on the outstretched hand, which causes dorsal displacement of the distal fragment. Intraarticular fractures have been classified and guidelines for treatment outlined. Closed reduction and cast immobilization is the traditional method of treatment for fractures of the distal radius; however, open reduction and internal fixation, external fixation, and, most recently, arthroscopic reduction with internal fixation are other methods that may be employed. The goal of treatment is to restore normal anatomy as closely as possible, particularly in the young athlete. In the athlete, it is important to obtain reduction by whatever means necessary to minimize radial shortening, radial inclination, and palmar inclination and to anatomically reduce any intraarticular component.

B. **Fracture of ulna.** The most common ulnar fracture is a nightstick fracture caused by a direct blow. These fractures are usually seen in hockey, lacrosse, or the martial arts. They are usually isolated fractures of the distal two-thirds of the bone and are stable. Immobilization in a Munster cast for 2 to 4 weeks followed by functional bracing is usually the treatment of choice. Stress fracture of the ulna has been reported in racquet sports players and baseball pitchers. Stress fracture should be suspected in cases of isolated specific tenderness on the ulna. Plain radiographs are frequently normal, and diagnosis is made by bone scan. These fractures may displace if the athlete continues to participate in sports. Treatment is rest until clinical and radiographic healing occurs. Displaced ulnar fractures are frequently seen in high-energy sports such as motor races and cycling and, occasionally, in contact sports. A Monteggia injury must be suspected in any displaced proximal ulnar fracture, and careful evaluation of the patient's elbow, radiographically and clinically, is indicated.

C. **Fracture of the scaphoid.** Fracture of the scaphoid is the most common and problematic fracture of the wrist in an athlete. The incidence of scaphoid fracture among college-level football players has been reported to be as high as 1% players per year.

   1. **History, physical examination, and radiographs.** The fracture usually occurs secondary to falls or contact with another player and has been described in football, soccer, boxing, and basketball. The mechanism of injury is usually forced hyperextension with the wrist in ulnar deviation. Scaphoid fractures are frequently misdiagnosed as "wrist sprains," and this results in a delayed diagnosis. Patients usually present with wrist pain localized to the radial aspect of the wrist. On physical examination, localized tenderness and swelling over the anatomic snuffbox may be noted. Radiographic assessment should include posteroanterior, lateral and a scaphoid views (anteroposterior view with 30 degrees of supination and ulnar deviation).
   2. **Classification and treatment.** For practical purposes, fractures of the scaphoid can be divided into acute nondisplaced stable fractures, displaced unstable fractures (including proximal third/proximal pole fractures), delayed union, and established nonunion.

      Acute nondisplaced fractures of the scaphoid may present a diagnostic challenge as the fracture line is frequently not visible on initial radiographs. In patients in whom the initial radiographs are negative and fracture of the scaphoid is still clinically suspected, a thumb spica splint should be applied and radiographs should be repeated in 2 weeks, when the fracture line may become visible. However, in an athlete, it is important to establish an early definitive diagnosis; to do this, a bone scan, 48 to 72 hr after injury, may be helpful. MRI scans may be of benefit but are expensive and should not be routinely ordered.

      Nondisplaced stable fractures are defined as fractures with less than 1 mm displacement and also as those fractures in which one cortex appears intact on a radiograph. Such a fracture may be treated by immobilization, with a union rate of 90% to 100%. The average time to union is usually 10 weeks if the fracture is treated acutely. If the diagnosis is delayed by more than 6 weeks, the healing time increases to 20 to 24 weeks. The optimum position of immobilization is slight radial deviation and palmar flexion at the wrist. A Munster-type cast may be used for 4 to 6 weeks, followed by a short arm thumb spica for 4 weeks. Some surgeons prefer to use a short arm thumb spica or a short arm cast from the outset.

Nondisplaced stable fractures in in-season athletes may present a problem if conventional treatment is carried out in that at least 10 to 12 weeks of sports participation is missed. Alternatives of treatment are (1) use of a playing cast for sports in which a cast is permitted and (2) surgery (open reduction and internal fixation—ORIF) followed by rehabilitation with an emphasis on regaining early ROM to facilitate early return to sports.

Although nondisplaced fractures of the scaphoid are usually treated by casting, ORIF using a Herbert screw may be used for patients with acute middle-third scaphoid fractures. This technique allows the athletes to return to sports as early as 5 to 7 weeks after the operation. We recommend that the treatment alternatives be discussed in detail with the athlete and family before making treatment decisions.

Acute displaced fractures are defined as fractures with 1 mm or greater displacement, more than 60 degrees of scapholunate angulation, or more than 15 degrees of lunocapitate angulation as seen on either plain radiographs or tomography. Potential for instability exists if the fracture line crosses both cortices. Acute displaced scaphoid fracture can be treated by closed reduction and cast immobilization if an acceptable reduction can be achieved and maintained. The union rate in unstable fractures treated by cast immobilization is 50% to 60%. If the fracture is diagnosed and treated early and union occurs, these fractures usually unite by 20 to 22 weeks. If the diagnosis is delayed, the union time is doubled and immobilization is of questionable value.

If an accurate reduction of the fracture cannot be obtained, other methods of treatment such as closed reduction and percutaneous pinning and ORIF should be considered. Immobilization following ORIF of the acute scaphoid fracture varies from 1 to 6 weeks, depending on the stability of fixation and the presence of associated injuries. Return to sports after an average of 7 to 8 weeks following ORIF is possible, although protective splinting is recommended for 2 to 3 months.

Ununited fractures of the scaphoid usually lead to progressive radiocarpal and intercarpal arthrosis. A symptomatic delayed or nonunion is an indication for surgery with bone grafting (with or without internal fixation) in order to obtain union. Union rates of 85% to 97% have been reported after grafting for stable scaphoid nonunions. Electrical stimulation has been proposed as an adjunct in the treatment of nonunion of the scaphoid fractures. Unfortunately, no prospective studies have been reported in the literature to support its efficacy.

Controversy still exists regarding the treatment of an ***asymptomatic delayed union or nonunion*** of scaphoid fracture. Bone grafting and internal fixation in a young athlete has been suggested based on natural history studies. The options of treatment must be discussed in detail with the athlete and his or her family.

Fractures of the proximal pole of the scaphoid have a higher incidence of delayed union, nonunion, and avascular necrosis. In patients with a nonunion following a fracture of the proximal pole of the scaphoid, bone grafting may be performed if the proximal fragment is large. However, if the proximal fragment is too small for adequate internal fixation and bone grafting, excision of the proximal fragment is performed and the resultant gap may be filled with a soft tissue such as capsule or tendon.

D. **Fracture of the hook of hamate.** Fracture of the hook of hamate is commonly seen in baseball players, tennis players, and golfers. It is felt that the fracture results from repetitive stresses with the bat, racquet, or golf club impinging on the hypothenar eminence.

1. **History, physical examination and investigations.** The diagnosis should be suspected in such an athlete (as mentioned above) presenting with ulnar wrist pain. On physical examination, tenderness over the hook of the hamate or dorsal aspect of the hamate may be elicited. Plain radiographs are usually negative. A carpal tunnel view or a 20-degree supinated oblique view may be helpful. Definitive diagnosis can be made by a bone or a CT scan.
2. **Treatment.** If this fracture is left untreated, the athlete may have persistent hypothenar pain and may sustain complications such as flexor tendon rupture or ulnar nerve dysfunction. Cast immobilization (from 6 to 12 weeks) may be used to obtain union. Our experience with immobilization even for incomplete fractures (as shown by CT scan) has been that all have failed to heal. Most authors recommend excision of the fractured hook fragment as the treatment of choice, with return to sports in an average of 7 weeks after surgery.

IV. Ulnocarpal Abutment Syndrome

Ulnocarpal abutment syndrome is common in sports involving repetitive flexion, extension, or radial and ulnar deviation activities or sports in which axial loading stresses are placed on the upper extremity.

Ulnocarpal abutment refers to impingement of the distal ulna on the ulnar aspect of the carpus primarily at the ulnar aspect of the lunate and lunotriquetral region.

Athletes are predisposed to ulnocarpal abutment syndrome if they have a positive ulnar variance, defined as a 1 to 2 mm increased length of the ulna versus the radius on a 0-degree rotation PA roentgenogram. Athletes may obtain a developmental positive ulnar deformity due to repetitive stresses on the distal radial physis, causing early closure of the physis and overgrowth of the distal ulna. This is most commonly seen in gymnasts.

The patients usually have diffuse ulnar wrist pain and tenderness in the ulnocarpal interval. Frequently a click is noted as a coexisting triangular fibrocartilage tear may be present.

A. **Radiographic findings.** Evaluation of this begins with a 0-degree rotation PA roentgenogram to look for a positive ulnar variance, as discussed above. Other studies such as wrist arthrography to evaluate the triangular fibrocartilage and the triquetrolunate articulation, which may also be secondarily affected by ulnocarpal abuttment. Bone scan and MRI may also be obtained to further evaluate pathology.

Wrist arthroscopy is an important diagnostic tool to evaluate chondromalacia of the lunate and lunotriquetral instability in cases of ulnocarpal abutment.

B. **Treatment.** Treatment of ulnocarpal abutment involves initially splinting and rest from the sport. If the athlete is unable to continue the sport, an ulnar shortening procedure (either of the Felden wafer type or a formal Milch type) may be indicated to relieve stresses at the ulnocarpal interval. The athlete may usually return to sports following such a procedure after rehabilitation period of 3 to 6 months. However, the fact that these procedures may be career-ending should be discussed with the athlete.

V. Kienböck's Disease

Fracture of the lunate is rare, although Kienböck's disease is not uncommon in an athlete. Kienböck's disease is essentially an avascular necrosis of the lunate. The precise cause of this condition and a universally accepted treatment are not yet well established. History of trauma may or may not be present. An association with Kienböck's disease and wrists with a negative ulnar variance has been reported. In such patients, the articular surface of the distal ulna is proximal to that of the distal radius. An athlete may present with wrist pain as well as decreased grip strength and ROM of the wrist.

A. **Radiographs.** In the early stages of the disease, plain radiographs may reveal no changes in the lunate, but a negative ulnar variance may be seen. In late stages of the disease, sclerosis, cyst formation, fragmentation, and collapse of the lunate with loss of carpal height and secondary degenerative changes in the wrist are seen.

B. **Treatment.** Treatment of Kienböck's disease is complex and depends upon the stage of disease and the degree of carpal collapse that has occurred at the time of diagnosis. Surgery (shortening of the radius or lengthening of the ulna) has proven effective in early cases (prior to collapse of the lunate) in patients with a negative ulnar variance.

In more advanced stages of the disease, treatment modalities include various types of intercarpal arthrodesis or excision of the lunate with either soft tissue interposition or silicone replacement arthroplasty. In patients with end-stage disease, salvage procedures such as proximal row carpectomy or wrist arthrodesis may be performed.

VI. Optional

A. **Protective splinting.** Protective splinting for injuries to the wrist and hand is an integral part of preparing athletes for a return to sports. With use of protective splinting, it is possible to allow an early return to sports while minimizing the risk of recurrent injury. Adequate rehabilitation should be undertaken before allowing athletes to return to sports. The three main factors that need to be considered in this regard are (1) the type and severity of the injury; (2) the type of sport, level of competition, and position played by the athlete; and (3) regulations governing the type of splinting allowed. Athletic trainers and physicians should familiarize themselves with local regulations concerning the use of protective splints because these regulations may vary among high schools and colleges as well as among school districts.

Rigid or semirigid splints may be used. Examples of the rigid types of splints used are orthoplast or other moldable firm materials, fiberglass casts, and metal splints. Semirigid splints include RTV-11, silicone rubber materials, 3M Scotch casts, and leather supports.

The reinjury rate from the use of both rigid and semirigid playing casts has been negligible. Results of a questionnaire circulated among National Football League (NFL) team physicians showed that no injuries to other individuals were attributable to the cast and there were no significant reinjuries to the protected part. A similar questionnaire returned by National Collegiate Athletics Association (NCAA) division I athletic trainers and physicians revealed that no injuries were sustained in athletes who played with a splint and no injuries to other players were caused by the use of the rigid playing cast. At the high school level, as of 1994, the National Federation of Official Football Rules state that rigid devices are allowed if covered by $^1/_2$ in. closed-cell foam. De Carlo and associates surveyed 148 high school football players who used RTV-11 casts while playing sports. Of the 87 patients responding to the survey, 85 reported good or excellent results with the use of RTV-11 cast.

The lion's paw leather splint is useful for the gymnast. It prevents maximum dorsiflexion of the wrist and cushions dorsiflexion stress. The Nirschl wrist brace may be used primarily for tennis players. It prevents the extremes of wrist motion and is an excellent device for the player returning to sports following an injury.

Acknowledgment

The authors thank Robyn Fitzgerald, RN, Research Coordinator at the Methodist Sports Medicine Center, Indianapolis, Indiana, for her editorial assistance on this manuscript.

Suggested Reading

De Carlo M, Darmelio J, Rettig AC, et al. Perfecting a playing cast for hand and wrist injuries. *Phys Sports Med* 1992; 20:95–104.

Melone CP Jr. Unstable fractures of the distal radius. In: DM Lichtman, ed. *The wrist and its disorders.* Philadelphia: WB Saunders, 1988:160–177.

Mooney JF III, Siegel DB, Koman LA. Ligamentous injuries of the wrist in athletes. *Clin Sports Med* 1992; 11:129–139.

Rettig AC, Adsit WS. Athletic injuries of the hand and wrist. In: LY Griffin, ed. *Orthopedic knowledge update: sports medicine.* Rosemont, IL: American Academy of Orthopaedic Surgeons, 1994:205–224.

Taleisnik J. Post-traumatic carpal instability. *Clin Orthop* 1980; 149:73–82.

44. THE WRIST AND HAND—SOFT TISSUES

Frank C. McCue III and Andrew M. Schuett

I. Triangular Fibrocartilage (TFC)

tears are difficult to diagnose because of their complicated anatomy. The TFC spans the lunate fossa from the radius to the ulna and up the edges of the ulnar wrist and fifth metacarpal. The TFC is considered part of the larger triangular fibrocartilage complex (TFCC), which includes the ulnar meniscus homologue, ulnar collateral ligament, dorsal and volar radioulnar ligaments, ulnotriquetral ligament, ulnolunate ligament, and extensor carpi ulnaris tendon sheath. In simple terms, the TFCC serves as a sling supporting the distal ulnar carpus and radius from the distal ulna. The TFCC is thickened along its volar and dorsal surfaces and it becomes thin in the lunar region. The central and radial aspects are known to be avascular and to heal poorly when injured. The peripheral region is vascular and portends better healing potential.

TFCC tears must be differentiated from radiocarpal and midcarpal complaints. A detailed history and physical examination can help localize the symptoms to the correct anatomic region.

The most common mechanism of injury involves wrist extension and hyperpronation of the forearm. History will usually include a fall on the outstretched hand, which initiates symptom production. The athlete should be encouraged to describe when and with what motion of the wrist the pain recurs. On physical examination, an attempt should be made to reproduce the exact position that localizes the pain.

In acute injuries, swelling, crepitance, instability of the ulnar head, and pain on volar compression of the ulna will be noted. In chronic injuries, these problems become more difficult to localize, and palpation tenderness may be the only clue to diagnosis. A "painful clunk" on passive repositioning of a dorsally subluxed ulna is often noted.

Radiographic evaluation should include the wrist and hand. Occasionally, the forearm and elbow will need to be seen. Wrist views consist of a true posteroanterior (PA) view with the shoulder abducted 90 degrees, elbow flexed to 90 degrees, and hand flat on the cassette. When this view is obtained appropriately, the radial and ulnar styloids should be at the extreme medial and lateral edges of the x-ray, with no overlap. Additionally, a lateral view of the wrist is obtained. The shoulder is positioned at 0 degrees abduction with the elbow flexed to 90 degrees and the thumb up. The cassette is positioned lateral to the wrist.

If plain films do not uncover an abnormality and the diagnosis is still suspected, computed tomography (CT) can be performed. The CT scan is the most reliable method of assessing for distal radioulnar joint congruence and avoids the rotational problems commonly seen in initial postinjury views of the wrist. Degenerative tears of the TFCC can be diagnosed via arthrography or magnetic resonance imaging (MRI). Direct visualization, via arthroscopy, is used when the above modalities are unsuccessful. In these instances, arthroscopic evaluation can be used as both a diagnostic and therapeutic procedure. It is especially helpful in the evaluation of synovitis and chondromalacia and it can confirm the ulnocarpal impaction syndrome. Bone scan has also been used to diagnose arthrosis in the wrist region.

Palmer has proposed a broad classification system of TFCC pathology with basic traumatic and degenerative categories. This scheme helps with treatment intervention. Green feels the athlete with an acute TFCC tear should be managed in a long arm cast for 4 to 6 weeks regardless of the time in the season. Injuries not responding to splints and nonsteroidal antinflammatory drugs (NSAIDs) should be treated with surgery. The procedure should address the specific function disrupted.

Generally, open or arthroscopic intervention should tend toward conservative TFCC debridement, especially with horizontal tears. Avulsions and midsubstance tears, which have been reapproximated, should be immobilized postoperatively for 4 to 6 weeks. Degenerative lesions—leading to ulnar impingement, radioulnar dissociation or ulnocarpal arthrosis—can be treated with ulnar shortening procedures.

II. Tendinitis

A. **DeQuervain's tenosynovitis** affects the abductor pollicis longus (APL) and the extensor pollicis brevis (EPB). This condition is usually associated with athletic or occupationally related repetitive hand and wrist motion. Physical examination can reveal a positive ***Finklestein's test*** (the thumb is flexed and abducted, followed by ulnar wrist deviation, producing pain over the first dorsal compartment at the wrist). In addition, pain and swelling may be elicited in the region of the radius without a provocative test. Generalized pain in the radial aspect of the wrist along with a positive Finklestein's test is highly suggestive of this entity.

Conservative management consists of rest, splinting, and NSAIDs. If the diagnosis is made early in the pathologic process, the chance of successful nonoperative treatment and return to sports is good. In more advanced and recalcitrant cases, steroid injection into the tendon sheath and rest can effect a cure. Steroid injection into the tendon can produce disruption. If the condition becomes chronic or does not respond to the above measures, surgical intervention becomes necessary. The procedure should include release of the EPB and APL hoods. The surgeon should look for possible anomalous anatomic variations that may be present in the APL. The most common cause of a poor surgical result is failure to release all slips of the APL tendon. Each slip must be identified and decompressed during the procedure.

B. **Extensor carpi ulnaris (ECU)** tendinitis results from inflammation within its fibroosseus canal at the wrist. Although not as common as DeQuervain's, it exists as a distinct pathologic entity. Anatomically, with forearm supination, the ECU tendon rests on the dorsal aspect of the forearm. Following pronation, the ECU tendon remains fixed to the ulnar aspect of the wrist and functions as a wrist adductor. When grasping objects, the wrist is stabilized by the ECU tendon. The ECU tendon inserts onto the fifth metacarpal. The canal of the sixth dorsal compartment is rather unyielding and, as in DeQuervain's, can have calcific deposits. When thickening of the canal does occur, a chronic stenosing tenosynovitis is produced. This requires surgical decompression. Fusiform enlargement of the tendon just distal to the site of decompression can be seen. Postoperatively, the time period until the patient becomes asymptomatic may vary. A trial of conservative therapy including rest, splinting, NSAIDs, and possibly steroid injections should be tried prior to surgical intervention.

C. **Flexor carpi ulnaris (FCU)** tendinitis is a relatively common entity. As in the case of DeQuervain's tenosynovitis, chronic repetitive trauma is the most common etiology. FCU tendinitis can occur bilaterally. Radiographic evaluation is usually noncontributory except in the small percentage of cases where calcification of the tendon may be present. Physical examination reveals pain with resisted flexion and ulnar deviation of the wrist. Occasionally, there is pain directly over the tendon on the palmar aspect of the wrist. Conservative treatment includes splint immobilization, avoidance of the aggravating activity, NSAIDs, and steroid injection. Most cases will improve with nonoperative management; however, recalcitrant cases require surgical intervention. Intraoperatively, a search for an offending calcium deposit or peritendonous adhesion is prudent. Occasionally, pisiform excision is required. If the FCU tendon is damaged or has been severed from its insertion, repair is required.

D. **Flexor carpi radialis (FCR)** tendinitis is less common than that of the FCU. Most commonly, the cause is repetitive trauma. Physical examination reveals tenderness and crepitus over the tendon. Pain is present on resisted flexion of the wrist. Nonoperative management, outlined above for FCU tendinitis, usually suffices. If a recalcitrant case of FCR tendinitis is encountered, surgical decompression of the fibroosseus tunnel is necessary.

E. **Extensor pollicis longus (EPL)** tendinitis may occur as an isolated entity. Usually, hypertrophic changes on the dorsal surface of the distal radius at Lister's tubercle precipitates the tenosynovitis. The dorsal exostosis can be a secondary manifestation of previous fracture of the distal radius. Attritional rupture of the EPL tendon may occur. EPL rupture produces the inability to extend the thumb at the interphalangeal joint. Radiographic evaluation usually shows the dorsal exostosis. It is best seen on the lateral view. Early surgical intervention directed toward excision of the dorsal bony prominence or EPL rerouting are the procedures of choice.

III. Nerve

A. **Carpal tunnel syndrome** is the most common compressive neuropathy associated with sporting activities. Any sport that involves repetitive motion or grasping with the hand can be contribute to its development. An increased incidence is noted especially in cyclists, throwers, and tennis players. A history of a fall producing wrist hyperextension or a Colles fracture may be significant. Many patients have associated flexor digit tenosynovitis. Symptoms include pain and paresthesias in the radial $3^1/_2$ fingers which frequently becomes worse at night. Pain may progress proximally to the shoulder. Chronic symptoms include weakness of pinch and grip. Pathognomonic clinical findings include a positive ***Tinel's sign*** over the median nerve at the wrist. This test is performed by tapping the median nerve as passes to the carpal canal on the palmar aspect of the transverse wrist crease. It produces a "shooting" sensation to the long and index fingers when positive. In addition, a positive ***Phalen's test*** is produced by palmar flexing the wrist to 60 degrees or more for 30 to 60 sec, recreating the patient's symptoms. When Tinel's test is inconclusive, a positive Phalen's test may be diagnostic. Other findings on physical examination include a mild flattening of the thenar eminence and decreased two-point discrimination in the median nerve distribution.

Electromyographic (EMG) and nerve conduction velocity (NCV) studies are considered the gold-standard tests for delayed median nerve conduction across the carpal tunnel. These tests are recommended prior to any surgical intervention.

Treatment may be conservative or surgical, depending on many factors including acuity, sport, hand dominance, symptoms, and severity. Conservative management includes avoidance of causative activities and splinting with the wrist in slight extension. Steroid injection into the carpal canal may also be beneficial in acute injuries. Most patients with symptoms due to repetitive trauma respond well to conservative treatment. Flexor tendon rupture due to poor technique is an avoidable iatrogenic complication. If the athlete continues to have sensory loss, symptom persistence, or muscle atrophy after 8 to 12 weeks of conservative therapy, surgery is necessary. Surgical release of the transverse carpal ligament via open incision or arthroscopy is also needed when conservative measures fail. Arthroscopic release should not be undertaken by the inexperienced arthroscopist. Various authors report good long-term results in 90% to 95% of cases treated via open techniques. Return to sports is guided by adequate return of hand and forearm strength along with abatement of symptoms. It is not unusual for symptoms to continue for up to 1 year after surgical release. The reason for this is not well understood at this time.

B. **Guyon's tunnel (cyclist's palsy) syndrome** is the ulnar nerve equivalent of median nerve compression at the wrist. It can be seen in conjunction with carpal tunnel syndrome and presents with paresthesias throughout all five fingers.

The ulnar nerve runs between the pisiform and hook of the hamate through Guyon's canal. The floor is formed by the transverse carpal ligament and the roof by the palmar fascia and palmaris brevis muscle. The mechanism of injury is thought to be direct compression on the ulnar nerve. This entity is commonly present among competitive cyclists. Physical examination will reveal paresthesias of the ulnar 1 1/2 digits with or without intrinsic muscle weakness and atrophy.

Associated causative conditions include ulnar artery aneurysms, fractures of the hook of the hamate, tumor, synovial cysts, and lipomas. Symptomatology depends on the point at which the ulnar nerve is compressed. Involvement of the deep terminal branch represents the most common form of ulnar nerve compression at the wrist. In this type, compression occurs distal to the hypothenar muscle branch. Physical examination reveals motor weakness to all the ulnar-innervated hand muscles except the hypothenars.

Two other forms of ulnar nerve compression at the wrist have been reported. One involves compression just proximal to Guyon's canal. Physical exam will include the above findings plus hypothenar muscle weakness. The second, less common variation is superficial terminal branch compression. This type can be seen with fractures of the hook of hamate and ulnar artery aneurysms, usually causing sensory loss only.

EMGs and NCVs help localize the exact site of compression and direct surgical intervention. Primary treatment should be avoidance of the symptom-producing activity. Cyclists may benefit from increased padding in their gloves and handlebars. When conservative treatment measures have failed or symptoms worsen, operative treatment is called for.

IV. Epiphysitis

occurs most commonly in the growth plate of the distal radius in gymnasts. Radiographs may show widening of the growth plate in the radius with haziness and breaking of the radial and volar aspects, pointing toward the epiphyseal plate. Cystic metaphyseal changes may also be seen. Some investigators feel that these changes are stress-related and may, in fact, be Salter-Harris type 1 or 5 fractures. Radiographic changes involving the distal ulnar growth plate have, in addition, been noted in some reports. Delayed skeletal maturation with development of a Madelung-type deformity has been discussed. This abnormality can be associated with positive ulnar variance, producing symptoms of secondary ulnar impingement.

Overuse is thought to produce delayed growth of the distal radius and, less commonly, the ulna. Development of wrist pain in the skeletally immature athlete accentuates the need for practical application of a conservative individualized training regimen. Any skeletally immature athlete with wrist pain and a suggestive history should undergo radiographic evaluation. Abnormality of the distal radial or ulnar growth plate should be treated with rest and immobilization for a minimum of 3 months. Evaluation of the elbow should be strongly considered in these cases.

Alternative cross-training techniques can be utilized during the period of relative wrist inactivity. When the patient is asymptomatic, a gradual return to the preinjury activity is advised. Serial radiographic and physical examination should be considered for up to 1 year after diagnosis and longer if a radiographic abnormality or pain persists.

V. Extensor Carpi Ulnaris Instability (ECU)

is characterized by a painful snap over the ulnodorsal aspect of the wrist with forearm rotation. Subluxation of the ECU tendon is rarely due to an acute injury. The usual mechanism of injury involves traumatic forearm hypersupination with or without ulnar deviation and palmar flexion; a meticulous history usually reveals the cause. ECU instability usually results from a tear in the extensor retinaculum over the sixth dorsal compartment. Most cases are caused by a single traumatic episode that occurred in the distant past. On physical examination, the wrist is placed in supination with ulnar deviation followed by wrist flexion, producing an audible snap. Pronation of the wrist relocates the tendon into its normal position. ECU instability occurs most often in tennis players, though it has been reported in golfers, weight lifters, bronco riders, and football players. ECU instability is usually evaluated as a subacute or chronic problem. Treatment consists of wrist immobilization in pronation and radial deviation for 3 to 4 weeks. If a significant history of recurrent subluxation is present or conservative treatment fails, operative intervention should be considered. Various surgical procedures have been described, including reconstruction of the extensor tendon sheath, removal of the ulnar ridge, and partial debridement of the sheath. Return to sports is possible in 4 to 8 weeks, depending on the type of surgery performed. Rehabilitation is directed toward initial postoperative control of pain and swelling. When the wound has healed active and active-assisted range-of-motion exercises should be started. Strengthening the wrist in resistive supination constitutes the final phase of the protocol.

Suggested Reading

Cabrera JM, McCue FC III. Nonosseous injuries of the elbow, forearm, and hand. *Clin Sports Med* 1986;6:681–699.

Green DP. *Operative hand surgery.* 3rd ed. Churchill-Livingstone, 1993;1598–1600.

Nicholas JA, Hershman EB. *The upper extremity in sports medicine,* 2nd ed. 1995; 478–481.

Palmer AK. Triangular fibrocartilage complex lesions: a classification, *J Hand Surg* 1989;14A:14–28.

Wood MB, Dobyns JH. Sports-related extraarticular wrist syndromes. *Clin Ortho* 1986;202:93–103.

45. THE HAND AND FINGERS

Charles P. Melone, Jr. and Sharon L. Hame

Trauma to the hand accounts for nearly one-third of all sports-related injuries. Frequently dismissed as trivial incidents, hand injuries are now recognized as a cause of major disability that can be prevented if prompt detection and precision treatment is rendered.

An accurate diagnosis begins with a precise history. Most patients initially report that they suffered a "jammed finger," a lay term that should be disregarded. An exact account of the event and the sport the athlete was engaged in helps the examiner define the injury. The clinical findings in hand injuries may include swelling, tenderness, and deformity making the diagnosis apparent. However, serious ligamentous injuries including dislocations may not present with obvious deformity. Meticulous examination including range-of-motion and stress testing will reveal subtle malrotations, angulations, and instabilities.

Radiographic evaluation is the key to an accurate diagnosis in bone and joint injuries to the hand. Posteroanterior, oblique, and lateral radiographs are essential to assess the extent of bone and joint displacement and angulation. Additionally, stress radiographs may demonstrate complete ligamentous disruption.

Most bone and joint injuries of the hand can be treated successfully by noninvasive techniques. However, injuries resulting in serious bone and ligament disruption such as fracture dislocations often require operative repair for preservation of bony alignment and joint stability. Injuries associated with soft tissue damage require prompt care, including soft tissue debridement and meticulous skin closure.

I. Metacarpal Fractures

A. **Anatomy.** The metacarpals are the long bones of the hand that articulate with the carpal bones proximally and the proximal phalanges distally at the metacarpophalangeal (MP) joint. The proximal phalanges provide the insertion for the MP joint's collateral ligaments, which are taut in flexion and relaxed in extension. The metacarpals are joined by the transverse carpal ligament and fan out like the spokes of a wheel. The dorsal and volar interosseus muscles originate from the shaft of the metacarpal and generate the deforming forces on the metacarpals when fractures occur.

B. **Classification.** Metacarpal fractures are categorized by both the level and configuration of the fracture plane. Accordingly, they can be classified as fractures involving the head, neck, shaft, and base of the bone with the fracture plane oriented in a transverse, oblique, or spiral pattern. Furthermore, they need to be defined as stable fractures with minimal displacement or unstable fractures characterized by excessive displacement or fragmentation. Whereas the stable fractures have an excellent prognosis for uncomplicated healing, requiring a 3 to 4 week period of splinting or cast immobilization, the unstable fractures often necessitate surgical treatment to restore normal skeletal alignment and ensure a favorable outcome. The nature of the sport the athlete participates in will determine the time the athlete may return. However, in general, it is recommended that the fracture be healed prior to splint-free participation.

1. **Metacarpal head fractures** most commonly occur in the second finger. Since they are intraarticular fractures disrupting the MP joint, they require anatomic reduction for optimal recovery. In some cases this can be accomplished with closed reduction and internal fixation, in others, open reduction and internal fixation is the only means of skeletal restitution.
2. **Metacarpal neck fractures** including those of the fifth metacarpal are traditionally termed ***boxer's** fractures* but rarely occur in professional

boxers. They tend to angulate dorsally, have volar comminution, and, as a result, are quite unstable. Fractures of the neck of second and third metacarpals necessitate an anatomic reduction to maintain function and cosmesis of the hand. Due to the compensatory motion at the base of the fourth and fifth metacarpals, an increased amount of dorsal angulation may be acceptable in neck fractures of the fourth and fifth metacarpals. Closed reduction and percutaneous pinning has been a consistently successful treatment for unstable angulated metacarpal neck fractures.

3. **Metacarpal shaft fractures** may be transverse, spiral, oblique, or comminuted. Transverse fractures commonly occur by a direct blow to the shaft. Dorsal angulation occurs secondary to the volar force exerted by the interosseus muscles. Spiral oblique fractures occur as a result of a torque force, with the finger acting as a lever arm. Consequently, they may shorten and malrotate. As a general rule, no angulation or rotation should be accepted; therefore, closed or open reduction with internal fixation is often required.
4. **Metacarpal base fractures** with the exception of the thumb metacarpal are usually stable. Slight malrotation, however, may lead to a large deformity at the finger and must be detected and corrected by reduction with internal fixation.

C. **Bennett's fracture-dislocation.** A Bennett's fracture is a fracture of the base of the thumb metacarpal that extends into the carpometacarpal joint. It characteristically comprises (1) a small, nondisplaced ulnar fragment still attached to the carpal trapezium by the deep ulnar ligament and (2) the metacarpal shaft displaced proximally by the pull of the abductor pollicis longus, attached to its base. This results in fracture displacement and joint subluxation. Athletes will complain of pain, swelling, and deformity at the base of the thumb. Because these fractures are very unstable, they require internal stabilization. Closed reduction is attempted; if this is successful, internal fixation is used to maintain the reduction. Unsuccessful attempts necessitate open reduction and internal fixation. Generally, athletes requiring use of the thumb may return to sports in 10 to 12 weeks. However, protective splinting may be required.

D. **Reverse Bennett's fracture (baby Bennett).** Fractures of the base of the fifth metacarpal deserve special consideration. The fracture fragments may be held in place by ligaments that attach to the fourth metacarpal and hamate. Any dorsal dislocation of the metacarpal must be identified. These fractures should be reduced and pinned, followed by 4 to 6 weeks of immobilization. Protection should continue for an additional 2 months, particularly while the patient is participating in athletic activities.

II. Phalangeal Fractures

A. **Fractures of the distal phalanges.** Distal phalangeal fractures can occur as tuft, shaft, or articular fractures. In general, they rarely require reduction or internal fixation. Tuft fractures are common and usually involve significant injury to the nail and nail bed. Subungual hematomas may occur and, if considerable, are optimally decompressed by removal of the nail. Nail bed injuries are also associated with phalangeal shaft fractures. Some of these fractures may require internal stabilization. Protective splints may be worn to ensure earlier return to sports for some athletes. Articular fractures may result in significant finger deformity and are included under joint injuries.

B. **Fractures of the middle and proximal phalanges**

1. **Classification.** Fractures of the middle and proximal phalanges are common in athletes. They may be divided into intra- and extraarticular types. Extraarticular fractures can be further subdivided into transverse, spiral or oblique, and comminuted fractures. Athletes will present with pain, tenderness, and deformity, including digital scissoring of the affected finger. Clinical examination as well as radiographs determine the stability of the fracture pattern.

2. **Treatment** of these fractures must be precise, as complications, especially residual joint stiffness, are common. Nondisplaced stable fractures can generally be treated with buddy taping to the adjacent finger. Unstable displaced fractures, commonly oblique or spiral, will require reduction, either closed or open, and internal fixation. Athletes may return to their sport without protective devices when fracture union is complete, after approximately 6 to 8 weeks. Comminuted fractures are associated with soft tissue injury and therefore lend themselves to external fixation. This allows for restoration of length and stability as well as healing of soft tissues.

C. **Condylar fractures** are articular fractures; they are common in athletes and often missed. Oblique radiographs are required to fully visualize the fracture and the amount of displacement. They can be divided into three types.

1. **Classification**
   a. **Type 1** is stable without displacement.
   b. **Type 2** is unicondylar and unstable.
   c. **Type 3** is bicondylar or comminuted.
2. **Treatment.** Displaced unicondylar fractures and bicondylar fractures are best treated operatively. They typically require open reduction and internal fixation.

III. Ligamentous Injuries and Dislocations

A. **Proximal interphalangeal (PIP) joints**

1. **Anatomy.** The stability of the PIP joint is provided by its articular anatomy and ligamentous structures. It is a hinge joint that allows an arc of motion of 100 degrees. The collateral ligaments, accessory collateral ligaments, and volar plate complex account for most of the joint's stability. These ligaments extend from a broad proximal origin and insert at the base of the middle phalanx. Additionally, the volar plate is reinforced by proximal extensions termed *check ligaments,* which impede hyperextension and also prevent rupture of the volar plate from its proximal phalangeal attachment.
2. **Collateral ligaments.** Injuries to the collateral ligaments may be partial or complete. Partial injuries show only mild laxity of the joint and a definite end point on stress testing. They may be treated with splinting in slight flexion until symptoms subside, followed by rehabilitation. No competition time will be lost if the athlete can be protected while participating. Complete ruptures show angular deformity or gross instability by gentle stress testing or subluxation on stress radiographs. These injuries are treated with prompt repair in an effort to minimize joint stiffness, residual instability, and reinjury. Chronic complete injury of a collateral ligament requires secondary repair or tendon graft reconstruction.
3. **Volar plate injury.** A volar plate injury should be suspected when a hyperextension injury results in pain, swelling, and tenderness at the volar aspect of the PIP joint. Clinical deformity and grossly abnormal radiographs are infrequent, whereas a small avulsion fracture detected on the lateral radiograph is a relatively common occurrence and is indicative of the injury. Splinting of the PIP joint in mild flexion, termed *extension block splinting,* coupled with early motion to prevent joint stiffness, has proved to be a highly successful treatment for these frequent injuries. Athletes may return to their sport unprotected when they are symptom-free. If such a lesion is left untreated, a swan-neck deformity may develop as a result of the joint's dorsal instability.
   a. **Dorsal dislocation** of the PIP joint without fracture, also known as a simple dislocation, can result from volar plate injuries. Excessive prominence of the middle phalanx on clinical examination and bayonet position of the phalanges on the lateral radiographs are the clas-

sic findings for this injury. The dislocation should be reduced after local block anesthesia by traction, mild hyperextension, and then direct pressure on the base of the middle phalanx. A stable reduction is obtained if a range of active motion of 20 to 90 degrees of flexion is achieved or no displacement occurs with gentle lateral stressing. Postreduction radiographs should be used to confirm the reduction. Once this has been done, the athlete is placed in an extension block splint for 3 weeks. Return to athletic participation is allowed after 3 weeks; however, buddy taping is suggested for continued protection of the joint.

b. **Dorsal fracture-dislocation.** When a hyperextension injury is combined with a compressive force, a ***dorsal fracture-dislocation*** of the PIP joint can occur. The stability of this injury is determined by the size of the fractured fragment at the base of the middle phalanx. Fragments involving less than one-third of the articular surface are considered stable and are treated as simple dislocations of the PIP joint with extension block splinting. Because the volar plate collateral ligament complex is severely disrupted in this injury and closed reduction is usually unsuccessful, fractures involving greater than one-third of the articular surface require open reduction and internal fixation. The minimum time to return to sports participation is approximately 6 weeks if surgery is required. Full-time buddy taping should continue until the end of the season. Clinical results are highly varied and decreased mobility of the joint can be expected.

4. **Volar PIP dislocations**

a. **Simple dislocations.** Unlike dorsal PIP dislocations, volar dislocations occur less frequently and are often overlooked. At close inspection, subtle malrotation of the finger may become evident. Furthermore, range-of-motion testing will demonstrate the athlete's inability to actively extend the PIP joint. Classically, the mechanism of injury involves a violent force applied to a flexed joint, resulting in rupture of a collateral ligament proximally followed by tearing of the extensor tendon's central slip at its insertion. Closed reduction is the treatment of choice. Splinting in extension is continued for approximately 6 weeks.

b. **Complex or rotatory dislocations.** In more violent injuries a second tear may also extend proximally between the central slip and the lateral band of the extensor mechanism adjacent to the ruptured collateral ligament. Consequently, the condyle of the proximal phalanx may protrude through the tear and cause volar displacement of the lateral band, which may become interposed between the proximal and middle phalanx, resulting in a ***complex or rotatory dislocation.*** Closed reduction is rarely successful; therefore open treatment is preferred. In the course of this, the lateral band can be dislodged atraumatically, the collateral ligaments and central slip repaired, and the joint located and pinned temporarily. The athlete is immobilized for 4 weeks. Following this, athletic participation is allowed with protection.

B. **Metacarpophalangeal (MP) joint**

1. **Anatomy.** The MP joint is shallow and condyloid in shape. It therefore depends on its collateral ligament–volar plate complex for stability. Its recessed position within the web space coupled with the protection afforded by adjacent fingers provides additional stability. The MP joint of the thumb, however, remains unprotected and is subject to frequent injury. Unlike that of the PIP joint, the volar plate of the MP joint permits hyperextension of the joint. It is thin proximally and not anchored by check ligaments. Sesamoid bones within the MP volar plate are found in the little finger, index finger, and thumb. Displacement of these small sesamoids within the MP joints as visualized on x-ray is a characteristic clue to a more serious dislocation.

2. **Collateral ligaments**
   a. **Thumb ulnar collateral ligament.** Although injury to the collateral ligament of the finger MP joints is uncommon, injury to the thumb's ulnar collateral ligament occurs frequently. Notoriously attributed to skiing, this injury occurs in all sports and is a result of forced abduction and dorsiflexion of the thumb at the MP joint. Most commonly a midsubstance tear, it is associated with injury to the dorsal capsule and the ulnar aspect of the volar plate as well as avulsion fractures of the ligamentous insertion at the volar base of the proximal phalanx.
      i. **Diagnosis.** The physical examination typically reveals swelling, tenderness, and the palpable mass of the torn collateral ligament at the ulnar aspect of the MP joint. A critical diagnostic distinction is that between the complete and partial or incomplete ligamentous disruption, since complete injuries usually require surgical repair whereas partial injuries generally heal with nonoperative treatment. Complete disruptions are distinguished by a difference of 30 degrees or more in lateral laxity between the injured and the uninjured thumb on comparative stress examinations. In addition, a 30% or greater subluxation of the joint on standardized stress radiography confirms the diagnosis of a complete tear.
      ii. **Treatment**
         (a) **Partial or incomplete tears** may be treated with 4 weeks of thumb spica cast immobilization followed by appropriate rehabilitation. Splinting is required during athletic activities to prevent excessive stress on the healing ligament.
         (b) **Complete tears.** Unlike incomplete tears, complete tears require early direct surgical repair. The ends of the disrupted ligament are prone to wide separation with interposition of adjacent soft tissue, particularly the adductor apponeurosis, as described by Stener. For most cases diagnosed within several weeks of injury, direct repair or ligament advancement to bone heals successfully. Athletes with chronic or irreparable ligamentous damage will require tendon graft reconstruction. Athletes should be immobilized for 4 to 6 weeks in a thumb spica cast. A splint is worn for an additional 2 weeks. Without protection, strenuous activities are not allowed for 10 to 12 weeks after surgery.
   b. **Radial Collateral ligament.** Although less frequent than tears of the ulnar collateral ligament, tears of the radial collateral ligaments of the thumb and finger MP joints do occur in the athlete. Injuries to the MP joints of the fingers occur with forced lateral deviation of the joint when in the flexed position. In this position the collateral ligaments are under maximum tension and vulnerable to rupture. Injury most commonly involves the radial collateral ligaments of the three ulnar fingers.
      i. **Diagnosis.** Clinically, patients have tenderness at the affected collateral ligament and pain with ulnar stress of the joint. If such an injury is suspected, radiographs of the injured joint should be carefully examined for avulsion fractures in the joint.
      ii. **Treatment.** For stable injuries, buddy taping the affected finger to the adjacent finger for 3 to 4 weeks allows for adequate range of motion and healing. Athletes can usually return to sports in several days if the finger is well protected. For injuries to the radial collateral ligament that result in obvious deformity, gross instability, or joint subluxation on the stress view, direct surgical repair of the ligament ensures the preservation of joint stability. Chronic cases may require delayed ligamentous repair or reconstruction.

3. **Dorsal dislocations.** Dorsal dislocations of the MP joint are caused by forced hyperextension of the digit, leading to rupture of the volar plate with interposition of its membranous portion between the dorsal metacarpal head and the volar base of the proximal phalanx. The taut medial and lateral structures prevent reduction. The index finger followed by the fifth finger are most commonly involved. The index finger's metacarpal head becomes entrapped by the lumbricals radially and the flexor tendons ulnarly. The fifth finger's MP joint is irreducible secondary to entrapment by the extensor digiti quinti and flexor digiti minimi ulnarly and the lumbricals and flexor tendons radially.
   a. **Classification.** Dorsal dislocations may be classified as simple or reducible and complex or irreducible.
      i. **Simple**
         (a) **Diagnosis.** In the simple type, the MP joint demonstrates a gross deformity with the proximal phalanx held in approximately 60–80 degrees of hyperextension. The volar plate, remaining with the proximal phalanx, is draped dorsally over the metacarpal head.
         (b) **Treatment.** A simple dislocation may be converted into a complex dislocation if the reduction technique is improper. No hyperextension or traction should be applied. Successful reduction is accomplished by first flexing the wrist and then applying steady pressure in a distal and volar direction over the dorsal base of the proximal phalanx. A short period of immobilization followed by active motion and buddy taping to prevent hyperextension has been very successful. Athletes may return to their sport when symptom free.
      ii. **Complex**
         (a) **Diagnosis.** In contrast to simple dislocations, complex dislocations demonstrate only a moderate extension deformity of the MP joint. The volarly displaced metacarpal head produces a palmar prominence and dorsal hollowing. Radiographs typically show a widened joint space. Visualization of sesamoid bones within the joint confirms the presence of volar plate interposition. Careful examination of the lateral radiograph may also reveal an osteochondral shearing fracture.
         (b) **Treatment.** Complex dislocations always require open reduction. The joint is approached volarly and the A1 pulley is released. The joint should then be immobilized in 30 degrees of flexion for 2 weeks, followed by a dorsal extension block splint for an additional 2 weeks. Free motion and return to sports with protection is allowed after 4 weeks. Recovery is most often complete; however, complications from this injury may include digital nerve damage, residual decrease in joint motion, and ultimately arthritis.
4. **Volar dislocation.** Volar dislocations of the MP joint are rare. They are typically irreducible and require open reduction and repair of disrupted soft tissue. Several causes of irreducibility have been described, including avulsion of the dorsal capsule from the proximal MP and avulsion of the volar plate at its distal insertion. Once the dislocation is reduced, early range-of-motion exercises are suggested.

IV. Tendon Injuries

A. **Mallet finger** is a common athletic injury, especially in sports such as softball, baseball, and basketball. The most common fingers involved are the long, ring, and small fingers. The injury results from a direct blow to the extended distal interphalangeal (DIP) joint, leading to disruption of the extensor tendon over the joint. Typically, forced flexion of the extended joint avulses the tendon with or without a small portion of bone.

1. **Diagnosis.** On physical examination, the DIP joint classically assumes a flexed position and full active extension is not possible. Full passive extension, however, is usually intact. As with all acute joint injuries, physical examination will reveal tenderness and swelling of the affected joint. Radiographs are essential for thorough evaluation to detect the presence of associated avulsion fractures, intraarticular fractures and, most importantly, subluxation of the joint.
2. **Classification.** Mallet fingers can be classified into four main types.
   a. **Type 1** results from blunt trauma with avulsion of the tendon with or without a small avulsion fracture.
   b. **Type 2** is a laceration of the tendon.
   c. **Type 3** involves a deep laceration.
   d. **Type 4** is characterized by articular fracture and is further categorized into several variations.
      i. The first is a transepiphyseal injury.
      ii. The second is caused by a hyperflexion force resulting in an articular fracture involving 20% to 50% of the articular surface.
      iii. The third and most severe subtype results from a hyperextensive force leading to an articular fracture involving more than 50% of the articular surface and volar subluxation of the joint.
3. **Treatment.** Management of a mallet finger is based on the size and displacement of the dorsal fracture fragment.
   a. **Type 1 injuries,** including those involving less than 20% of the articular surface, are successfully treated with splinting of the DIP joint in extension. Care must be taken not to splint the joint in too much extension because skin necrosis may result. Furthermore, splinting may be external, with off-the-shelf or custom-made extension splints, or internal, by means of transarticular K-wire that allows continuation of some activities. Continuous splinting for 8 weeks ensures healing in a majority of cases. Athletes may return to their sport with a well-secured splint if they do not require active motion of the DIP joint.
   b. **Type 2 and 3** injuries are open injuries and require irrigation and debridement with repair of the tendon. Type 2 may be repaired with a figure-eight stitch, which includes both the tendon and the skin, followed by splinting for 6 to 8 weeks. Type 3 injuries require meticulous soft tissue repair. Return to sports may be dictated by the condition of the soft tissue injury.
   c. **Type 4.** The treatment goal of type 4 injuries is restoration of articular congruity. Transepiphyseal fractures must be adequately reduced and splinted. Internal fixation may be required if the fracture is unstable. Mallet fingers with significant fracture fragments and palmar subluxation of the distal phalanx require open reduction and internal fixation with interosseus wiring to restore joint congruity. Temporary transarticular internal fixation of the joint is also employed as a method of internal protective splinting. The wire is removed at 4 weeks and physical therapy is begun.
   d. **Untreated or chronic mallet fingers** may develop a swan-neck deformity as a result of relaxation of the volar plate and dorsal subluxation of the lateral bands. If the deformity is flexible, splinting may be attempted. If this fails, surgical intervention is warranted to prevent further deformity of the finger. Surgical procedures include release of the central slip or reconstruction of the oblique retinacular ligament. For chronic fixed deformities, arthrodesis of the DIP joint is indicated as well as reconstruction of the oblique retinacular ligament. Athletes should have these treated in the off season.

B. **Rupture of the flexor tendon (jersey finger).** Rupture or avulsion of the flexor digitorum profundus at its insertion on the distal phalanx, frequently termed *jersey finger,* most commonly occurs in the ring finger and is typically caused by grasping the pants or jersey of an opposing player. As the finger is forcibly extended, the flexor digitorum profundus tendon contracts with excessive tension and ruptures at its distal attachment.

1. **Classification.** These injuries have been classified into three different types.
   a. **Type 1.** The disrupted tendon retracts into the palm and a serious interruption of tendon blood supply occurs.
   b. **Type 2.** The tendon retracts to the level of the PIP joint.
   c. **Type 3.** A bony fragment is avulsed with the tendon and is tethered at the A4 pulley adjacent to the DIP joint.
2. **Treatment.** Type 1 avulsions require early repair, within 7 to 10 days of the injury, so that tendon integrity and circulation can be successfully restored. Since type 2 avulsions maintain some blood supply through both the intact long vinculum and the perfusion afforded by the intact tendon sheath, successful repair may be accomplished as late as 3 to 6 weeks after injury. Prompt repair, however, is recommended to prevent further retraction of the tendon and conversion of the type 2 into the more serious type 1 injury. As with type 2 injuries, blood supply is maintained in type 3 avulsions. These avulsion fractures require open reduction and internal fixation as well as volar plate repair. The repaired tendon must be protected for 6 to 8 weeks. However, athletes should not expect to return to their sports for at least 3 months.

C. **Boutonniere deformity (extensor mechanism rupture).** A boutonniere deformity may result from direct trauma or acute forced flexion of the PIP joint with opposed active extension. The central slip of the extensor mechanism is ruptured at its insertion on the base of the middle phalanx.

1. **Diagnosis**
   a. **Acute.** In an acute injury the athlete will present with PIP joint swelling, pain, and decreased active terminal extension of the PIP joint. This injury must be differentiated from sprain or dislocation of the PIP joint, since treatment is entirely different. Although radiographs are usually normal, avulsion fractures with the attached central slip occasionally occur and are a clearly visible sign of acute injury.
   b. **Chronic.** In the chronic setting, the classic boutonniere deformity is characterized by excessive flexion at the PIP joint and hyperextension at the DIP joint. This occurs secondarily to progressive proximal retraction of the central slip with volar displacement of the extensor mechanism's lateral bands and unopposed tension of the flexor digitorum sublimus. Secondary contractures of the capsular structures ultimately occur and result in a fixed deformity.
2. **Treatment.** The goal of treatment is to prevent progressive, destructive joint deformity.
   a. **Acute** injuries, once recognized, should be splinted, with the PIP joint immobilized in full extension and the DIP joint free for active motion for a period of 6 to 8 weeks. If a large avulsion fracture is present, open reduction and internal fixation are required. If the athlete is not a ball handler, he or she may return to his or her sport early.
   b. **Chronic** deformities have been successfully treated with serial splints or finger casts; however, if correction is not accomplished in three to six months, operative treatment may prove necessary.

D. **Dislocation of the extensor digitorum communis tendon at the MP joint** is uncommon in the athlete. It may result from a direct trauma to the flexed MP joint or a flexion ulnar deviation force applied to the involved finger. This disrupts the sagittal band of the extensor hood, which maintains the position of the extensor tendon centrally at the MP joint, leading to dislocation of the tendon. The long finger is most commonly involved, as is the radial aspect of the joint.

1. **Diagnosis.** The athlete will present with swelling and inability to extend fully at the MP joint. The tendon may also be palpated between the two metacarpal heads.
2. **Treatment.** Initial treatment may consist of splinting; however, if reduction cannot be maintained, sagittal band repair is indicated. In chronic cases, reconstruction procedures may be required. The joint should be immobilized postoperatively for 4 to 6 weeks. Return to athletic activities is possible during this time if protection can be maintained.

E. **Boxer's knuckle or complete disruption of the extensor mechanism** is usually caused by isolated or repetitive blunt trauma and typically involves the MP joint of the long finger secondary to its prominence when a fist is made. The lesion is most commonly characterized by a vertical tear, either radially or ulnarly, in the sagittal band of the extensor hood adjacent to the central tendon; less frequently, the central tendon splits longitudinally. In more extensive lesions, a massive capsular disruption can also occur.

1. **Diagnosis.** The boxer presents with pain, profound joint swelling, and incomplete or weak extension of the affected finger at the MP joint. A palpable, exquisitely tender tissue defect in the extensor mechanism may also be present, as well as dislocation or subluxation of the central tendon.
2. **Treatment.** Direct surgical repair and realignment of the central tendon is usually adequate and successful. Augmentation with tendon slips is rarely indicated. Athletes require immobilization for 6 weeks postoperatively. Punching is not allowed until the hand demonstrates normal, pain-free range of motion and normal strength—usually 4 months.

Suggested Reading

Melone C. Joint injuries of the fingers and thumb. *Emerg Med Clin North Am* 1985; 3:319–331.

Melone C. Complex joint injuries of the hand. In: Petrone FA, ed. *AAOS symposium on upper extremity injuries in athletes.* St Louis: Mosby, 1986:142–169.

Pyne J, Adams B. Hand tendon injuries in athletes. *Clin Sports Med* 1992; 11:833–850.

Rettig A. Closed tendon injuries of the hand and wrist in the athlete. *Clin Sports Med* 1992; 11:77–99.

46. THE SPINE AND LOW BACK

Robert G. Watkins

I. Low Back Strain

A. **History.** Mechanical low back pain that appears with bending and moving, increases with activity, decreases with rest, and may be worse when the patient is sitting in a seat that is inappropriately designed. The pain may or may not be associated with a specific injury.

There may be pain that appears only when the patient is bending forward or making certain motions. No radicular pain is associated with the back pain, but there may be referred pain on the fronts of the thighs and on through to the sacroiliac (SI) joint's lateral trochanteric and lateral pelvic areas. Certain stretching or pelvic flexion exercises or back extension exercises may relieve the symptoms temporarily.

B. **Physical examination.** The patient shows back pain with bending, twisting, or mechanical motions of the spine. There is negative straight-leg raising and negative Cram test (see Appendix 6) and neurologic signs are normal.

C. **Diagnostic studies.** X-rays are ***normal,*** as can be magnetic resonance imaging (MRI). The MRI may show evidence of degenerative disc disease.

D. **Nonoperative treatment.** Attempt to identify sources of the patient's irritation, such as a badly designed office chair or car seat. Use of a lumbar roll and a different type of car seat may relieve the mechanism of injury. Begin the trunk stabilization program (see Appendix 5) for overall strengthening.

E. **Operative treatment.** There is no operative treatment for this condition. Occasionally facet rhizotomies, epidurals, or facet blocks may be indicated on somewhat more persistent problems and when there are difficulties getting the patient into rehabilitation.

F. **Rehabilitation.** Correction of the environmental causes of low back strain is the key to an effective rehabilitation program, along with patient education on the causes and prevention of low back pain.

Begin the trunk stabilization program (see Appendix 5) for overall strengthening. Instruct the patient in the mechanics of spine function, what kinds of motions or activities to avoid to keep from aggravating the condition, and the role of sitting posture in causing it. Begin posture-correction exercises. Selective stretching exercises that relieve the symptoms, such as standing and arching the back backward, can be practiced many times during the day to augment the organized stabilization and aerobic conditioning programs.

II. Annular Tear in Intervertebral Disc

A. **History.** Upon suffering an acute rotatory injury, the athlete senses a "pop" in the back along with a sudden, severe, intense reflex back spasm and pain. The athlete often collapses to the ground and may even have to be mobilized by ambulance. There may be associated bilateral leg symptoms and acute back spasms that persist. Coughing, sneezing, straining, or anything that increases intradiscal pressure may reproduce the symptoms. There can be intense referred pain into the SI joint and burning in the pelvic and lateral trochanteric areas. The pain and spasm requires bed rest and relief of intradiscal pressure.

B. **Physical examination.** The patient has back pain with straight-leg raising, which can often be as little as 10 degrees. Any motion of the back or any dural stretching produces severe back pain, and there may be intense inflammatory changes in the spinal canal that produce neurological symptoms. Severe back pain and palpable spasm are the predominant features.

Examination may also reveal anterior spinal tenderness when the area is palpated through the abdomen. Lumbar flexion produces back pain. A simple modified sit-up may produce severe back pain, an indication of a more compressive type lesion. Placing the patient prone and doing a simple rotation maneuver on one side of the pelvis may reproduce a significant amount of back pain with that rotation. These tests indicate a rotatory annular injury. But the history of the injury alone is often more than enough to demonstrate the rotatory nature of the annular injury.

C. **Diagnostic studies.** ***X-rays*** appear normal and do not reveal a lesion. ***MRI*** may demonstrate disc degeneration or be normal. But careful observation of MRI may demonstrate the annular tear by an actual disruption in the annular pattern. It is possible to have an acute annular tear of an intervertebral disc and a normal MRI. Symmetric or asymmetric bulging may be present at the injured segment. If multiple segments are degenerated, however, MRI will not reveal the symptomatic segment with any accuracy. The amount of time it takes for an annular disruption to present with a loss of T2-weighted signal has been hypothesized to be 3 to 4 months, but the exact time is unknown.

The harsh effects of the annular tear are, in part, secondary to the chemical neuritis that results from the emission of fluid through the disrupted annulus. The reflex spasm is mediated through the sinuvertebral nerve to the posterior primary ramus and to the posterior musculature.

D. **Nonoperative treatment.** Muscle spasms should be treated as a symptom rather than as the cause of the problem, much as a fever is treated as a symptom of an infection. Local modalities of ***ice*** and ***bupivacaine HCl (Marcaine)/steroid injection*** can temporarily relieve symptoms, while muscular relaxants are of questionable efficacy in relieving muscle spasm.

The underlying cause of muscle spasms is inflammation secondary to the injury, and aggressive ***antiinflammatory*** means are the basis for nonoperative treatment of an annular tear and its resulting symptoms. The severity of the symptoms determines the aggressiveness of the diagnostic and therapeutic plan. Patients with severe symptoms are treated with aggressive antiinflammatory techniques, such as *methylprednisolone* (**Medrol Dose Pak**), a large dose of *indomethacin* (***Indocin***), and ***epidural injections.*** Occasionally ***facet injections*** and ***rhizotomies*** may be warranted.

As soon as it is prudent to do so, get the patient into ***physical therapy*** and a rehabilitation program. There may be no alternative to bed rest initially for a patient with severe involvement, but after that the time otherwise spent in severe pain and stiffness could be better spent in a rehabilitation program. Early use of antiinflammatory techniques, stabilization techniques, trunk strengthening, and training decreases the ultimate time of disability. Strong antiinflammatory measures followed by trunk stabilization and neutral position training is the key to bringing a severely symptomatic spine back to health.

E. **Operative treatment.** Surgery is ***rare*** for this condition. Percutaneous discectomy decreases intradiscal pressure only temporarily, and since neither laminectomy nor discectomy should produce any beneficial effect for an acute annular tear, the role of surgery is limited.

If a chronic situation develops, it may be treated with discography to identify the segment, but an ***interbody fusion*** should be performed only after a complete and properly performed nonoperative program has been exhausted and the patient demonstrates sufficient morbidity to justify surgery.

F. **Rehabilitation.** Proper rehabilitation consists of ***aerobic conditioning*** and the ***trunk stabilization program,*** followed by return to function (see Appendix 5).

III. Herniated Disc

Sciatica may be characterized pathologically as nerve root tension, compression, inflammatory neuritis, and peripheral nerve entrapment.

Nerve root tension can be caused by a disc herniation whereby the nerve root is being stretched around and over the herniation; stretching the nerve by SLR, neck flexion, foot dorsiflexion, or cram test may produce pain in the ipsilateral or contralateral leg. There is an element of inflammation involved in nerve root tension, and an inflamed nerve can be exquisitely sensitive to increases in nerve root tension.

Compressive pathology, such as that seen with spinal stenosis, is suspected when patients present with leg pain secondary to standing and walking. Upright posture produces narrowing of the spinal canal, and spinal extension produces relative narrowing, while flexion increases the spatial capacity of the spinal canal. The act of altering the status of the spinal canal through standing or walking, therefore, produces leg pain, which may be associated with a herniation. Since the obstructive pathology may predominate even when nerve root tension is present, straight-leg raising is typically not as positive under these circumstances as in the case of nerve root tension. Certainly the patient may have varying degrees of neuroinflammation and neuritis.

Severe inflammatory neuritis due to an annular tear with or without herniation can sometimes release intradiscal chemicals and produce a low-pH intradiscal fluid. This may result in searing leg pain and a radiating dermatomal distribution of pain, possibly with a neurological deficit. The action of the intradiscal substances produces symptoms that very closely mimic disc herniation even when there is none. Chemical neuritis has a good prognosis overall, but the course may be quite protracted and frustrating to people who present with no herniation.

Peripheral nerve entrapments can present with sciatica, as in the case of disc herniation. Compressive pathology anywhere along the course of the nerve can produce pain anywhere along that nerve. Entrapment of the sciatic nerve anywhere from the pelvis to the tarsal tunnel can produce radiating pain over the whole leg as well as sciatic notch tenderness. Usually the history lacks the component of strong back pain initial to many disc herniations. Piriformis syndrome can occur from a congenital band, injury to the area, or impingement of the nerve by the fascia of the hamstring origin.

A. **Clinical history.** The onset of discogenic injuries may occur either through compression or through the more common mechanism of torsion. Reaching to grab something while turning at the waist, for example, causes the body's upper mass to exert torque on the annular fibers of the disc, which can produce a radial tear in the annulus and, subsequently, herniation.

   Herniation typically presents with an intense inflammatory back pain that radiates into the SI joint and upper buttocks. It evolves during the most common natural history for this condition, from a situation in which as much as 90% of the pain is located in the back to one in which up to 90% of the pain presents as leg pain.

   Common to a disc herniation are both radiculitis, in which pain radiates in the distribution of a radicular nerve, and radiculopathy, in which there is radiating pain plus neurological deficit. Pain location varies from an initial intense back distress to very severe leg pain. But it is leg pain that is the hallmark of a herniated disc, though at times the patient may present with significant neurological deficit, with the intense pain having resolved itself.

B. **Physical examination.** Characteristics of disc herniation are increased pain with coughing, sneezing, or the Valsalva maneuver and radicular pain with neck flexion or foot dorsiflexion. Herniations usually present with leg pain either when sitting or standing and walking.

   A back examination typically shows a lateral shift, loss of range of motion, pain with bending motions, and/or pain that may be worse with flexion or extension. Straight-leg raising (SLR) is tested sitting and supine. Distribution of pain in a dermatomal pattern is typically reproduced with SLR, and patients with sitting pain are more likely to have more prominent SLR. Supine SLR produces more lumbar rotation and may be more painful than SLR while sitting. SLR is positive when it reproduces leg pain. There may be back pain only with SLR, and that should be noted.

SLR is additionally enhanced by checking for such positive stretch signs as foot dorsiflexion or neck flexion. Test muscle strength for dorsiflexion, plantarflexion, knee extension, foot and toe flexion, and extension for inversion and eversion. Sensory examination will test for pinprick, light touch, and fibratory sense—loss of which may be indicative of peripheral neuropathy. A positive Cram or bowstring test (see Appendix 5) is the most sensitive test for sciatica if this produces pain up or down the leg.

Reflexes checked are knee jerk, ankle jerk, and posterior tibial reflex. Posterior tibial reflex, if brisk on one side and absent on the other, can be indicative of an L5 root disturbance. The L5 root can affect the Achilles tendon but it is predominantly SI, while L3 and L4 radiculopathy can decrease the patellar reflex.

Sciatica is typically located in the back, in the paraspinous area and sciatic notch, buttocks, or leg. Pressure in the sciatic notch producing radiating leg pain has been referred to as a **Spurling test.** The reverse SLR test is done with the patient on his or her side and extension of the hip to neutral, then flexion of the knee. Reproduction of anterior thigh pain is indicative of an upper lumbar radiculitis.

C. **Diagnostic studies.** MRI or contrast computed tomography (CT) scan should be the first choice for imaging in patients with suspected lumbar disc herniation. Both have been shown to be more informative than myelography. ***MRI*** permits the identification of a disc herniation, spinal stenosis, disc degeneration, intradural tumors, and metastatic disease to bones of the spine. The typical presentation is a dark disc space indicative of loss of water content with extrusion of discogenic material asymmetrically into the spinal canal. Nerve root displacement, free soft tissue fragments in the canal, or small, strategically placed herniations in the area of the stenosis are demonstrable on the MRI. ***CT with or without contrast*** may demonstrate the same asymmetrical soft tissue protrusion in the spinal canal. ***Electromyography (EMG)*** may indicate which nerve is irritated by denervation and fibrillation changes in the muscle supplied by that nerve. ***Bone scan*** is usually negative, as opposed to the differential diagnosis of acute spondylotic defect. ***Discography*** and ***CT discograms*** can demonstrate protrusion of intradiscal content into the spinal canal. To distinguish this from an annular tear and collection of dye, the mass should be demonstrable on a plain MRI or CT scan. ***Selective nerve root blocks*** may reproduce the pain of a radiculopathy and relieve the pain. It therefore has both therapeutic and diagnostic value when used to identify which nerve is the source of the problem.

D. **Nonoperative treatment.** Spontaneous recovery from disc herniation is well known and is an important aspect of treatment strategy. The chance that a disc herniation will be cured nonoperatively within 90 days is excellent. Among the approaches to nonoperative treatment are the following: (1) ***nonsteroidal anti-inflammatory drugs,*** the strongest being indomethacin (Indocin SR) and the mildest over-the-counter medications; (2) ***methylprednisolone*** (Medrol Dose Pak); (3) ***epidural injections,*** facet blocks, nerve root blocks; (4) ***ice***; (5) ***rest***; and (6) ***physical therapy.*** We start trunk stabilization (see Appendix 5) as soon as the patient, on anti-inflammatory medication, can tolerate a trip to the physical therapist. Other methods include ***acupuncture*** and ***manipulation.***

E. **Operative treatment.** While long-term outcomes for both standard discectomy and conservative treatment appear to be about the same, discectomy offers better short-term outcomes. Disc herniations with spinal stenosis and claudication symptoms may require epidurals. Even with injections, however, there is a good chance that surgery will be necessary; if this is the case, though, surgery is simplified when nonoperative treatment has improved trunk function.

Among the various surgical possibilities are (1) *microscopic lumbar discectomy*—initial treatment of a disc herniation and sciatica with a microscopic lumbar discectomy produces an 85% to 90% cure of the herniation's symptoms; (2) *endoscopic discectomy,* both through the interlaminar area and through the foramen, which offers good results with a 1-cm incision; (3) *hemilaminectomy, medial facetectomy,* or *foraminotomy*; (4) *percutaneous discectomy* after discal therapy; and (5) *enzymatic intradiscal treatment.*

F. **Rehabilitation.** ***Trunk stabilization,*** with a heavy emphasis on ***aerobic conditioning,*** again is the bedrock of treatment, since the speed and success of return to function depends on the levels of stabilization obtained (see Appendix 5). For example, with resolution of symptoms, a level 2 stabilization should be able to bring about return to daily activity and to mild exercise for level 3 to 4 stabilization, including golf and even more strenuous sports.

G. **Follow-up.** Typical follow-up is for a year from the surgery.

IV. Facet Joint Syndrome

A. **Anatomy.** The facet joint is made up of two articular surfaces: the inferior facet, which is dorsal and medial, and the superior facet, which is volar and lateral. It is a synovial joint with articular cartilage, joint fluid, and a joint capsule.

The disc and the two facet joints are part of a three-joint complex making up one neuromotion segment (a neuromotion segment being defined as the disc, two facet joints, ligaments, nerves, and vessels composing one vertebral segment, such as the L4-L5 joint or L5 neuromotion segment). The joint is innervated by the posterior primary rami of the spinal nerve of that segment. Additionally, the posterior primary rami of each segment may branch cephalad and caudad and contribute to the innervation of more than one facet joint.

B. **Pathomechanics.** There is an increase in the impingement of facet joint articular surfaces in extension and rotation. The orientation of the facet joint affects rotation of the lumbar spine. The more coronal-facing facet joint allows more rotation, whereas a parasagittal facet joint always allows less.

Adaptive changes of osteoarthritis to repeated rotatory stresses in the lumbar spine produce deformity of the facet joint, consisting of enlargement of osteophytes and the coronal portion of the joint. The coronal medial aspects of the joint enlarges to produce a J-shaped orientation.

Facet trophism has been implicated in producing abnormal rotatory stresses of a neuromotion segment. That is, if one facet joint has a coronal orientation, the other parasagittal. There will be increased rotation toward the coronal joint, producing asymmetric stresses on the intervertebral disc.

The facet joint may contribute to spinal stenosis by enlarging medially. It can trap the traversing nerve root of the neuromotion section against the marginal osteophytes of the disc space medial to the medial wall of the pedicle. With degeneration, the superior facet may migrate cephalad, producing impingement of the exiting nerve root at the intervertebral foramen. The upper migration of the superior facet pinches the exiting nerve against the pedicle above.

It is generally felt that symptomatic spinal stenosis requires motion between two different vertebrae. In both of these instances, the motion of the impingement medially and laterally is affected by motion in the two vertebrae of the neuromotion section, such as L4 and L5. Additionally, there is motion in the neurological structures of the spine and inflammation contributing to symptoms.

The facet joint syndrome arises when rotation or extension produces injury to a joint. The fibers of the annulus of the disc are the main restraint to abnormal motion in the facet joint. Injury to the annulus of the disc may produce excessive segment rotation and motion, producing articular impingement and articular impaction of the articular surfaces of the facet joint and repeated cartilaginous injury.

C. **Clinical history.** The strain of repetitive rotation in one direction, as can occur with an annular tear and repeated stress, as in a golfer's swing, may produce joint changes. Chronic repeated rotation may produce deformity of the arch of the lamina, deformity of the facet joint's articular surfaces, and annular bulging.

The patient presents with pain predominantly with rotation and extension in the back. There may be referred facet joint pain across the posterior ilium SI joint, and lateral pelvis to the greater trochanteric area. Leg pain has been produced by facet joint injection and relieved with facet joint block. This pain is felt to be referred pain and not direct nerve root impingement.

D. **Differential diagnosis** includes (1) spondylitic defect—any patient with pain on extension and rotation must be evaluated for a spondylitic defect in the pars interarticularis; (2) facet joint fracture—seen in major league baseball pitchers and other athletes—careful use of bone scan and MRI can diagnose this; and (3) annular injury. It is felt that a significant injury to the facet joint requires, at the least, annular laxity or injury, whether the injury is acute or chronic. Some annular injuries may produce pain in extension and rotation. Neoplasms of the posterior column may produce posterior column pain. Usually this will be of an unrelentingly severe and non-mechanical nature to the mechanical pain.

E. **Physical examination.** There is pain in the back, the referred area, or both. There is pain with extension and rotation. The neurological exam is negative, as are nerve tension signs. There is possibly increased bone scan warmth in the facet.

F. **Nonoperative treatment.** ***Facet joint block*** consists of injections into the articular capsule and blocking the sensory posterior primary ramus at the facet joint capsule. Relief of the pain with the facet joint block may lead to facet rhizotomy, radiofrequency, or electrocautery.

G. **Operative treatment.** There is ***no surgical treatment*** per se other than treating the entire neuromotion segment.

H. **Rehabilitation.** We use the ***trunk stabilization program*** (see Appendix 5) for restoring strength to the patient with facet syndrome. Flexion exercises will not hurt the segment, but placing the spine in the slight flexion that occurs with trunk training can be an excellent way of restoring strength and stability to the spine.

V. Spondylolisthesis

A. **History.** Spondylolisthesis is the gradual displacement of one vertebra on another vertebral or sacral segment. It is thought to be a congenital predisposition to an acute stress fracture acquired in adolescence. It is classified as congenital (dysplastic), isthmic (spondylolytic), traumatic, degenerative, pathological, and postsurgical. In sports medicine, we deal primarily with the congenital, traumatic, and isthmic types.

Spondylolysis (a fracture) and spondylolisthesis (the slippage) have a higher incidence within the athletic population than in the general population (a 13.5% incidence among athletes versus 4% to 7% in the general population and up to 18% in gymnasts). In fact, these kinds of fractures represent the most common serious athletic injury to the lower back, with gymnasts, weight lifters, and football players at highest risk. For those involved in professional sports, these two conditions represent common causes of back and leg pain.

The system used to grade spondylolisthesis relates to measurements of the articular surface of S1: grade 1 is 25% of the S1 articular surface; grade 2 is 50%; grade 3 is 75%, and grade 4 is 100%, with grade 5 being severe angulation of the front of S1.

Early signs of a predisposition to progression of the deformity are as follows:

1. Observation of the problem at ages 9 or 10
2. Doming of S1
3. Congenital spina bifida occulta of S1

It is rare for cases observed in the late teens or adulthood to ever show progression. The clinical history of spondylolisthesis in an adolescent athlete may consist of

1. An episode of acute back pain of temporary duration and of mild to moderate severity.
2. No acute episode but rather a mechanical backache; patients presenting with their first episode of back pain sometimes are found to have a grade 1 or 2 spondylolisthesis.
3. Deformity with no prior history of pain occurring during childhood—for example, a patient with heart-shaped buttocks, a thin waist, and posture that is indicative of a significant spondylolisthesis or spinal apoptosis. (However, the heart-shaped buttocks and loss of waist seen with spinal apoptosis are rare. Patients often present simply as an acute back injury.)

B. **Physical examination.** Typical signs are pain with extension and hamstring tightness, which are believed to be secondary to nerve irritation. Also, spondylolisthesis can often be felt by palpating the spine's processes at the level of the olisthesis. There may be a very prominent process with some depression cephalad to that prominent area if spondylolisthesis is present. During the examination, the patient may complain of mechanical back pain with lumbar motion.

C. **Diagnostic studies.** ***Plain x-ray*** will demonstrate the condition if the posterior laminar line is carefully observed for vertebral offset (olisthesis) which may be indicative of (1) congenital spondylolisthesis, in which no spinal defects are seen, or (2) an acquired spondylolisthesis, in which the spinal defect may be observed on the oblique x-ray when looking for the neck of the "Scotty dog." In children, however, oblique views may or may not demonstrate the defect, whereas an elongated, intact pars in a child or adolescent may accompany spinal olisthesis. A certain amount of experience is necessary when one is looking for an abnormal pars: the exact ring on the Scotty dog may not be visualized, and observation of the spondylitic defect on anteroposterior (AP) film is difficult because of the often prominent radiolucency produced by the cephalad tip of the superior facet.

The best study for diagnosing the type of spondylolisthesis is provided by ***CT.*** The key to reading a CT scan on transverse sections is to read the sequential cuts and look for the intact pars, not for the defect, which often looks like a facet joint. There should be an intact pars at each level. If there is not, then what could appear to be a facet joint may actually be a spondylitic defect.

The ***parasagittal CT*** and the ***parasagittal MRI*** are best for diagnosing the degree of olisthesis. Certain signs can be observed on the parasagittal sections by looking for an intact bone between each of the joints. With experience, the presence of a grade 1 spondylolisthesis can be diagnosed on a transverse section because there is an increased space behind the affected vertebrae.

Careful observation of the intervertebral foramen in the case of any olisthesis may demonstrate foraminal obstruction. With L5-S1 spondylolisthesis the most common radiculopathy presents at the exiting L5 nerve root. However, there may be traction on the S1 nerve root and a good deal of recess obstruction at the level of the olisthy, as, for example, the L5 nerve root and L4-5 in spondylitic spondylolisthesis or degenerative spondylolisthesis.

D. **Nonoperative treatment.** We treat spondylolysis/spondylolisthesis and degenerative spondylolisthesis nonoperatively using the same ***trunk stabilization program*** (see Appendix 5) we employ with a patient with an annular injury, with or without sciatica, because the program's methods for strengthening the neutral position, with no particular emphasis on flexion or extension, is completely compatible with spondylolisthesis. Therefore, ***epidurals blocking the defect,*** spinal ***nerve root blocks, methylpred-***

nisolone, and nonsteroidal antiinflammatories are all used to help the patient get into the rehabilitation as soon as feasible.

Beginning trunk motion, which the program does not get into until the neutral position has been adequately strengthened, is done to tolerance. Therefore, the presence or absence of spondylolisthesis is not a major factor in our rehabilitation program, nor does it change the necessary sequence of strengthening exercises.

E. **Operative treatment.** Whether symptoms are radicular or mechanical low back pain, operations at the spondylitic spondylolisthetic level should include a ***spinal fusion.*** We avoid using decompressive techniques only at the spondylolisthetic level because they are not likely to have as much success as the nonoperative program.

Patients with an increasing olisthy, uncontrolled pain, neurologic symptoms, or severe hamstring tightness are candidates for surgical intervention. Fusion at L5-S1 at an early age is certainly compatible with a long, successful career in athletics, and fusion in the younger patient (age 16 to 22) at L5-S1 should not be a major impediment to successful athletic performance or longevity of career. For the older athlete, however, recovering from a spinal fusion can be difficult, prolonged, and can interfere with career development. The effect on athletic performance of a spinal fusion at L4-5 the subsequent strain at the levels above and below the midsegment fusion of that type is unknown, but one could hypothesize it would have an effect on adjacent levels. Every effort is made, therefore, to treat the athlete with spondylolisthesis nonoperatively before resorting to surgery.

A recent poll of National Football League (NFL) doctors asked whether they felt that grade 1 spondylolisthesis would affect for the worse their evaluation of potential career performance in a football player. They replied, 27 to 1, that they believed it would. The one dissenting vote was this author's. The results of this poll may reflect either a greater breadth of experience among the 27 or this author's favorable experience with an aggressive, nonoperative rehabilitation program.

F. **Rehabilitation.** The patient should complete level V of the trunk stabilization program (see Appendix 5). Sports-specific exercises will help the injured athlete gradually to return to sports. Since some techniques used in sports may put undue strain on the spine, patients should be reevaluated and, if possible, reeducated through coaching. To protect their back, the athlete should maintain a proper stabilization and conditioning program for an indefinite time following return to sports, work on sport-specific stabilization training techniques, and work gradually back into practice first and then play.

G. **Follow-up.** Reevaluate the rehabilitation program as it develops into the exercise program. Check that the patient is continuing the program and has developed no bad habits. Continuance of the program should result in fewer and fewer attacks of decreasing severity.

VI. Spondylolysis

Athletically acquired spondylosis is a stress fracture through the pars interarticularis, that area of a vertebra between the superior and inferior articular facets.

A. **History.** Athletic activities requiring lumbar extension and rotation can put the spine—the immature spine in particular—at risk for developing spondylolysis. This can be gradual or sudden, sometimes with a bilateral presentation, but usually unilateral (though it can start in one side and switch to the other). Most prominent in adolescent athletes, it also occurs commonly in young adults playing at professional levels. In throwing athletes, it generally appears on the side of the body opposite the throwing arm.

Typically, pain intensity is most severe at the onset of spondylolysis and is at its worst with extension, though torsion and flexion will also cause pain in the affected area. After some gradual improvement, the severity of the pain will level off but it will become more generalized, being produced by nearly all other types of mechanical activity; pain upon sitting is common, for example. Pain will also likely be reproduced when the athlete performs the primary physical movements appropriate to his or her particular sport (e.g., shooting for the hockey player, batting for the baseball player, performing specific maneuvers for the gymnast, hurling the javelin for the javelin thrower, and rowing for the sculler). There may be periods of improvement during which the pain vanishes with the activities of daily living but returns when the athlete returns to his or her sport. Additionally, several months after relief from the initial injury, the opposite side may fracture and become painful.

B. **Physical examination.** In the general population, the majority of patients with spondylolysis and spondylolisthesis are asymptomatic, but athletes will typically note pain with certain activities during training or during a game. Neurological status is intact. Motion, especially extension and rotation, and possibly flexion, produces pain. There will also be a decrease in range of motion in extension, and there may be associated radicular pain in the thigh and posterior buttocks. Symptoms will be predominantly unilateral, found anywhere between the SI joint area to the sciatic notch. Straight leg raising produces back pain, and a Cram test will be negative.

C. **Diagnostic studies.** A ***bone scan*** and ***single-photon-emission computed tomography (SPECT) scan*** is mandated in the case of every adolescent athlete or professional athlete who sustains a new onset of low back pain lasting more than a month. Should the scan prove negative, an ***MRI*** may then be obtained. While diagnosis of an acute fracture is within the scope of a properly conducted MRI, the diagnostician who mistakenly relies only on MRI, failing first to do a bone scan, risks failure to diagnose what is possibly an acute spondylitic defect.

   If the bone scan is positive, a ***CT scan*** should be done and evaluated to more clearly demonstrate the spondylitic defect. Look on the CT scan for the exact location of the hot spot. Further evaluation should proceed by identifying all of the intact pars interarticularis, since looking for just the fracture may result in misinterpretation of the fracture as the facet joint. Identifying an intact, nonfractured pars at every level is an approach that will clearly reveal any fracture in the pars. The ability to identify an intact pars on the transverse section of the CT scan as well as on the parasagittal section enables the diagnostician to gather evidence vital to making a proper diagnosis. An intact pars may be hot on the scan prior to development of the fracture. An EMG should be negative.

D. **Nonoperative treatment.** Most patients will rid themselves of their pain simply by ceasing play in their sport for a period of time, limiting their daily living activities, and using such simple assistive devices as a ***lumbosacral roll.*** Others may need to use such devices as ***lumbosacral corset*** or binder, while some may require a ***lumbosacral orthosis*** or a cast with pantaloon. In any event, nonsurgical treatment should institute that amount of ***rest*** necessary to eliminate or reduce symptoms. ***Antiinflammatory medications*** may also be needed.

   Once the pain has been significantly eased, the ***trunk stabilization program*** (see Appendix 5) should be started and should progress as symptoms drop away and the patient's ability to perform the exercises properly improves. When the patient can perform specific levels of the program and is pain-free, he or she may return to sports.

E. **Operative treatment.** Several methods may be used for acute repair of a spondylolytic defect. These include grafting, the Scott wiring technique, or the Mosier hook-and-screw technique.

   Repair of a spondylolytic defect can be performed through a small midline incision by dissecting down the lamina, identifying the pseudarthrosis, opening the capsule pseudarthrosis, and identifying the particular surface of both the caudad and the cephalad articular false facet. After identifying the transverse process and the cephalad facet joint, a 2.0 oscillating drill is used to drill from the insertion point on the midportion of the caudal edge of the lamina to a point just cephalad to the transverse process across the false joint. The proximal hole is overdrilled and a lay screw is placed across the defect.

F. **Rehabilitation.** The trunk stabilization program (see Appendix 5).
G. **Follow-up.** No further follow-up is necessary when there is no pain and the patient is functioning at full performance. If pain continues, repeat the bone scan and CT scan.

Suggested Reading

Alexander MJL. Biomechanical aspects of lumbar spine injuries in athletes: a review. *Can J Appl Sport Sci* 1985;10:1–20.

Bozdech Z, Dufek P. Spondylolisthesis in young gymnasts. *Acta Uni Carolinae Med* 1986;32:4–9.

Mooney V. Differential diagnosis of low back disorders: principles of classification. In: Frymoyer JW, ed. *The adult spine,* New York: Raven Press, 1991:1551–1566.

Ross F, Dragoni S. Lumbar spondylolisthesis and sports: the radiologic findings and statistical considerations. *Radiol Med (Italy)* 1994;87:397–400.

Watkins RG, Campbell DR. Sports Medicine in the older athlete: the older athlete after lumbar spine surgery. *Clin Sports Med* 1991;10:391–399.

47. INJURIES TO THE PELVIS, GROIN, AND BUTTOCK

Per A. F. H. Renström

Problems affecting the groin and pelvis are common in sports such as fencing, hurdling, horseback riding, ice hockey, and soccer. Adolescents can sustain injuries to the pelvic region such as avulsion fractures and apophysitis. Adult athletes usually have problems with overuse injuries, but injuries such as hip pointers, muscle strain, and fractures can occur. The areas most susceptible to injury in the pelvic region are the pubic symphysis, the pubic rami, and the areas lateral to the sacroiliac joints.

I. Anatomy

The pelvic girdle includes three fundamental parts: the ilium, ischium, and pubis, all of which form a portion of the acetabulum or hip socket. The pelvic girdle also includes the sacrum—a fusion of five vertebrae and the coccyx unifying the terminal three to five rudimentary vertebral bodies. There is little motion across the joints of the pelvis and no muscle action on these joints. The pelvis functions primarily as a weight-bearing connection between the lower extremities and the trunk.

II. History

The athlete can sustain trauma such as an avulsion fracture or a strain. The history is then characterized by a sudden pain, like the stabbing of a knife in that region. The injured athlete cannot continue to perform in his or her sport but can often put weight on the leg and walk straight forward. A sudden direct trauma to the area characterizes contusion types of injury. Pain often increases over time as the hematoma develops. There maybe an early complaint of a limitation of hip motion and a painful limp. Overuse injuries such as stress fractures are characterized by a low-grade ache and pain during activity.

A. **Type and location of pain**
   1. Pain that is sudden and occurs in combination with a trauma is often caused by a fracture or a muscle tear.
   2. Pain associated with some kind of trauma and that gradually increases with time is often a contusion injury with a developing hematoma.
   3. Pain aggravated by physical activity can be of a chronic nature, indicating mechanical joint problems—such as osteitis pubis or sacroiliac joint problems—or an injury of the muscle-tendon junction.
   4. An avulsion fracture or hip pointer often causes pain localized to the iliac spine.
   5. Pain in the groin with radiation down the leg is often characterized by aching during and after activity and is caused by soft tissue injuries.

B. **Functional activities.** The injured athlete shows decreased function. He or she can, however, often walk with careful weight bearing, although perhaps with a limp. Such patients may have problems in performing pelvic bending activities such as putting on a stocking or crossing the legs. If there is a major fracture, weight bearing is usually not possible.

III. Physical Examination

A. **Gait.** The athlete should be observed when walking. There is often a limp present. Alignment should be inspected.

B. **Patient standing**
   1. Leg-length discrepancy should be evaluated.
   2. Pelvic alignment. should be checked.
   3. With the patient standing on one leg, pain and the Trendelenburg sign should be evaluated.

C. **Patient supine**
 1. Location of tenderness should be evaluated carefully. The maximum point of tenderness is often the anatomic site of the injury.
 2. Palpate the groin area for soft tissue injuries and hernia.
 3. Evaluate active and passive hip range of motion.
 4. The hip abductors, adductors, extensors, and flexors should be evaluated with resistive tests. Pain on these tests gives an indication of the muscle group involved. Muscle strength can also be evaluated in this way.
 5. Pain on hip rotation indicates an intraarticular lesion.

D. **Patient prone**
 1. Palpate the lumbosacral and gluteal areas to find any source of pain.
 2. Evaluate hip extensor strength.

IV. Laboratory Studies

A. **Plain radiographs** should include an anteroposterior view of the pelvis. A lateral view of the hip on the affected side should also be included to exclude injuries. If lumbosacral disease is suspected, views of the lumbosacral spine should be obtained. If the patient is an adolescent, views of the contralateral side should be obtained for comparison, so as to evaluate the degree of skeletal maturity and the status of the normal apophysis.

B. **Bone scans** can be indicated if there is pain during activity as the pelvis is not an uncommon location for stress fractures.

C. **Computed tomography (CT) or magnetic resonance imaging (MRI)** is sometimes needed to evaluate the sacroiliac joints, hip joints and pubic region, especially as the pelvis is subjected to tumors of different kinds. A magnetic resonance arthrogram (MRA) can give valuable information about intraarticular hip lesions.

D. **Blood studies** are sometimes indicated (e.g., sedimentation rate and white blood cell count with a differential, uric acid and rheumatoid factor).

V. Treatment Options

A. ***Prevention*** including proper warming up and stretching, especially of the hip adductors, is essential and should be included in every training session.

B. In the acute phase after an injury, rest, immobilization if possible, cold, and elevation can be applied. ***Crutches*** are often recommended during the initial phase. Once the diagnosis is established, treatment can start, but it should be well planned.

C. **Antiinflammatory** medication can be used for a short period especially during the first 3 weeks (except the first 1 to 2 days) and may relieve the symptoms. It is often effective against morning stiffness. It can however, mask the seriousness of an injury and should not be taken before an athletic event.

D. **Muscle exercises** can and should usually be initiated early, which means within 3 to 5 days after a muscle tendon injury. Fractures should, of course, be excluded first. The initial exercise program should start with careful isometric contractions without resistance followed by isometric contractions against resistance, the limit being pain. Dynamic exercises can gradually be increasingly used. Advice by a physical therapist or a trainer is recommended.

E. **Stretching** should start as early as possible. Be careful if there is an avulsion fracture or major trauma involved.

F. **Local steroid injections** can sometimes be indicated in chronic bursitis syndromes and chronic overuse injuries. Such an injection should be combined with 5 to 7 days of rest. A steroid injection should never be given into the tendon itself.

G. **Surgical intervention** is occasionally indicated. If a major bone fragment is significantly displaced, surgery can be discussed. In chronic overuse injuries where conservative treatment has failed, surgery is often helpful.

H. **Return to sport** varies according to the injury. Athletes with avulsion fractures can often return to sports within 2 to 3 months. The return to sports is often much quicker after an acute soft tissue injury. Return within weeks after the injury is often possible.

Return to sports after a chronic injury may take a long time; the rehabilitation time for a chronic muscle-tendon injury in the groin may be more than 6 to 8 months.

V. Differential Diagnosis

A. **Pelvic fractures.** Pelvic fractures differ from simple avulsion injuries due to unstable open fractures of the pelvic ring. Each fracture has its specific pattern of associated injuries, treatment, rehabilitation, and outcome.

1. **Major pelvic fractures**—such as avulsion fractures, fractures of the pubis or ischium, fracture of the wing of the ilium, fracture of the sacrum, and fracture or dislocation of the coccyx—can occur without a break in continuity of the pelvic ring. There can also be a single break or double breaks in the pelvic ring.

   Physical signs commonly associated with pelvic fractures are as follows:
   a. **Destot's sign**—a large superficial hematoma formation beneath the inguinal ligament or in the scrotum
   b. **Roux's sign**—decrease in the distance from the greater trochanter to the pubis on the affected side
   c. **Earle's sign**—a bony prominence or large hematoma with associated tenderness on rectal examination

   The following maneuvers can be performed in an athlete with suspected pelvic injury:
   a. **Posterior pressure** exerted on the iliac crest of the supine patient.
   b. **Iliac wings** compressed with direct pressure in a lateral to medial direction.
   c. **Direct downward pressure** placed on the pubic symphysis. If pain is noted, a pelvic fracture should be suspected.

2. **Avulsion fractures** are usually treated conservatively, but surgery is occasionally needed. Fractures in adolescents occur from any of the muscle or tendon insertions in the groin and pelvic area. Clinical examination will reveal localized pain and tenderness and the history usually includes muscular trauma. The function of the involved muscle tendon attachment will be painful and active resistive motion will cause pain to the area involved. Radiographic examination will establish the diagnosis. Different locations are as follows:
   a. **Traction injury to the anterior superior iliac spines,** due to trauma to the sartorius muscle during jumping or running. The trauma occurs when the hip is extended and the knees are flexed. Active flexion or abduction of the affected thigh will elicit pain.
   b. **Avulsion of the anterior inferior iliac spine** due to contraction of the rectus femoris muscle in kicking the ball in soccer. Active flexion of the hip causes pain.
   c. **Avulsions of the ischial apophysis.** These occur in athletes between the ages of 15 and 25 years. Avulsion is caused by maximal hamstring contraction with the pelvis fixed in flexion and the knee in extension. Gymnastics and hurdling are common causes. A sudden onset of pain and tenderness at the ischial tuberosity is common, as is discomfort while the patient is sitting and getting up from a sitting position. Extension of the hip against resistance will produce pain.
   d. Injuries to the iliac crest are often called ***hip pointers.*** Avulsion injury can occur as well as contusion in sports such as soccer and football. There are pain and tenderness over the iliac crest, and hip abduction against resistance will elicit pain. The treatment of avulsion fractures is usually conservative. If a large fragment is avulsed with a large gap, surgical reduction may be needed.

3. **Stress fractures** in the inferior pubic bone are common, but they may also occur in the femoral neck and shaft. They are seen after a sudden

change in training routines or repetitive loading in runners and joggers. When exercise or motion of the hip joint elicits pain or if pain is experienced after exercise, the examiner should not be satisfied with a negative radiograph but should order a bone scan. This may be positive after 2 to 8 days and will confirm the diagnosis.

The treatment is rest until activities can be carried out without pain. Swimming pool activities and sometimes biking are beneficial to maintain function. Stress fractures of the femoral neck need special attention and care as there is a risk of full fracture. Surgery may therefore be indicated. Specialist advice is always recommended.

4. **Coccygeal fractures** can occur when the athlete falls in a sitting position and sustains a direct blow to the coccyx. This injury can occur in football but is most common in horseback riding. Local tenderness characterizes it. It can be very painful when the patient is walking and sitting but is not really disabling. Radiographs will confirm the diagnosis. The treatment is avoidance of painful activities. A doughnut-shaped pillow can relieve some pain.

B. **Inflammatory conditions of the pelvic joint**

1. **Inflammatory conditions such as sacroiliitis** are seen in outdoor winter sports. Sacroiliitis can also be a symptom of a general disease such as rheumatoid arthritis or part of a syndrome such as Morbus Bechterew. Pain and/or discomfort may radiate out into the groin, to the hip joint, or to the thigh. Changes in the sacroiliac joints may be present without associated pain. The symptoms include pain during motion and stiffness, often most pronounced in the morning. There may be long intervals without symptoms. The diagnosis is made by clinical examination and with the aid of a CT scan or MRI. The treatment comprises anti-inflammatory medication and rest from abuse.
2. **Osteitis pubis** can cause pain localized to the pubic bone. Inflammation characterizes this injury, which is due to mechanical strain from trauma, abnormal motion, or shear stress in the pubic region. This lesion can occur with or without pubic instability. It is common in soccer, ice hockey, and football players but is also seen in runners and weight lifters. The pain may radiate down along the medial aspect of the thigh but also proximally to the abdomen. Passive abduction and resisted active adduction can cause pain. There may be tenderness over the region of the pubic bone.

   Plain radiographs can show bony changes 2 to 3 weeks after an onset of symptoms. These include symmetrical bone absorption, widening of the pubic symphysis, and sclerosis along the bone. Occasionally, there may be radiographic changes in the pubic bone but no reports from the athlete of any problems. A steroid injection can be given with the aid of fluoroscopy. Surgery is rarely indicated. Return to sports is gradual and is usually possible after 4 to 8 months on average. Although this injury is usually self-limited, the associated discomfort can last for a long time. Surgery may eventually be needed.

C. **Muscle tendon injuries of the pelvic ring.** The insertion of the abdominal muscles on the iliac ring, the gluteal muscles from the ilium to the insertion on the proximal femur, the origin of the adductors on the pubis and the insertion of the iliopsoas at the lesser trochanter can all be subjected to injury. These injuries are usually caused by a violent muscle contraction during an excessively forceful stretch. These soft tissue injuries can be acute, subchronic, and chronic.

1. The most common groin injuries with pain radiating up to the pelvic area involve the muscle tendon units of the adductor longus. Other muscle tendon units involved include the rectus femoris, rectus abdominis, and iliopsoas. History, local tenderness, and pain on resistive tests confirm the diagnosis of these injuries. Treatment includes a gradually increased exercise program.

2. External oblique abdominal strains of the pelvis can occur by forceful contraction of the abdominal muscles while the trunk is forced to the contralateral side. This occurs in football, ice hockey, and soccer. To some degree there is a detachment of the abdominal muscles from the insertion along the anterior and internal portions of the iliac crest. There is some pain at the time of injury and, on the day after, there is difficulty in straightening the trunk. Other strain injuries can cause local tenderness along the iliac crest or the superior rim of the inner tables, e.g., sartorius, tensor fascia lata, etc. Active flexion to the opposite side will cause pain. The treatment is conservative with a gradually increased exercise program.

D. **Contusion injuries through the pelvic region**

1. These injuries occur where there are bony prominences such as the greater trochanter, ischial tuberosity, and pubic rami. A direct blow to the iliac crest is called a ***hip pointer.*** It is combined with the formation of a subperiosteal hematoma, which may cause disability. The symptoms are the same as when there is a fracture. Deep contusions with significant hemorrhage may occur and may occasionally be complicated by the formation of a myositis ossificans. Early treatment includes ice, compression, and rest. Careful stretching can start early. Strengthening exercise should wait until function has returned. Be aware of the risk for reinjury.
2. Contusion of the sciatic nerve can occasionally result after a blow to the buttock resulting in pain in the buttock and extending through the back and distally.

E. **Bursitis.** Bursitis can occur in any of the many bursae in the pelvic region such as the ischial, iliopectineal, and trochanteric bursae. Bursitis most commonly arises as a result of friction.

1. **Iliopectineal bursitis** located anterior to the hip joint and behind the iliopsoas can cause pain radiating up to the pelvic region causing limping. In a position of hip flexion and external rotation the athlete has some relief.
2. **Hemorrhagic bursitis.** Posttraumatic bursitis can also occur. A direct blow or contusion may cause hemorrhagic bursitis secondary to hematoma formation in the bursa. This condition may lead to scarring, adhesions, and calcification and cause chronic bursitis. This sequence of events commonly occurs with superficial trochanteric bursitis.
3. **Ischial bursitis** can occur after a blow to the ischial tuberosity, with pain and tenderness in that region.

   The treatment of bursitis is rest, ice, and compression. Anti-inflammatory medication can be of value. Cortisone injections may be used in the chronic stage. If chronic pain is present, surgery may be indicated, with removal of the bursa.

F. **Hamstring syndrome.** Pain in the sitting position characterizes this syndrome, with local tenderness around the ischial tuberosity. Sciatic nerve irritation is produced due to compression by tendinous structures within the hamstring muscle. Conservative therapy with a gradually increased exercise program may be successful but can take a long time. Surgery is occasionally needed.

G. **Hernia is one of the most common causes of pain in the groin region.** Pain during physical activity or coughing should lead to a visit to the general surgeon.

H. **Other disorders causing pain.** Urinary infection can cause pain radiating to the pelvic region. Gynecologic disorders may cause pain radiating to the groin. Other diseases causing pain in this area include rheumatoid arthritis, spondylitis, Reiter's syndrome, gout, and so on. Bone infections causing pelvic pain may include osteomyelitis and tuberculosis, but these conditions are rare. The treatment depends on the diagnosis.

I. **Tumors.** Tumors in the pelvic region may include osteochondroma, chondrosarcoma, malignant osteosarcoma, and others. Persistent pain in the pelvic or groin region should be carefully investigated to exclude a tumor. A radiologic examination should be included at an early stage in patients with diffuse pelvic or groin pain. MRI or CT usually confirms the diagnosis. The treatment depends on the diagnosis. It is often recommended that patients with long-lasting, diffuse pain be referred to a specialist.

Suggested Reading

Renstrom P. Groin injuries. *Clin Sports Med* 1992;11:679–904.

48. HIP INJURIES

Cato T. Laurencin and Michael T. Rowland

Introduction

Hip injuries in adolescents and adults are relatively common. They encompass a wide variety of disorders. The type of injury an individual may sustain depends on his or her physiologic age and general physical condition as well as the amount of force applied. The hip joint transmits the forces of weight bearing from the appendicular skeleton to the axial skeleton. Studies have demonstrated that up to 6.4 times the body weight can be transmitted through the hip with walking. These forces may be many times greater with high-impact activities such as running and contact sports.

Anatomy

It is important to understand normal skeletal growth of the hip in the pediatric and adolescent population. At birth, there is a single proximal femoral epiphyseal growth plate. The medial portion of this becomes the subcapital epiphyseal plate and the lateral portion becomes the greater trochanteric epiphyseal plate. A third epiphyseal plate develops at the lesser trochanter. Secondary ossification centers appear at distinct ages. Fusion of epiphyseal plates also occurs in an expected order.

The anatomy of the proximal femur changes during development. The neck-shaft angle decreases from 155 degrees at birth to 130 degrees at maturity. Femoral anteversion decreases from 40 degrees to 15 degrees in females and 10 degrees in males.

The physiologic properties of the physis are also important. Interdigitations in the physeal plate resist shear forces. The vascular supply to the femoral head and acetabulum changes during development. At birth, the primary blood supply to the femoral head is through metaphyseal vessels: the medial and lateral circumflex arteries. By 4 years of age, the cartilaginous physeal plate blocks metaphyseal blood from reaching the femoral head. The retinacular vessel system surrounding the proximal femur penetrates the capsule and becomes the primary blood supply to the head. The artery of the ligamentum teres has minimal contribution to the femoral head until 8 years of age. It eventually carries approximately 20% of the blood supply in adulthood. The acetabulum forms from three ossification centers (the ilium, ishium, and pubis), which fuse at 16 to 18 years of age. The blood supply to the triradiate cartilage must remain uninterrupted for normal acetabular development to occur.

Assessment

The athlete with a hip injury may present with acute complaints requiring immediate care or with chronic complaints necessitating diagnosis and treatment. In cases of acute injuries sustained on the playing field, a rapid assessment of the athlete must be performed. If obvious deformity of the lower extremity is present, this indicates either femoral fracture or hip dislocation. Reduction of fractures or dislocations should not be performed on the field unless neurovascular compromise is present. The extremity should be stabilized and the athlete transferred to an emergency center.

The athlete may present in the office with complaints of long-standing pain or irritation that limits athletic participation. A careful history and full physical examination will usually reveal the underlying pathology. The physician must be aware that hip pain may be secondary to pathology in another anatomic location.

Classification

A number of classification systems have been used. For simplicity, injuries about the hip can be divided into two groups: those affecting bone and cartilage and those affecting soft tissues.

Specific Injuries

I. Bone and Cartilage Injuries

A. **Avulsion fractures.** Apophyseal avulsion fractures may occur at any open physis in adolescents. They most often occur at the anterior superior iliac spine, the ischium, the lesser trochanter, the anterior inferior iliac spine, and the iliac crest. Avulsion of the greater trochanter is exceedingly rare. Avulsion fractures are more common than tendinous ruptures in skeletally immature athletes, as the physis is the weakest link. Commonly involved athletes include sprinters, jumpers, gymnasts, soccer players, and football players. The mechanism of injury is usually intense, violent muscle contraction, but it may be secondary to overstretching of a muscle. In the skeletally mature athlete, this would likely cause a muscular strain. External trauma rarely causes avulsion fractures. The common age group is between 14 and 17. Avulsion injuries have been more common in males; however, this is less predominant as female athletic participation increases.

1. **Presentation.** The athlete presents with pain, localized tenderness and swelling, and limited motion at the site of injury. Pain may be severe. In avulsions of the lesser trochanter, the hip may be held in mild adduction and internal rotation. The patient will be unable to flex the hip when in a seated position—a positive Ludloff sign. The hip position in greater trochanteric avulsion is slight abduction and flexion. The Trendelenburg sign will be positive. Appropriate radiographs confirm the diagnosis. Chronic avulsion injuries have been described and are thought to be secondary to repetitive traction injuries leading to apophyseal displacement. These athletes present with chronic pain in the affected area, which limits athletic activity.
2. **Treatment.** Initial treatment is with bed rest, ice, analgesics, and placing the limb in a position to reduce tension in the affected muscle. A five-step program for treatment and rehabilitation is useful, in the following stages: (1) Rest in the relaxed position, ice, and analgesia—48 to 72 hr; (2) gradual increase in musculotendinous excursion as pain resolves—72 hr to 1 week; (3) start of a resistive exercise program after full range of motion is achieved—1 to 3 weeks; (4) integration of the musculotendinous unit with other muscles once 50% strength has been obtained—3 to 4 weeks, during which the reinjury rate is greatest; and (5) return to competitive sports only when full strength and integration have recovered 4 to 6 weeks. Isometric strengthening is used in the early phases, resistive isokinetic strengthening is used in late phases. Painful fibrous union or nonunion may occur, limiting athletic participation. Some authors recommend surgical intervention if displacement is greater than 2 cm, especially in greater trochanteric avulsions, to prevent a painful nonunion.

B. **Epiphyseal injuries.** Acute physeal fractures of the proximal femur and acetabulum are rare in sports. They are caused by significant trauma and may represent some other pathological process. Acute fractures of the capital femoral epiphysis are associated with a high rate of avascular necrosis. The most common hip disorder in adolescents is slipped capital femoral epiphysis (SCFE). This rarely occurs as an acute injury during sports. SCFE is felt to be secondary to chronic microtrauma to the physis under normal conditions during the adolescent growth spurt. SCFE is more common in heavy males. It rarely occurs in boys younger than age 11 or girls younger than 9. It may be associated with hypothyroidism or renal osteodystrophy. It is bilateral 50% of the time.

1. **Presentation.** The athlete with an acute slip is in severe pain, which is exacerbated with movement of the affected hip. The leg is flexed and externally rotated. Diagnosis is confirmed with anteroposterior (AP) and lateral hip radiographs.
2. **Treatment.** The first goal of treatment is stabilization of the femoral head. The risk of avascular necrosis and malunion increase as displace-

ment worsens. Fixation with smooth pins or cannulated screws is urgently performed. One attempt at closed reduction of an acute slip is recommended. If this fails, open reduction may be performed. Reduction of chronic slips may be associated with a higher rate of avascular necrosis. The patient is maintained with no weight bearing for 4 to 6 weeks postoperatively; however, range-of-motion exercise is encouraged. Progressive weight bearing and activity are allowed for 6 additional weeks. Slips of 45 degrees are associated with limited flexion, significant external rotational deformity, and risk of osteoarthritis.

C. **Hip dislocations.** Hip dislocations are infrequent in competitive sports, as significant trauma is required. In children, hip dislocations are more common than hip fractures. They occur most commonly in the early adolescent age group. Most dislocations are posterior.

1. **Presentation.** The involved extremity is held in flexion, adduction, and internal rotation with posterior dislocations. If the dislocation is anterior, the leg is extended, abducted, and externally rotated. A careful neurovascular examination of the leg is required prior to reduction, as sciatic nerve injury may be present. Attention must be paid to the ipsilateral knee, as it may also be injured. Radiographs are obtained to assess for any associated fracture. A computed tomography (CT) scan may be helpful when clinically indicated.

2. **Treatment.** A hip dislocation is an orthopaedic emergency. Closed reduction under light sedation is usually accomplished. Postreduction radiographs are required to make sure that a concentric reduction is obtained. Intraarticular fragments or an inverted limbus may prevent a concentric reduction. Open reduction or hip arthroscopy may be necessary to remove osteochondral loose bodies or an inverted limbus.

   Postreduction treatment varies depending on the surgeon's preference. Light traction for 3 to 7 days is recommended; however, a longer course of traction may be necessary if open reduction was required. The patient is maintatined with no weight bearing for 3 to 4 weeks followed by protected weight bearing for 3 additional weeks. Rehabilitation with strengthening and range-of-motion exercises are performed for 6 more weeks. Full activity is allowed once full strength and range of motion are recovered. The major complication of hip dislocation is avascular necrosis (AVN), reported at 10% incidence. Factors influencing the development of AVN are delay in reduction, severity of injury to the hip joint, and age greater than 5. Follow-up hip radiographs are obtained every 3 months for 1 year and then every 6 months for 2 years. A bone scan and magnetic resonance imaging (MRI) can be useful to follow potential avascular necrosis.

D. **Fractures of the femoral neck.** Acute fractures through the femoral neck are infrequent in sports. They occur as a result of severe trauma and account for approximately 50% of pediatric hip fractures.

1. **Presentation.** The patient will have severe pain in the affected hip or groin that worsens with movement. The leg may be externally rotated and shortened or have a normal appearance. Radiographs confirm the diagnosis.

2. **Treatment.** These fractures require urgent operative anatomic reduction and internal fixation. If the patient is skeletally immature, hardware should not cross the physis. Postoperative treatment includes early motion, no weight bearing for 4 to 6 weeks, followed by 6 weeks of partial weight bearing.

E. **Stress fractures.** Stress fractures of the femoral neck are the result of repetitive microtrauma. They commonly occur in recruits to the armed forces or track and field athletes. These fractures can be divided into two main types, distraction and compression. The distraction type occurs as a transverse fracture involving the superior portion of the femoral neck. This area is under tension and displacement may occur. Distraction fractures are more common in adults. The compression type involves the inferomedial femoral neck. This region is under compression and displacement is less frequent; however, a varus deformity may develop. The compression type is seen more often in children.

1. **Presentation.** The athlete presents with a complaint of persistent groin pain, which is exacerbated with activity. Physical examination may demonstrate mild groin tenderness and limited flexion and internal rotation. If initial radiographs are normal, maintain the patient without weight bearing and obtain repeat radiographs and a technetium bone scan.
2. **Treatment.** Once the diagnosis has been made, all athletic activity is terminated to prevent acute displacement of the fracture. If the fracture is the distraction type, internal fixation with threaded pins is recommended, as displacement may arise. If it is the compression type, limitation of activity is all that is usually necessary. Both fractures are treated with protected weight bearing until radiographs demonstrate evidence of healing or bone scan is negative. Bicycling and swimming are permitted. When light activities and range of motion are pain-free, in 4 to 6 weeks, aggressive physical therapy is begun to recondition the extremity. A gradual return to competitive sports is allowed once full strength has returned in 2 to 3 months.

II. Soft Tissue Injuries

A. **Bursitis.** Bursitis is a common cause of lower extremity pain in patients of all ages and activity levels. Patients typically complain of pain that is exacerbated by activity. Symptoms may arise acutely following a single traumatic event or gradually secondary to chronic overuse. Localization of pain may be difficult, as many bursae are deep in tissue and surrounded by structures. Lower extremity bursitis is common in running athletes.

Two types of bursae have been described; constant and adventitial. Constant bursae are saclike endothelium-lined structures that develop during normal embryonic growth. They are found between tendon and bone or skin, allowing for smooth gliding of tendons over areas of high friction. Synovial cells are present that secrete collagen, proteoglycan, and enzymatic proteins, which act as lubricants. Adventitial bursae develop secondary to myxomatous degeneration of fibrous tissues at areas of stress between structures. No endothelial cells or synovial fluid is present. Both types can be involved in acute or chronic bursitis.

Bursitis may develop following trauma, crystal deposition, or infection. Inflammatory bursitis occurs following repetitive subacute injury to the bursae. Trauma leads to local vasodilatation and increased vascular permeability into the bursae. The influx of proteins and fluid stimulates an inflammatory response. Greater trauma may lead to hemorrhage into the bursae. Significant swelling and pain ensue, with subsequent limitation of joint motion.

1. **Presentation.** The athlete will commonly give a history of repetitive injury or describe a single traumatic event. Physical examination demonstrates tenderness, swelling, erythema, and warmth over the involved bursae. Active range of motion and strength may be limited secondary to pain. Chronic bursitis may lead to disuse atrophy. Radiographs may be of assistance, as osteophytes or bony pathology will be demonstrated. Aspiration should be performed if infection is suspected.
2. **Treatment** Treatment guidelines include two parts. The first is suppression of the inflammatory response and pain. The second is rehabilitation and prevention of recurrence. The treatment plan should include protection, relative rest, ice, compression, elevation, medication, and modalities (PRICEMM). Nonsteroidal antiinflammatory drugs (NSAIDs) are the pharmacologic agents of choice. Intrabursal injection with a corticosteroid gives excellent antiinflammatory relief. Injections should be

reserved for patients who have failed a trial of conservative therapy and should be administered no more than three times in one year. Rehabilitation of the involved area is extremely important. Symmetrical strengthening of adjacent muscles reduces friction in the bursae.

3. **Locations.** The *ischiogluteal bursa* lies over the ischial tuberosity deep to the gluteus maximus. Chronic, continuous pressure from prolonged sitting causes injury to this area, leading to inflammation of the bursae, It is described as "weaver's bottom." Patients complain of pain with sitting or walking. Palpation of the ischial tuberosity is painful. Discomfort is aggravated with passive hip flexion and resisted extension. Treatment includes a padded seat cushion and PRICEMM.

   The *greater trochanter* has up to three bursae. Bursitis may develop following direct trauma, overuse, or mechanical factors such as shortened hip abductors or external rotators and increased varus angulation of the hip. Patients complain of aching, lateral hip pain that may radiate to the buttocks or knee. The greater trochanter is tender, especially inferiorly or posteriorly. The pain is often worse at night. Resisted hip abduction and external rotation exacerbate the pain. Treatment includes PRICEMM and local steroid injections if symptoms are not improving.

B. **Snapping-hip syndrome.** The snapping-hip syndrome may occur in athletes in any sport. Two separate physiologic conditions have been described; *iliotibial band syndrome* and *psoas tendon syndrome.* The first is irritation of the greater trochanteric bursae by the iliotibial band; this has been described as the *external snapping-hip syndrome.* The latter is the result of tenosynovitis of the iliopsoas tendon at its insertion on the lesser trochanter or catching of the iliopsoas tendon as it passes over the iliopectineal eminence. This has been described as the *internal snapping-hip syndrome.*

1. **Iliotibial band syndrome**
   a. **Presentation.** The athlete will complain of a snapping sensation with discomfort laterally over the greater trochanter. Some report feeling that the hip dislocates. The greater trochanter may be tender. Symptoms of snapping are reproduced with hip flexion, adduction, and internal rotation. The Ober test is often positive (inability to adduct the affected hip in extension) (see Appendix 6).
   b. **Treatment.** Conservative therapy consist of rest, NSAIDs, and iliotibial band stretching. The athlete may return to sports when he or she is asymptomatic, in 2 to 6 weeks. In cases of failure of conservative therapy, surgical release of the iliotibial band can be considered.
2. **Psoas tendon syndrome**
   a. **Presentation.** The athlete describes a snapping sensation in the groin or anterior hip. Hip abduction with external rotation reproduces symptoms. Diagnosis may be facilitated by iliopsoas bursography with cineradiography.
   b. **Treatment.** This consists of a nonsurgical program of NSAIDs and abduction and external rotation hip stretching. Ultrasound therapy may be beneficial. Sports are allowed when symptoms have resolved, in 2 to 6 weeks. Surgical release of the iliopsoas tendon is occasionally indicated.

C. **Piriformis syndrome.** Piriformis syndrome is a rare condition that can cause sciatic nerve injury. The symptoms develop due to compression of the sciatic nerve as it exits deep to the piriformis muscle posteriorly.

1. **Presentation.** Patients have pain and symptoms in the sciatic distribution similar to those of a radiculopathy. Pain is exacerbated by athletic activity or sitting. Examination reveals buttock tenderness, pain over the piriformis fossa, and pain with sustained hip flexion, adduction, and internal rotation. Freiberg's sign, pain with passive internal rotation of the hip, is positive, as is Pace's sign, pain and weakness on resisted abduction and external rotation of the thigh. CT, MRI, or electrodiagnostic studies may be helpful in the diagnosis.

2. **Treatment.** Initial treatment is conservative, with stretching, ultrasound, NSAIDs, and corticosteroid injections. Return to activity is allowed once symptoms resolve, in 2 to 6 weeks. Surgical exploration and decompression of the sciatic nerve by transecting the piriformis tendon is indicated if conservative treatment fails.

D. **Hamstring syndrome.** Hamstring syndrome has recently been described. The clinical presentation is similar to that of piriformis syndrome. The sciatic nerve becomes entrapped by a fibrous band between the biceps and semitendinosis muscles.

1. **Presentation.** The athlete will complain of pain in the lower gluteal region, which radiates down the posterior thigh to the popliteal fossa. Symptoms occur with sitting, stretching, or running. Rapid active hip flexion may elicit pain. Passive hamstring stretching may also cause symptoms. Examination reveals ischial tuberosity tenderness.
2. **Treatment.** Conservative therapy with stretching and NSAIDs is initiated. If this fails, surgical exploration with release of the fibrous band usually relieves symptoms.

E. **Neurologic conditions**

1. **Meralgia paresthetica.** Meralgia paresthetica occurs secondary to compression of the lateral femoral cutaneous nerve. The nerve passes beneath the inguinal ligament inferior and medial to the anterior superior iliac spine and exits the fascia lata a few centimeters distal to the inguinal ligament.
   a. **Presentation.** Patients complain of pain, paresthesias, and numbness in the lateral thigh, which limits physical activity. Motor strength should be preserved. In children, involvement is bilateral 50% of the time and typical body habitus is thin and muscular. In adults, bilateral involvement is rare and body habitus is obese. Tinel's sign is positive with percussion just inferomedial to the anterior superior iliac spine. Diagnosis can be confirmed with a local nerve block.
   b. **Treatment.** Conservative expectant treatment is the standard. Surgical decompression of the lateral femoral cutaneous nerve is indicated in cases of severe pain or in refractory cases.
2. **Iliacus hematoma syndrome.** Compression of the femoral nerve by hematoma formation in the iliac fossa results in the iliacus hematoma syndrome. This occurs most often in patients with a coagulation disorder. It is rare in athletes; however, it most often occurs in gymnasts through mechanisms that are poorly understood.
   a. **Presentation.** Symptoms consist of paresthesias over the anterior thigh and anteromedial leg with giving out of the knee. Examination of the extremity reveals weak or absent quadriceps strength and a diminished knee-jerk reflex. The psoas stretch test will be negative. The iliac fossa may be tender, with evidence of a mass and ecchymosis. Diagnosis is best made with MRI.
   b. **Treatment.** Treatment is evacuation of the hematoma, either via aspiration or open drainage. Full neurologic recovery is expected.

Suggested Reading

Butcher JD, Salzman KL, Wade LA. Lower extremity bursitis. *Am Fam Physician* 1996;53:2317–2324.

Paletta GA, Andrish JT. Injuries about the hip and pelvis in the young athlete. *Clin Sports Med* 1995;14:591–628.

49. THE GROIN AND THIGH

Barry P. Boden and William E. Garrett

I. Anatomy and Function

Skeletal muscle constitutes the single largest tissue mass in the body, making up 40% to 45% of the total body weight. The primary function of skeletal muscle is to provide joint movement and locomotion. The muscle fiber is the basic structural element of skeletal muscle. Muscle fiber originates from tendon or bone and courses across one or more joints to insert into bone via a tendon.

The fiber's arrangement and length are important factors in determining the contractile properties of the muscle. Muscle fibers may run parallel or oblique to the long axis of the muscle. Oblique fiber arrangements are referred to as *unipennate, bipennate,* or *multipennate.* Pennation permits production of increased force by packing a large number of fibers into a smaller cross-sectional area. The total amount and speed of shortening is related to the length of the muscle fiber. A muscle which produces large force output over a small range of motion, such as the deltoid, would contain short muscle fibers arranged in a pennated fashion. In contrast, a muscle needed for small force production over a large range of motion, such as the biceps, would contain long muscle fibers arranged in a parallel fashion.

Muscle fibers are composed of four major structural proteins: *myosin, actin, tropomyosin,* and *troponin.* Myosin or thick filaments contain projections capable of binding to the actin or thin filaments and hydrolyzing adenosine triphosphate (ATP). Tropomyosin and troponin are located on the thin filaments and prevent the myosin cross bridges from binding. Electrical impulses or action potentials in the muscles cause the release of calcium from the sarcoplasmic reticulum. Calcium induces a conformational change in the troponin and tropomyosin and allows the myosin cross bridges to attach to the thin filaments. The energy stored in ATP provides the chemical energy to cycle cross bridges and generate force in muscle.

A. **Fiber types.** The ability of the myosin ATPase to hydrolyze ATP can serve to classify muscle fibers into slow oxidative or fast glycolytic types and their subdivisions. Although muscles are often designated as slow-oxidative or fast-glycolytic, most muscles contain a mixture of fiber types.
   1. **Type I** or slow-oxidative fibers are extremely resistant to fatigue. Most type I muscles, such as the soleus, have a postural role and are located close to the bony skeleton.
   2. **Type II** or fast-glycolytic fibers, such as the gastrocnemius, are fatigue-sensitive but supply speed and power. They are often situated in a more superficial location. Type II fibers are further subdivided into types IIA, IIB, IIC, and IIM. As the fiber types develop faster contractions, they become more fatigue-sensitive.

II. Muscle Injury

A. **Prevalence.** Muscle injury is usually cited as the most frequent injury in sports.

B. **Etiology.** Although the exact mechanism of muscle injury remains unknown, there are several factors that may predispose muscle to injury. Muscle tears usually occur when the muscle is undergoing an eccentric or lengthening contraction. Type II fast-twitch muscles are prone to injury during eccentric contractions due to the large forces produced by the contractile element in addition to the extrinsic forces stretching the muscle. Muscles that cross two joints are subject to more stretch and are susceptible to injury.

"Two-joint" muscles that are frequently injured include the hamstrings, the rectus femoris, and the medial head of the gastrocnemius.

C. **Classification.** Indirect muscle injury may be divided into three distinct categories. It is best to wait 24 hr to allow the injury to declare itself prior to classification.

1. **Delayed-onset muscle soreness** (DOMS) is the most common type of muscle injury and is defined as generalized muscular pain that occurs 1 to 2 days after intense, eccentric exercise. Histological changes have been identified in muscle fibers throughout the muscle and not specifically at the musculotendinous junction. Clinically, muscle swelling and weakness may persist for 3 to 5 days. Strength loss may be up to 50% immediately postexercise. DOMS is usually not associated with any long-term morbidity. The structural abnormalities that accompany DOMS include Z-band streaming, A-band disruption, and myofibril misalignment.
2. **Incomplete or partial muscle strain injuries** present as more focal pain noted as an acute event during exercise and often result in significant morbidity. The vulnerable site in partial muscle strain injury is the musculotendinous junction. The failure occurs in the muscle fibers within several millimeters of the junction.
3. **Complete muscle ruptures** are recognized by a palpable defect in the muscle. Retraction of the muscle may be seen with attempts at muscle contraction. In the skeletally immature child, avulsion fractures are more common than complete muscle tears.

D. **History.** DOMS is a common problem following unaccustomed, intense exercise and is characterized by pain and weakness beginning several hours after exercise and peaking at 1 to 3 days. Partial and complete muscle injuries are marked by immediate pain following a powerful muscle contraction.

E. **Physical examination.** There are few findings on physical examination of DOMS other than pain and occasional weakness. In partial and complete muscle injury, swelling and subcutaneous ecchymosis may be detected after the injury. Unlike direct muscle contusions, where bleeding often occurs within the muscle belly, the bleeding in indirect muscle injuries escapes through the perimysium and fascia to the subcutaneous space. Often the ecchymosis is not visible for several days.

F. **Special Tests.** Intramuscular enzymes often reveal increased levels of creatine kinase, myoglobin, and lactate dehydrogenase. Diagnosis is based on clinical findings rather than biopsy or serological studies.

G. **Radiography.** Magnetic resonance imaging (MRI) has been found to be the most effective adjunctive study to localize free-fluid levels and hemorrhage in partial or complete muscle injuries. MRI predictably reveals injury at the myotendinous junction. Fluid collects at the disruption site and dissects along the epimysium, occasionally breaking through to the interfascial regions or subcutaneous space. Muscle tissue remote from the myotendinous junction also demonstrates changes in MRI signal consistent with edema and inflammation.

Some centers have had success diagnosing muscle injury with the use of ultrasonography. This technique may be helpful in imaging superficial muscles that are not covered by excessive subcutaneous fat.

H. **Treatment.** Present treatment strategies are often based more on clinical protocols than on scientific data. Initial treatment of all muscle injuries consists of ice and elevation. Heat modalities are usually avoided. Athletes with DOMS may be rapidly advanced to isokinetics, running, and sport-specific training. Those with partial and complete injuries must be advanced at a much slower pace. Local injection of steroids, application of dimethylsulfoxide (DMSO), and use of hyperbaric oxygen chambers have not proven to be beneficial. Surgical intervention is reserved for complete ruptures within the tendon or at the tendon-bone junction.

I. **Criteria for return to sports.** The athlete should not be allowed to return to sports until isokinetic testing reveals function within 10% of normal at slow and fast speeds. Satisfactory restoration of flexibility and endurance and a trial run of the specific sport should be achieved prior to game participation.

J. **Prevention.** Stretching, warm-up, and strength training are the cornerstones of preventing muscle injury. Muscles are often injured during eccentric contractions while they are resisting stretch. Therefore, flexible muscles may be protected from injury by being able to stretch further before injury. Static stretching at a slow speed is recommended over ballistic stretching. In addition, proper warm-up elevates muscle temperature and increases the amount of muscle elongation prior to rupture. Muscles are prone to injury when they are fatigued and can absorb less energy. Strength training through eccentric exercises may allow muscles to absorb more energy prior to failure.

III. Quadriceps Strains.

The rectus femoris is the most frequently injured muscle of the quadriceps mechanism. The muscle crosses two joints, has a high percentage of type II muscle fibers, and acts in an eccentric manner to decelerate motions at the hip and knee. Injuries are common in sports requiring sprinting or kicking, such as soccer.

A. **Anatomy.** The rectus femoris has two tendinous origins. The direct head originates off the anteroinferior iliac crest, while the indirect head arises from the superior acetabular ridge. Recent cadaveric studies have revealed that the tendon of the direct head is anterior and superficial, coursing along one-third the length of the muscle. The tendon of the indirect head initially lies in the posteromedial aspect of the muscle-tendon unit. As it progresses distally along the muscle, the tendon flattens out, rotates laterally, and migrates to the middle of the muscle belly. The tendon terminates in the middle of the muscle belly at the distal third of the muscle-tendon unit.

B. **Classification.** Significant disruption of the rectus femoris muscle may occur at two separate sites. The first injury occurs where the distal muscle fibers are disrupted from the quadriceps tendon. A more recently described injury occurs in the proximal belly substance at the musculotendinous junction of the indirect head. In skeletally immature children, the epiphyseal plate is weaker than the musculotendinous unit and avulsion of the tendon off the anterior inferior iliac crest may occur.

C. **Physical examination.** Complete disruption of the muscle fibers from the distal tendon results in proximal retraction of the entire muscle belly and an obvious asymmetry with the contralateral quadriceps mechanism. In contrast, the mass seen with proximal intrasubstance tears is less obvious and migrates distally toward the quadriceps tendon.

D. **Diagnostic tests.** MRI can be helpful in differentiating the two injuries. In the distal tendon tears, the abnormal signal is located more posteriorly within the muscle in the region of the posterior fascia and distal tendon of insertion. With the proximal intrasubstance tears, MRI reveals a "bull's-eye" lesion (high-intensity signal surrounding a low intensity area) centered about the deep tendon of the indirect head.

E. **Differential.** The intrasubstance lesion can be differentiated from a neoplastic lesion by T2-weighted MRI.

F. **Treatment.** Because no symptoms or functional deficits are associated with distal tears, nonoperative therapy is usually successful. The remaining quadriceps muscles will compensate for the rectus femoris. Intrasubstance lesions should also be treated conservatively. However, with chronic strain injury, the two tendons may function independently, causing refractory symptoms.

IV. Hamstring Injuries

are the most common muscle strains of the thigh and frequently occur in sprinters, participants in kicking sports, and water skiers.

A. **Anatomy.** All of the hamstring muscles with the exception of the short head of the biceps femoris cross two joints. Imaging studies have shown that injury can occur in any of the hamstring muscles, with the long head of the biceps femoris probably being the most common. The proximal and distal tendons of the long head of the biceps extend beyond the midpoint of the muscle, overlapping each other.

B. **Etiology.** In addition to spanning two joints, the hip and knee, the long head of the biceps femoris has a large percentage of type II fibers. The hamstrings are subject to high levels of tension, produced by the type II fibers and the extrinsic stretch, which make them prone to injury during vigorous athletic activities.

C. **History.** Often the athlete experiences prodromal symptoms of pain and stiffness in the muscle prior to the injury. The clinical history of a strain consists of acute pain in the posterior thigh during a sprint or kicking event. Less commonly, the proximal hamstring tendons are avulsed off the ischial tuberosity with or without a piece of bone. These avulsion injuries may occur in skeletally immature athletes or in adults exposed to a violent stretching force. In the novice water skier, the injury typically occurs during takeoff if the knees are locked. The skis are tilted upward, dorsiflexing the ankle, and the boat accelerates to pull the hips into extreme hip flexion. With proper training, the skier should be able to prevent this type of injury by maintaining a crouched position during takeoff. Among expert water skiers, the injury is typically due to a violent fall.

D. **Physical examination.** DOMS and partial muscle strains are characterized by pain near the muscle tendon junctions of the hamstrings. Occasionally ecchymosis and swelling may be present in partial strains. In a complete avulsion, a palpable defect may be present just distal to the ischial tuberosity. Ecchymosis may track subcutaneously to the ankle. Even with complete ruptures at the ischium, the patient maintains the ability to flex the knee because of the short head of the biceps femoris.

E. **Imaging.** Plain radiographs can rule out a bony avulsion of the ischium. Although computed tomography (CT) and magnetic resonance imaging (MRI) have contributed to the understanding of these injuries, a thorough history and physical examination usually suffice.

F. **Natural history.** Midhamstring muscle strains have a reported recurrence rate of 20% to 25%. This high recurrence rate may be related to scar formation from the original injury.

G. **Treatment.** Partial strains at the musculotendinous junction of the long head of the biceps are best treated conservatively with ice and elevation followed by stretching, strengthening, and sport-specific training. Treatment of complete avulsions in adults is somewhat controversial. The natural history of conservatively treated avulsions is far worse than that of a routine hamstring strain.

V. Adductors

A. **Anatomy.** Of the five adductor muscles, the adductor longus is the most frequently injured. The tendon of the adductor longus can be palpated subcutaneously in the groin region near its origin on the pubic bone.

B. **History.** The mechanism of injury may be overuse or trauma. Acute injuries are common in soccer, when the adductor muscles lengthen to prevent hyperabduction during a kicking maneuver.

C. **Physical examination.** In addition to local tenderness, partial strains may be accompanied by ecchymosis in the medial midthigh. A complete rupture may be diagnosed by a palpable defect in the muscle, inability to contract the muscle, and/or asymmetry as compared with the contour of the opposite groin. In adductor muscle strains, pain is reproduced by resisting adduction of the leg. Abdominal strains can be distinguished from adductor injuries by the presence of symptoms while the patient is performing sit-ups against minimal resistance.

D. **Differential.** Hip joint pathology, osteitis pubis, hernias, nerve entrapment, and rectus abdominis muscle strains may all mimic adductor muscle injuries.

E. **Treatment.** The majority of adductor injuries can be successfully managed with conservative therapy. Several authors have reported good results with an adductor tenotomy and excision of scar tissue for chronic, refractory cases.

VI. Quadriceps Contusions

In addition to indirect mechanisms, muscles may be injured by direct blows.

A. **History.** Athletes usually report a specific traumatic event in which an external object such as a knee or a helmet impacted the anterior thigh. These injuries are common in contact sports such as football, rugby, and the martial arts.

B. **Physical examination.** The severity of the contusion is often underestimated initially. Localized pain, swelling, and loss of knee flexion are typical symptoms. In severe thigh contusions, a sympathetic knee effusion may develop.

C. **Classification.** Mild contusions are diagnosed by knee motion greater than 90 degrees and no alteration in gait. Moderate contusion are characterized by total knee motion of 45 to 90 degrees and an antalgic gait. Severe contusions are exquisitely tender, have less than 45 degrees of motion, and are associated with a severe limp.

D. **Treatment.** The goal of therapy is to limit swelling, hemorrhage, and subsequent formation of scar tissue. Early treatment consists of ice, elevation, and compression to minimize hemorrhage. Nonsteroidal antiinflammatory drugs (NSAIDs) such as indocin may relieve pain and diminish the incidence of myositis ossificans. Immediate immobilization of the knee in flexion also helps to control swelling and stretch the quadriceps. This is followed by range-of-motion exercises, concentrating on flexion. Once 120 degrees of pain-free knee motion is achieved, functional rehabilitation is commenced. Emphasis on early immobilization in flexion combined with flexion exercises has dramatically reduced the disability caused by moderate and severe contusions.

E. **Complications.** Restoration of motion is often the limiting factor in regaining normal function. Hemorrhage into the thigh can result in fibrosis and scarring within the quadriceps mechanism, leading to a loss of flexion even after pain resolves.

VII. Myositis Ossificans (MO) may develop in 10% to 20% of thigh contusions.

A. **Etiology.** Pathologic findings have revealed that most of the tissue damage occurs deep within the vastus intermedius as it is crushed against the bone by blunt trauma. Intramembranous bone formation probably develops from metaplasia of the reparative scar tissue cells to osteoblastic cells. The MO may become severe enough to act as a check rein to prevent knee flexion.

B. **Risk factors** for the development of MO include knee range of motion <120 degrees at classification, a previous quadriceps injury, a sympathetic knee effusion, and delayed treatment.

C. **Diagnostic tests.** Radiographic evidence of MO first presents by 3 to 4 weeks after injury. Bone scanning may demonstrate the lesion several weeks prior to plain radiographs. Creatine kinase levels, although elevated, are inaccurate in predicting the formation of MO.

D. **Natural history.** By 3 to 6 months, the mass matures into cancellous bone and often stabilizes or resolves.

E. **Treatment.** Early treatment to limit swelling and hemorrhage minimizes the incidence of MO. Once MO is formed, most athletes do not develop any disability. If symptoms persist, excision of the heterotopic bone is recommended. The bone should never be resected prior to maturity of the mass, otherwise recurrence is likely.

VIII. Hernia

Direct, indirect, and femoral hernias are well-known entities in the medical community. Another condition that must be considered in the differential of groin pain is pubalgia.

A. **Etiology.** The condition is characterized by a weakness or defect near the pubic insertion of the rectus abdominus and internal oblique muscles. It is thought that the repetitive stresses of sprinting and kicking result in microtears of the pelvic floor musculature.

B. **History.** Athletic pubalgia may be seen in elite or professional-level athletes who participate in intense daily exercise. Initially pain is localized to the inguinal area; but with vigorous exercise, it may radiate into the lower abdomen, testicles, or medial thigh. Strenuous exercise such as sprinting and hard kicking may exacerbate the symptoms.

C. **Physical examination.** Findings include tenderness at the pubic tubercle and pain with resisted hip flexion and internal rotation. Symptoms are similar to those of a direct inguinal hernia, but the presence of a palpable hernia mass is rare.

D. **Treatment.** Conservative therapy consists of rest, antiinflammatory medications, and light muscle-strengthening exercises. Often nonoperative therapy is only temporarily effective and many athletes develop recurrent symptoms upon return to competition. For those who fail a 3- to 6-month trial of conservative therapy, a Bassini herniorrhaphy may be indicated. Good results have been reported using this procedure and most athletes are able to return to full competition by 4 to 6 months postsurgery.

IX. Femoral Shaft Stress Fractures

Stress fractures are fatigue fractures of bone secondary to repetitive forces. In a review of over 300 athletes with a stress fracture, femoral stress fractures were found to be the fourth most common bone injured (7%) after the tibia (48%), tarsals (25%), and metatarsals (9%). Femoral shaft stress fractures are overuse injuries commonly found in military recruits and long-distance runners.

A. **Anatomy.** Femoral shaft stress fractures are usually located on the medial, compression side of the femur at the junction of the proximal and middle thirds of the femoral shaft.

B. **Etiology.** Stress fractures may occur when there is an imbalance between bone injury and bone remodeling. The exact mechanism responsible for initiating stress fractures remains unclear. One theory holds that excessive forces are transmitted to the bone when the surrounding muscles become fatigued. In contrast, another theory states that highly concentrated muscle forces act across a localized area of bone to cause mechanical insults above the stress-bearing capacity of the bone.

Systemic factors such as nutritional deficiencies, metabolic disorders, hormonal abnormalities, or sleep deprivation may contribute to the onset of a stress fracture. Due to the increased susceptibility of stress fractures in women, it is important to investigate intrinsic factors in this group of athletes. Many female athletes, especially those participating in gymnastics, figure-skating, and cross-country running, may develop eating disorders during puberty to maintain their muscular, petite, body image. Others have delayed menarche or menstrual irregularities due to the intensity of exercise. A low-estrogenic state leads to a decrease in bone mineral density and an increased risk of stress fractures.

C. **History.** Athletes often provide a history of an abrupt increase in the duration, intensity, or frequency of physical activity. Symptoms are often vague and limited to a deep ache in the thigh or groin region. Quite often the pain is difficult to localize due to the overlying musculature.

D. **Radiographic findings** are delayed from 2 to 4 weeks after the onset of pain. Due to the paucity of clinical findings and the delay in radiographic findings, scintigraphy has proved valuable in confirming the presence of a stress fracture within 3-5 days.

E. **Treatment.** The majority of femoral shaft stress fractures are related to training errors and can be treated by a period of rest followed by gradual resumption of activity. The initial treatment involves a period of cessation of all impact activities. Amenorrhea or metabolic abnormalities should be included in the differential and treated appropriately.

Suggested Reading

Brunet ME, Hontas RB. The thigh. In: DeLee JC, Drez D, eds. *Orthopaedic sports medicine: principles and practice*. Philadelphia: W.B. Saunders, 1994:1086–1112.

Hasselman, CT, Best TM, Hughes C IV, et al. An explanation for various rectus femoris strain injuries using previously undescribed muscle architecture. *Am J Sports Med* 1995; 23:493–499.

Ryan JB, Wheeler JH, Hopkinson WJ, et al. Quadriceps contusions: West Point update. *Am J Sports Med* 1991; 19:299–304.

Taylor DC, Meyers WC, Moylan JA, et al. Inguinal hernias and pubalgia. *Am J Sports Med* 1991;19:239–242.

50. KNEE-LIGAMENTS

John A. Bergfeld and Marc R. Safran

Knee ligament injuries are among the most common (medial collateral ligament) and significant (anterior cruciate ligament) as well as potentially disabling (multiple ligaments) injuries sustained during athletic activities. Early diagnosis and treatment may reduce long-term morbidity and return the athlete to sports sooner. Though magnetic resonance imaging (MRI) has aided in the diagnosis of knee ligament injuries, most of these injuries can be diagnosed by history and physical examination alone, particularly if the knee can be examined immediately after injury (on the field). The immediate management of isolated knee ligament injuries includes ice to reduce swelling in the knee, quadriceps strengthening (straight leg raises, quad sets) to reduce the disuse atrophy and atrophy associated with large intraarticular swelling, range-of-motion exercises, and crutches for ambulation until the athlete is able to walk without a limp. A hinged knee brace may also be useful, particularly for collateral ligament injuries.

I. Anatomy

There are four main ligaments in the knee. The medial collateral ligament (MCL) runs from the medial femoral epicondyle to the proximal medial tibia, sending a deep band to the medial meniscus. It is the main ligament resisting valgus stress to the knee. The lateral collateral ligament (LCL) is an extraarticular ligament that runs from the lateral femoral epicondyle, just posterior to the popliteus origin, to the fibular head. It is the primary stabilizer resisting varus force. The anterior cruciate ligament (ACL) and posterior cruciate ligament (PCL) are considered extraarticular though they are within the notch of the knee running from the femur to the tibia. The ACL originates on the posteromedial wall of the lateral femoral condyle and inserts onto the tibial eminence, resisting anterior tibial translation. The PCL originates on the anterolateral wall of the medial femoral condyle and inserts slightly distal to the articular surface of the posterior tibial plateau; it primarily resists posterior tibial translation. The capsule of the knee has thickenings of functional significance. The posteromedial knee capsule contributes oblique fibers from the superficial medial collateral ligament; often this is called the posteromedial corner or posterior oblique ligament (POL). The posterolateral corner of the knee includes capsular thickenings and other ligamentous tissues known as the popliteal-fibular ligament. Together, this area is known as the posterolateral corner.

II. Classification of Ligament Sprains

The classification of ligament sprains depends on the extent of tear and degree of abnormal laxity that results. A *grade I* sprain results in pain and tenderness along the ligaments (MCL and LCL) due to microscopic tearing and hemorrhage but no abnormal laxity to stress testing as compared with the other knee and a firm end point. A *grade II* sprain is a partial tear with partial loss of function of the ligament as determined by a slight amount of increased translation to stress testing (3 to 5 mm). A firm end point is noted. A *grade III* sprain is a complete tear of the ligament. Stress testing reveals 5 mm more of joint translation than that of the contralateral (normal) knee. There is no firm end point with stress testing

III. Medial Collateral Ligament

The MCL is the most commonly injured ligament about the knee. Injuries of the MCL rarely causes any long-term problems provided that the full range of motion is restored. These injuries may occur in any part of the ligament.

A. **Etiology.** Sprains of the MCL are often caused by a blow to the lateral knee, particularly while weight bearing and the foot is planted. Noncontact mechanisms include valgus or valgus-rotation types of injuries.

B. **History.** The athlete will give a history consistent with the mechanism described above. He or she will complain of medial knee pain, particularly with valgus stress, and occasionally weight bearing. The patient may say that the knee "bent inward." Rarely, the patient will note a "pop" at the time of injury, but more commonly a tearing or pulling sensation on the medial aspect of the knee is noted. There may be some swelling at the site of injury (over the MCL), with ecchymosis developing 1 to 3 days following injury. With lesser degrees of injury, the athlete may be able to continue playing, seeking evaluation only after the game or during an intermission.

C. **Physical Examination.** This will reveal tenderness along the MCL. The patient may walk with a limp and the knee partially flexed, particularly if seen a few days following the injury. An effusion may be absent in isolated MCL injuries. There will be tenderness over the ligament and there may be laxity with valgus stress testing (see appendix 6) as the ligament is tested in 20 to 30 degrees of flexion. Valgus stress testing should reproduce or accentuate the patient's knee pain. Assessment of laxity in full extension is also important. Laxity in full extension may be indicative of injury to the posteromedial capsule and signifies a more significant injury, and care should be taken to evaluate for concomitant ACL and PCL injury. The severity of the pain does not correlate to the severity of the sprain.

D. **Diagnostic Tests.** Plain radiographs are required to rule out associated injury or fracture. In the acute setting, anteroposterior, lateral, oblique, and Merchant views of the patella radiographs are obtained. In the subacute or chronic situation, a 45-degree flexion weight-bearing posteroanterior view should be added.

E. **Special Tests.** If the physical examination is difficult to perform or if damage to other intra-articular structures is suspected, an MRI may be helpful to confirm the full extent of injury.

F. **Natural History.** Isolated MCL injuries generally heal, regardless of the degree of injury. Athletes with injuries involving the femoral origin tend to have a higher incidence of knee stiffness. Additionally, proximal MCL injuries tend to heal with more residual laxity as compared with injuries involving the tibial insertion.

G. **Prevention.** The prevention of MCL sprains is a controversial topic. The general feeling is that prophylactic knee bracing is only minimally effective in preventing an initial injury, though a functional brace with medial and lateral stays may reduce the risk of reinjury for contact sports.

H. **Treatment Options.** With new research showing the detrimental effects of immobilization on injured and healing ligaments, immobilization of MCL sprains has fallen out of favor. Further, isolated MCL tears heal well without surgery, regardless of the degree of injury, patient's age, or activity level. Usually some residual laxity can be elicited on examination after a grade II or III injury because the ligament may heal in a lengthened state, but this has little effect on knee function.

I. **Recommended Treatment.** This depends on the stability of the joint. Grades I and II MCL sprains are treated symptomatically with or without a rehabilitation brace. Isolated grade III MCL sprains are unstable with valgus stress and are treated with a hinged rehabilitation knee brace for 4 to 6 weeks. This program allows for early motion and reduced stiffness while the inflammation resolves. Ice and cold compression may help initially. Isometric exercises of the quadriceps and hamstrings help reduce disuse atrophy. Stationary cycling at low resistance is helpful for maintaining and gaining motion. Assistive devices are useful for ambulation until the athlete can fully extend the knee without an extensor lag and can walk without a limp.

J. **Return to Sports.** The patient can return to full athletic activity when the ligament is no longer tender, there is no pain to valgus stress, laxity to valgus stress testing is minimal or no residual, and there is full range of motion, good strength, normal endurance, and full functional use.

IV. Lateral Collateral Ligament

This is the least commonly injured knee ligament. Injury of the LCL more often occurs in conjunction with other ligamentous injuries of the knee. Isolated injury to this ligament in athletes is uncommon because a direct blow to the medial side of the knee is an unusual occurrence in sports.

A. **Etiology.** Sprains of the LCL are usually the result of a direct varus stress to the knee, generally with the foot planted and the knee in extension. Varus stress to the knee may also occur during the stance phase of gait, with sudden imbalance and shift of the center of gravity away from the side of injury resulting in tension on the lateral structures of the knee. The varus injury to the knee often involves a rotational component. Straight varus injuries result in LCL injuries. These tend to be tears from the fibular head (with or without avulsion) but may occur anywhere in the LCL.

B. **History.** The athlete may note the above mechanism of injury. He or she may have heard or felt a pop in the knee and noted lateral knee pain.

C. **Physical Examination.** Acutely, there is tenderness along the lateral aspect of the knee. The athlete may walk with a limp or, in chronic cases, there may be a lateral thrust in stance phase. An intraarticular effusion may be present, signifying a capsular injury or an associated meniscal or chondral lesion. Because the LCL is extraarticular, isolated LCL injuries do not commonly result in an effusion of the knee. The ligament can usually be palpated with the knee in the "figure four" position (while the patient is seated, the foot of the injured knee is placed on the contralateral knee). The ligament feels like a taut band from the fibular head to the lateral femoral epicondyle. When it is injured, the ability to palpate this ligament is diminished. Neurovascular examination is important, since peroneal nerve injuries are commonly associated with LCL injuries. Laxity to varus stress is assessed in 30 degrees of knee flexion and in full extension (see appendix 6). Since LCL tears commonly occur in conjunction with other knee ligament injuries, a complete knee ligament assessment is important, as with any knee injury, paying special attention to injuries of the PCL, ACL, and posterolateral corner (see Appendix 6).

D. **Diagnostic Tests.** Plain radiographs are needed to look for avulsion fractures of the fibular head as well as to rule out associated injury or fracture. In the acute setting, anteroposterior, lateral, and Merchant views of the patella as well as oblique radiographs are obtained. In the subacute or chronic situation, a posteroanterior radiograph with 45-degree flexion weight bearing is added.

E. **Special Tests.** If the physical examination is difficult to perform or if damage to other structures is suspected (posterolateral corner, ACL, PCL, menisci, etc.), an MRI may be helpful to confirm the full extent of injury.

F. **Natural History.** For isolated LCL injuries, this has yet to be determined. There are only a few studies with limited numbers of subjects with isolated LCL disruptions. Severe straight lateral instability with more than 10 mm of lateral joint opening as compared with the contralateral knee usually implies injury to the ACL and/or PCL. It appears that truly isolated LCL injuries do well with nonoperative treatment.

G. **Prevention.** The prevention of LCL sprains is a controversial topic. The general feeling is that prophylactic knee bracing is ineffective in preventing an initial injury.

H. **Treatment Options.** With new research showing the detrimental effects of immobilization on injured and healing ligaments, immobilization of LCL sprains has fallen out of favor. Further, isolated low-grade LCL tears are felt to heal well without surgery. Isolated grade III LCL injury does not occur. Thus grade III LCL injuries are surgically repaired with the associated injured structures. Displaced bony avulsions are usually treated with surgical reduction and fixation.

I. **Recommended Treatment.** This depends on the stability of the joint. Grades I and II LCL sprains are treated symptomatically with or without a rehabilitation brace. A hinged rehabilitation knee brace for 4 to 6 weeks may be of benefit. This program allows for early motion and reduced stiffness while the inflammation resolves. Ice and cold compression may help early. Isometric exercises of the quadriceps and hamstrings help reduce disuse atrophy. Stationary cycling at low resistance is helpful for maintaining and gaining motion. Assistive devices are useful for ambulation until the athlete can fully extend the knee without an extensor lag and can walk without a limp.

Surgical management for grade III LCL injuries is recommended for those patients who have varus abnormal laxity, for those with a bony avulsion that is displaced 3 mm or more, or combined ligament injury.

J. **Return to Sports.** This occurs when the ligamentous pain to palpation resolves and there is no pain to varus stress, minimal or no residual laxity to varus stress testing, full range of motion, good strength and endurance, and full functional use. For those undergoing bony fixation, this may be 3 months or longer, while repair for acute or chronic varus abnormal laxity may require 6 months of postoperative rehabilitation.

V. Anterior Cruciate Ligament

The ACL is the primary stabilizer for resisting anterior translation of the tibia on the femur. It also serves as a secondary stabilizer to resist internal rotation of the tibia on the femur as well as varus and valgus rotation. The ACL is one of the most commonly injured ligaments in the knee.

A. **Etiology.** The ACL may be injured by contact or noncontact mechanisms. Pathomechanics include a valgus force applied to a flexed, externally rotated knee with the foot planted or hyperextension often combined with internal rotation. This common mechanism occurs when the athlete is landing from a jump. Less common mechanisms of injury include hyperflexion or a direct valgus force. The direct valgus force often produces combined MCL and ACL injuries, commonly with meniscal tears. Injuries of the ACL occur as the result of sports such as basketball, soccer, and football that place a high demand on the knee through jumping, pivoting, and hard cutting forces as well as direct contact. The majority of ruptures occur in the midsubstance of the ligament.

B. **History.** The athlete will often recall hearing or feeling a "pop" in the knee at the time of injury and will note intraarticular swelling within 2 to 6 hr of the time of injury. The injury is usually disabling and the athlete is unable to continue playing. Skiers usually have to be helped from the slopes by the ski patrol. The patient may complain of knee instability or giving way.

C. **Physical Examination.** This will vary based on the time from injury. Acutely there is large knee swelling, whereas a chronic ACL tear may or may not have an effusion. The patient may walk with a limp. The Lachman test is the easiest and most reproducible indicator of a torn ACL (see Appendix 6). The patient must be relaxed, as hamstring contraction or spasticity may reduce the anterior translation of the test (see Appendix 6). Excessive anterior translation of the tibia on the femur at 30 degrees of knee flexion with a soft or lack of a firm end point is indicative of a torn ACL. The pivot shift maneuver is a useful confirmatory test; however, patient guarding with an acute injury may not allow the examiner to perform this test. Range of motion may be limited by the large effusion or associated injury to the MCL or a displaced meniscal tear. A complete knee examination is necessary to rule out associated injuries, such as damage to the MCL, meniscal tears, patellar dislocations, etc. Note that a patellar dislocation can easily be confused with an acute ACL injury.

D. **Diagnostic Tests.** Plain radiographs are required to rule out associated injury or fracture. In the acute setting, anteroposterior, lateral, merchant views of the patella and occasionally oblique radiographs are obtained. In the subacute or chronic situation, posteroanterior views with 45-degree flexion weight bearing are obtained. The Segond sign is a lateral capsular avulsion fracture with a small fleck of bone pulled off the lateral tibia. This is pathognomonic for an ACL tear.

E. **Special Tests.** If the physical examination is difficult to perform or if damage to other intraarticular structures is suspected, a repeat physical examination as the acute reaction settles down is usually of benefit. In addition, an *MRI* may be helpful to determine the full extent of injury. If a patient elects to undergo surgery, an MRI is not necessary. The MRI is useful to assess meniscal tears and document of bone bruises and injury to the articular cartilage for the patient who would prefer not to undergo reconstruction. An MRI is not necessary to make the diagnosis; a carefully performed physical examination will give the diagnosis in over 90% of cases. The *KT-1000* knee ligament arthrometer can be useful to quantify and document the amount of knee laxity. A manual maximum side-to-side difference of more than 3 mm (as compared with a normal contralateral knee) is diagnostic of an ACL tear. In the acute setting, *joint aspiration* will reveal a bloody effusion. If this is present, there is an approximately 85% likelihood that the patient has sustained an ACL tear. Again, a patellar subluxation or dislocation may be confused with an ACL tear.

F. **Natural History.** In the case of isolated ACL injuries, this is still unclear. The torn ACL does not heal, and ACL deficiency leads to combined anterior and rotatory abnormal laxity, resulting in functional disability. This can occur with activities of daily living in some; with sports activities such as running (deceleration), cutting, and jumping in others; and with no functional instability in others still. Repetitive episodes of giving way may result in meniscal tears and damage to the articular cartilage, which can result in posttraumatic arthritis. Debate exists as to whether isolated ACL tears will result in joint degeneration. A direct relationship exists between future episodes of giving way and activity level (amount of time in high demand sports), but many patients can return to sports at a *less* stressful level of activity.

G. **Prevention.** This is a controversial topic. Prophylactic knee bracing is ineffective in preventing an injury to the ACL, though some surgeons do use functional braces for variable periods of time after ACL reconstruction to protect the healing ACL graft. Proprioceptive education, strengthening, and proper technique may play a role in prevention of knee ligament injuries.

H. **Treatment Options.** Grade I or II ACL tears may be treated nonoperatively provided that there is a good end point on examination. Unfortunately, these are very rare injuries. Grade III ACL tears may be treated with activity modification, bracing, and rehabilitation or surgical reconstruction. Many techniques of ACL reconstruction exist, but all rely on replacing the torn ACL with a graft from another location (central third patellar tendon or hamstrings) or from a cadaveric donor (allograft patellar tendon or Achilles tendon).

I. **Recommended Treatment.** This depends on the stability of the joint. To return to high-level sports, the athlete usually requires an ACL reconstruction for grade III injuries. However, treatment must be individualized based on the athlete's goals, expectations, and disability. Combined injuries to the ACL and MCL are usually an indication to reconstruct the ACL. Further, in the young athlete with a concomitant meniscal tear that is reparable (as opposed to an irreparable tear that requires excision), the meniscal repair should be performed with an ACL reconstruction to enhance the likelihood that the meniscus will heal. Tears of the ACL in skeletally immature athletes are usually treated nonoperatively initially. If functional instability persists after rehabilitation, consideration is then given to reconstruction. Rehabilitation of ACL tears concentrates on reduction of effusion, regaining full range of motion, exercise to regain muscle control and strength (particularly in the hamstrings), functional training, bracing, and patient education, including avoidance of high-risk activities involving stop/cut/change of direction.

J. **Return to Sports.** This occurs when there is no pain and when full range of motion, good strength and endurance, and full functional use have been restored. This usually requires 6 to 9 months following an ACL reconstruction, and 3 to 6 months for nonoperatively treated knees.

VI. Posterior Cruciate Ligament

The PCL is the largest and strongest ligament in the knee. It resists posterior translation of the tibia on the femur and serves to control hyperextension of the knee. The true incidence of PCL tears is unknown, though it is thought to account for 3 to 20% of all significant knee injuries. Our understanding of the PCL and the consequences of rupture lag behind that of the ACL and MCL.

A. **Etiology.** The PCL requires a large force to rupture it. The mechanism of most athletic injuries is a fall on the flexed knee with the foot plantarflexed. This imparts a posteriorly directed force on the proximal tibia, which ruptures the taut ligament (like the dashboard injury in car accidents). Another mechanism of injury to the PCL is a downwardly directed force applied to the thigh while the knee is hyperflexed, as when landing from a jump. Hyperflexion of the knee without a direct blow to the tibia can also result in an isolated PCL injury. Other mechanisms of injury can result in injury to the PCL, but these often cause injury to other ligaments as well. Forced hyperextension can injure the PCL, but generally this also results in injury to associated capsular structures as well as the ACL. A posteriorly directed force applied to the anteromedial tibia with the knee in hyperextension may also cause injury to the posterolateral corner and results in lateral and posterolateral instability. Significant varus or valgus stress injures the PCL only after the appropriate collateral ligament is injured.

B. **History.** The athlete will give a history consistent with a mechanism as described above. An intraarticular swelling is often noted within 2 to 6 hr of the time of injury, though it is usually less than that seen with an anterior cruciate ligament tear. The athlete may or may not be able to continue playing that day, though he or she will have difficulty competing for the next few weeks. Occasionally, these injuries are felt to be minor events. Athletes who present several months after injury may complain of patellofemoral pain and occasionally of instability.

C. **Physical examination** will vary based on the time from injury. Acutely there may or may not be much knee swelling, whereas a chronic PCL tear usually does not have an effusion. The patient may walk with a limp. A posterior sag of the tibia on the femur may be noted by looking from the lateral side of the knee with the patient supine and the hip and knee flexed and relaxed (see Appendix 6). The posterior drawer is the easiest, most reproducible, accurate, and sensitive indicator of a torn PCL (see Appendix 6). The patient must be relaxed, as quadriceps contraction or spasticity may reduce the posterior sag and hamstring contraction may accentuate the posterior sag of the tibia, reducing the posterior translation of the drawer test. The reverse pivot shift maneuver is a useful confirmatory test if there is associated posterolateral capsular injury; however, patient guarding may not allow the examiner to perform this test (see Appendix 6). The quadriceps active test may also be useful in making the diagnosis of PCL injury (see Appendix 6). Range of motion may be limited by effusion or associated injury to the MCL or a displaced meniscal tear. Because of the great amount of force necessary to tear the PCL, a complete knee examination is necessary to rule out associated injuries, such as MCL, meniscal tears, posterolateral corner injury, and so on, though associated chondral fracture and meniscal injury are less common than with ACL tears. A grade III injury is identified by a excessive posterior translation (greater than 10 mm) during the posterior drawer test with a soft end point or none and a positive reverse pivot shift maneuver. A partial or isolated PCL injury is indicated by (1) abnormal posterior laxity less than 10 mm, (2) decreasing abnormal posterior laxity with internal rotation of the tibia, (3) no rotatory abnormal laxity greater than 5 to 10 degrees, and (4) no significant varus or valgus abnormal laxity.

D. **Diagnostic Tests.** Plain radiographs are required to rule out associated injury or fracture. In the acute setting, anteroposterior, lateral, and merchant views of the patella are obtained. In the subacute or chronic situation, a posteroanterior 45-degree flexion weight-bearing view is added. A lateral radiograph is mandatory to assess for posterior tibial avulsion fracture, which is not uncommonly seen in the skeletally immature athlete.

E. **Special Tests.** If the physical examination is difficult to perform or if damage to other intraarticular structures is suspected, an *MRI* may be helpful to determine the full extent of injury. The MRI or computed tomography (CT) scan can reveal a nondisplaced or minimally displaced fracture of the posterior tibia. If a patient elects to undergo surgery, an MRI is not necessary. But the MRI is useful to assess meniscal tears and to document bone bruises for those patients who would prefer to avoid reconstruction. The *KT-1000* knee ligament arthrometer can be useful to quantify and document the amount of knee laxity. In the acute setting, *joint aspiration* may or may not reveal a bloody effusion (as opposed to the ACL injury, which almost always involves a bloody effusion). The presence of fat globules suggests a fracture.

F. **Natural History.** In the case of isolated PCL injuries, this is beginning to be clarified. Some patients experience almost no functional limitation and compete at high-level athletics, whereas others are severely limited during activities of daily living. Some investigators have shown that people adapt functionally to the PCL deficiency over 3 to 8 months, then do well for 15 to 20 years. After this time, it is felt that many progress to develop degenerative change within the medial compartment and patellofemoral joints of the knee. This progression to functional adaptation and to arthritic change has yet to be shown by others. A recent landmark study confirms that 90% of isolated PCL injuries do well clinically in spite of persistent abnormal laxity. Thus, the PCL injury differs from the ACL injury. Quadriceps strength has been shown in some studies to correlate with good knee function following PCL injury. It does appear that some PCL injuries heal in a lengthened position.

G. **Prevention.** This is unclear. As with other knee injuries, proper technique, strength, and proprioceptive training may help to reduce the incidence of PCL sprains.

H. **Treatment Options.** Isolated PCL tears are treated nonoperatively, since many athletes do well with this injury. Grade III PCL tears may be treated with activity modification, rehabilitation, or reconstruction. Many techniques of PCL reconstruction exist, but all rely on replacing the torn PCL with a graft from another location (central third patellar tendon or hamstrings) or from a cadaveric donor (allograft patellar tendon or Achilles tendon). Due to the complexity of the PCL anatomy, surgical reconstruction rarely restores normal laxity to the knee and thus rarely restores completely normal kinematics. Displaced bony avulsions are usually treated acutely with open reduction and internal fixation.

I. **Recommended Treatment.** This depends on the stability of the joint. Most grade I and II isolated PCL tears are treated nonoperatively with ice to reduce effusion, crutches to assist in ambulation until the patient can ambulate without a limp, strength training (emphasizing quadriceps strength), and range-of-motion exercises. Grade III PCL injuries are more controversial. If the injury is outside the previously described physical examination for isolated PCL injury, there is concomitant capsular or ligament injury and reconstruction is indicated. Further, acute displaced bony avulsions are treated with open reduction and internal fixation. Chronic, *symptomatic* PCL tears are treated with reconstruction if the athlete has failed an adequate rehabilitation program. Patient education is important for nonoperatively treated patients due to the tendency to develop posttraumatic changes in the patellofemoral and medial tibiofemoral compartments of the knee. Patients should avoid activities that cause pain and swelling of the knee as well as repetitive activities that involve high loading of these joints, as this may accelerate the degenerative process.

J. **Return to Sports.** This occurs when there is no pain and when full range of motion, good strength and endurance (within 90% of the contralateral quadriceps), and full functional use have been recovered. This usually requires 9 to 12 months following a PCL reconstruction and 1 to 2 months for nonoperatively treated knees.

VII. Knee Dislocation and the Multiple-Ligament-Injured Knee

Knee dislocations and other less severe multiple ligamentous injuries make up approximately 20% of all grade III knee ligament injuries. Other than combined ACL-MCL injuries, combined ligamentous injuries account for less than 2% of injuries to knee ligaments. Frequent two-ligament injury combinations include ACL-MCL, PCL-MCL, ACL-LCL, PCL-posterolateral corner, ACL-posterolateral corner, and ACL-PCL. To dislocate the knee, usually three ligaments must be torn (usually both cruciates and one collateral). Neurovascular injuries must be considered in all multiple-ligament injuries but occur more commonly after knee dislocation and less commonly in a knee in which only two ligaments are injured (except for LCL injuries).

A. **Etiology.** A person may dislocate the knee simply by stepping in a hole and hyperextending the knee, adding a rotational component to the isolated ligamentous injury mechanism (ACL-MCL) or continuing the force to cause further injury after an isolated ligament injury (such as continued hyperextension to tear the ACL then the PCL). Dislocations can also occur from a high-energy blow to the knee. A posteriorly directed force applied to the anteromedial tibia with the knee in hyperextension may cause injury to the PCL and posterolateral corner, resulting in lateral and posterolateral instability. Significant varus or valgus stress injury injures the ACL or PCL only after the appropriate collateral ligament is injured.

B. **History.** The athlete will often give a history of significant trauma, though, as noted above, it may be trivial. An intraarticular swelling within 2 to 6 hr of the time of injury is often noted, though it may not be large owing to often associated capsular injuries. The athlete will note hearing one or more "pops" in the knee and usually cannot continue sports participation. A deformity may be noted if the knee is dislocated and not reduced spontaneously.

C. **Physical Examination.** This will vary based the type of injury. A thorough examination is necessary to assess each ligament: varus and valgus stress tests to evaluate the collateral ligaments, the Lachman test and pivot shift to assess the ACL, the posterior drawer to evaluate the PCL. The Dial test helps evaluate the posterolateral corner, and the hyperextension-recurvatum test confirms the presence of a combined injury to the PCL-posterolateral corner. Neurovascular examination is of importance immediately after injury. Popliteal artery disruption occurs in 20% to 40% of all knee dislocations (it is highest with posterior knee dislocation), with a high incidence of amputations, particularly if the arterial injury is not recognized. Nerve injury, particularly involving the peroneal nerve, occurs in 20% to 30% of all knee dislocations, particularly with LCL and posterolateral corner injuries. Associated meniscal tears and chondral fractures are not common with knee dislocations. Neurovascular injuries are less common in knees with two ligaments injured.

D. **Classification.** This is based on the position of the tibia with relation to the femur: anterior, posterior, medial, lateral, and rotatory. The specific ligaments injured are graded as above.

E. **Diagnostic Tests.** Plain radiographs are required to rule out associated injury or fracture. In the acute setting, anteroposterior, lateral, and oblique radiographs are obtained. In the subacute or chronic situation, flexion weight-bearing posteroanterior, lateral, and sunrise views are obtained.

F. **Special Tests.** An ***MRI*** is helpful to determine the full extent of injury to assess intra and extra-articular structures. An ***angiogram*** is useful to assess the popliteal artery in knee dislocations. Even if a pulse is palpated, there may be an intimal tear that may disrupt blood flow in a delayed fashion. The ***KT-1000*** knee ligament arthrometer can be useful to quantify and document the amount of knee laxity of the ACL and PCL. ***Stress radiographs*** may be useful to quantify varus and valgus laxity.

G. **Natural History.** With regard to knee dislocations and multiple-ligament-injured knees, this is unknown owing to the uncommon nature of these injuries as well as to the many types of dislocations and mechanisms of injury (high- versus low-velocity) that can occur. It is known that if a vascular injury is left untreated for more than 8 hr, there is an 86% amputation rate. Associated nerve injury has a guarded prognosis for recovery regardless of treatment. The development of instability, loss of motion, and arthritis is unclear. The level of function in patients with multiple ligamentous injuries is worse than in those with an isolated ligamentous injury.

H. **Prevention.** Proper technique as well as strength and proprioceptive training may help to reduce knee injury.

I. **Treatment Options.** These include nonoperative approaches with functional bracing and aggressive rehabilitation. Properly timed surgical repair or reconstruction of all or some or the ligaments in the hands of an experience orthopaedic surgeon has the best chance of an optimal result.

J. **Recommended treatment** depends on the patients' goals, the ligaments injured, associated injuries, and the surgeon's comfort with the procedures. In repair, all vascular injuries take priority and represent true surgical emergencies. An unreducible knee dislocation is also a true surgical emergency. For knee injuries and dislocations involving multiple ligaments, injured properly timed surgical intervention (repair or reconstruction) is generally recommended to help regain stability to the knee and allow for early, aggressive rehabilitation to regain as much motion and strength as possible. Further, it is felt that the enhanced stability may reduce the risk of delayed arthritis.

K. **Return to Sports**

This occurs when there is no pain and a return to full range of motion, good strength and endurance (within 90% of the contralateral quadriceps), and full functional use. This varies with the injury and associated injuries. *Some athletes may never return to sports following a knee dislocation, depending on the associated injuries and demands of the sport.* The combined ligamentous injuries involving a cruciate and collateral ligament usually allow return to sport in the same time frame as that for cruciate reconstruction. Injuries of the posterolateral corner usually require 9 to 12 months of recovery before return to sports can occur.

Suggested Reading

Daniel DM, Stone ML, Dobson BE, et al. Fate of the ACL injured patient: a prospective outcome study. *Am J Sports Med* 1994; 22: 632–644.

Dejour H, Walch G, Peyrot J, Eberhard P. The natural history of rupture of the PCL. *French J Orthop Surg* 1988; 2: 112–120.

DeLee JC, Riley MB, Rockwood CA. Acute straight lateral instability of the knee. *Am J Sports Med* 1983; 11: 404–411.

Indelicato PA, Hermansdorfer J, Huegel M. Non-operative management of complete tears of the MCL of the knee in intercollegiate football players. *Clin Orthop Rel Res* 1990; 256: 174–177.

Irrgang JJ, Safran MR, Fu FH. The Knee: ligamentous and meniscal injuries. In: Zachazewski JE, Magee DJ, Quillen WS eds. *Athletic injuries and rehabilitation.* Philadelphia: WB Saunders, 1996.

Shelbourne KD, Patel D. Natural history of acute isolated non-operatively treated posterior cruciate ligament injuries of the knee: a prospective study. Presented at the 64th Annual Meeting of the AAOS, San Francisco, CA, February 1997.

Shelbourne KD, Porter DA, Clingman JA, et al. Low-velocity knee dislocation. *Orthop Rev* 1991; 20: 995–1004.

Veltri DM, Warren RF. Isolated and combined PCL injuries. *J Am Acad Orthop Surg* 1993; 1: 67–75.

51. KNEE-CARTILAGE

Christopher D. Harner and Ronald A. Navarro

I. Meniscus

A. Tears

1. **Anatomy.** The menisci are two crescent-shaped wedges of fibrocartilage between the femoral condyles and the tibial plateau. The outer border is attached to the adjacent capsule and tibia (coronary ligament). The meniscus is thickest peripherally and tapers centrally. There are anterior and posterior bony anchors that resist extrusion of the meniscus due to body weight. The peripheral 10% to 30% of the meniscus is generally its vascular zone and is supplied by branches from the medial and lateral geniculate arteries. Circumferential and radial fibers in the meniscus resist hoop and shear stresses, respectively. The medial meniscus is less mobile than the lateral meniscus. The menisci increase joint congruity and stability.
2. **Types.** Tears have been classified on the basis of their location in relation to the peripherally based blood supply (and healing potential). The meniscus is divided into circumferential thirds, with tears in the peripheral third considered to be within the vascular or *red-red zone.* Because of its proximity to the arterial supply, the greatest healing potential exists in this zone. Tears in the avascular central or *white-white zone* have limited healing potential unless special techniques are used. Tears in the middle or *red-white zone* have intermediate healing potential. Tears can also be classified based on their orientation and have been described as *longitudinal, radial, horizontal,* or *oblique. Complex* tears are combinations of these. Terms that have been used to describe the appearance of different types of tears include *bucket-handle, flap,* and *parrot-beak.* The interchangeable use of all of the above terms can be confusing. The length, specific location, and tear pattern should always be documented for clarity.
3. **Etiology.** Disruption of the collagen fibrils within the meniscus can occur as a result of acute injury or the degeneration that is typical with aging. Because there is a relative paucity of radially oriented fibers, the meniscus is susceptible to shearing forces, which tend to split it in longitudinal or horizontal directions. Longitudinal tears account for 50% to 90% of tears in young patients and horizontal cleavage tears make up a majority of the degenerative tears seen in older patients. Radial and flap tears transect the circumferential fibers of collagen. This requires increased force or compromised meniscal integrity; as such, these tears are less commonly encountered.
4. **Incidence.** The prevalence of an acutely torn meniscus approximates 61 per 100,000. Cadaveric studies have revealed degenerative tears in 60% of specimens at the age of 65. Sports-related meniscal injuries account for only one-third of all athletic injuries in one study. With respect to athletes involved in football and basketball, however, meniscal pathology accounted for the greatest number of injuries. The male–female ratio is 2.5:1. The medial meniscus is more commonly injured than the lateral (three times as often). Disruption of the anterior cruciate ligament (ACL) is the most common associated injury. Lateral meniscal tears are seen in association with acute ACL injuries, while medial meniscal tears are seen most commonly with chronic ACL injuries.
5. **History.** To be ascertained are the mechanism of injury, symptoms occurring immediately after the injury, time elapsed since the injury,

and residual symptoms. The most common scenario leading to meniscal injury is that of sudden onset of knee pain following a twisting injury or rapid change in direction. An effusion typically forms over a 24-hr period. An immediate hemarthrosis may occur with a tear in the vascular periphery of the meniscus, but this should also raise the suspicion of an ACL injury. Knee locking or an inability to extend the knee after it has been in a flexed position due to a mechanical block is most often seen in patients with a bucket-handle tear. Pain, recurrent effusion, and discomfort with stair climbing are common signs in patients with chronic meniscal injuries but should also raise suspicions of patellofemoral pathology.

6. **Physical Examination.** Joint-line tenderness, specifically when localized to the posteromedial or posterolateral joint line, has been shown to be the most sensitive clinical sign of a torn meniscus. Pain is often exacerbated by hyperflexion. Various provocative tests that manipulate the knee into a position that subluxes the meniscus have been described to elicit symptoms associated with a torn meniscus: the *McMurray test, Helfet maneuver, Steinmann test, Apley grind test, squat test,* and *duck-walk test.* The McMurray or flexion McMurray test is shown in appendix 6. Examination for effusion and quadriceps atrophy should also be performed. Examination for knee instability is essential if meniscal pathology is found because of the strong association between meniscal and cruciate injuries.
7. **Diagnostic Tests.** Plain radiographs should be performed on all patients with suspected intraarticular pathology to exclude fractures, bony lesions, and capsular injuries, such as the lateral capsular sign. This should include AP, lateral, Merchant and 45-degree posteroanterior flexion weight-bearing views for optimal evaluation of degenerative changes.
8. **Special Tests.** Although double-contrast arthrography was traditionally the workhorse for radiographic evaluation of torn menisci, more recently magnetic resonance imaging (MRI) has become the most frequently used diagnostic test. MRI is noninvasive, with accuracy for tears greater than 90%. MRI can also exclude other sources of knee pain and allows evaluation of the cruciate ligaments. In experienced hands, a careful clinical diagnosis may be all that is required. Arthroscopy is considered the gold standard for diagnosis of meniscal tears. All portions of the meniscus should be visualized.
9. **Natural History.** This may be one of spontaneous healing or cessation of symptoms without healing, but at the cost of lifestyle changes. However, many patients will continue to have recurrent effusions with episodes of locking and/or pain.
10. **Treatment.** A trial of rest and protected weight bearing is indicated for most patients. Most patients will be refractory to nonoperative treatment and should be offered arthroscopy. Because of the well-known association between meniscectomy and degenerative arthritic change, attempts to preserve or repair the meniscus should be the main priority. For patients with persistent symptoms, arthroscopy is performed to assess and treat the meniscus. Stable tears may be observed or rasped to promote healing, while unstable tears can be partially resected or repaired. Stable tears are defined as partial-thickness splits, minor inner-rim tears, degenerative tears in a knee with osteoarthritis, and tears of the peripheral rim that are less than 10 mm in length and displace less than 2 to 3 mm when probed. Complex tears and tears in the avascular zone of the meniscus are resected, always with an attempt to leave a stable meniscal rim. Vertical longitudinal tears that are within 5 mm of the meniscocapsular junction and long tears of the peripheral rim that are displacable are repaired. Techniques for arthroscopic meniscal repair include inside-out, outside-in, and all-inside repairs.

Application of each technique is usually a matter of the surgeon's individual preference. Autogenous fibrin clot, rasping, and, to a lesser degree, vascular tunnels and synovial flaps all have been used to enhance the healing of meniscal repairs.

11. **Return to Play.** Range-of-motion exercises and weight bearing as tolerated in a brace in full extension are begun immediately. Strengthening is begun with straight leg raising and quads sets initially. The patient is weaned from the brace to a neoprene sleeve for comfort and slow progression of strengthening is done over the next 2 months. In the final stages of rehabilitation, athletes should perform sport-specific functional strengthening. Proprioceptive sense can be enhanced by exercising on surfaces of different resilience. Return to competition varies greatly with each athlete's specific meniscal surgery and progress in therapy, but it is usually possible in 3 (partial meniscectomy) to 6 months (meniscal repair).

B. **Discoid**

This meniscal anomaly is seen uncommonly. The name refers to the abnormal rounded shape of the normally crescent-shaped meniscus. This anomaly can be symptomatic, usually presenting first in younger age groups.

1. **Anatomy.** The discoid meniscus is usually encountered in the lateral compartment. Medial discoid menisci are very rare. The true discoid meniscus is oval or disc-shaped and has varied coverage of the tibial plateau. A variant also exists that is more normal in shape but lacks posterior meniscotibial ligamentous attachment and occasionally has a hypertrophied posterior horn.
2. **Types.** Watanabe has classified the discoid meniscus into (a) incomplete, (b) complete, and (c) Wrisberg types. The incomplete and complete types differ in the amount of tibial plateau that is covered by the abnormally disc-shaped meniscus with a normal posterior coronary ligamentous attachment. The Wrisberg type is usually fairly normal in size and shape but lacks a posterior meniscotibial attachment. Its only posterior attachment is usually via the ligament of Wrisberg, hence the name. The posterior attachment can vary, so this type has been described as a meniscal variant with absence of the posterior coronary ligament.
3. **Etiology.** The etiology is unknown but various congenital and developmental theories have been proposed.
4. **Incidence.** A range of 0.4% to 5% incidence of lateral discoid meniscus types (a and b above) in Caucasian populations has been found, while Asian studies have revealed an incidence of 8.1% to 26%. The incidence of the lateral Wrisberg type varies as well, with an incidence of 0% to 2% seen in Caucasian populations and 0% to 3.1% in Asian populations. Medial discoid meniscus is rare and has been reported to vary from 0% to 0.3% in different studies. Less than a 10% incidence of bilaterality has been reported.
5. **History.** The age at presentation of incomplete and complete types tends to be somewhat greater than with the Wrisberg type, and the lesion often presents as an incidental findings at the time of arthroscopy for other reasons. If the incomplete and complete types involve a tear of the meniscal substance, signs and symptoms specific to any meniscal tear predominate. The *snapping-knee syndrome* presents most commonly in children with the Wrisberg type. This syndrome consists of pain in the affected compartment, audible clunking with knee range-of-motion exercise, and absence of any history of trauma to the affected knee. In general, symptoms in children are often vague and inconclusive, and a high index of suspicion for meniscal pathology must always be maintained. Adults can present with any of the three types of discoid menisci.
6. **Physical Examination.** Joint-line tenderness is usually present and frequently a loud clunk is audible, visible, and sometimes palpable during

the last 15 to 20 degrees of extension in the flexed knee. Occasionally a flexion contracture is the only presenting sign. Atrophy of the thigh, joint effusion, and synovial thickening are less common. If a tear is present, provocative meniscal symptoms can be elicited. At times, forced hyperextension of the knee may elicit pain on the lateral aspect of the joint.

7. **Diagnostic Tests.** Plain radiographs are usually normal, but a variety of findings have been described. A widened tibiofemoral joint line, cupping of the lateral tibial plateau, hypoplasia of the lateral tibial spine, and a high-riding fibular head can be seen. Later squaring of the lateral femoral condyle, osteochondritis dissecans of the lateral femoral condyle, secondary osteoarthrosis, and loose bodies have all been described.
8. **Special Tests.** Contrast arthrography has generally been replaced by MRI. Criteria for MRI diagnosis of an incomplete or complete discoid meniscus include (a) anterior and posterior horns, which are seen to be in continuity on three continuous sagittal images (5-mm cuts); (b) transverse width of the meniscus greater than 14 mm on coronal cuts; and (c) elongated appearance of the meniscus on axial 3-D volume MRI.
9. **Differential Diagnosis.** This includes meniscal cysts, congenital subluxation of the tibiofemoral joint, abnormal movement of the popliteus tendon, snapping of the tendons about the knee, subluxation or dislocation of the proximal tibiofibular joint or of the patellofemoral joint, osteochondritis dissecans, and chondromalacia patella.
10. **Natural History.** Because a majority of the patients are asymptomatic and the process is discovered incidentally during arthroscopy for other pathology, the natural history is unclear. Such asymptomatic patients usually proceed uneventfully through life without need for intervention. Patients with tears or snapping syndrome of the discoid meniscus will continue to be symptomatic. It is unclear how many patients progress to degenerative changes in the affected compartment because so many of the patients are asymptomatic.
11. **Treatment Options.** Symptomatic knees are treated with arthroscopy, which begins with a systematic assessment of the knee joint.
    a. **Incomplete or Complete Discoid Meniscus plus/minus Tear.** A thorough evaluation for a tear should be carried out. If no tear is present, then observation is recommended, as a high rate of reoperation has been reported following surgical treatment of intact discoid menisci. If a tear is present, arthroscopic saucerization is recommended.
    b. **Wrisberg Discoid Meniscus.** An arthroscopic suture repair of the meniscus back to the peripheral capsule should be attempted. Open meniscal reduction may be required if the meniscus is markedly displaced.
12. **Return to Play.** Same as for partial meniscectomy or meniscal repair.

C. **Meniscal Cysts**

1. **Anatomy.** Cysts are uncommon extensions of the lateral meniscus. The medial meniscus is less commonly involved; cysts are generally associated with a degenerative meniscal tear. Usually, they are found immediately anterior and proximal to the head of the fibula. They are firm and as a rule, fixed to the capsular tissue. They contain clear, gelatinous material and are usually multilocular.
2. **Definitions.** A *popliteal* or *Baker's cyst* is a distended *bursa* located in the popliteal space. The semimembranosus bursa is most prone to develop symptoms. It is located in the popliteal fossa between the semimembranosus tendon and the medial head of the gastrocnemius tendon. These cysts can also be associated with intraarticular pathology, including meniscal tears. Although, etiologically, the initiation of this lesion is different from that of a true meniscal cyst, treatment and prognosis are similar.

3. **Etiology.** Cysts usually develop following trauma. The lateral central meniscus is thicker and subject to reduced peripheral vascularity caused by its separation from the capsule by the popliteus tendon and thus is most prone to degeneration. Degeneration leads to weakening of the meniscal tissue. A gelatinous cyst forms, which presents externally through the capsular region of least resistance. Susceptibility to tearing is heightened in the setting of degeneration.
4. **History.** Cysts are usually painful, with activity accentuating symptoms. If a tear is present, the classic signs of meniscal tears are also present.
5. **Physical Examination.** Often the cyst is palpable; most commonly it is more prominent with the knee in flexion and less prominent with the knee in extension. Cysts may disappear when the knee is in flexion. Effusion may be present.
6. **Diagnostic Tests.** Large, untreated cysts of the lateral meniscus can erode the tibial condyle just inferior to the lateral margin of the articular cartilage and may produce a radiographically visible defect. MRI and arthrography can confirm the clinical diagnosis.
7. **Treatment Options.** Conservative treatment including antiinflammatory medications and steroid injections can be tried. If symptoms persist, surgical intervention is warranted. Arthroscopic evaluation should thoroughly assess for meniscal tears. If this lesion is evaluated early in its course, a meniscal tear may not be present and open cyst excision should be performed with repair of the meniscosynovial junction. If meniscal cleavage tears are encountered during arthroscopy, an arthroscopic partial meniscectomy is required. A peripheral rim of meniscus is best retained. Usually the cyst is decompressed during the arthroscopic procedure and does not require a separate incision. If it has not been decompressed during the meniscal work, needle aspiration and corticosteroid injection are advised.
8. **Return to Play.** If the meniscosynovial junction was repaired, range-of-motion exercises and weight bearing as tolerated without extensive cutting or running should be employed for approximately 4 to 6 weeks. Thereafter, a progressive rehabilitation program should begin to increase strength, with graduated running and cutting. Any procedures that require meniscectomy, either partial or subtotal, should employ the rehabilitation protocols already stated for these procedures.

II. Osteochondral Lesions

A. Osteochondritis Dissecans (OCD)

This is a lesion of bone and articular cartilage of uncertain etiology that results in a separation of varying amounts of subchondral bone and overlying articular cartilage. The lesion may be partially attached or may become loose. Osteochondroses occur throughout the body, but this discussion covers the specific entity of OCD of the femoral condyle.

1. **Anatomy.** The lesion is usually located on the non-weight-bearing lateral aspect of the medial femoral condyle. Lateral lesions are likely to be located in the central area of the condyle. The lateral femoral trochlea is involved in a minor number of patients, usually adults.
2. **Types.** Different classification schemes have been used to describe OCD. These classifications are usually based on a description of the fragment location, size, extent of involvement, and degree of separation. These classifications are helpful in planning treatment. The categories include *(a) in situ, (b) early separation, (c) incomplete detachment, and (d) complete detachment.* Some authors believe that a juvenile form of OCD (JOCD) exists, which has a better prognosis than the adult form. JOCD is distinguished by its presence in patients with open growth plates.
3. **Etiology.** The cause is controversial, but OCD is generally thought to be the result of cumulative stress to the subchondral bone, resulting in subchondral stress fractures.

4. **Incidence.** JOCD has a peak appearance in early adolescence with a male predominance of 4:1. It is rare in children under 10 years of age. Bilaterality has been reported to range between 20% and 30%. The exact incidence of adult OCD is unknown.
5. **History.** Patients complain of pain, stiffness, and swelling. Sensations of locking, catching and giving way can develop. Loose bodies can form after fragment separation, with symptomatology specific to this entity.
6. **Physical Examination.** Knee range of motion, quadriceps atrophy, and weakness should be assessed. Any effusion should be documented and occasionally a loose body or defect can be palpated. Some patients may have a positive *Wilson's sign* (pain with internal rotation and extension of the knee that is relieved with external rotation).
7. **Diagnostic Tests.** OCD is seen classically on radiographs as a well-circumscribed area of subchondral bone separated from the remaining femoral condyle by a crescent-shaped radiolucent line. The posterolateral aspect of the medial femoral condyle (most common area) is best imaged by flexion weight-bearing views.
8. **Special Tests.** Nuclear imaging may be beneficial in describing subtle lesions and may have a role in documenting the course of this process. Bone scans have also been used to predict the vascularity of the bone bed and suitability for repair in surgical staging. MRI has been shown to be useful in evaluating the mechanical stability of these lesions by providing an assessment of the integrity of the overlying cartilage. Diagnostic arthroscopy is usually required for this purpose in older individuals.
9. **Natural History.** JOCD patients appear not to suffer long-term complications associated with the original lesion, while adult OCD patients show progression to early degenerative joint disease.
10. **Treatment Options.** In patients with JOCD without a loose body, initial treatment should be nonoperative, as the prognosis is generally good. Surgical indications are discussed below. In OCD, an earlier progression to arthroscopic evaluation and management is usually undertaken.
    a. **Recommended Treatment**
        i. **Conservative.** Conservative measures include the use of crutches for 4 to 6 weeks, especially in JOCD. Casts, braces, and prolonged avoidance of weight bearing are not used routinely. Once the patient is symptom-free, crutches are discarded; some have used bone scans to follow the lesion every 2 months until healing. During this time competitive sports are eliminated. As healing progresses, recreational cycling, swimming, and lower extremity strength training are added as long as the patient remains asymptomatic.
        ii. **Surgical.** When surgical treatment is undertaken, it is usually because of failure of conservative measures in a patient with an otherwise stable lesion or because the lesion is partially detached or loose. Surgery is indicated when (a) the fragment becomes detached or unstable while the patient is under treatment, (b) there are persistent symptoms in a compliant patient, (c) there is persistently elevated or worsening scintigraphic activity while the patient is being followed with nuclear medicine studies, and (d) the patient is approaching epiphyseal closure. Criterion a is an absolute indication, as is a combination of criteria c, d, and e. If the articular cartilage is intact via MRI or at arthroscopy and scintigraphic osseous repair activity is present, arthroscopic nonarticular retrograde drilling is performed using image intensification and drill guides. If intact articular cartilage is present but repair activity is absent, concomitant bone grafting is required. If the articular cartilage is softened or unstable and there is good scan activity, curettage and base preparation,

drilling, grafting, and internal fixation should be performed, usually via an open approach. If there is poor scan activity in this setting, grafting and internal fixation may be less successful. Partially detached or loose fragments should be internally fixed if they are in the weight-bearing area. Autograft or osteochondral allograft replacement may be necessary if there is no alternative to removal of the fragment from the weight-bearing area or if the other surgical methods fail. In the non-weight-bearing area, removal of the fragment or loose body is an option.

11. **Return to Play.** If drilling is the only procedure on a stable lesion, the patient is allowed to progress to weight bearing as tolerated. If internal fixation is used for partially detached fragments or loose bodies, range-of-motion exercise is begun immediately but avoidance of weight bearing is necessary for 1.5 to 3 months. The same time period is used for convalescence after autograft or osteochondral allograft replacement. Clinical examination, radiographs, and bone scans can be used at bimonthly intervals to follow progression to healing. Swimming and biking are excellent alternative sports in the rehabilitation period. Return to active sports must be judged on a case-by-case basis according to the patient's age, fragment stability, and previous treatment.

B. **Chondral Injuries and Osteochondral Fracture.**
This injury is troublesome due to the limited healing potential of the defects. The avascularity of articular cartilage prevents a vascular response when there is cartilage injury alone. When the subchondral bone is injured, the inflammatory response produces mainly fibrocartilaginous tissue. This tissue is composed of mostly type I collagen rather than type II collagen seen in normal articular cartilage. The type I fibrocartilage is not durable and has been associated with eventual osteoarthritic degeneration.

1. **Types.** Most chondral injuries are in the weight-bearing area of the articular cartilage and usually in the medial compartment. The six types of changes are identified: *(a) linear, (b) stellate, (c) flap, (d) crater, (e) fibrillated, and (f) degraded.* Osteochondral injuries can occur anywhere in the knee, but they usually involve the medial facet of the patella or the lateral femoral condyle. Many surgeons describe acute chondral lesions as Outerbridge outlined: grade I, softening, swelling; grade II, fragmentation and fissuring less than 1/2 in. in diameter; grade III, fragmentation and fissuring greater than 1/2 in. in diameter; grade IV, subchondral bone exposure. Osteochondral injuries are best described by location, size, and depth.
2. **Etiology.** Osteochondral fractures of the knee are usually restricted to the femoral condyles and the patella. The tibial articular surface is spared in most cases. Patellofemoral osteochondral injuries are most often the result of a patellar dislocation. Impaction, avulsion, shearing, and rotational forces in direct trauma (as opposed to OCD lesions) are the most common causes of injury to femoral articular cartilage. Exogenous fractures secondary to direct trauma can also occur. The tibial spine has been hypothesized to play a role in the production of these injuries. In younger patients, the cartilaginous tidemark is not fully developed. As the hyaline articular cartilage has firm attachment to the subchondral bone, the shearing forces are transmitted to the weaker subchondral cancellous bone.
3. **Incidence.** Osteochondral fractures tend to occur mainly in adolescents. Where the patellofemoral articulation is concerned, the incidence closely follows that of recurrent patellar instability.
4. **History.** Torsional traumatic or patellofemoral instability mechanisms are usually described by the injured patient. Most patients present with pain and effusion. These injuries can mimic meniscal and synovial injuries. The pain can either be localized or diffuse, and locking and crepitus can occur.

5. **Physical Examination.** Joint-line tenderness and patellar facet tenderness predominate and an effusion is usually present. Because of the torsional mechanism required for femoral condylar lesions, they are often associated with tears of the anterior cruciate ligament, meniscus, and parapatellar ligament.
6. **Diagnostic Tests.** Arthrocentesis of hemarthrosis can reveal the presence of fat globules, indicating a fracture. Radiographic findings are usually normal if only a chondral injury has occurred. With osteochondral injuries, the bony component of the injury is visible radiographically. Anteroposterior, lateral, flexion weight-bearing, and patellar sunrise views are necessary to visualize the injury.
7. **Special Tests.** Arthrography and CT have been used in the past, but MRI has the ability to detect chondral defects as small as 3 mm. Osteochondral fractures are readily apparent on T2-weighted images, especially when an effusion is present. The effusion fills the defect and creates endogenous contrast. Frequently the chondral injuries remain undiagnosed until diagnostic arthroscopy is utilized.
8. **Natural History.** It appears that lacerations of the superficial cartilage will heal by the synthesis of new matrix by functioning chondrocytes. Deeper chondral injuries and osteochondral fractures fare less well if left untreated. The progression to degenerative change has been hypothesized in humans and proven in animal models.
9. **Treatment Options.** A conservative regimen of decreased weight bearing, ice, antiinflammatory medication, and continued range-of-motion exercises should be tried. If symptoms continue for more than 4 to 6 weeks, it is reasonable to consider an arthroscopic evaluation. Loose pieces of articular cartilage should be removed unless they contain in excess of 25 % of the joint surface. Screws, pins, and fibrin adhesive materials have been used to promote fixation and healing in the setting of large fragments that require repair. Microfractures created with special awls or drilling have been advocated to allow adhesion of subsequent blood clot to an intact subchondral plate. Some believe that drill-associated heat necrosis impedes tissue healing. Autograft, osteochondral allograft replacement, or autologous chondrocyte transplantation may be necessary if there is no alternative to removal of a large fragment from the weight-bearing area.
10. **Return to Play.** Same as for OCD/JOCD lesions.

Suggested Reading

Cahill BR. Osteochondritis dissicans of the knee: treatment of juvenile and adult forms. *J Am Acad Orthop Surg* 1995; 3:237.

Fu FH, Baratz M. Meniscal injuries. In:DeLee, Drez, eds. *Orthopaedic sports Medicine,* vol 2. Philadelphia: WB Saunders, 1994:1146–1162.

Lopez RA. Arthroscopic management of cysts of the lateral meniscus. *J Arthrosc* 1990; 6:156.

Neuschwander DC. Discoid meniscus. *Op Tech Orthop* 1995; 5:78.

Rodrigo JJ, Steadman JR, Silliman JF. Osteoarticular injuries of the knee. In:Chapman MW, ed. *Operative orthopaedics,* vol 3, 2nd ed. Philadelphia: Lippincott, 1993:2077–2082.

52. UNCOMMON CAUSES OF KNEE PAIN IN THE ATHLETE

Freddie H. Fu and Marc R. Safran

Relatively uncommon sources of knee pain in the athlete are becoming more common and more commonly recognized as our population ages and as recreational sports continue to become more popular. These problems include Hoffa's disease, semimembranosus tendinitis, pes anserinus syndrome, tibial collateral ligament bursitis, popliteus tendinitis, iliotibial band syndrome, fabella syndrome, and proximal tibiofibular joint instability. Other uncommon causes of knee pain that must be ruled out but are beyond the scope of this section include tumors (benign and malignant), reflex sympathetic dystrophy (causalgia), osteonecrosis, and infection.

The knee problems discussed in this chapter are uncommon. Thus the literature lacks data on the true incidence of these entities. Most of these knee problems are soft tissue overuse injuries with normal radiographs except as specifically noted.

The ***initial treatment*** is the same for each of these problems including ***rest*** from the offending or inciting activity (relative rest), ***ice*** for 15 to 20 min at a time, ***modalities*** such as ultrasound, whirlpool, iontophoresis, phonophoresis and transcutaneous electrical nerve stimulation (TENS), and ***nonsteroidal antiinflammatory drugs*** (NSAIDs). More specific treatment recommendations and surgical indications are listed under each entity.

I. Anterior Knee Pain

A. ***Hoffa's disease,*** also known as infrapatellar fat-pad syndrome, fat-pad syndrome, and synovial lipomatosis, is characterized by hypertrophy and inflammation of the infrapatellar fat pad. This problem is typically caused by direct trauma (a blow to the anterior knee) or to repeated injury to the infrapatellar fat pad during activities that require maximal, repetitive extenstion/hypertension of the knee. The fat pad becomes caught and compressed between the femoral condyles and the tibial plateau upon extension of the knee, resulting in anterior knee pain. This problem is most often seen with sports involving jumping or kicking.

1. **History.** There are no specific pathognomonic symptoms. Most athletes will note pain below the inferior pole of the patella, which is often exacerbated by physical activity or knee extension.
2. **Physical Examination.** Swelling is identified on either side of the patellar ligament. Tenderness can be elicited with palpation of the fat pad deep to the patellar ligament or along its edge. Occasionally, there will be swelling or recurrent effusions of the knee. Anterior pain can be reproduced with passive knee hyperextension (bounce test).
3. **Special Tests.** An injection of a small amount of lidocaine into the inflamed fat pad will confirm the diagnosis by reducing the pain shortly after the injection.
4. **Prevention.** Shoe heel lifts my reduce or prevent knee hyperextension and thus prevent repetitive injury to the fat pad.
5. **Treatment.** In addition to the initial treatment listed in the introduction, an injection of a corticosteroid preparation (1 ml of a corticosteroid mixed with 3 ml 1% lidocaine) into the fat pad will reduce inflammation. Heel lifts can be used to prevent entrapment and thus reinjury of the fat pad by preventing knee hyperextension. Surgical resection of the fat pad is reserved for cases that do not respond to conservative measures within 6 months.
6. **Return to sports** is based on the athlete's symptoms. A heel lift may allow the athlete to return to sports while preventing further fat-pad injury.

II. Medial Knee Pain

A. **Semimembranosus tendinitis** is usually associated with other overuse knee disorders, mostly degenerative medial meniscal tears or chondromalacia of the patella, but it may also occur as an isolated syndrome. It is seen most commonly from repetitive loading or overloading of the musculotendinous unit in middle-aged endurance athletes. In the nonathlete it usually results from compensation for other knee problems. It is most often seen in distance runners, triathletes, race walkers, or persons involved in activities such as bending, lifting, or climbing.

1. **History.** Athletes with this entity complain of pain located at the very posteromedial corner of the knee immediately below the joint line that is most noticeable during or after strenuous activities. The pain is insidious in onset and progressive without treatment.
2. **Physical Examination.** Tenderness is palpated along the anterior medial tendon of the semimembranosus immediately below the knee and at the insertion of the posterior medial tendon on the posteromedial tibial condyle. This tenderness is accentuated by flexing the knee to 90 degrees and externally rotating the lower leg maximally. Assessment for foot hyperpronation and hip anteversion is important, since these are predisposing factors.
3. **Special Tests.** A bone scan may show increased uptake at the semimembranosus insertion on the posteromedial corner of the proximal tibia.
4. **Treatment.** In addition to the treatments listed in the introduction, it is also important to stretch and strengthen the hamstrings. Resistant cases may be treated with an injection of a corticosteroid preparation (1 ml of a corticosteroid mixed with 5 ml of 1% lidocaine) into the tendinous sheath around the semimembranosus. Surgery is indicated for isolated tendinitis (that is not associated with an intraarticular cause) after failing 6 months of conservative treatment. This chronic, recalcitrant, isolated tendinitis is treated with surgical exploration, drilling of the insertion site, and semimembranosus transfer. For those with secondary semimembranosus tendinitis, surgical correction of the underlying intraarticular pathology is indicated if conservative treatment fails to eliminate or reduce the symptoms within 6 weeks.
5. **Return to sports** should not occur until the athlete is asymptomatic. This varies depending on the severity of the tendinitis and the duration of symptoms. The great majority of patients respond to conservative treatment within 6 months and many within the first month.

B. **Pes anserinus syndrome** (tendinitis and bursitis) is found most commonly in long-distance runners, though it my also occur in sports that involve pivoting, cutting, jumping, and deceleration. It is more common in long-distance runners and in those just beginning a training program, though it may occur in athletes of any level. It is usually caused by overuse friction or by a direct contusion. Exacerbating factors include incorrect training techniques (excessive hill running, no or incorrect stretching, recent large increases in mileage, and inadequate time for rest between workouts), tightness of the hamstring muscles, valgus knees, and excessive external rotation of the lower leg. It is also common in conjunction with osteoarthritis in the elderly.

1. **Anatomy.** The pes anserinus is the tendinous insertion of the sartorius, gracilis, and semitendinosus muscles onto the anteromedial aspect of the proximal tibia just below the flare of the condyle. A bursa lies between these tendons and the medial collateral ligament, 5 to 6 cm below the anteromedial joint line.
2. **History.** These athletes complain of pain that is insidious in onset and gradually intensifies as the activity is continued. They note the pain is over the proximal tibial metaphysis about 5 to 6 cm below the joint line, though it may radiate along the joint line; it extends along the course of the hamstring tendons posteromedially.

3. **Physical Examination.** There is localized tenderness in the proximal medial tibia (5 to 6 cm below the joint line) that often extends posteromedially to the insertion of the semimembranosus tendon. Slight swelling and crepitus on the medial side of the knee at the level of the tibial tubercle is often seen. Athletes should be examined for excessive hamstring tightness, excessive femoral anteversion, genu valgum, and excessive external tibial torsion, as these are predisposing anatomical findings.
4. **Radiographs** are normal in cases not associated with arthritis.
5. **Prevention.** Runners should reduce mileage, shorten stride length, gain and maintain hamstring flexibility, and allow adequate rest between workouts. Orthotics may be helpful for excessive heel or knee valgus.
6. **Treatment.** In addition to the initial treatment listed in the introduction, an injection of a corticosteroid preparation (1 ml of a corticosteroid mixed with 5 to 9 ml of 1% lidocaine) into the bursa may be of benefit in resolving of the bursitis. Conditioning of the hamstring and quadriceps muscles is important, including isometric exercise and stretching, with progression to resistance exercises as symptoms allow. Orthotics with inner heel wedges can be of benefit for those with excessive knee or heel valgus. Surgical excision of the bursa in an athlete is indicated only with multiple recurrences of an extremely large or chronically inflamed bursa. Surgery is elective and is rarely indicated in the general population.
7. **Return to sports** may occur when the athlete is asymptomatic. Premature return may result in recurrence and eventually a chronically inflamed bursa.

C. **Tibial collateral ligament bursitis** results in pain at the medial joint line that is not associated with meniscal tears or mechanical symptoms. The cause of this bursitis is unclear, but it is more often found in runners, tennis players, swimmers, and cyclists.

1. **Anatomy.** Five bursae deep to the medial collateral ligament assist the ligament in gliding over the medial meniscus and medial tibial condyle.
2. **History.** These athletes note pain at the medial joint line at the level of the tibial (medial) collateral ligament. These patients have no mechanical symptoms of the knee locking or giving way.
3. **Physical Examination.** The athlete may have a palpable tender enlargement beneath the medial collateral ligament at the medial joint line. This pain is most often exacerbated by valgus stress to the knee. Pain may also be increased by knee extension/hyperextension or external rotation of the leg.
4. **Special Tests.** The diagnosis may be confirmed by a bursal injection of lidocaine with temporary relief of pain and symptoms. A magnetic resonance imaging (MRI) study may show the inflamed bursa.
5. **Treatment.** In addition to the initial treatment listed in the introduction, an injection of a corticosteroid preparation (1 ml of a corticosteroid mixed with 3 ml of 1% lidocaine) into the bursa can be both diagnostic and therapeutic. A rehabilitation program emphasizing quadriceps strengthening is also important. Surgery is rarely needed. If chronic, severe symptoms persist, excision of the bursa may be necessary.
6. **Return to Sports.** The majority of athletes improve with conservative treatment within 1 to 2 months and may return to sports when they are asymptomatic.

III. Lateral Knee Pain

A. **Popliteus tendinitis** results in posterolateral or lateral knee pain particularly associated with downhill running and with hyperpronation of the foot. This entity is based on overuse of the popliteus muscle as it functions to decelerate and internally rotate the tibia. Thus, it most commonly afflicts people involved in downhill walking or running, those who run on banked terrain, and those with hyperpronation of the foot causing external rotation of the tibia.

1. **Anatomy.** The popliteus has a wide insertion on the posterior tibia above the soleal line. It courses superolaterally and anteriorly under the arcuate ligament, becoming tendinous about 1 cm distal to the joint line. The tendon passes through the popliteal hiatus and through the joint to its bony origin on the lateral femoral condyle anterior to the lateral collateral ligament.
2. **History.** These athletes typically note insidious onset of lateral or posterolateral knee pain without history of acute injury. The pain occurs mainly during weight bearing with knee flexion between 15 and 30 degrees or during the early part of the swing phase of gait. The athlete notes that once pain develops, the onset is sudden after running a particular distance, forcing the athlete to discontinue running. Often a history can be obtained that reveals a recent abrupt change in training schedule or terrain.
3. **Physical Examination.** The physical examination is often normal unless the tendinitis is chronic or the athlete is seen immediately after activity. In these cases, there is tenderness localized over or along the popliteus origin. Pain may be elicited with Garrick's test (see appendix 6) and with passive external rotation of the affected leg.
4. **Treatment.** The management of acute cases begins with the relative rest, ice, NSAIDs, and the modalities outlined above. Muscle conditioning, including hamstring and quadriceps stretching and strengthening, is also important. Modification of training techniques such as running uphill and changing the side of the road or direction on the track is beneficial. Orthotics may be of benefit for the athlete with hyperpronated feet. Persistent cases are treated with an injection of a corticosteroid preparation (1 ml of a corticosteroid mixed with 3 ml of 1% lidocaine) into the peritendinous tissues, taking care not to inject into the popliteus tendon or lateral collateral ligament. Further, it may help to impose further activity restrictions. Arthroscopy or MRI may be indicated if associated meniscal pathology, ligament or tendon rupture, is suspected.
5. **Return to Sports.** Symptoms usually resolve within 10 to 14 days, when gradual return to running may begin. More severe cases may take up to 6 weeks to resolve.

B. **Iliotibial band syndrome** is an overuse injury (tendinitis or bursitis) caused by excessive friction between the iliotibial band and the lateral femoral epicondylar eminence. It occurs most often in long-distance runners, cyclists, and other athletes performing activities involving repetitive knee flexion. Training errors and abrupt changes in intensity, duration, and/or frequency of training are major causes of this syndrome. Many anatomical factors may also predispose an athlete to developing this problem.

1. **Anatomy.** The iliotibial tract originates proximally near the greater trochanter from the fascia of the tensor, gluteus maximus, and gluteus medius. As it passes distally, it remains in contact with the lateral intermuscular septum of the thigh muscles and inserts into a tubercle on the lateral tibial condyle. In extension, the iliotibial band lies anterior to the lateral epicondyle of the femur, and it passes over the condyle during flexion greater than 30 degrees.
2. **History.** The usual history is one of pain that initially develops only after a long run and may improve after the runner has warmed up. The athlete notes lateral knee pain during activity that may radiate proximally or distally. In more severe and chronic cases, the athlete complains of pain while running. The farther the distance run, the more severe the pain and subsequent disability. The pain may limit the activity at a certain point and the athlete will have to stop. Pain is initiated or exacerbated by running on banked surfaces or hills. Running downhill or climbing stairs may aggravate the symptoms and is most intense at heel strike while attempting to decelerate the limb.

3. **Physical Examination.** There is localized tenderness over the lateral epicondyle 2 to 3 cm proximal to the lateral joint line. Occasionally, soft tissue swelling or crepitus is present. Pain can be produced with the Nobel compression test (see appendix 6) and single-limb stance knee-bend test (see appendix). Anatomic factors that predispose to the development of this syndrome include excessive tightness of the iliotibial band, excessive foot pronation, genu varum, an abnormally prominent lateral femoral epicondyle, and internal tibial torsion. Excessive iliotibial band tightness should be assessed by Ober's test (see Appendix 6). Effusion of the knee joint and tenderness of the popliteus tendon are absent.
4. **Special Tests.** Ultrasound or MRI can confirm the diagnosis.
5. **Treatment.** Treatment of the acute iliotibial band syndrome includes the initial treatment listed in the introduction, while an injection of a corticosteroid preparation (1 ml of a corticosteroid mixed with 3 to 5 ml of 1% lidocaine) into the bursa can be both diagnostic and therapeutic. A rehabilitation program emphasizing stretching of the iliotibial band is imperative in cases of iliotibial band tightness. Alterations in training are beneficial in those cases where this is a major etiological factor. Wedge orthotics may be helpful for a tight iliotibial band, while a rigid orthotic may be helpful for excessive pronation. If symptoms persist despite these measures, total restriction of activity for 4 to 6 weeks is necessary. Surgery is rarely indicated for this problem. In chronic cases where 6 months of conservative therapy has failed, bursectomy and lateral fascial/tendon resection may relieve symptoms effectively.
6. **Return to Sports.** Most athletes will respond to nonoperative management and can return to sports when they are free of pain.

C. **Fabella syndrome** produces pain in the posterolateral knee due to inflammation of the fabella. This condition occurs most frequently in late adolescence but is seen in older patients as well. Several theories regarding the etiology exist: roughening of the articular surface, tendinitis from irritation by the sesamoid, and synovial irritation from either of the above. Also postulated as causes are direct trauma, overuse syndrome/repeated microtrauma, and arthritic changes in the fabella. Excessive functioning of the lateral head of the gastrocnemius muscle, especially during the beginning stages of knee flexion and during external rotation of the lower leg immediately before full extension, is also thought to be related to the pathogenesis of this syndrome.

1. **Anatomy.** The fabella is a sesamoid bone located in the tendinous portion of the lateral gastrocnemius muscle directly posterior to the lateral femoral condyle. The anterior surface of the fabella articulates with the posterior portion of the lateral femoral condyle. A fabella is present in 10% to 18% of the normal population.
2. **History** reveals a gradual onset of a sharp, intermittent pain localized to the posterolateral knee, though it may radiate down the leg.
3. **Physical Examination.** There usually is tenderness localized over the fabella. The pain is elicited by moving the fabella transversely when the knee is extended or slightly flexed.
4. **Special Tests.** Injection with a local anesthetic to confirm the diagnosis.
5. **Radiographs** of the knee are normal. In adolescents, the fabella may not yet be ossified, even though it can be symptomatic.
6. **Treatment.** The initial treatment is as listed in the introduction, while recalcitrant cases may benefit from an injection of a corticosteroid preparation (1 ml of a corticosteroid mixed with 3 to 5 ml of 1% lidocaine). Conservative measures should be continued for at least 6 months before surgical excision is considered. However, the majority of patients do require surgical excision.
7. **Return to sports** may occur when the athlete is asymptomatic. This may be up to 6 months in those treated surgically.

D. **Proximal Tibiofibular Joint Instability.** Anterolateral dislocation is the most common type of proximal tibiofibular dislocation, occurring in about

90% of the patients, and is especially common in athletics. The most common mechanism resulting in anterolateral instability of the proximal tibiofibular joint is falling on a flexed, adducted leg with the ankle inverted. Reports of this problem have been noted in soccer, football, distance jumping, wrestling, gymnastics, basketball, jet skiing, horseback riding, skiing (water and snow), rugby, baseball, judo, and volleyball.

1. **Anatomy.** The proximal tibiofibular joint is an inherently stable diarthrodial joint that is separate and distinct from the knee joint. The proximal fibula sits behind the lateral tibial condyle in a sulcus and is maintained there in part by the anterior bony prominence of the tibia. The joint capsule is reinforced by ligamentous and tendinous structures.
2. **History.** The athlete will note some significant trauma to the knee, usually a fall into the "hurdler's" position, with the knee flexed, foot adducted, and ankle inverted. They will complain of lateral knee pain, though occasionally they may also have ankle pain. This may vary from disabling pain and inability to bear weight or move the knee to only a slight discomfort. Athletes with this problem note that their knee will sometimes either give out quickly or simply lock. They will have no complaints of knee effusion, though they may note lateral knee swelling or a mass.
3. **Physical Examination.** A mass or prominence of the lateral knee is usually identified below the tibial plateau. It is usually tender, and small amounts of swelling and ecchymosis are often noted around the proximal fibula. The proximal fibula is mobile when the knee is examined in hyperflexion. Occasionally, ankle dorsi- and plantarflexion result in lateral knee pain. It is imperative to examine the peroneal nerve (motor and sensory function), as this nerve may be injured with proximal tibiofibular dislocation.
4. **Radiographs.** Anteroposterior radiographs reveal the fibular head to be laterally displaced and the proximal interosseous space to be widened. Bilateral knee radiographs are of benefit for comparison, since the findings are subtle and often missed. Lateral radiographs show an increased overlap of the fibula on the tibia. Radiographs should also be assessed for fractures of the fibula, avulsions, and abnormal calcification.
5. **Treatment.** Treatment involves closed reduction (done with the knee in hyperflexion) of the dislocation. Immobilization and bracing are not necessary, since this is an inherently stable joint. Relative rest from sports, running, and squatting; ice; and NSAIDs are helpful in the first few days after the reduction. Strengthening of the hamstrings (biceps femoris) may help reduce the likelihood of recurrent dislocations. Surgical reconstruction is reserved for those with recurrent proximal fibular dislocations.
6. **Return to sports** may occur when the athlete is asymptomatic, usually within 1 to 2 weeks of reduction.

Suggested Reading

Holmes JC, Pruitt AL, Whalen NJ. Iliotibial band syndrome in cyclists. *Am J Sports Med* 1993; 21:419–424.

Kerlan RK, Glousman RE. Tibial collateral ligament bursitis. *Am J Sports Med* 1988; 16:344–346.

Larsson LG, Baum J. The syndrome of anserina bursitis: an overlooked diagnosis. *Arthritis Rheum* 1985; 28:1062–1065.

Mayfield GW. Popliteus tendon tenosynovitis. *Am J Sports Med* 1977; 5:31–36.

Ray JM, Clancy WG Jr, Lemon RA. Semimembranosus tendinitis: an overlooked cause of medial knee pain. *Am J Sports Med* 1988; 16:347–351.

Safran MR, Fu FH. Isolated post-traumatic recurrent proximal tibiofibular joint instability: a new technique of reconstruction. *Am J Knee Surg* 1994; 7:141–147.

Safran MR, Fu FH. Uncommon causes of knee pain in the athlete. *Orthop Clin North Am* 1995; 26:547–560.

Weiner DS, McNab I. The fabella syndrome: an update. *J. Pediatr Orthop* 1982; 2:405–408.

53. KNEE-PATELLOFEMORAL

John P. Fulkerson

I. Anatomic Considerations

The patellofemoral joint is composed of the patella itself, a sesamoid bone invested in the extensor mechanism/quadriceps tendon (the retinacular support structure around the patella), the trochlea (which is the groove into which the patella fits), and the knee joint itself, with the synovium and synovial fluid within it.

A. **Patella.** The patella is enclosed within the quadriceps extensor tendon. Articular cartilage on the patella is very thick, as substantial stress is transmitted through it. The medial facet is convex and the lateral facet is concave. There is also an "odd facet," which articulates only in full flexion of the knee.

B. **Patellar Tendon.** A tendon distal to the patella, the patellar tendon is a thick structure that connects the quadriceps extensor mechanism to the tibia at the tibial tubercle.

C. **Lateral Retinaculum.** The lateral retinaculum is composed of two main layers—the superficial and deep transverse layers. It connects the patella to the iliotibial band on the lateral side of the knee.

D. **Medial Retinaculum.** The medial retinaculum is composed of tendinous tissue, including the medial patellofemoral ligament, which supports the patella and helps prevent lateral dislocation.

E. **Central Quadriceps Tendon.** Above the patella is the central quadriceps tendon, which contains a confluence of the quadriceps muscles, including the vastus lateralis, rectus femoris, vastus intermedius, and vastus medialis. The central quadriceps tendon provides proximal support to the patella.

II. Definitions

A. **Dislocation.** The patella is dislocated if it is displaced completely out of the trochlea. Most dislocations occur laterally.

B. **Subluxation.** Subluxation of the patella is a transient displacement of the patella from its normal location within the trochlear groove. Subluxation involves displacing the patella short of complete dislocation.

C. **Tilt.** The patella is tilted when it is rotated out its coronal plane in the center of the trochlea. This rotatory displacement can occur with or without subluxation of the patella.

D. **Plica.** There are numerous synovial folds within the knee joint, particularly the *medial infrapatellar plica,* which can cause snapping and pain in the patellofemoral joint.

E. **Apophysitis.** This is irritation or inflammation of a growth area at the point of tendon insertion. With regard to the patellofemoral joint, it is possible to have an apophysitis at either end of the patellar tendon. Proximally, this is referred to as *Sinding-Larsen-Johansson syndrome*; distally, at the tibial tuberosity level, an apophysitis is referred to as *Osgood-Schlatter's disease.*

F. **Chondromalacia.** This term simply means soft cartilage, nothing more. Chondromalacia indicates deterioration of cartilage, which may be manifest as crepitation or cracking. This term does not describe any specific syndrome and does not necessarily define a source of pain.

III. History

A. **Mode of Onset**

1. **Traumatic.** A fall onto the knee or a dashboard type of injury can cause true articular or retinacular damage around the knee. A fall onto the knee during sports usually occurs with the knee flexed. Because of this, proximal articular cartilage of the patella is usually damaged, as this is the part of the patella that articulates with the knee in flexion. A crush of patellar articular cartilage can cause irreversible joint damage and painful clicking within the knee joint, which can impair athletic participation.

2. **Spontaneous.** Athletes with underlying malalignment of the patellar extensor mechanism can have abnormal mechanics of the patellofemoral joint, such that there is strain of the structure supporting the patella and overload on the patella, usually the lateral facet. Typically, malalignment of the extensor mechanism results in lateral overload (excessive lateral pressure syndrome). Lateral subluxation and/or tilt of the patella will similarly cause *deficient* contact stress on the medial patella, particularly the distal medial patella, where articular cartilage may also break down owing to deficient contact stress on the cartilage and resulting excessive shear.
3. **Referred.** It is important to recognize that pain in the anterior knee can occur as a result of referred pain from the hip or back. Also, in cyclists, overuse or compartment syndrome in the quadriceps muscle can refer pain to the anterior knee.
4. **Traumatic Dislocation of the Patella.** Usually this is an obvious event in which the patella becomes displaced laterally onto the lateral side of the knee. Nonetheless, there can be a transient dislocation of the patella with a feeling of the "knee going out of place." It is not uncommon to confuse a patellar dislocation with a tear of the anterior cruciate ligament. Some patients who have a lateral patellar dislocation will think that the patella went medially because they feel the medial condyle and mistake it for the patella.

B. **Character of the Pain.** In discussing a patellofemoral problem with an athlete, it is important to know whether the pain started during physical activity and whether the pain is sharp, dull, associated with numbness, related to crepitus in the knee, transient, or continuous. Most of all, the examiner should try to find out whether the pain is related to the patellofemoral articulation or whether it is emanating from support structures around the patella, suggesting overuse or strain of the retinacular or tendinous supports.

C. **Effusion.** If there is fluid in the knee joint related to patellofemoral pain, this suggests either synovial inflammation or true articular damage with loose cartilage causing irritation within the knee. Most retinacular overuse problems will not cause effusion. Therefore, in most cases, effusion indicates an intraarticular problem.

D. **Previous Surgery.** It is important to know whether the athlete has had any previous surgery on the knee, including arthroscopy. It is possible to have a neuroma at any incision, site of injury, or arthroscopy portal. All of these areas should be examined.

E. **Past Medical History.** One should ask the athlete whether there is any history of arthritis in the family and whether there has been any previous problem with the knee. Also, it is useful to know if there is any psoriasis, colitis, rheumatoid arthritis, or osteoarthritis in the family.

IV. Physical Examination

A. The athlete should be examined both supine and prone. During the *supine examination,* the knee should be taken through a range of motion with a hand on the patella to see whether there is crepitus (noise in the patellofemoral joint). If the pain bothering the athlete occurs upon compression of the patella and is simultaneous with crepitus, it may be due to softening of the articular cartilage (chondromalacia) or breakdown on the patella or trochlea. One must remember that painful crepitus may occur when a pathological plica catches in the patellofemoral joint.

1. The patellofemoral joint should be observed to see if the patella looks tilted laterally and whether there is any fluid in the joint. The skin is examined for evidence of trauma or reflex sympathetic dystrophy.
2. The patellofemoral joint and the knee is palpated (with the knee extended) to see if there is fluid or blood within the joint.
3. The retinacular structure is palpated medially and laterally to see if there is any specific area of tenderness. It is important also to palpate the entire

retinacular structure, including the central quadriceps tendon and the patellar tendon. Particularly in athletes, retinacular strain or traumatic tendinitis is common. In the skeletally immature athlete, the apophysis where the patellar tendon inserts into the tibia must be palpated as well as the origin of the patellar tendon for evidence of apophysitis.

4. The examiner should watch the patella track while flexing and extending the knee to see if there is a "J sign," in which the patella comes from an abnormally lateral position and falls into the trochlea abruptly upon flexion of the knee. This denotes lateral positioning of the patella.

B. **Prone Examination.** The examiner looks for quadriceps tightness by flexing both knees as fully as possible with the athlete prone. This may suggest that stretching of this area will be important to prevent further problems. With the athlete prone, the hips are rotated internally and externally to see if there is any limitation suggesting a problem that might originate from the hip region. If there is limitation of hip rotation, the examiner should suggest an x-ray of the hip.

C. With the athlete standing, the examiner looks to see if there is any asymmetry of muscle; while the athlete is slowly bending the knees, the examiner watches tracking of the patella to see if the patella drops gradually and directly into the trochlea of the femur upon knee flexion. The athlete's feet are examined with the athlete standing to see if there is excessive pronation, which might benefit from orthotics. Finally, any abrasions or bruises—which might suggest direct injury to the anterior knee—are noted.

V. Radiographs

It is usually best to obtain anteroposterior and lateral views of the knee as well as an axial view of the patellofemoral joint. The Merchant axial view with the knee flexed either 30 or 45 degrees is most useful. Axial views with the knee flexed more than 45 degrees are less useful and less accurate for picking up more subtle malalignment problems. A true lateral with the posterior condyles superimposed is extremely useful and permits the examiner to evaluate the morphology of the trochlea as well as rotation of the patella out of its normal plane. Some experience is necessary to evaluate precise lateral radiographs accurately.

VI. Special Studies

A. **Computed Tomography (CT).** This modality is very useful when there are questions regarding the presence or degree of patella malalignment. *Precise* midpatellar transverse images taken at 0, 15, 30, and 45 degrees of knee flexion (patient's normal standing alignment reproduced in the scanner), with the posterior femoral condyles included in the images, will provide useful information. The patella should be centered in the trochlea (without tilt) by 15 degrees of knee flexion. The patella is tilted if the angle formed by lines along the lateral patella facet and the posterior condyles is *less than* 12 degrees. [This is the patellar tilt angle or (PTA)].

B. **Magnetic Resonance Imaging (MRI).** This modality is helpful for evaluating the condition of patellar or trochlear articular cartilage and for evaluating soft tissue structures. Tendon injury or tendinosis may be noted on MRI, as well as some pathologic plicae, hemangiomata, cartilage loose bodies, meniscus injury, and hypertrophic synovium. MRI, however, has been less useful for evaluating alignment than CT.

C. **Scintigraphic Imaging.** The technetium 99 bone scan is useful in particularly difficult cases when documentation of subchondral bone activity will help in the treatment. The bone scan may differentiate chondroosseous damage of the trochlea versus the patella and may also help differentiate proximal/distal and medial/lateral lesions.

VII. Treatment Overview

A. **Dislocation.** In acute dislocation, once the patella is relocated, one will recommend arthroscopic intervention and reconstruction of any clear osteochondral damage. If there is no evidence of osteochondral injury and the patella is satisfactorily located, one should aspirate the knee of any hemarthrosis and immobilize the joint in extension for 10 to 14 days to encourage medial soft tissue healing in first-time dislocators. The clinician should recognize, however, that osteochondral damage can seriously limit subsequent athletic participation, and early replacement of significant fragments (those with bone attached) should be encouraged.

Following recurrent patellar dislocation, most athletes will need realignment of the extensor mechanism, preferably at the tibial tubercle level, to gain long-term patellofemoral stability. This will usually be done after the patient has gained both motion and strength subsequent to the acute injury. If there is a significant distal or distal/medial articular lesion, anteromedial tibial tubercle transfer may be most appropriate.

Return to Sport. This may occur at 4 to 6 months if the athlete wears a knee sleeve with the patella cut out.

B. **Subluxation.** Most patients with minor subluxation of the patella can be treated nonoperatively with quadriceps strengthening, patellar taping, bracing, orthotics, and modification of body mechanics if necessary. If recurrent patellar subluxation limits day-to-day activities or important athletic activities, tibial tubercle transfer and lateral release will sometimes become necessary.

C. **Tilt.** In some patients with minor degrees of tilt, patellar taping, quadriceps strengthening, lateral retinacular stretching, and body mechanics or orthotics may be sufficient. If there is definite, objective patellar tilt and the patient remains disabled despite a full trial (at least 6 to 8 weeks, but usually 3 to 4 months of nonoperative treatment), lateral retinacular release may be extremely helpful and can sometimes render a patient asymptomatic with full return to athletics. If there is a *distal* articular lesion of the patella, particularly on the medial aspect of the patella, anteromedial tibial tubercle transfer may be necessary in selected patients.

D. **Plica.** Stretching of a symptomatic plica and injection with corticosteroid may relieve symptoms in some patients. If a pathological plica remains persistently symptomatic (more than 6 to 8 weeks); simple arthroscopic resection of the plica is indicated.

E. **Apophysitis.** The majority of patients with apophysitis around the knee will improve with time, modified or restricted athletic activity, and symptomatic treatment. Some patients who have failed conservating treatment and have pain with activities of daily living require cast immobilization for 6 to 8 weeks, but surgery is rarely indicated unless there is a symptomatic apophyseal fragment that remains symptomatic following skeletal maturity.

F. **Chondromalacia.** In most cases, it will be best not to think in terms of treating "chondromalacia." Instead, one should identify sources of pain and treat these specifically. If there is a specific flap of loose articular cartilage causing pain, this may require arthroscopic resection. In most cases, it will be necessary to identify an underlying malalignment (tilt and/or subluxation) and treat this specifically to avoid further articular cartilage problems. In most patients with articular cartilage softening, nonoperative treatment including modified activity, taping, bracing, straight-leg quadriceps strengthening, and symptomatic measures will eventually lead to improvement. In resistant cases, the underlying cause must be treated when possible or pressure on deficient articular cartilage relieved by tibial tubercle transfer and/or anteriorization.

VIII. Arthroscopy

A. **Indications.** Arthroscopy of the patellofemoral joint gives important confirmatory information regarding the presence, location, and extent of articular lesions. It is rare, however, to do patellofemoral arthroscopy for diagnosis alone. Most of the time, arthroscopy will be done immediately prior to definitive surgery to be sure that patellar alignment and lesions are appropriate for the procedure selected.

B. **Technique.** The arthroscope is best introduced into a superior portal with the patient supine on an operating room table. The author prefers a superomedial portal, two finger breadths above the patella, and a second inferolateral portal for probing and for arthroscopy of the rest of the knee.

C. **Findings.** The patella, trochlea, and related structures must be fully examined. Every articular lesion is quantified as to *size, degree of cartilage breakdown* (soft versus flaps versus fibrillation versus exposed bone), and *location.* The Outerbridge Classification is useful when details and location of lesions are also given. In the Outerbridge Classification, soft cartilage is grade 1, fibrillated on an area under 1/2 in. in diameter is grade 2, fibrillated over an area larger than 1/2 in. in diameter is grade 3, and exposed bone is grade 4.

The surgeon must also describe how the patella enters the trochlea and whether there is evidence of patellar tilt or subluxation. At 60 mm Hg pressure, the patella, when viewed with an arthroscope, will normally be centered without tilt by 45 degrees knee flexion.

IX. Treatment Specifics

A. **Nonoperative.** The basic program should include stretching of the hamstrings and quadriceps, antiinflammatory medication as indicated, mobilization of the patella, quadriceps strengthening (avoiding pressure on areas of chondromalacia), patellar taping (McConnell technique), bracing, progression to improved aerobic fitness, and maintenance of a home program after initial symptoms subside.

B. **Operative**

1. **Lateral Release.** This is most appropriate for patients with documented patellar *tilt* when there is little or not evidence of patellar cartilage disruption. Lateral release is not generally helpful when there has been direct trauma to the patella unless there is associated tilt. The lateral retinacular release may be done arthroscopically or open, with generally similar results. Open release does provide some advantages, however. Open lateral release allows optimal visualization of the patella, maximal hemostasis, and direct release of tight structures. Either technique is acceptable. Early range-of-motion exercise should be encouraged, but return to vigorous athletics is unusual in less than 3 to 4 months.
2. **Vastus Medialis Imbrication.** This technique, together with lateral release, can correct *lateral subluxation* of the patella but carries some potential risk for increasing articulating loads on the medial patella. It is most useful in the *skeletally immature* patient when tibial tubercle transfer must be avoided. Properly done, this technique is also appropriate for adult patients as long as medial overtightening is avoided.
3. **Medial Tubercle Transfer.** Using a technique such as the Trillat procedure, the tibial tubercle may be transferred directly medial on a pedicle of bone, securing the transferred bone pedicle with cortical screws. This technique is the most reliable way to correct a lateral patellar tracking vector. Early range-of-motion exercise and protected weight bearing on crutches for 6 weeks should be encouraged; return to sports is not usually possible for 6 months.
4. **Anteromedial Tibial Tubercle Transfer.** An oblique osteotomy deep to the tibial tubercle allows anteromedial transfer of the extensor mechanism when there is cartilage breakdown on the lateral and/or distal aspects of the patella. As in the Trillat procedure, secure fixation with cortical bone screws will permit early motion, but return to vigorous athletics may not be possible for 6 months or more.
5. **Arthroscopic Patellar Debridement.** In some people there is symptomatic loose cartilage on the patella that may benefit from resection of the fibrillated fragments of cartilage. This is more common after direct injury to the patella and is not generally appropriate as an isolated procedure when there is an underlying malalignment causing cartilage damage. In that case, the alignment should be corrected to reduce abnormal pressure distribution on the patella.

X. Prognosis

Most athletes with patellofemoral pain or instability will respond to nonoperative care and return to sports in 6 to 12 weeks with brace support. Some of these problems, however, remain chronic and require surgery. When treatment is accurately administered by a skilled therapist or surgeon, most athletes will ultimately return to their sport. Delays in return to sport can be substantial in some cases. In more severe cases, it maybe necessary to restrict an athlete for up to a year from the onset of symptoms when there is cartilage damage related to extensor mechanism malalignment. If there is advanced cartilage damage to the patella or trochlea, return to vigorous athletics may not be possible in some cases.

Suggested Reading

Fulkerson J. *Disorders of the patellofemoral joint.* Third Edition. Baltimore: Williams & Wilkins, 1997.

54. THE LEG

Robert A. Pedowitz and Anthony J. Saglimbeni

I. The Leg

A. Anatomy

The tibia and fibula serve as a rigid link between the ankle and knee. These bones are surrounded by soft tissues, which provide motion and stability for the thigh, ankle, and foot. The four prominent compartments of the leg (anterior, lateral, superficial posterior, and deep posterior) are defined by nonelastic osseofascial boundaries; within each compartment lie specific muscles, nerves, and vessels.

B. Define the Problem

Leg disorders frequently interfere with sports participation and performance. Certain acute injuries, such as fractures and contusions, are covered elsewhere in this manual. "Shin splints" are well known to athletes and care providers; however, this nonspecific diagnosis should be avoided because it does not guide evaluation or treatment of the usual causes of shin pain. Acute and chronic leg disorders often reflect training errors. Avoidance of injury is facilitated by awareness of these common overuse disorders.

C. History

The time course and mechanism of injury should be explored in detail. It is important to probe for changes in training routine, shoe wear, or running surface. History of prior injury in the affected or contralateral limb should be elicited. The pattern of pain should be documented in detail. For example, stress fractures are usually associated with immediate pain upon exercise. Chronic compartment syndrome typically produces pain after a relatively reproducible period of exertion. In contrast, tendinitis may become particularly painful a day or so after strenuous activity. A history of back pain or vascular disease should be excluded, particularly in older patients, because neurogenic or vascular claudication may present as exertional leg pain.

D. Physical Examination

The leg should be observed for evidence of focal deformity, swelling, or ecchymosis. Active and passive knee and ankle range of motion should be documented; pain with passive stretch may reflect muscle ischemia or myotendinous injury. Focal tenderness may guide diagnosis. For posteromedial leg pain, carefully palpate the tibia, tibial periosteum, and muscle bellies of the deep posterior compartment in an attempt to differentiate stress fracture, periostalgia, and chronic compartment syndrome, respectively. Muscle hernias (more common with chronic compartment syndrome) may be more apparent with muscle contraction—for example, during a heel or toe rise. Thompson's test should be performed to rule out Achilles rupture (see below). Muscle strength testing may elicit pain related to tendinitis or muscle strain injury. Neurovascular examination and sciatic nerve stretch tests may implicate a referred etiology of leg pain.

E. Diagnostic Tests

The history and physical examination usually establish the diagnosis; however, adjunctive tests may help to sort through the differential diagnosis. Although plain radiographs generally demonstrate overt tibial or fibular fracture, stress fractures are usually not visualized initially. In about half of the cases, plain films never demonstrate the fine lucency or sclerosis of a stress fracture. A three-phase bone scan may demonstrate focally increased activity (i.e., stress fracture) or diffusely increased uptake (i.e., medial tibial periostalgia). The bone scan may also help to pick up unusual diagnoses, such as osteoid osteoma or occult infection. Magnetic resonance imaging (MRI) is very sensitive and specific for stress fractures and for acute and chronic musculotendinous abnormalities and should play an important adjunctive role as techniques become more cost-effective. Electromyograms and nerve conduction studies are quite specific but not completely sensitive for confirmation of a nerve entrapment disorder. In the appropriate setting, direct measurement of intracompartmental pressure should be used to confirm a chronic compartment syndrome. Noninvasive vascular studies and advanced spinal imaging may be helpful in some cases.

II. Specifc Diagnoses

The following discussion focuses upon the specific presentation, evaluation, and treatment of common leg disorders in athletes.

A. Exertional Leg Pain

It is useful to have a structured approach to differential diagnosis of exertional leg pain. Physical examination findings are often nonspecific in athletes with exertional leg pain. Specific diagnostic tests are usually directed by assessment of the history of injury and the pattern of pain production. The differential diagnosis should include stress fracture, chronic compartment syndrome, and periostalgia. Neurogenic or vascular claudication should also be considered in some athletes with exertional leg pain.

1. **Stress fractures (insufficiency feature)** are usually caused by increased and/or altered physical activity that exceeds the bone's tolerance for cyclic stress. Stress fractures may also occur with normal physiologic loads in pathologic bone—for example, with osteopenic bone in ammenorrheic or postmenopausal women. A history of increased training duration or intensity, changes of running surface or shoe wear, and history of prior stress fracture should be explored. With stress fractures, athletes usually describe leg pain that is present upon initiation of activity and increases during exercise. Pain is generally minimal when the athlete is not bearing weight. The bone may be tender to palpation, and there may be local induration related to a periosteal healing response. Radiographs are usually nondiagnostic initially, but lucency may become apparent within a few weeks. Plain films may never show abnormalities in up to 50% of patients. Three-phase radionuclide imaging is a very sensitive but less specific. MRI may become the diagnostic method of choice but is currently relatively expensive.

   Treatment of stress fractures should focus on limitation of activity in order to facilitate healing. Activities that cause more than mild pain should be avoided. Training should be gradual and progressive, with careful attention to the factors that caused the initial problem. Aerobic fitness can usually be maintained by nonimpact training. In recalcitrant cases, surgery may help to stimulate a healing response (drilling or bone grafting) and/or stabilize the bone (intramedullary nail). In the midshaft of the tibia, anterior cortical stress fractures are particularly prone to delayed union or overt fracture; in this case dense radiolucency without callus formation warrants assertive activity restriction and perhaps earlier surgical intervention.

2. **Compartment syndromes** are due to elevation of intracompartmental pressure, which interferes with microvascular flow and causes tissue ischemia and pain. Acute compartment syndromes are caused either by increased intracompartmental contents (i.e., swelling or bleeding related to trauma) or by decreased compartmental volume (i.e., external constriction from a cast). A full-blown acute compartment syndrome is a surgical emergency that requires immediate fasciotomy in order to avoid permanent ischemic contracture. In contrast, chronic compartment syndrome (CCS) involves elevation of intramuscular pressure and pain during exercise with return to baseline after exercise. The basic etiology of CCS is poorly understood. In some cases, muscle hypertrophy with increased training probably exceeds the compartment's inherent volume. In other athletes, fascial thickening or an anatomic variant may predispose to CCS.

Athletes with CCS often describe onset of leg pain after a relatively consistent exercise interval (i.e., 4 min after the start of a run). A sensation of pressure, fullness, or ache may be described; however, a history of sharp or stabbing pain does not rule out CCS. Numbness or weakness—for example foot drop—may be appreciated. Typically, the intense pain subsides within minutes after cessation of exercise, although milder pain may persist for hours to days. Physical examination findings are nondiagnostic in CCS. However, muscle hernia (palpable defects in the fascia) are more common in CCS patients than in others.

Definitive diagnosis of CCS currently requires direct measurement of intramuscular pressure using small pressure catheters that are positioned percutaneously. Intramuscular pressures may be measured before, during, and after exercise. Measurement of during-exercise pressures is technically difficult and requires a system with high-frequency response. Various diagnostic pressure criteria are described in the literature, and accurate diagnosis requires good understanding of the limitations and characteristics of specific measurement techniques. CCS patients may have elevated intramuscular pressure at rest before exercise. These patients usually demonstrate increased pressure in the early period after exercise (1 to 5 min), with delayed return to baseline values (greater than 6 min recovery).

CCS usually does not respond to conservative therapy. Some patients choose to limit their activity in order to avoid exertional pain. Most athletes choose decompressive fasciotomy in order to return to high-level sports participation; this procedure is usually effective when the diagnosis is accurate.

3. **Medial periostalgia** is more accurate and descriptive than the commonly used, wastebasket diagnosis of "shin splints." Medial periostalgia is very common and quite debilitating. The clinical history often mimics the setting of stress fractures—that is, marked increase of activity or sudden change of training routine. However, athletes with medial tibial periostalgia often describe leg pain that is present without weight bearing and persists after cessation of exercise. Some patients note exquisite tenderness along the inside of the shin.

   Physical examination may help to distinguish periostalgia from tibial stress fracture. With medial periostalgia, the periosteum tends to be tender over a broad zone (i.e., the middle third of the tibia) as opposed to the point tenderness associated with a stress fracture. Careful palpation may demonstrate periosteal thickening and induration just posterior and medial to the tibial cortex. Plain radiographs are frequently negative, but they may show periosteal thickening. Definitive diagnosis can be confirmed with a bone scan, which usually demonstrates diffusely increased uptake along the medial tibia (as opposed to the focal abnormality of a stress fracture).

   Medial periostalgia usually responds to nonoperative treatments, including rest, training modification, stretching, ice massage, nonsteroidal antiinflammatory drugs (NSAIDs), orthotics, or taping. In severe or recalcitrant cases, surgery consists of local exploration and periosteal cauterization. The procedure is usually effective; however, it is not clear whether its success is due to the local decompressive fasciotomy required for bone exposure, stimulation of periosteal healing by scar formation, denervation of the pain-causing tissue by cauterization, or the fact that patients are forced to rest and rehabilitate for a defined period afar surgery.

B. **Achilles Tendinitis and Rupture**

1. *Anatomy*

   The Achilles tendon is formed by the merging tendons of the gastrocnemius and soleus muscles. The gastrocnemius heads originate from the femoral condyles and the soleus originates from its broad attachment to the posterior tibia and fibula. The Achilles tendon inserts onto the calcaneus. The tendon is encased by a paratenon sheath and is relatively hypovascular 4 to 5 cm proximal to the calcaneal insertion.

2. *Definition*

Achilles tendinitis is inflammation of the Achilles tendon or, more commonly, the paratenon. This is usually an overuse injury and commonly results from an increased intensity of activity, a change in playing surface, or a change in footwear.

Complete Achilles tendon tears usually occur 4 to 5 cm proximal to the calcaneus (where blood flow is poorest), through regions of preexisting tendon degeneration. This occurs most commonly in the 30- to 50-year-old "weekend warrior."

3. *Etiology and Mechanism of Injury*
   a. Risk factors for tendinitis include new-onset activities, an increased level of intensity of old activities, surface changes, and altered footwear (i.e., lower heels than usual). Hyperpronation may contribute. Runners, gymnasts, cyclists, and volleyball players are among the most commonly affected athletes.
   b. Achilles rupture typically involves forced dorsiflexion against active plantarflexion of the ankle. This occurs most commonly in the sports of basketball, diving, and tennis.
4. *History*
   a. With tendinitis, athletes complains of Achilles pain that is worst with onset of activity, often disappearing with continued activity and again accentuated after exercise. Some patients complain of pain on awakening. There is usually no history of trauma.
   b. With Achilles rupture, the patient typically reports a sudden exertional pain or "pop" in the posterior leg during exertion, sometimes thinking that he or she was kicked or cut in the heel. The patient may reveal a history of prior heel cord pain and/or corticosteroid injections to the area, increasing the risk of such an injury.
5. *Physical Examination*
   a. **Tendinitis.** The exam may show swelling or erythema along the area of the Achilles tendon. There is usually tenderness to palpation in the area 2 to 5 cm proximal to the calcaneus. Passive plantarflexion and dorsiflexion may be accompanied by crepitus along the Achilles tendon. Thickening of the Achilles tendon may be palpable (see Appendix 6). Passive ankle dorsiflexion is usually limited and active resisted plantarflexion may increase the pain.
   b. **Rupture.** The region may be swollen with a palpable defect. Passive dorsiflexion may be increased. Plantarflexion strength is usually diminished with a decreased ability to toe rise. These signs may be absent because other muscles—such as tibialis posterior, toe flexors, and peroneals—may substitute for the torn Achilles tendon. The Thompson test is usually positive with a complete Achilles tendon rupture and its results should be compared with those from the opposite, noninjured leg (see appendix 6).
6. *Diagnostic Tests*

Diagnostic studies are not usually necessary, but plain radiographs may show tendinous calcification in chronic cases. Ultrasound or MRI may show incomplete tears of the tendon and may be used to rule out complete tears when suspected.

7. *Prevention*

Correction of hyperpronation, avoidance of hill running, and low-heeled shoes, as well as a gradual increase in the intensity of workouts, will go a long way to avoiding Achilles tendinitis and decreasing the frequency of exacerbation. A regular program of heel-cord stretching is particularly important.

8. *Treatment Options*
   a. **Tendinitis.** Treatment is mostly conservative, but any predisposing anatomic variations must be corrected first. As with any overuse injury, a period of relative rest is essential to break the cycle. Uphill

running and uneven surfaces should be avoided. Other conservative measures include ice and NSAIDs. A heel lift up to 15 mm will decrease the degree of dorsiflexion and thus the tension on the tendon. Tape, orthotic bracing, or night splints may help limit dorsiflexion as well. Severe cases may indicate a 4- to 6-week period of rest in a short-leg walking cast.

Rehabilitation should focus on heel-cord stretching and strengthening of the ankle musculature. Corticosteroid injection is not recommended because the weakened tendon may be predisposed to rupture. Iontophoresis and phonophoresis can be beneficial. In chronic cases, surgical debridement of inflamed paratenon or degenerative tendon may provide relief.

b. **Rupture.** Treatment options include conservative therapy with equinus casting and open repair (a long-standing controversy). Conservative therapy starts with long-leg casting with the knee at 45 degrees and gravity equinus for 4 weeks. This is followed by a 4-week period in a short-leg walking cast with gravity equinus. A 1-in. heel lift should then be used for at least 4 weeks; the lift may gradually be eliminated over the ensuing months. Progressive stretching and strengthening should be initiated when casting is completed. This method is often advocated for the less active or more elderly patient.

Open repair with reapproximation of the torn ends of the tendon is associated with a lower incidence of rerupture as well as less loss of strength. Postoperative therapy has moved to early mobilization and rehabilitation. This is the recommended procedure for the younger and more active individual.

9. *Return to Play*

Return to play should be gradual to avoid relapse. Full activity requires pain-free range of motion with good strength. Heel lifts, taping, or bracing may help resist dorsiflexion and facilitate rehabilitation.

C. **Tennis Leg (Medial Head Gastrocnemius Tear)**

1. *Anatomy*

The medial head of the gastrocnemius muscle originates from the medial femoral condyle posteriorly and merges with the lateral head and eventually the Achilles tendon, inserting into the calcaneus.

2. *Definition*

Tennis leg is a tear or strain of the medial head of the gastrocnemius muscle at the myotendinous junction. The differential diagnosis includes a ruptured or inflamed Baker's cyst, plantaris tendon rupture, and Achilles rupture.

3. *Etiology and Mechanism of Injury*

Typically this involves an explosive activation of the leg while the athlete is in complete knee extension and ankle dorsiflexion. It can also occur while he or she is lifting a heavy object with terminal toe and foot plantarflexion or with hill running.

4. *History*

These patients are usually middle-aged recreational athletes. They often complain of a sharp pain in the medial calf occurring with an explosive leg activation. The patient describes a sensation of being kicked or struck sharply. For this reason, the injury has been referred to as a "snap of a whip."

5. *Physical Examination*

Ecchymosis and swelling may be present at the site of local tenderness or may spread distally into the foot. Tenderness is noted at the proximal muscle-tendon junction of the medial gastrocnemius. Active ankle plantarflexion is usually painful.

6. *Diagnostic Studies*

The diagnosis is usually made clinically. MRI or ultrasound will show myotendinous disruption and local hemorrhage/edema.

7. *Prevention*
   Prevention should focus upon warm-up, stretching, and muscle strengthening.
8. *Treatment*
   Treatment is conservative and starts with (RICE) therapy. An Ace wrap, neoprene sleeve, or shoe lift may provide some comfort during return to sports. Severe tears can be splinted in a short leg cast or cast boot with the ankle in a neutral position for 2 to 3 weeks. Stretching and strengthening should be initiated as soon as pain starts to resolve.
9. *Return to Play*
   Return to play should be based upon recovery of strength and range of motion. This is an extremely variable period and may range from 1 to 12 weeks.

D. **Peroneal Nerve Entrapment**

1. *Anatomy*
   The common peroneal nerve comes from the bifurcation of the sciatic nerve above the popliteal fossa. It courses across the lateral head of the gastrocnemius, medial to the biceps tendon, and then divides into the superficial and deep peroneal nerves. The common peroneal nerve is particularly vulnerable as it courses around the fibular head superficially. The deep peroneal nerve travels through the anterior compartment of the leg. In the ankle, the nerve passes beneath the extensor retinaculum.
2. *Definition*
   The common peroneal nerve is usually compressed at the fibular head, resulting in foot drop. Compression of the deep peroneal nerve results in dorsal foot pain and sensory loss in the web space between the first and second toes.
3. *Etiology and Mechanism of Injury*
   The most common mechanism of injury is direct trauma to the common peroneal nerve along its superficial course. Rarely, however, fracture callus, local inflammation, or tumor in the area of the fibular head can produce a nerve entrapment syndrome. Deep peroneal nerve injury may be attributed to the use of very tight fitting footwear. One common situation is the use of new or rented ski boots or improperly fitted cast boots.
4. *History*
   The athlete may complain of numbness or tingling over the anterolateral leg, foot, or first web space. He or she may describe foot drop or weakness of ankle dorsiflexion and/or eversion. There may be a history of trauma or a prolonged period of sitting in the "Indian" position. Pain may be exacerbated by running. There may also be a history of recurrent ankle sprains.
5. *Physical Examination*
   a. **Common Peroneal Nerve.** The physical exam may reveal ecchymosis or swelling at the point of trauma. The region may be tender, and percussion may result in a positive Tinel's sign (referred dysesthesia). Neurologic testing may demonstrate weakness on dorsiflexion and/or eversion and a focal sensory deficit in the anterolateral leg.
   b. **Deep Peroneal Nerve.** In severe cases, atrophy may be noted in the extensor digitorum brevis. Sensory testing shows a deficit between the first two toes, and motor testing may show weakness of the toe dorsiflexors. Pain can be provoked by ankle dorsiflexion and plantarflexion.
6. *Diagnostic Studies*
   Plain radiographs are helpful to rule out tumor or fracture at the fibular head. Electromyography and studies of nerve conduction velocity may differentiate lumbar or sciatic radiculopathy and may help isolate the specific location of nerve entrapment.

7. *Treatment*
   Treatment is usually conservative and is focused on the underlying cause. Orthotic bracing may help stabilize the area while the patient is walking and avoid extrinsic pressure to the area. Inspection of footwear is essential and changes may make for an easy solution. Progressive motor loss or persistent pain may require decompression.
8. *Return to Play*
   Once sensation returns and strength is normal, the athlete may return to participation. Many athletes will play despite this problem. In severe cases, gradual return to play can be initiated after a period of rest.

Suggested Reading

Detmer DE, Sharpe K, Sufit RL, Girdley FM. Chronic compartment syndrome: diagnosis, management, and outcomes. *Am J Sports Med* 1985; 13:162–170.

Pedowitz RA, Hargens AR, Mubarak SJ, Gershuni DH. Modified criteria for objective diagnosis of chronic compartment syndrome of the leg. *Am J Sports Med* 1990; 18:35–40.

Mandelbaum BR, Myerson MS, Forster R. Achilles tendon ruptures: a new method of repair, early range of motion, and functional rehabilitation. *Am J Sports Med* 1996; 23:392–395.

55. THE ANKLE

William G. Hamilton

I. Anatomy

The ankle joint is shaped like a carpenter's mortise formed by the medial malleolus, the tibial plafond, and the lateral malleolus containing the dome of the talus. It has 15 to 20 degrees of dorsiflexion and 35 to 40 degrees of plantarflexion. The mortise is held together by the syndesmosis (the anterior and posterior tibiofibular ligaments) holding the fibula in the sigmoid notch of the tibia. The dome of the talus within the mortise is shaped like the segment of a cone with its apex on the medial side. It is wider anteriorly and laterally. This makes the medial ligament complex (the deltoid ligament) compact and relatively stable but leaves the lateral ligament complex—the anterior talofibular ligament (ATFL), calcaneofibular ligament (CFL), and posterior talofibular ligament (PTFL)—like the spokes of a wheel radiating outward from the lateral malleolus and potentially unstable. The critical angle between the ATFL and CFL is quite variable (70 to 140 degrees). This, along with generalized ligamentous laxity and the cavovarus foot, makes some ankles more potentially unstable than others.

A. **The anatomic structures** around the ankle are as follows:
   1. **Medial.** The posterior tibial tendon, the flexor digitorum longus, the neurovascular bundle, and the flexor hallucis longus. (The mnemonic for these—tibial tendon, digitorum longus, and hallucis longus—is "Tom, Dick, and Harry.")
   2. **Lateral.** The peroneus brevis and longus tendons and the sural nerve.
   3. **Anterior.** The anterior tibial tendon, the extensor hallucis longus, the neurovascular bundle, the extensor digitorum longus and the peroneus tertius ("Tom, Harry, and Dick").
   4. **Posterior.** The Achilles tendon, the os trigonum or the trigonal (Stieda's) process.

B. **The subtalar (ST) joint.** The talus rides "side saddle" on the os calcis beneath it. The longitudinal axis of the talus is in line with the first metatarsal while that of the os calcis is in line with the fifth metatarsal. The ligaments stabilizing the ST joint are:
   1. **Medial.** The superficial portion of the deltoid ligament.
   2. **Anterior.** The talonavicular and calcaneocuboid joints and their ligaments.
   3. **Lateral.** The CFL, the lateral branches of the extensor retinaculum, the cervical ligament, the lateral talocalcaneal ligament, and the interosseus talocalcaneal ligament.
   4. **Posterior.** The posterior talocalcaneal ligament.

   In 80% of people the ST joint is *helical,* so motion here occurs in three planes:

   Eversion ↔ inversion, anterior glide ↔ posterior glide,
   internal rotation ↔ external rotation

   Therefore, instabilities involving the ST joint (grade III ankle sprains) are *complex and triplanar.*

II. Biomechanics

The tibiotalar (talocrural) joint, the subtalar joint, and midtarsal joints with their ligaments work in concert and must be considered as one unit. The subtalar joint is the key to the biomechanics of the foot and ankle. It must *evert* at heel strike to unlock the foot/ankle complex, making it flexible to absorb energy. It must *invert* at toe-off to lock the joints for rigidity and efficient transfer of power from the Achilles mechanism through the ankle and forefoot. This motion is limited (5 degrees of eversion and 15 degrees of inversion) but is absolutely essential for normal function, especially in high-performance athletics. Anything that interferes with or reduces this motion—such as arthritis, a tarsal coalition, or arthrofibrosis—will cause dysfunction of the entire foot/ankle complex. This loss of motion should be looked for carefully during the physical examination.

III. Specific Injuries

A. **Sprains.** The sprained ankle is the most common injury in sports that involve running and jumping. (An injury to a ligament is a *sprain*—an injury to a tendon or muscle is a *strain.*) Ankle sprains occur 1 per 10,000 people per day. They represented 25% to 50% of injuries in running sports, and 10% to 30% of these sprains develop chronic symptoms. Ligamentous injuries are classified (after O'Donoghue) as follows: grade I, a minor tear with no instability; grade II, a partial tear with moderate instability; and grade III, a complete tear with gross instability. Some 90% of ankle sprains are lateral, whereas 10% are medial.

1. **Lateral ankle sprains** usually occur when the ankle is plantarflexed, during loading or unloading. (The ankle is 80% stable with all ligaments sectioned when loaded in neutral.) In the plantarflexed position, the ATFL is vertical and under tension; it is usually damaged first. If the stress continues, it tears completely, followed by rupture of the CFL. Isolated tears of the CFL can occur if the inversion stress happens when the ankle is dorsiflexed, but they are rare.

   a. **Evaluation of the acute sprain.** Presenting history: A twisting injury to the ankle. Questions: Did you fall to the ground? Were you able to get up and walk on it? Have you had other injuries to this ankle? (Is this "one of many" or the first time?) Were you taken to an emergency department and did they take x-rays? What did they show and how were you treated—soft cast, ace bandage, etc.?

   b. **Physical examination.** Swelling, ecchymosis, and tenderness around the lateral malleolus. Look for tenderness at the proximal fibula, a Maisonneuve fracture. At the midfibula, look for a high ankle fracture. Use the "squeeze" or "West Point" test to find a syndesmosis injury. At the anterior syndesmosis, look for the "high" ankle sprain. In the sinus tarsi, look for ATFL injury. On the lateral malleolus look for possible fracture instead of sprain. At the tip of the malleolus, look for CFL injury or avulsion fracture. On the posterior malleolus, look for a Shepherd's fracture of the posterior process or peroneal subluxation. At the anterior process of the calcaneus, look for an avulsion fracture. Finally, at the base of fifth metatarsal, look for a tubercle fracture. The anterior drawer sign, done in 10 to 15 degrees of plantarflexion, will usually reveal the degree of the injury. Standard anteroposterior (AP), mortise, and lateral views of the ankle and, if needed, an AP view of the foot should be taken based on the physical exam. Stress x-rays are optional.

   c. **Classification** of lateral ankle sprains—see Table 55-1.

   d. **Treatment** of acute sprains.

      i. **RICE** (rest, ice, compression, and elevation). Weight bearing as tolerated with support (air-cast or cam walker), with cane or crutches if necessary. Cast immobilization (in slight dorsiflexion) is rarely used except for some grade III injuries. The overall prognosis is good, even with grade III sprains. Open repair of acute grade III sprains is usually not indicated; most will do well without surgery, those that do not can be reconstructed later.

      ii. **Range-of-motion exercises,** weight bearing as tolerated with taping or support (aircast), toe raises, and peroneal strengthening (in full plantarflexion!) are implemented as tolerated.

Table 55-1. Classification of lateral ankle sprains

Injury	Usual pathology	Physical examination and x-ray*
Grade I	Partial tear of ATFL	Normal drawer sign Normal talar tilt
Grade II	Torn ATFL (CFL intact)	2+ Drawer sign (<5mm) Mild talar tilt (<10 degrees)
Grade III	Torn ATFL and CFL	3+ Drawer sign (>10 mm) 3+ Talar tilt (>15 degrees)

*The talar-tilt x-ray performed in *plantarflexion* will show laxity of the ATFL; performed in *dorsiflexion,* it will show laxity in the CFL.

iii. **Return to sports** when pain and swelling are minimal and *the peroneals are strong.*

e. **The "hidden injury."** The acute ankle sprain can be accompanied by other injuries that may fail to heal and cause symptoms later. Patients should be examined carefully for the following: malleolar or epiphyseal injury, the Maisonneuve fracture (disruption of the deltoid and syndesmotic ligaments with fracture of the proximal fibula), the "high" ankle sprain (partial tear of the anterior tibiofibular ligament), fracture of the lateral process of the talus (the "snow boarder's fracture"), anterior process fracture of the os calcis, posterior process fracture (Shepherd's fracture), fibular avulsion fracture, osteochondral fracture of the talus, cuboid subluxation or fracture, and fracture of the fifth metatarsal.

2. **Medial ankle sprains.** Deltoid ligament injuries are rarer than lateral ones (5% to 10 %) because the ligament is much stronger and more compact. The diagnosis can usually be made on the basis of the physical examination. If disruption is suspected, a reverse talar tilt stress film can be obtained to see if there is significant instability. *Be certain that there are no fractures present before performing this test* and look for associated injuries—e.g., lesions of the medial talar dome.
   a. **Presentation.** A valgus-pronation injury, tenderness and ecchymosis around the medial malleolus.
   b. **Treatment** is similar to that for lateral sprains. Grades I and II require protection and early rehabilitation. Grade III call for immobilization for 6 to 8 weeks or, rarely, open repair. Medial injuries that "don't heal" should be worked up for talar dome lesions, posterior tibial tendon injuries, or medial malleolar pathology.
3. **Syndesmotic or "high" ankle sprain.** This is a partial tear of the anterior tibiofibular ligament. It presents with tenderness over the anterior syndesmosis and pain on external rotation of the tibia with the ankle in dorsiflexion. If there is a possibility that significant injury has taken place, weight-bearing x-rays and stress films in dorsiflexion–external rotation should be taken. (This may require a local anesthetic.) The athlete should be warned of this injury because it can take much longer to heal than a "regular" ankle sprain. At times it can fail to heal (after more than 3 months) and may require a corticosteroid injection or even surgical exploration. Synovial hernias through the anterior tibiofibular ligament have been reported here. If the entire syndesmosis has been disrupted, then open reduction and internal fixation (ORIF) with a lag screw placed just above the syndesmosis should be performed, with the ankle held in slight dorsiflexion so that the mortise is not closed too tightly.

B. **Tibiotalar instability.** "Chronic" ankle sprains are usually described as *functional* or *mechanical.*

1. ***Functional*** **instability** is motion beyond voluntary control but not exceeding the physiologic range of the joint—i.e., subjective "giving way."
2. ***Mechanical*** **instability** is motion beyond the physiologic range—i.e., objective looseness. Greater than 50% of functionally unstable ankles are also mechanically unstable. Grade I ankle sprains do not usually result in significant instabilities. Grade II injuries with rupture of the ATFL result in mildly increased anterior, rotatory, and inversion laxity, but if peroneal strength is normal, recovery is usually complete. The CFL is a major stabilizer of the subtalar joint and, when it is torn in grade III sprains, a combined fibiotalar and subtalar instability will result. In addition, *rotatory* laxity will also be present and can be symptomatic in "turning" athletes (dancers, gymnasts, and skaters) (see Sec. III.G).
3. **The "sprained ankle that won't heal."** Most sprains (even grade III) will heal uneventfully with rehabilitation. The degree of the injury usually governs the healing time. Symptoms that persist for more than 3 months can be a diagnostic challenge. Look for the following: residual peroneal weakness, a very common cause of late symptoms; rotatory instability, especially in "turning" athletes; posterior impingement, on the os trigonum, trigonal (Stieda's) process, or soft tissue (the "posterior pseudomeniscus"); Shepherd's (posterior talar process) fracture; peroneal pathology (partial tears or rents); FHL tendinitis; problems around the tip of the fibula, such as soft tissue entrapment (the "meniscoid" lesion), avulsion fractures (usually the insertion of the CFL), a symptomatic os subfibulare, possibly present since birth but not symptomatic prior to the sprain; fracture of the lateral process of the talus (the "snow boarder's fracture"), fracture of the anterior process of the os calcis (the origin of the extensor digitorum brevis), or the sinus tarsi syndrome.

C. **The peroneal tendons**

1. **Acute subluxation.** The peroneal tendons can shift over the posterior edge of the lateral malleolus when an inversion sprain occurs, causing rents or longitudinal tears in the peroneus brevis that may be symptomatic after the sprain heals. These splits are often diagnosed poorly on magnetic resonance imaging (MRI).
   a. **Presentation.** Persistent tenderness and swelling over the peroneal sheath in the region of the peroneal retinaculi should be a sign that the problem is present. The diagnosis can be confirmed by injecting of lidocaine into the peroneal sheath. *Corticosteroid injections are not effective and should not be used here.*
   b. **Treatment.** Persistent dysfunction (greater than 3 months) is an indication for surgical exploration and repair or partial excision of the affected tendon (usually the peroneus brevis). If chronic instability is present, this can be combined with a ligament reconstruction using the split in the peroneus brevis to harvest a graft for the repair.
2. **Acute dislocation.** Peroneal dislocation usually occurs with a forceful dorsiflexion of the foot and ankle against resistance, as in a ski boot. The injury is often mistaken for a lateral ankle sprain. Patients with a shallow peroneal groove are may be predisposed to this injury.
   a. **Treatment.**
      i. **Nonsurgical.** The incidence of recurrent subluxation following the acute episode is extremely high when not treated in a short leg cast with *no weight bearing* for 6 weeks. This form of treatment yields better than 50% satisfactory results. Rarely, the dislocation can go unrecognized and untreated and the patient presents much later with the peroneal tendons running asymptomatically down the anterior aspect of the lateral malleolus. This is best left alone.

ii. **Surgical.** Because of the uncertain prognosis with conservative treatment, many sports medicine surgeons recommend primary repair of the acute injury. The superior peroneal retinaculum is usually torn from its insertion on the outer portion of the posterior lateral malleolus. The tendons usually dissect the insertion of the retinaculum off the bone and slide under the periosteum over the lateral malleolus. The acute repair consists of suturing the avulsed retinaculum back into place at its anatomic location.

3. **Chronic subluxation.** Recurrent subluxation is a common sequela to acute dislocation. Conservative measures such as bracing or strengthening are usually futile. Unless there is a contraindication, surgery is the best treatment for recurrent subluxation. If there is a contraindication to surgery, the condition is should be treated by "benign neglect."
   a. **Surgical treatment.** There are several options:
      i. **Restore the normal anatomy** by reattaching the retinaculum to its normal insertion, usually in a small groove with pull-through sutures in the bone. (This procedure is analogous to the modified Bröstrom procedure for laxity in the anterior ankle ligaments). If the groove behind the fibula is shallow, it should be deepened with a gouge or burr. It is not necessary to attempt to resurface the raw area.
      ii. **A sliding bone graft** may be taken from the superficial portion of the malleolus and shifted or rotated posteriorly and distally and then held in place by small screws.
      iii. **The peroneal tendons may be rerouted** under the calcaneofibular ligament by osteotomy of the tip of the fibula, by removing the calcaneal insertion of the ATFL with a bone plug and replacing the plug in the calcaneus with a screw, or by dividing the peroneal tendons and then suturing them back together.
      iv. An outmoded procedure involves harvesting a strip from the from lateral portion of the Achilles tendon, leaving the distal insertion intact, and suturing the proximal end to the posterior fibula to hold the tendons in place. This operation can produce unacceptable stiffness and loss of motion in the ankle and is *not* recommended.

4. **Peroneal rupture.** If these ruptures are diagnosed when they occur, surgical repair with Kessler-type sutures to restore normal anatomy should be attempted. Those found later (after more than 4 to 6 weeks) usually cannot be repaired primarily and reconstruction must be performed.
   a. **Rupture of the peroneus brevis** is rare. Usually it is associated with trauma (e.g., being hit by a hockey puck or by having had repeated injections of cortisone into a partial rupture). Reconstruction of the peroneus brevis can be done using all or a portion of the peroneus longus. If the stump of the peroneus brevis is long enough, it can be sutured to the tip of the fibula, as in the Evans ankle ligament reconstruction.
   b. **Ruptures of the peroneus longus** usually occur distally at the level of the os peroneum adjacent to the cuboid; (the painful os peroneum or POP syndrome). If the rupture occurs distal to or through the os peroneum, proximal migration of the os can often be seen on the lateral x-ray. Reconstruction of the peroneus longus involves sewing the proximal end of the torn peroneus longus tendon into the peroneus brevis.
   c. **When both peroneals are missing,** the peroneus brevis can be reconstructed using the FHL tendon after a tunnel has been created with a Hunter rod.

5. **Peroneal tendinitis.** This is often due to a partial rupture or longitudinal tear in the tendon. Posterior ankle pain due to posterior impinge-

ment, an os trigonum or a Shepherd's fracture is frequently misdiagnosed as peroneal tendinitis. (Posterior impingement is differentiated from peroneal, FHL, and Achilles pathology by the *plantarflexion sign*: forced plantarflexion will cause pain specifically with posterior impingement but not with other conditions.)

D. **The posterior tibial tendon**

1. **Tendinitis.** Posterior tibial tendinitis may be acute, chronic, or recurrent. It is typically seen as an overuse syndrome in pronated runners. The diagnosis should be obvious on physical examination but can be confirmed by lidocaine injection into the tendon sheath. The tendon may be strained above the retinaculum, at the distal end of the retinaculum, or at its insertion in the plantar medial tarsal navicular.

   a. **Acute tendinitis** should be treated by modified activities, physical therapy modalities, and non-steroidal antiinflammatory drugs (NSAIDs), but these should be used only as part of an overall treatment program and not as a "quick fix." If the runner is pronated, orthoses should be ordered to correct the pronation during running activities. The condition can be difficult to differentiate from a painful accessory navicular bone. Posterior tibial tendinitis in obese, middle-aged females is a different disease from that seen in a young athlete. (In the older patient, it is often a precursor to attenuation and eventual rupture and should be treated aggressively.)

   b. **Chronic and recurrent tendinitis.** Acute tendinitis that fails to heal and becomes chronic or recurrent is often a sign of rents or partial ruptures of the tendon. These will need an MRI study and surgical exploration if present. Steroid injections here should be avoided.

   c. **Rupture of the posterior tibial tendon** is extremely rare in healthy athletes unless the tendon has been injected with corticosteroids or lacerated. When such a rupture occurs, it should be surgically repaired to prevent collapse of the arch. If the tendon is irreparable, it should be reconstructed with the (FDL) tendon, but this may not prevent collapse later.

   d. **Acute subluxation of the posterior tibial tendon** is very rare. The best results are obtained when early surgical repair of the torn posterior tibial retinaculum is performed, as in acute repair of dislocated peroneal tendons, otherwise the retinaculum will have to be reconstructed with a periosteal flap.

E. **Anterior impingement.** This is the "footballer's ankle." The cambium layer of the periosteum has osteogenic potential and, when disturbed, either by traction or impingement, can form bone spurs. Anterior osteophyte formation is common in the older athlete, especially if he or she has a cavus foot or ligament laxity. The osteophytes can fracture, leaving loose bodies in the anterior joint.

1. **Physical examination.** The diagnosis is usually obvious—loss of dorsiflexion and anterior ankle pain with dorsiflexion, as in landing from a jump or running uphill. It can be confirmed with a weight- bearing lateral x-ray in maximum dorsiflexion.

2. **Conservative treatment** usually involves heel lifts (in order to open up the front of the ankle and relieve the impingement) and modified activities—i.e., "don't do what hurts."

3. **Operative treatment.** There are many different classifications of anterior ankle impingement, often related to the size of the lesions. The author's classification is related to the surgical implications for treatment.

   a. **Type I.** The osteophytes are primarily on the lip of the tibia (most amenable to arthroscopic debridement).

   b. **Type II.** The osteophytes are primarily on the neck of the talus, usually in the capsular insertion. It can be difficult and time-consuming to these with the arthroscope, because the capsule must be taken down from the neck of the talus in order to visualize the pathology.

c. **Type III.** Osteophytes are present on both the tibia and the neck of the talus (making it quite difficult to do an adequate cleanout with the arthroscope). The author's preference, for types II and III, is a small anterior medial arthrotomy using a head lamp, small osteotomes, and Kerrison rongeurs.

F. **Nerve entrapments**

1. **The tarsal tunnel syndrome** is characterized by dysesthesias and neuralgic pains on the undersurface of the forefoot in the distribution of the posterior tibial nerve. The symptoms are often exacerbated by pronation.

   a. **Diagnosis.** The true syndrome usually has a positive Tinel's sign and a space-occupying lesion on the MRI study, usually a ganglion, varicosity, lipoma, or, rarely, a neurolemmoma. FHL tendinitis or the posterior impingement syndrome can be mistaken for the tarsal tunnel syndrome. At times the entrapment occurs lower, where the medial and lateral plantar nerves enter the fascia of the abductor hallucis muscle.

   b. **Treatment.** Orthoses or medial heel wedges can be helpful. If a space-occupying lesion is present, surgery is usually needed. The dissection should be carried down in the plane between the medial malleolus and the neurovascular bundle and should go distally into the abductor hallucis fascia.

2. **The anterior tarsal tunnel syndrome.** Entrapment of the deep peroneal nerve can occur on the dorsum of the forefoot as the nerve passes under the extensor retinaculum.

   a. **Diagnosis.** This syndrome is characterized by hypesthesia in the first web space and a positive Tinel's sign at the point of entrapment. Frequently the cause is an osteophyte, which can be seen on a lateral x-ray.

   b. **Treatment.** A mild form of this condition is common in the athlete with a cavus foot who uses sneakers or ski boots, etc., that are too tightly laced and therefore press tightly over the dorsum of the instep. In these cases, conservative treatment with moleskin on the tongue of the sneaker or relief of the pressure of the boot will usually correct the problem. If conservative treatments fail, surgical removal of the osteophyte and lysis of the nerve can relieve the symptoms.

G. **Subtalar Instability.** The calcaneofibular ligament (CFL) is a major stabilizer of the subtalar joint and, when it is stretched or attenuated, as in grade III lateral sprains, a combination of tibiotalar and subtalar instability will be present. In the vast majority of lateral ankle sprains, the inversion occurs in plantarflexion, tearing the ATFL first and the CFL second. In the rare instance when the ankle is dorsiflexed and then inverted, the CFL can be torn, leaving the ATFL intact and resulting in a pure subtalar instability. It is characterized by apparent functional instability (giving way in an ankle with minimal anterior drawer). The true nature of the mechanical instability will not be apparent on physical examination, and the standard talar tilt x-rays may be normal.

1. **Diagnosis.** The diagnosis can be made with a stress Broden's view of the subtalar joint. In this view, the subtalar joint under stress should open only a few millimeters at most. Anything more than that is positive. In 80% of people, the subtalar joint is helical, so subtalar instability is multiplaner: varus/valgus; anterior/posterior, and rotational.

2. **Treatment.** Peroneal strengthening and bracing will often control the symptoms. If surgery is needed, the operative procedure to correct subtalar instability must restore the function of the CFL and ATFL if they are attenuated. The author's preferred technique is the Gould modifica-

tion of the Bröstrom procedure. If heel varus is present, it must be corrected with a valgus osteotomy.

H. **Osteochondritis dissecans (OCD).** There are two types; spontaneous and posttraumatic. Spontaneous OCD usually presents as painless swelling in teenage athletes with no history of significant trauma. Traumatic OCD lesions are usually associated with lateral ankle sprains and tend to be crush lesions of the medial talar dome and chip fractures of the lateral talar dome. The classic locations are posteromedial and anterolateral (though the lesions are not invariably found in these locations). Symptoms usually begin when the surface of the articular cartilage is fractured.
   1. **Diagnosis.** X-rays and MRI or computed tomography (CT) scan will usually reveal the extent of the lesion.
   2. **Treatment.** These lesions are usually not discovered until they are symptomatic, and once symptoms begin, conservative treatment is usually not effective. Immobilization will usually provide temporary relief. Lateral lesions of the talar dome are very amenable to arthroscopic curettage and drilling. Lesions of the medial talar dome are more difficult to correct with the arthroscope. They can be very large and posterior in location. These lesions are often best approached with a medial malleolar osteotomy. Simple drilling of soft, intact lesions usually does not work. It is best to curette and then drill such lesions. The overall prognosis is good.

I. **Uncommon problems**
   1. **The posterior-process fracture** (Shepherd's fracture) typically occurs when a woman in high heels catches the heel of her shoe going downstairs and sustains an abrupt plantarflexion sprain, fracturing the posterolateral (Stieda's) process of the talus or dislodging a previously asymptomatic os trigonum. The patient has pain when the ankle is dorsiflexed.
      a. **Diagnosis.** There will be tenderness behind the fibula and forced passive plantarflexion, the *plantarflexion sign,* will be markedly positive. A hairline fracture can be difficult to see on the x-ray, but the bone scan will be positive.
      b. **Treatment.** Immobilization in a walking boot or cam walker for 4 to 6 weeks until the symptoms subside.
   2. **The posterior impingement syndrome** is common in ballet dancers and "equinus athletes"—i.e., ice skaters, gymnasts, etc. It presents as posterior or posterolateral ankle pain increased with forced plantarflexion and is often mistaken for peroneal tendinitis.
      a. **Diagnosis.** The x-rays show an os trigonum or a trigonal process and, on rare occasions, only soft tissue impingement. There will be localized tenderness behind the fibula and the "plantarflexion sign" will be positive. In dancers, this condition may be accompanied by FHL tendinitis medially—"dancer's tendinitis."
      b. **Treatment.** This comprises modified activities, immobilization, if necessary, and cortisone injections (FHL lesions medially should *not* be injected.) Surgical removal is recommended if conservative therapy fails after 3 or 4 months.
   3. **Tarsal coalition** (The "peroneal spastic" flat foot) presents with subtalar pain and peroneal spasm. The symptoms are increased with running, jumping, or walking on uneven ground and are decreased by immobilization, but they tend to recur. Coalitions usually become symptomatic in the teens and early adulthood and may be bony, cartilaginous, or fibrous. The lesion most commonly involves the naviculocalcaneal articulation, next the talocalcaneal (middle facet) joint, and, on rare occasions, the talonavicular and naviculocuboid joints.
      a. **Diagnosis.** On physical examination there is decreased or absent subtalar motion. Regular x-rays, including an oblique x-ray of the foot, will often show a naviculocalcaneal bar. The Harris or "ski

jump" view will show middle-facet lesions. In subtle conditions, CT scans and MRIs can be useful. A diagnostic injection of local anesthetic will confirm the diagnosis.

b. **Treatment.** In young patients, the lesion can be taken down surgically. A wide resection should be used, with interposed muscle or fascia to prevent regrowth. Coalitions often tend to re-form and subtalar motion will not be normal, even after a take down, because the subtalar joint never moved or formed normally. Older patients or those with failed resections will often require fusion of the affected joints.

4. **The sinus tarsi syndrome** is characterized by pain and localized tenderness deep in the sinus tarsi, usually following lateral ankle or midfoot sprains. It is exacerbated by lunging and pronation and is usually caused by soft tissue entrapment, by osteophyte formation, or a bone chip. It can be difficult to differentiate from the subluxed cuboid. X-rays, MRIs, and CT scans are usually normal. A bone scan may show mild increased uptake.
   a. **The diagnosis** is usually made by the history and physical examination but can be confirmed by injecting lidocaine into the trigger point in the sinus tarsi.
   b. **Treatment.** If the pain is relieved by the liocaine, then a corticosteroid injection will often be very effective. On rare occasions, surgical exploration and cleanout may be indicated if symptoms persist in spite of conservative treatment (modified activities, arch supports with medial heel wedges).
5. **The subtalar syndrome.** Pain can be coming from the subtalar joint rather than the sinus tarsi. This can be due to instability or derangement.
   a. **Diagnosis.** The two can usually be differentiated by the history, physical examination, and lidocaine injection. The sinus tarsi syndrome is characterized by pain without instability, whereas the subtalar syndrome usually presents with both pain and either giving way or marked stiffness.
   b. **Treatment** usually involves peroneal strengthening and bracing (Aircast or Swedo) for the instability. Orthoses can sometimes be effective.

Suggested Reading

Clanton TO, Schon LC. Athletic injuries to the soft tissues of the foot and ankle. In: Mann RA, Coughlin MJ, eds. *Surgery of the foot and ankle,* 6th ed. St Louis: Mosby, 1993.

Greenfield G, Stanish WD. Tendinitis and tendon ruptures. *Op Tech Sports Med* 1994;2:9–17.

Hamilton WG. Foot and ankle injuries in dancers. *Clin Sports Med* 1988;7:143–173.

Hamilton WG. *Traumatic disorders of the ankle.* New York: Springer-Verlag, 1984.

Renstrom PAFH. Persistently painful sprained ankle. *J Am Acad Orthop Surg* 1994;2:270–280.

56. THE FOOT

G. James Sammarco and Frank G. Russo-Alesi

I. Fractures

The foot and ankle are subjected to a variety of forces during sports. The ankle may experience forces greater than five times body weight during leaping maneuvers. These forces are transmitted through the bones of the foot and their ligamentous supporting structures. Fractures may occur in any of these bones. A high index of suspicion, thorough history, understanding of the mechanism of injury, and complete physical examination are essential in making a diagnosis. Weight-bearing x-rays are usually sufficient to confirm the diagnosis. Stress fractures are common in athletes and should be suspected when a history of chronic pain is present. These injuries also may involve any bone.

II. Tarsal Fractures

Hindfoot injuries are common in athletes participating in distance running and leaping activities where repetitive high-impact loads are part of the event. They may take the form of stress fractures and "bone bruises" as well as acute displaced intra- or extra-articular fractures.

A. **Stress fractures.** These injuries occur in the calcaneus, navicular, talus, and cuboid bones. They typically result from repetitive forces. A prodrome of symptoms—including a dull, aching pain in the hindfoot with occasional sharp lancinating pain for a period of 2 weeks to several months (especially in dancers)—may be present. Onset is insidious and usually occurs shortly after activity begins. Pain increases gradually with repeated practices and games.

1. **History and physical examination.** Nonspecific tenderness in the hindfoot may be localized to the calcaneal tuberosity or other tarsal bones, which may be difficult to differentiate from retrocalcaneal bursitis, Achilles tendinitis, posterior ankle impingement, and plantar fasciitis. Pain may be experienced in the talonavicular region or the lateral aspect of the foot at the cuboid. Rarely is there any outward sign of fracture.
2. **Diagnostic tests.** Depending on the duration of symptoms and the time of onset of symptoms, plain x-rays may reveal the subchondral radiodensity diagnostic of a healing stress fracture. In the calcaneus, they are usually parallel to the posterior facet or through the posterior tuberosity. Talar stress fractures are often parallel to the talonavicular joint. Early in the course of symptoms, plain x-rays may not reveal a stress response; a technetium bone scan is then indicated. Increased uptake in the involved bone indicates a positive scan. Magnetic resonance imaging (MRI) may reveal localized bone edema or the fracture in difficult cases.
3. **Treatment.** Restricting activities that produce symptoms for up to 6 weeks is usually adequate treatment for calcaneal, navicular, and cuboid stress fractures. Cast immobilization initially for 2 weeks is beneficial in reducing pain. Rehabilitation includes cross training with cycling in addition to hydrotherapy. This allows the athlete to maintain strength and flexibility during the healing phase. Stress fractures of the navicular and the cuboid may take considerably longer to heal. Assess union by clinical exam, computed tomography (CT), or plain tomography. Resumption of athletics may take place 12 to 18 weeks after nonoperative treatment. Delayed union, which occurs after 12 weeks of treatment, may require surgery. Displacement and/or frank nonunion is treated by internal fixation and may be augmented by bone grafting. After healing, a semirigid orthosis is prescribed before the athlete is allowed to return to sports.

4. **Return to sports** is permitted after symptoms resolve. There may still be x-ray evidence of a healing stress response. Weight-bearing and impact-loading activities should be resumed slowly in a controlled rehabilitation program to prevent recurrence.

B. **Osteochondral fractures.** A lesion of the talar dome occurs as a result of an inversion injury. The lateral ankle ligament complex usually remains intact, but the lesion has been be associated with chronic lateral ligamentous laxity. It occurs most frequently along the anterolateral or posteromedial ridge of the talar dome's articular surface.

1. **Physical examination.** Symptoms include pain present at extremes of motion and especially with forced eversion and inversion. Occasionally a fragment is displaced and a loose body may be palpable and cause locking. Mild synovitis and ankle swelling occur. The ankle should be checked for instability with forced inversion of the hindfoot and be compared with the uninjured contralateral side. The anterior drawer test (see Appendix 6) checks the integrity of the anterior talofibular ligament. Testing the ankle for continuity of the calcaneofibular ligament is done with the talar tilt test (see Appendix 6).
2. **Diagnostic tests.** Anteroposterior (AP), lateral, and mortise x-rays of the ankle often reveal the lesion. It may be difficult to determine whether the lesion is subluxed from its bed on standard x-rays, in addition to the status of the articular cartilage. Magnetic resonance imaging (MRI) or computed tomography (CT) is helpful in defining the extent of articular involvement.
3. **Treatment.** Acute nondisplaced osteochondral fractures are treated with a cast boot for 6 weeks and partial weight bearing with crutches. Range-of-motion exercises and a gradual return to weight-bearing activities are then prescribed. If large, displaced fragments require anatomic reduction and fixation. If the fragment is small, excision with drilling of the bed is recommended. Associated chronic instability of the lateral ligament requires reconstruction of the lateral ligament in addition to treatment of the talar dome lesion.

C. **Fractures of the talar lateral process** at the subtalar joint of the ankle. This injury is caused by hindfoot inversion associated with dorsiflexion or plantarflexion and compression. Diagnosis requires a high index of suspicion. Moreover, despite appropriate diagnosis and treatment, even nondisplaced fractures can become a chronic source of lateral ankle pain and contribute to subtalar arthrosis.

1. **History and physical examination.** There is tenderness in the area of the anterior talofibular ligament (ATFL) and calcaneofibular ligament (CFL). There is pain with inversion and eversion, which is localized just distal to the lateral malleolus. Local edema and hematoma or ecchymosis may be seen. The fracture may be mistaken for a lateral ankle sprain.
2. **Diagnostic tests.** Plain x-rays reveal a fracture at the inferolateral border of the talus at the posterior joint facet of the subtalar joint. An AP x-ray with the foot 45 degrees internally rotated and plantarflexed may also help visualize it. In order to assess the amount of displacement, a CT scan is recommended.
3. **Treatment.** The size of the fragment, degree of comminution, and extent of joint involvement are important in determining treatment. Fractures with small fragments that are minimally displaced are immobilized for 4 weeks. Larger fragments with significant joint involvement require open reduction and internal fixation and if comminuted, excision of the fragments is indicated. After immobilization of 4 weeks, range-of-motion exercises are begun. If the fragments have been excised, early motion is mandatory. If the fixation is adequate, early range-of-motion exercise is instituted with protected weight bearing. Return to sports through a rehabilitation program is permitted.

D. **Fractures of the anterior process of the calcaneus.** The anterior process or "parrot beak" articulates with the talus via the anterior facet of the subtalar joint and the calcaneocuboid joint inferiorly. Multiple soft tissue attachments play a role in displacing this fracture. The mechanism of injury is inversion and plantarflexion, resulting in avulsion fracture.

1. **History and physical examination.** The point of maximum tenderness is just distal to the sinus tarsi at the dorsal calcaneocuboid joint. There may be associated swelling and ecchymosis. Pain is produced with motion of Chopart's joint.
2. **Diagnostic tests.** Oblique or lateral x-rays of the foot best demonstrate this fracture. Occasionally, CT may be necessary to assess the degree of articular involvement. This fracture may be mistaken for an ankle sprain and is occasionally called a "sprain fracture."
3. **Treatment.** Small fragments with minimal joint involvement are treated with a cast boot. Range-of-motion exercise is started after 4 weeks. Larger fragments with articular incongruity greater than 2 mm are treated surgically with open reduction and internal fixation. Comminuted fragments are excised. Some 50% of patients will continue to have residual pain for an indefinite period of time. Posttraumatic arthritis of the calcaneocuboid joint may require arthrodesis if symptoms persist.

III. Metatarsal Fractures

The forefoot transfers ground-reaction forces to the midfoot during sprinting and jumping. It also is subjected to a variety of torques and shear forces that frequently cause both bony and soft tissue injuries.

A. **Stress fractures.** The second metatarsal is most commonly affected because of its length in relation to the other metatarsals and also to the fact that it is the most rigid ray in the foot. This injury may be associated with hallux valgus due to a transfer lesion. A stress fracture—i.e., march fracture—which occurs at the neck is usually due to poor conditioning. More proximal fractures tend to occur in the conditioned athlete or dancer. They can occasionally extend to become intraarticular and may also occur in the other metatarsals, though with less frequency.

1. **History and physical examination.** The athlete describes a dull, nonspecific forefoot pain prodrome at the end of activity, which then becomes apparent earlier after the onset of activity. Tenderness along the metatarsal becomes more localized with time and a fullness is palpable overlying the fracture.
2. **Diagnostic tests.** If symptoms have been present for less than 1 month, plain x-rays of the foot are unreliable and a technetium bone scan is indicated. Increased uptake is evident on the delayed phase of the scan at the fracture site. This should not be confused with a synovitis, which shows more distal uptake on both sides of the metatarsophalangeal joint.
3. **Treatment.** Rest and a stiff-soled shoe are mandatory. Cross training to maintain strength and flexibility is indicated after the fracture is healed. Treatment is complete when pain subsides and radiological union is evident. Custom-molded orthotics should be considered in athletes with recurrent stress fractures.

B. **The Jones fracture.** Acute and chronic fractures of the proximal fifth metatarsal metaphysis are common in athletes. Some 75% occur in athletes between the ages of 15 and 21 years. Fractures tend to be prevalent in males and in patients with either cavus or planus deformities. These injuries occur while the athlete is pivoting internally or externally on the ball of the foot, and they occur earlier in the athletic season, after a period of inactivity. The Jones fracture should not be confused with an avulsion fracture of the fifth metatarsal styloid—an intraarticular injury resulting from inversion injury. The Jones fracture is notorious for nonunion and can lead to chronic pain and disability. When the injury is acute, it is the result of a sudden forceful load to the forefoot beneath the fifth metatarsal head. This occurs more commonly in unconditioned athletes. The chronic fracture may occur following an acute event after a prodrome of pain for at least 2 weeks.

1. **History and physical examination.** The foot is tender along its lateral border, and pain is produced with forceful manipulation of the forefoot. There may also be associated swelling in the vicinity of the proximal metatarsal, depending on the duration of symptoms.
2. **Diagnostic tests.** Initial AP, lateral, and oblique x-rays may be unremarkable; at 2 weeks, however, films may reveal the "dreaded black line" representing an incomplete fracture extending from the lateral inferior cortex in a dorsomedial direction. The fracture line occurs approximately three-fourths of an inch distal to the styloid of the metatarsal. The chronic fracture demonstrates some degree of medullary narrowing and sclerosis, which may completely obliterate the canal.
3. **Treatment.** Acute fractures without evidence of medullary sclerosis are treated in a short leg cast with no weight bearing for 6 weeks. Resumption of activities is based upon radiographic union and absence of pain. A chronic Jones fracture requires prolonged immobilization, which may take from 2 to 12 months or more to heal. This is often not practical and surgery may be indicated. Intramedullary compression screw fixation with debridement of the sclerotic canal is recommended. Bone grafting is an adjunct to be considered in addition to intramedullary fixation, especially when there is nonunion. This is then followed by immobilization in a non-weight-bearing cast until the fracture has healed (usually 2 to 3 months).

C. **The "Dancer's fracture."** This is an acute spiral fracture at the distal half of the fifth metatarsal shaft and neck. It is the most common acute fracture of the foot in dancers, typically occurring when the dancer loses balance while in the demi-pointe position and rolls over the lateral forefoot.

1. **Physical examination.** Tenderness is noted along the lateral border of the foot distal to the fifth metatarsal tuberosity. Edema and ecchymosis is present at the fracture site.
2. **Diagnostic tests.** X-rays reveal a spiral fracture of the distal shaft into the neck but rarely involving the metatarsal head.
3. **Treatment.** Initially, a non-weight bearing cast boot is in order. This is replaced with a stiff-soled shoe and partial weight bearing as symptoms permit, usually within 2 weeks. The fracture typically heals in 6 to 8 weeks but may take as long as 5 months. A gradual return to sports is permitted after the fracture unites. During the healing process, cross training may be performed to maintain strength and flexibility.

IV. Lisfranc's Fracture-Dislocations and Midfoot Sprains

Injuries to the midfoot vary considerably. Supporting structures—including the bones, ligaments, and muscle—are responsible for maintenance of the longitudinal and transverse arches of the foot. This complex anatomy permits shock absorption and load transmission from the forefoot to the hindfoot and ankle. Injuries may result from forefoot flexion associated with rotation. Impact from another player may result in a direct compression injury. This injury is notorious for eluding diagnosis and may be the source of undiagnosed chronic midfoot pain. A high index of suspicion and detailed history and physical examination with attention to weight-bearing x-rays is helpful in making the diagnosis.

A. **History and physical examination.** Particular attention to the mechanism of injury is important. Moderate or severe pain with weight bearing is characteristic. The pain is described as sharp in character and may be either plantar, medial, or dorsal. Swelling is usually present. There is exquisite tenderness to palpation at the tarsometatarsal joint. The bones are held by a rigid keystone at the second tarsometatarsal joint, so that ligamentous injuries are associated with chip fractures and slight subluxation of the metatarsals.

B. **Diagnostic tests.** Weight-bearing views of the foot including AP, lateral, and oblique projections are necessary. Particular attention is addressed to the first and second metatarsals to determine if diastasis is present. This may indicate an injury to Lisfranc's ligament or isolated first-to-second metatarsal sprain. More obvious fracture-dislocations from high-impact loads reveal overriding metatarsals at the tarsometatarsal joint. The second metatarsal should always be aligned with the middle cuneiform on the AP x-ray. In the subtle injury where articular step-off is not apparent, a CT scan may be helpful in determining the amount of articular misalignment. If there is any question regarding the alignment of the midfoot, comparison views of the uninvolved foot are helpful in determining bony alignment.

C. **Treatment.** The acute nondisplaced injury is treated with ice, rest, compression, and elevation. Limited weight bearing with crutches is permitted. A minor ligamentous sprain with a stable joint requires only a supportive brace and symptomatic medication. Return to sports is permitted when the pain subsides. Restricted weight bearing is recommended for up to 6 weeks. A brace or taping is prescribed as needed. A stiff-soled shoe and orthosis may be necessary. Unstable injuries with diastasis of the first-to-second metatarsal interval require closed reduction with pin or screws to reduce displacement. An associated fracture should be reduced and fixed open with either K wires or screws. Non-weight bearing cast immobilization for 4 to 6 weeks is recommended. It is not uncommon to have chronic pain after this injury. A good reduction is related to the long-term functional outcome and prognosis. Occasionally, chronic symptoms require arthrodesis, which may preclude future athletics.

V. Heel Pain

Injury to the athlete's heel is a common source of pain. The anatomy is complex, with a multitude of muscles, cushioning pads, and ligamentous attachments including the Achilles tendon and plantar fascia, which are frequently the sites of injury and pain. The heel pad, constructed so as to cushion heel strike, may be damaged or simply wear out. Several nerves and tendons adjacent to the calcaneus may also be injured. These conditions are typically related to overuse or improper training. The etiologies are varied.

A history of the inciting event and training technique is essential. Male athletes should also be questioned about any history of sexually transmitted diseases, so as to rule out the possibility of Reiter's syndrome. An understanding of the hindfoot's anatomy and biomechanics is also necessary in making the correct diagnosis.

A. **Heel pain syndrome.** The most common site of heel pain is the medial calcaneal tuberosity. This is the site of origin of the plantar fascia and flexor digitorum brevis, quadratus plantae, and abductor hallucis muscles. The first branch of the lateral plantar nerve (nerve to the abductor digiti quinti) may be entrapped as it passes beneath the medial border of the plantar fascia. This overuse phenomenon is commonly seen in runners and results from repetitive heel impact along with hyperextension of the toes. This places tension on the plantar fascia at its insertion and results in microtears at the fascial origin and an inflammatory response. Microscopic tissue degeneration can occur and a calcaneal spur maybe seen on lateral x-ray of the heel, at the origin of the flexor digitorum brevis.

1. **History and physical examination.** The plantar heel pain initially occurs after a period of activity and eventually occurs earlier and earlier after onset of activity. Pain at rest occurs later. Pain occurs with the first few steps in the morning. The point of maximum tenderness is directly over the medial calcaneal tuberosity and plantar fascia. Contracture of the Achilles tendon is a common associated finding. Lateral calcaneal pain is often suggestive of peroneas tendon injury.
2. **Diagnostic tests.** The lateral x-ray of the calcaneus rules out stress fractures or tumor. A plantar calcaneal spur extending distally from the plantar tuberosity may be present. In unclear cases, without specific classic findings, a technetium bone scan may reveal increased uptake in

the vicinity of the plantar fascial origin, which will aid in diagnosis of stress reaction in the bone at the attachment of the plantar fascia or a frank stress fracture. An MRI will rule out peroneas brevis or longos tears in difficult cases of lateral heel pain.

3. **Treatment.** Nonoperative treatment is successful in 95% of patients. However, it is not uncommon for symptoms to persist up to 12 months. Stretching of the heel cord and plantar fascia two to three times a day is recommended. Non steroidal antiinflammatory drugs (NSAIDs) and contrast baths are also helpful. Silastic heel inserts, 1/8 in. medial heel wedges or shoe lifts may be of benefit. In refractory cases, a night splint is a useful adjunct. A single steroid injection at the plantar fascia origin can relieve pain. But 95% of patients with plantar fascia heal without surgery within 15 months. Despite a thorough trial of nonoperative measures, surgery, including a partial plantar fasciectomy, may be necessary. This is usually combined with release of the nerve to the abductor digiti quinti and occasionally heel spur excision. Return to sports is permitted when symptoms resolve. The distance runner should decrease the distance and duration of the workout and cross training should be performed during the course of treatment. This helps maintain strength and flexibility during convalescence.

B. **Entrapment of the first branch of the lateral plantar nerve** (nerve to the abductor digiti quinti) may account for 20% of chronic heel pain. It is particularly common in athletes who spend a lot of time with the foot plantarflexed, such sprinters, ballet dancers, and figure skaters. This nerve is responsible for the motor innervation of the abductor digiti quinti as well as for innervating the periosteum of the medial calcaneal tuberosity, the long plantar ligament, and the flexor digitorum brevis. Entrapment occurs between the deep fascia of the abductor hallucis and the medial head of the quadratus plantae origin or between the calcaneal spur and the long plantar ligament. Inflammatory changes associated with heel pain syndrome may cause a secondary entrapment of the nerve.

1. **History and physical therapy.** Morning pain is not as prevalent as with heel pain syndrome. The point of maximum tenderness is where the nerve passes beneath the deep fascia of the abductor hallucis muscle. This is slightly more dorsal than the tenderness at the medial calcaneal tuberosity in heel pain syndrome. Percussion over the posterior tibial nerve behind the medial malleolus may help determine if a more proximal nerve entrapment is present. A low back examination to rule out radiculopathy is also necessary.
2. **Diagnostic tests.** Although electromyography (EMG) and nerve conduction velocities are useful in excluding radiculopathy and tarsal tunnel syndrome, two potential sources of chronic heel pain, these studies are rarely positive for entrapment of the first branch of the lateral plantar nerve.
3. **Treatment.** Rest, ice, heel cushions, and longitudinal arch supports to prevent excess pronation of the forefoot are utilized alone or in combination. Stretching of the Achilles tendon and plantar fascia are important treatment modalities. Refractory cases of greater than 12 months, duration are treated surgically with neurolysis. With adequate and complete neurolysis, good to excellent results can be expected in up to 90% of patients. Removal of the heel spur, if present, may eliminate a potential cause of entrapment.

C. **Heel compression syndrome.** Also referred to as *fat-pad atrophy,* can be debilitating to the running athlete. The specialized adipose tissue of the heel is rich in monoglycerides and is anchored to the calcaneus and plantar fascia via a network of fibrous septae. This imparts shock-absorption properties and helps the heel to resist shear forces. The heel fat pad slowly deteriorates after the third decade. Decreased collagen, elastic tissue, water, and overall thickness may be a potential source of pain in the seasoned runner.

1. **History and physical examination.** The pain is described as diffuse plantar heel pain and is aggravated by running on hard surfaces or in a shoe with poor shock-absorption capacity at the heel. Tenderness is central and diffuse and the underlying bone may be palpable. There is no radiation of pain and the plantar fascia is usually not tender.
2. **Diagnostic tests.** Plain x-rays of the heel rule out a stress fracture or intraosseous lesion. A bone scan may be required to rule out stress reaction.
3. **Treatment.** Cushion heel cups, a more shock-absorbent shoe with a rounded heel, and changing to a softer running surface are helpful. A heel lift serves to transfer weight anteriorly, decreasing forces at the heel. Athletic modifications to pain-free activities and cross training are utilized during recovery. The athlete should be counseled that this may be a chronic problem.

D. **Superior heel pain.** The differential diagnosis of superior heel pain includes retrocalcaneal bursitis, Achilles insertional tendinitis, and peritendinitis. Enlargement of the superior posterior bursal prominence of the calcaneus with associated inflammation of the surrounding tissues is referred to as *Haglund's disease.*

1. **History and physical examination.** Pain is experienced with activity and especially with plantarflexion as the shoe's heel counter presses on the inflamed upper border of the calcaneus and the associated soft tissues. Retrocalcaneal bursitis is characterized by edema and tenderness anterior to the Achilles tendon just above its insertion onto the calcaneus. In Haglund's disease, a firm palpable tender soft tissue mass and bony prominence are noted anterior to the Achilles tendon. Often the skin in this region is erythematous and edematous. Insertional tendinitis is noted for tenderness distal to the retrocalcaneal bursa and is in the midline of the heel at the tendon attachment to the bone. Occasionally firm nodules may be palpable, which represent focal areas of scarring and degeneration within the tendon (tendinosis).
2. **Diagnostic tests.** A lateral plain film of the calcaneus may reveal calcification within the Achilles tendon and at its insertion. In Haglund's deformity, the superoposterior aspect of the calcaneus or bursal projection is hypertrophied.
3. **Treatment.** A heel lift of 1 in. to move the loads on the foot forward in the shoe and decrease pressure of the shoe counter on the inflamed posterosuperior heel, can be effective. A portion of the shoe counter may be removed to reduce pressure in the heel. The athlete is encouraged to wear an open-back street shoe when not active in sports. NSAIDs and ice are useful adjuncts. Steroid injections are not routinely recommended because of the potential for skin and soft tissue atrophy as well as the possibility of tendon rupture. Stretching of the Achilles tendon is prescribed, along with strengthening exercises. Often, reducing mileage per run along with a pre- and postactivity stretching and icing will reduce symptoms. Occasionally, a cast boot is necessary to treat a recalcitrant case while maintaining cross-training activities. Surgery is indicated for recalcitrant cases that fail adequate nonoperative treatment for at least 3 months. The operation is directed at the specific underlying pathology, only removing the small area of bone and scar which is tender on clinical examination, (less is more).

VI. The Great Toe

The great toe can be a significant source of symptoms. In addition to common toenail problems, arthritis of the metatarsophalangeal joint can result in hallux rigidus. Bunions may be cause of significant pain and result in secondary problems such as transfer lesions. Injury to the plantar plate and sesamoids also are also common in high-demand athletes.

A. **Hallux rigidus.** This condition results from arthritis of the first metatarsophalangeal joint, with the development of periarticular osteophytes. As a result, there is limited painful dorsiflexion secondary to impingement of the osteophytes on the metatarsal head and on the dorsal base of the proximal phalanx. Several factors are implicated in the etiology. These include a flattened metatarsal head, long first ray, pes planus, and a pronated forefoot. In addition to the pain created by impingement, pain is produced by pressure from the shoe. This relative joint stiffness and pain may result in an abnormal gait with shift of weight bearing to the lateral aspect of the foot and a resultant transfer lesion.

1. **History and physical examination.** Symptom onset is usually insidious, without antecedent trauma. Occasionally, a history of a turf-toe injury may be present. Pain with dorsiflexion of the metatarsophalangeal joint is present in running and jumping sports. A bony tender prominence is palpable dorsally and occasionally laterally at the joint. Active and passive joint motion is markedly diminished and associated with pain.
2. **Treatment.** Conservative measures include stiff-soled shoes, custom full-insole orthotics with a Morton's extension, or a rocker-bottom sole to limit dorsiflexion at the hallux metatarsophalangeal (MTP) joint. The athlete must be aware that although these will often alleviate or improve symptoms, they may hamper athletic performance. A wider toe box and adhesive padded "donuts" alleviate pressure of the overlying shoe on the osteophytes. Failure of nonoperative care is not uncommon. Surgical options include cheilectomy, arthroplasty, and MTP arthrodesis. In the presence of adequate articular cartilage in the joint, strong consideration should be given to cheilectomy, which preserves an adequate amount of dorsiflexion for the athlete to engage in running and jumping events. Mobilization of the sesamoids is occasionally necessary to obtain adequate dorsiflexion. Sixty percent of the motion obtained at surgery may be lost in the postoperative period. If more motion is required at the time of surgery, consideration may be given to a dorsal closing wedge osteotomy of the proximal phalanx. Arthrodesis is a reliable long-term surgical option that can be successful in selected athletes. The exception is the dancer who must have dorsiflexion of the first MTP joint.
3. **Return to sports.** Following cheilectomy, early motion at 10 days post operation is recommended. After 4 weeks, gradual return to weight-bearing exercises, including running and jumping, is permitted as tolerated. If an arthrodesis is performed, adequate radiographic healing is necessary prior to the resumption of sports. A rocker-bottom sole or an orthosis with a Morton's extension helps to distribute loads across the joint.

VII. Bunions

The incidence of bunions in the athlete is no greater than that in the general population.

A. **History and physical examination.** Age of onset of deformity and the status of the bunion during athletics indicates whether the condition is progressive. Assessment of planus or cavus foot deformity is also necessary, as this may contribute to the symptoms. Range of motion of the hallux MTP joint should be checked to assess for associated rigidity. Symptoms include pain at the medial eminence from to direct pressure of a shoe or from the bunion itself. Adolescent bunion is often quite painful and may effect performance.

B. **Diagnostic tests.** AP, lateral, and oblique weight-bearing x-rays are necessary to demonstrate the extent of deformity. Measurement of the intermetatarsal angle between the first and second rays as well as hallux valgus angle and sesamoid subluxation is important. The lateral x-ray will reveal cavus or planus deformity. In adolescents the dista metatarsal articular angle is an important indicator in determining the severity and risk of recurrance following surgery.

C. **Treatment.** Pain and progression are the two main indicators for treatment. Efforts are aimed at nonoperative modalities to alleviate pain and return the athlete back to a tolerable asymptomatic state. An adequate shoe toe box of sufficient width to accommodate the forefoot is prescribed. Off-the-shelf arch supports or custom-molded orthotics with a longitudinal arch support help prevent excess pronation. A Morton's extension orthosis provides relief in the patient with a short first ray. Spacers between the first and second toes also provide some relief. Surgical intervention is indicated if symptoms progress despite conservative measures or if the deformity increases. Surgical options are based on the degree, location, and various components of the deformity. Soft tissue surgery may result in stiffness in the first MTP joint and affect overall athletic performance. The Keller procedure and prosthetic implants are not recommended in the athlete.

VIII. Turf Toe

As a result of the use of synthetic athletic surfaces as well as grass surfaces, more sophisticated and flexible footwear is required by the athlete. The great toe is subjected to significant stresses during running and jumping. Turf toe is a common condition in linemen who crouch. As the first MTP joint is hyperextended during rapid and explosive push-off, injury to the plantar plate can occur. This also is caused when another player lands on the back of the athlete's foot, further hyperextending the MTP joint. This injury has been graded: grade I injury, a mild sprain; grade II injury, a partial tear of the capsuloligamentous complex; and grade III, a complete tear of the capsuloligamentous complex associated with metatarsal head articular injury. It differs from tripping injury which is caused by hyperflexion of the great toe.

A. **History and physical examination.** The patient describes a hyperextension injury to the first MTP joint, as described above. There is usually mild diffuse swelling, especially on the plantar aspect of the MTP joint. With higher-grade injuries there may be more significant swelling and ecchymosis with significant pain and decreased range of motion, especially dorsiflexion. A sesamoid fracture can also occur.

B. **Diagnostic tests.** X-rays of the great toe are usually normal but may reveal bone chips surrounding the metatarsal head. These are typically associated with grade III injuries.

C. **Treatment.** The initial treatment includes rest, ice, compression, and elevation. Contrast baths with progressive range of motion and NSAIDs are helpful. In the case of the grade I injury, the athlete may continue to play with a stiff-soled shoe, which restricts dorsiflexion to between 25 and 30 degrees. In a grade II injury, the player can be expected to lose 1 to 2 weeks during the convalescent and rehabilitation period. Taping is necessary upon resumption of activity to limit dorsiflexion (Appendix 2, Fig. 4). A stiff-soled shoe or a steel plate in the sole is necessary to further limit dorsiflexion and to allow resumption of activities. Grade III injuries require 3 to 6 weeks of healing and time off from sports. Surgery may be necessary if conservative measure fail. Removal of loose bodies and repair or excision of sesamoid fracture fragments may be necessary. If the plantar plate has been avulsed from the proximal phalanx, reattachment is required. The potential late sequelae of the turf toe, even appropriately treated, includes a hallux valgus or rigidus.

IX. Toenail Problems

The toenails protect the toes from pressure on the forefoot and from trauma. Conditions that develop in the nail present with severe, disabling pain, limiting performance. The great toe is most commonly involved. There are many causes, including hereditary factors, trauma, improper nail trimming, and nail plate malformation.

A. **Ingrown toe nail (onychocryptosis)**

1. **History and physical examination.** There is a long history of swelling along the medial or lateral border of the great toe. Often the athlete self-treats this problem and it becomes chronic. Swelling and erythema are present, as well as exquisite tenderness. The infection can involve the pulp of the toe. Subungual purulence may be present. Hallux valgus forces the great toe laterally often pinching it between the second toe and shoe.
2. **Diagnostic studies.** X-rays rule out the rare case of osteomyelitis.
3. **Treatment.** Nonoperative treatment is appropriate. This includes proper nail trimming, warm soaks, and topical antibiotics. If there is an abnormal nail plate with mild deformity, debridement of the granulation tissue and oral antibiotics and soaks are prescribed. A grossly

deformed to nail and a recurrent deformity with chronic granulation tissue may require a partial, removal of the nail and nail bed ablation, removing 20% of the nail and its germinal area. With conservative treatment, the athlete returns to sports in 5 to 10 days. If partial nail bed ablation is performed 3 weeks is required to heal. Although phenol may be used, it is not advocated because it is associated with a higher recurrence rate. Surgical ablation of the nail bed is preferred.

B. **Subungual hematoma.** This condition is also known as "black toe" and is common among tennis players, joggers, and skiers. It results from hemorrhage between the nail plate and the nail bed secondary to separation of these two structures after repeated contact of the shoe against the nail. The nail bed appears dark blue or black.

1. **History and physical examination.** Discomfort is noted under the nail after exercise. The hematoma may not appear for several days after the activity, but a small blood clot beneath the nail plate appears. The patient is asymptomatic by this time.
2. **Diagnostic tests.** X-rays are not helpful.
3. **Treatment.** An adequate toe box and proper trimming of the nails is usually adequate treatment. An acute subungual hematoma that is painful requires the nail bed to be decompressed with a large-bore needle drilled through the dorsum of the nail plate. Occasionally the nail may be lost. This lesion disappears as the nail plate grows distally. If the blackened nail does not clear up, however, suspect a subungual melanoma or glomus tumor and proceed with appropriate workup.

X. Nerve Injuries and Neuromas

Nerve entrapment may cause significant pain. The athlete describes symptoms consistent with dysesthesias or paresthesias in the foot. Associated systemic disease—such as diabetes mellitus, thyroid disorders, and other cause of peripheral neuropathy—should be considered. Psychological disorders and nutritional defects may also present with symptoms of neuritis. Ill-fitting or worn shoes with minimal padding and shock absorption qualities also cause nerve-related symptoms.

A. **Interdigital neuroma.** Morton's neuroma, as it also called, commonly affects one interspace and is usually unilateral. The male and female athletes are equally affected, as opposed to the nonathletic population, wherein females predominate. The most common location is the web space between the third and fourth toes.

1. **History and physical examination.** Symptoms begin as vague forefoot pain. These progress to neuritic symptoms, including burning and numbness between the third and fourth metatarsal heads that may radiate into the toes and to other toes as well. These symptoms are present during or after activities. Eventually the athlete has pain with walking. Medial-lateral compression of the metatarsal heads may reproduce the symptoms with a palpable click. Dorsoplantar compression in the web space between the third and fourth metatarsal heads reproduces pain. It is uncommon to have more than a single neuroma present.
2. **Diagnostic studies.** AP, lateral, and oblique views of the foot are typically negative. A selective injection of 1% lidocaine into the affected web space may be diagnostic if symptoms resolve. A bone scan will rule out synovitis or stress fracture in cases with atypical symptoms.
3. **Treatment.** Initially modification of training techniques including cross training with less impact of the forefoot may help alleviate symptoms. A metatarsal pad is placed just proximal to the metatarsal heads to help alleviate pressure on the forefoot. An orthosis with metatarsal pad at the affected interspace may relieve symptoms. NSAIDs are also effective. If the symptoms fail to resolve over several months, surgery may be considered. Following resection of the neuroma, return to sports requires as long as 8 weeks. The patient is allowed to bear weight within 2 weeks and progresses to power walking within 4 weeks after surgery.

B. **Jogger's foot.** Medial plantar nerve entrapment typically occurs in the region of the knot of Henry. It affects males more commonly than females and is common in distance runners. It also may be associated with chronic lateral ankle instability, excess forefoot abduction, heel valgus, and hyperpronation. Occasionally, it may be caused by an excessively high arch support.

1. **History and physical examination.** The athlete describes pain along the medial arch that radiates distal to the medial toes and occasionally proximally to the ankle. The pain is worse after running on level ground. Burning and paresthesia is noted along the medial arch beneath the navicular tuberosity. Pain may be elicited with forced heel valgus and forefoot abduction. Standing on tiptoes also may elicit pain.
2. **Diagnostic tests.** AP, lateral, and oblique weight-bearing x-rays of the foot may reveal an accessory navicular. Midfoot arthritis must also be ruled out. Stress fracture of the navicular or first metatarsal may be visible. EMG and nerve conduction velocities rule out more proximal nerve entrapment, including a radiculopathy, tarsal tunnel syndrome, or a peripheral neuropathy.
3. **Treatment.** A medial longitudinal arch support to prevent or decrease hyperpronation of the forefoot may be effective. In addition, NSAIDs and cross training may be beneficial. If these measures fail, one should consider surgical neurolysis of the medial plantar nerve. If surgical neurolysis is undertaken, a portion of the naviculocuneiform ligament is usually released. Training is permitted 6 weeks postoperatively with a custom-molded orthosis.

XI. Corns

There are two varieties of corns. Hard corns result from tight shoes and are most common along the lateral aspect of the fifth toe at the condyle of the dorsal aspect of the proximal interphalangeal joint, associated occasionally with hammertoe. Soft corns occur on toes between bony prominences at the point of contact between the lateral base of the proximal phalanx of the fourth toe and the medial condyle of the proximal phalanx of the fifth toe. They also occur between the second and third toes.

A. **History and physical examination.** With either of these lesions, pain with a callosity overlying the area of discomfort is present. Occasionally, there may be breakdown of the skin, cellulitis, and abscess, especially with soft corn. Shoes may be too tight in the toe box. The clavus beneath a metatarsal head may be exquisitely tender.

B. **Diagnostic studies.** X-rays of the foot aid in determining the presence of bony prominence underlying the lesion.

C. **Treatment of hard corns.** Protective padding in the form of an adhesive donut may be adequate. A shoe with a wider toe box is helpful. Shaving or sanding of the callosity helps reduce symptoms. If nonoperative measures fail, surgical treatment including removal of the underlying bony prominence is usually effective. If a hammertoe is present, surgical correction is necessary to solve the underlying problem.

D. **Treatment of soft corns.** Padding between the toes where the soft corn is present is adequate. It allows the moisture to evaporate and the skin to dry. A wider toe box can be helpful. Shaving the callosity, although difficult, also relieves symptoms. Removal of the adjacent bony prominences ("kissing osteophytes") between the involved toes is an effective surgical option. With either hard or soft corns, resumption of activities can be undertaken within 4 weeks postoperatively.

Suggested Reading

Baxter DE, Donald E. *The foot and ankle in sport.* St Louis: Mosby, 1994.

Heckman JD. *Instructional course lectures:* vol 42, sec III. *The lower extremity in sports.* Rosemont, IL: American Academy of Orthopaedic Surgeons, 1993.

Mann RA, Coughlin MJ. *Surgery of the foot and ankle,* 6th ed. St Louis: Mosby, 1993.

Sammarco GJ. *Rehabilitation of the foot and ankle.* St Louis: Mosby, 1995.

PART XI. **FACE/ENT/DENTAL**

57. MAXILLOFACIAL INJURIES

John Downs

Maxillofacial injuries have accounted for less than 10% of all the injuries sustained in the intercollegiate environment. This is probably related to the use of facial protection in contact sports such as football, ice hockey, and lacrosse.

Although infrequent, facial injuries can be of great importance. The face is the initial site of respiration and nutrition, and the individual's presentation to the world depends largely on his or her face.

Anatomic Considerations

The skin of the neck, scalp, and face is thin and pliable. It is firmly attached to the underlying cartilage of the external ear and nose, but the subcutaneous tissue is generally loose and fatty, with an excellent blood supply. The facial muscles are subcutaneous voluntary muscles, which arise from bones or fascia and insert into skin. When the overlying soft tissue of the facial skeleton is subjected to trauma, laceration, abrasion, and/or contusion can result. The same soft tissue helps to determine the kind, manner, and degree of displacement of facial fracture.

The orbits, nasal region, maxillae, mandible, and forehead are prominent bony features. These prominences protect some vital structures when subjected to trauma and can suffer fracture.

Facial Injuries

The establishment and control of an adequate airway is the top priority in maxillofacial trauma. Soft tissue bleeding can usually be controlled by direct pressure. Nasal packing may be necessary to control epistaxsis resulting from trauma.

Lacerations can be apparent, but careful examination of the wound is always necessary to determine injury to nerves, salivary and lacrimal ducts, eyes, and facial bones.

Signs of underlying facial fractures are (1) asymmetry of bony prominences, (2) palpable defects of mandibular or orbital margins, (3) malocclusion, (4) mobility of alveolar arches, (5) infraorbital anesthesia, (6) ecchymosis, (7) diplopia, and (8) subconjunctival hemorrhage. Any question of underlying facial fractures should be answered by standard radiographic examination of facial bones and special studies (laminograms, computed tomography) as indicated. Evidence of underlying facial fractures requires consultation with the appropriate surgical specialist.

Examination of an injured eye includes testing of visual acuity and range of motion; inspection of lids; oblique illumination of the conjunctiveae, cornea, anterior chamber, pupil, iris, and lens; and intraocular examination. Immediate referral to an ophthalmologist is required by hyphema; corneal injuries; injuries to the lens, choroid, macula, and/or retina; and lacerations involving the lacrimal apparatus, tarsal plates, and globe.

Principles of Wound Care and Soft Tissue Repair

Most sports injury wounds are "clean" (less than 12 hr old with minimal contamination) and may be closed primarily. In cases of gross contamination, delay in closure after debridment is an acceptable approach.

Using universal precautions, abrasions should be thoroughly cleaned using surgical sponges and the wound left uncovered. Antibacterial ointments may be used.

Again using universal precautions, the first step in primary closure of a laceration is preparation of the area with povidone-iodine (Betadine). It may be necessary to use local anesthesia at this stage to reduce the patient's discomfort. Use lidocaine HCl 1% or 2% with epinephrine 1:2,000,000 in highly vascular areas. Inject slowly, using a 25- to 26- gauge needle. Avoid use of vasoconstrictors directly in the areas of the nose and ear, where the overlying cutaneous structures are very tight. The toxic dose of lidocaine is approximately 7 mg/kg.

Sterile-drape the area to prevent contamination of surgical instruments and suture materials.

Irrigate the wound, with debridment of necrotic tissue and removal of debris. Hemostasis should be achieved with ligation of bleeders or electrocautery. Hematomas are to be *avoided.*

Do a careful, layered closure of the underlying tissue with the greatest strength (fascia and dermis) using absorbable suture material. Atraumatic needles, atraumatic handling of tissue, and avoidance of placing needless subcutaneous sutures all enhance eventual closure, healing, and wound appearance.

Use nonabsorbable monofilament suture material; avoid braided suture for skin closure. A suture of size 6-0 or 7-0 is appropriate for the delicate tissue of the face. Closure should be effected without tension to achieve the best possible result.

A pressure dressing may be used, but an antibacterial ointment applied to the wound surface will prevent crusting and drying of the wound.

Sutures should be removed at 5 days. Adhesive strips may be applied for several more days for wound support.

Principles of Management of Facial Fractures

The principles of good management of facial fractures comprise reduction and immobilization with return to normal function and appearance.

Facial fractures have been classified as stable and unstable, displaced and nondisplaced. Stable facial fractures are the majority of fractures encountered. These fractures usually require no reduction but may require stabilization for healing.

Nondisplaced stable mandibular and maxillary fractures can be stabilized using intermaxillary wiring.

Nondisplaced stable nasal fractures require no reduction but will need some protective device prior to return to competition.

Displaced nonstable fractures of the facial skeleton will require operative intervention. Fracture of the zygomatic-orbital complex will require an open reduction and stabilization with intraosseous wires or miniplates. Some blowout fractures of the orbit may require graft support of the orbital floor.

Displaced stable fractures of the zygomatic process may be elevated to normal position and are stable for healing.

Open reduction of nonstable displaced fractures of the maxilla and mandible may require a combination of intermaxillary wiring, interosseous wiring, or miniplates.

Displaced nasal fractures after reduction may require some nasal packing for control of epistaxis and support of the nasal bone.

Return to competition following reduction and stabilization of facial fractures is dependent upon the stability of the fractures, healing, and availability of protective devices.

The surgeon must make individualized decisions based upon her or his best judgment.

Suggested Reading

Coverse KM. *Kazankian and Converse's surgical treatment of facial fractures,* 4th ed. Baltimore: Williams & Wilkins.

Dingman RO, Natvig P. *Surgery of facial fractures.* Philadelphia: WB Saunders.

Rowe N, Kiley HC. *Fractures of the facial skeleton.* Edinburgh: E&S Livingstone.

Journal of Oral and Maxillofacial Surgery

58. THE EAR, NOSE, AND THROAT

Jeffrey W. Bailet

Sports-related injuries frequently involve the ear, nose, and—less commonly—upper aerodigestive tract structures. This chapter attempts to categorize these injuries and should serve as a quick reference guide to their management in the field and will aid in determining when individuals should be referred for otolaryngologic evaluation and treatment.

I. Ear Injuries

Injuries to the ear can be anatomically subdivided into three regions: ***the external ear,*** comprising the pinna, lobule, and external auditory canal; ***the middle ear,*** which includes the tympanic membrane and ossicles; and ***the inner ear,*** which consists of the cochlea and vestibular system.

A. **The external ear**

1. **Lacerations.** The pinna of the external ear is the most commonly injured site, given that it protrudes from the lateral face and is relatively unprotected. Lacerations or partial avulsion of the pinna occur from torsion or sharp trauma to the ear and are especially common among rugby players, wrestlers, and boxers. Fortunately the pinna has an excellent blood supply, allowing for sound healing and resistance to infection.
   a. **Repair.** The goal in repairing lacerations is to preserve all viable tissue and to ensure that all exposed cartilage is covered with overlying skin.
      i. **Irrigation and debridement,** if necessary, should be carried out prior to closure. Partially detached portions of the ear should be reapproximated.
      ii. **Cartilage lacerations** should be repaired with absorbable suture.
      iii. **Daily cleaning** of the suture line and any associated abrasions with hydrogen peroxide followed by application of an antibiotic ointment should be done to prevent excessive crusting.
      iv. **A bandaged dressing** is usually not necessary, but if one is required, it should be nonadhesive.
      v. **Oral antistaphylococcal antibiotics** should be administered to prevent infection.
      vi. **Adequate healing** usually occurs within a week to 10 days. During this period, patients are instructed to avoid activities that may result in reinjury of the ear. Lightly taping a paper or plastic foam cup over the ear at night usually prevents sleeping on the ear, which should be avoided until the wound has healed.
   b. **Complete avulsion of the pinna** is fortunately uncommon.
      i. **The avulsed segment** should be carefully wrapped in saline-moistened gauze, sealed in a plastic container, and then placed on ice. This allows for cooling but not freezing of the detached auricle.
      ii. **Successful primary reattachment** is possible depending on the extent of damage to the ear and if it can be accomplished within 2 to 3 hr from the time of injury.
2. **Auricular hematomas** of the pinna occur commonly among wrestlers and boxers.
   a. **Pathophysiology**
      i. **Caused by blunt trauma** that creates a shearing force, separating the auricular perichondrium from the underlying cartilage and causing the subperichondrial space to fill with blood.

Without its own intrinsic blood supply, auricular cartilage is dependent on the overlying perichondrium for nutrients.

ii. **Separation of the perichondrium** from the underlying cartilage can result in cartilage necrosis and increased risk of infection leading to permanent disfigurement. The ***"cauliflower ear"*** deformity results from resorption of necrotic cartilage. Less severe deformities, such as residual thickening of the pinna, are the result of replacement of the unevacuated clot by fibrosis.

b. **Treatment**

i. **Needle aspiration** of auricular hematomas followed by a pressure dressing, although still used by some practitioners, usually results in the recurrence of the hematoma.

ii. **The preferred treatment option** involves incision and drainage of the hematoma and reapposing the perichondrial layers using through-and-through monofilament sutures placed over dental rolls or rubber battens. This method allows for good compression of the wound and prevents reaccumulation of blood or serum in the potential space.

(a) The sutures should be left in place for a minimum of a week.

(b) An antistaphylococcal antibiotic should be prescribed.

(c) Opinions are divided regarding whether an athlete may resume wrestling during this period, but limited competition with protective headgear usually does not disrupt the healing process.

3. **External otitis** or "swimmer's ear" is a common complication among individuals who spend considerable time in the water, such as swimmers and divers.

a. **Etiology** is typically bacterial, with ***Pseudomonas*** **or** ***Staphylococcus*** being the most common bacteria responsible for the infection. ***Overzealous use of a Q-tip*** to dry or scratch the ear canal often exacerbates the condition.

b. **Treatment**

i. **Keep the ear dry** when showering, which can be accomplished by placing a cotton ball into the ear canal and coating its outer surface with petroleum jelly.

ii. **An antibiotic corticosteroid drop** should be used until the infection clears, which usually occurs within a week to 10 days.

iii. **Individuals should be referred to an otolaryngologist** for:

(a) **Removal of cerumen and epithelial debris**

(b) **possible placement of a wick for canal wall edema,** which ensures that the topical medication will reach the infected canal wall epithelium.

iv. **Oral antibiotics** may also be necessary in ***severe infections*** associated with preauricular cellulitis or trismus.

v. **Diabetics** should be followed closely, given the risk of developing ***malignant external otitis,*** a severe infection involving the skull base, and ***should be referred*** for an otolaryngology evaluation if they have severe infections initially or fail to respond to therapy.

vi. **Swimming should be avoided** until the infection clears, but cotton impregnated with petroleum jelly can be used in limited situations if the infection is mild. These individuals should flush the ear out with an acetic acid solution, such as Domeboro or Acetasol drops, immediately after exiting the water.

vii. **Diving** with any type of plug should be avoided so as to prevent barotrauma to the external ear canal and middle-ear structures.

viii. **Custom swimmer's plugs used** while swimming or showering are effective at preventing infections in individuals who are prone to develop recurrent external otitis.

ix. **Divers** who suffer from recurrent infections can coat their ear canals protectively with a silicon oil, such as Dow Corning 200-lb fluid or silicote spray to prevent infection.

4. **Frostbite** injuries to the pinna, although uncommon, can occur during winter sport activities, including Nordic or Alpine skiing and snowboarding.
   a. **Etiology.** Frostbite occurs when temperatures drop below freezing and the resultant disruption of sensory input from auricular skin prevents the individual from sensing the impending injury. Ice formation within the extracellular space results in cellular dehydration and necrosis of involved tissue.
   b. **Treatment** should include:
      i. **Rapid rewarming** of the ear using moist cotton pledgets at a temperature of 38° to 42°C (100.4° to 107.6°F) as soon as possible.
      ii. **Avoid** placing the ear under a heat lamp or rubbing it with snow, which only serves to worsen the injury.
      iii. The resultant ***formation of bullae, necrosis, and associated erythema*** may last for months following the injury and may require the use of cream for superficial infections.
      iv. **Dressings** of any kind are usually avoided.

B. **The middle ear**

1. **Perforation of the tympanic membrane**
   a. **Etiology**
      i. **Compressive forces** that occur in association with simultaneous occlusion of the ear canal, as from a slap or blow to the side of the head.
      ii. **Water-jet injuries,** resulting in tearing of the tympanic membrane, can occur while the athlete is water skiing, when his or her ear comes in contact with the water surface at high speeds. This high-energy injury can also result in ossicular or inner ear damage; therefore a greater degree of associated hearing loss may be expected.
      iii. **Barotrauma** from swimming or diving may also result in rupture of the tympanic membrane. With water injuries, infection with resultant otorrhea is more likely, due to contamination of the middle ear.
   b. **Treatment**
      i. **Dry-ear precautions** should be used regardless of the mechanism of injury. Petroleum jelly applied to a cotton ball after it is inserted into the ear canal, as described previously, is effective at preventing water from entering the middle-ear space.
      ii. **An oral antibiotic** should be prescribed if otorrhea develops.
      iii. **Limited use of a topical antibiotic corticosteroid drop** is probably indicated despite the somewhat controversial potential for ototoxicity.
   c. **Outcome.** Approximately 90% of traumatic perforations heal spontaneously within 4 to 8 weeks. A membrane may fail to heal due to
      i. The development of infection
      ii. Torn membrane edges curled into the middle ear space
      iii. Defects too large for the healing epithelium to bridge
   d. **Referral to an otolaryngologist** is warranted if the tympanic membrane fails to heal, persistent infection develops, or associated vertigo occurs, suggesting the presence of an inner-ear injury.
2. **Ossicular chain injury** is usually the result of a high-energy head injury; therefore referral for further medical evaluation is commonly made, since there are generally associated injuries of equal or greater severity.

a. **Clinical findings** suggestive of an ossicular injury may include
   i. A ruptured tympanic membrane
   ii. The presence of a hemotympanum
   iii. A significant hearing loss
   iv. A displaced ossicle seen on physical evaluation
b. **Treatment** should include an otolaryngologic evaluation with audiometric testing. If the tympanic membrane is ruptured, the ear should be kept dry, as previously described.

3. **Middle-ear barotrauma** is a common complaint among scuba divers. It is the result of an inability to equalize the pressure within the middle ear, usually due to eustachian tube dysfunction. This phenomenon commonly occurs on descent and can happen in just a few feet of water.
   a. **Symptoms** include hearing loss and dizziness; the diver may suffer severe otalgia or a ruptured tympanic membrane if the descent is not halted.
   b. **On clinical examination,** the tympanic membrane may appear hyperemic and a hemotympanum may be present.
   c. **Treatment** is beyond the scope of this text, but divers should refrain from returning to the water until they have received medical clearance.
   d. **Prevention** includes the use of topical nasal and systemic decongestants in combination with serial autoinflation of the middle-ear space beginning on the surface and proceeding throughout the dive. Failure to take adequate precautions to prevent middle-ear barotrauma may result in permanent hearing loss; therefore preventative measures are routinely included in diver certification courses.

C. **Inner-ear injuries,** although rarely associated with sports injuries, can occur from severe head injuries usually associated with excessive speeds. Inner-ear barotrauma is also possible and is sometimes experienced by scuba divers.
   1. **Symptoms** suggestive of an inner-ear injury include ***marked hearing loss, vertigo, otalgia, facial weakness or paralysis, and bloody or cerebrospinal fluid otorrhea.***
   2. **Clinical signs** include a ***hemotympanum,*** a ***bulging or ruptured tympanic membrane,*** *or a* ***lacerated external auditory canal*** associated with basilar skull fractures.
   3. **Treatment** of more severe associated injuries take precedence, but ***otolaryngologic evaluation is essential*** once the patient is stabilized.
   4. **Prevention** of inner-ear injuries includes using an adequate protective helmet and sound judgment when excessive speed or the possibility of sustaining a head injury exists. Divers need to perform serial autoinflation of the middle-ear space, as previously described. Suspicion of inner ear injuries mandates otolaryngologic referral.

II. Nasal Injuries

A. **Nasal fractures** are common in many contact sports, since the nose is relatively unprotected.
   1. **Symptoms**
      a. **Severe pain**
      b. **Transient epistaxis**
      c. **Nasal congestion**
   2. **Clinical findings**
      a. Rapid edema of the nasal bridge
      b. Deviation of the nasal dorsum is present in displaced fractures
      c. Associated periorbital ecchymosis often develops within 12 to 24 hr.
   3. **Treatment**
      a. **Intranasal inspection** of the nasal septum to rule out the presence of a ***septal hematoma*** should be carried out at the time of the injury.

b. **Nasal x-rays,** although not mandatory, are often obtained for documentation for insurance purposes.
c. **Ice packs** may be used for the first 24 hr to aid in minimizing nasal edema.
d. **Topical nasal steroid sprays** may help speed the resolution of intranasal edema.
e. **Immediate otolaryngologic evaluation** is often **not required**, but reasons for referral include presence of a ***septal hematoma, persistent epistaxis, obvious nasal deformity,*** or ***persistent nasal congestion.***
f. **Closed nasal reduction** within the first week is often successful for minimal or moderate displacement of the nasal dorsum. An associated deviated nasal septum, which often results in persistent nasal obstruction, can frequently be medialized enough to improve nasal airflow via this same closed procedure. An external nasal cast is applied to maintain the reduction, and occasionally intranasal splinting is used following drainage of septal hematomas or correction of a severely deviated septum. The cast is removed within 1 week, and oral antistaphylococcal antibiotics are used while intranasal packs are in place to prevent infection.
g. **Nondisplaced fractures** usually do not warrant treatment; however, all individuals should be cautioned about using glasses, which may cause a permanent nasal dorsal depression if worn within 2 weeks of the injury.
h. **Vigorous nose blowing** or twisting of the nose in any way should be avoided until adequate mending of the fracture occurs, usually within 10 days to 2 weeks.
i. **Protective nasal splints** or face shields can be utilized to prevent reinjury if the individual desires to resume sporting activities.

B. **Epistaxis** is usually self-limited and generally requires no medical intervention.

1. **Etiologies** include trauma, platelet dysfunction (such as that due to the use of aspirin or other NSAIDs), hypertension, or excessive drying of the nasal mucosa resulting in friability of surface blood vessels, usually along the anterior septum.
2. Regardless of the etiology, most nasal bleeding occurs within the anterior portion of the nose and therefore ***can be controlled*** by applying firm, direct pressure to the anterior nose just below the nasal bones. This constant pinching of the nose should be performed for 10 min by the clock. If bleeding persists, a topical nasal decongestant spray such as oxymetazoline can be applied, followed by another round of continuous firm pressure for an additional 15 min. If bleeding persists, supportive measures should be initiated, as in any patient who is hemorrhaging, including adequate venous access and fluid resuscitation, and the patient should be transported to a medical facility emergently for further treatment.
3. **Prevention of recurrent epistaxis** relies on correcting the underlying etiology. Antihypertensive agents may be necessary. Stopping the aspirin or NSAIDs is recommended for up to 2 weeks to allow for normalization of platelet function. Excessive drying of the nasal mucosa, commonly seen in athletes during the winter when the air is especially dry, can be prevented by using a topical saline nasal spray several times during the day, using a humidifier at night, and applying an antibacterial ointment to the nasal septum twice a day. If recurrent epistaxis still persists after the above measures are implemented, referral for an otolaryngology evaluation is warranted, where vessel cauterization can be accomplished and other etiologies such as the presence of a nasal tumor can be ruled out.

III. Laryngeal and Neck Injuries

A. **Laryngeal fracture.** Blunt trauma to the anterior neck can occur in contact sports such as football, rugby, and ice hockey. If enough force is involved, fracture of the laryngeal skeleton can occur. Additional cervical structures can be injured, including the pharynx and esophagus.

1. **Symptoms** may be relatively minor or absent immediately following the injury. As complications stemming from the injury evolve, hoarseness, dysphagia or odynophagia, dyspnea, or hemoptysis may develop. Mild bruising or abrasions of the anterior neck or loss of the thyroid cartilage prominence may be the only clinical signs to suggest the severity of the injury. Subcutaneous emphysema is an ominous sign, suggesting disruption of the endolarynx, pharynx, or esophagus and demands emergent medical attention.
2. **Early detection** of laryngeal injuries can prevent serious complications—most importantly, airway obstruction from laryngeal edema or hematoma, respiratory arrest, or mediastinal abscess. Late complications include laryngeal stenosis, arytenoid dislocation, or vocal cord paralysis. Manipulation of the airway may compound the injury, but individuals who have rapid onset of severe airway obstruction may need intubation or emergent cricothyrotomy if intubation is unsuccessful. If the possibility of a laryngeal or pharyngoesophageal injury exists, rapid evaluation in an emergency department is essential and is often lifesaving.

B. **Vessel injuries.** Damage to cervical vessels resulting from blunt neck trauma is extremely rare because of their compliance. Injured vessels include the vertebral, basilar, and, less commonly, carotid arteries. Often the only injury from blunt trauma is an endothelial tear, and the only signs suggestive of vessel injury are neurologic deficits resulting from thromboembolic events. Unfortunately, symptoms may develop weeks later and can be fatal. When an individual develops neurologic symptoms following cervical trauma, immediate medical evaluation is warranted.

Suggested Reading

Dickey LS. Diving injuries. J Emerg Med 1984; 1:249–269.

Frenguelli A et al. Head and neck trauma in sporting activities: review of 208 cases. J Craniomaxillofacial Surg 1991; 19:178–181.

Kizer, KW. Medical hazards of water skiing douch. Ann Emerg Med 1980; 9:268–269.

Lacher A, Blitzer A. The traumatized auricle—care, salvage, and reconstruction. Otol Clin North Am 1982; 15:225–239.

Singer DE et al. Otitis externa. Ann Otol Rhinol Laryngol 1952; 61:317–330.

Votey S, Dudley JP: Emergency ear, nose, and throat procedures. *Emerg Med Clin North Am* 1989; 7:117–154.

59. THE EYE

John B. Jeffers

I. Introduction

An estimated 43,659 sports and recreational product-related eye injuries were treated in hospital emergency rooms in 1994 (United States Consumer Product Safety Commission). This number did not include athletes who were examined by personal physicians; this therefore, is a gross underestimate. The important message: Some 90% of sports-related eye injuries are ***preventable!***

II. Sports with the Highest Frequency of Injuries

A. Baseball: struck by ball while batting, line drive, flyball, "bad hop"
B. Basketball: fingers or elbows
C. Pool sports: fingers or elbows
D. Racquet/court sports: usually ball, occasionally racquet

III. Sports with the Highest Frequency of Eye Injuries by Age Group

A. 5 to 14 years of age: baseball (Little League age group)
B. 15 to 24 years of age: basketball
C. 25 to 64 years of age: basketball

IV. Preparticipation Evaluation: History and Complete Eye Examination

A. Refractive error?
   1. Glasses or contact lenses
   2. Highly nearsighted—potential for retinal detachment
   3. History of refractive surgery (i.e., radial keratotomy weakens cornea)
B. Strabismus (i.e., crossed eyes)
   1. Amblyopia ("lazy eye")
C. Intraocular surgery (i.e., cataract extraction, repair or retinal detachment) or eye trauma (traumatic hyphema, laceration of globe).

V. Sports-Related Risk to the Eyes

Sports-related injuries are traditionally categorized as being related to contact (collision) or noncontact sports. This classification is inappropriate with regard to eye injuries; racquetball or squash are considered noncontact sports but have a high incidence of eye injuries because they are played in a confined area with close encounters among the participants. Potentially devastating eye injuries may occur from either a fast-moving missile (ball) or a racquet. The sports listed by eye injury risk are as follows:

A. **Low-risk sports.** Swimming, track and field, cross country, cycling, tennis (singles)
B. **High-risk sports.** Hockey (ice or street), football, baseball, basketball, softball, tennis (doubles), racquet sports (racquetball, squash, "handball," badminton), water polo, fencing, men's lacrosse
C. **Very high risk sports.** Boxing, wrestling, full-contact martial arts

VI. Mechanisms of Eye Injury

Eye injuries may be ***blunt or sharp*** in nature. The ***sharp*** type injury may result in lacerations of the lid or globe, possibly related to the shattering of eyeglasses (eyewear should be appropriate for the particular sport). Fingernails forcibly jabbed into the eye may be cause a laceration (especially with a basketball). The majority of eye injuries are of a ***blunt*** nature. The most common would be edema and ecchymosis of the eyelids, orbital fracture, corneal abrasion, traumatic iritis, traumatic hyphema, or commotio retinae (edema).

When a contusion force impacts the globe, there is a sudden decrease in the anteroposterior diameter and an increase in the equatorial diameter. Shock waves traverse the globe, resulting in an increase in the intraorbital pressure. This distortion of the globe may result in the tearing of intraocular or intraorbital tissues, which often results in hemorrhage. When the intraorbital pressure is increased, the walls that are thinner (i.e., floor and medial walls) may break, resulting in a ***blowout fracture.*** A floor fracture may result from a severe impact on the inferior rim of the orbit, which results in buckling. Extraocular tissues may become entrapped in fractures sites, resulting in limitation of motion of the eye and therefore diplopia. If the floor fracture site is large, there may be a sinking of tissues, resulting in enophthalmus (sunken eye). ***General rule;*** the more intraocular damage, the less orbital damage, and visa versa.

VII. Potential for Serious Eye Injury: Danger Signs and Symptoms

A. Sudden loss or decrease of vision
B. Loss of field of vision (complete or partial)
C. Pain on movement of the eye
D. Photophobia ("light sensitivity")
E. Diplopia* (versus "ghost image")
F. Protrusion of one eye
G. "Lightning flashes," especially with large "floaters"
H. Irregularly shaped pupil
I. Foreign-body sensation
J. "Red eye"
K. Blood in the anterior chamber
L. "Halos" around lights

VIII. Functionally One-Eyed Athletes

It is imperative the functionally one-eyed athlete be identified prior to participation. The ***most common cause*** is amblyopia; other causes may include prior trauma, eye disease, or surgery resulting in scarring and opaque media (congenital cataract). ***Definition:*** the weaker eye is worse than 20/40 (best corrected); the stronger eye corrects to 20/40 or better.

Damage to the stronger eye due to a serious sports-related injury would result in a serious alteration in an athlete's lifestyle (i.e. work, sports, driving,† etc.). The functionally one-eyed athlete may participate in a number of sports as long as the appropriate, well-fitted protective eyewear (polycarbonate lenses 3 mm thick at the center in a molded frame) is worn. Exceptions are boxing, wrestling, or full-contact martial arts. Polycarbonate eye protection (2 mm thick) must be strongly recommended during ***all waking hours*** as well!

IX. Most Common Types of Sports-Related Eye Injuries

A. "Black eye" (edema/ecchymosis)
B. Corneal abrasion
C. Traumatic iritis
D. Traumatic hyphema
E. Orbital fracture
F. Commotio Retinae (edema of retina)

X. Evaluation of the Player with Eye Injury on Field or Court

A. Brief history: determine etiologic agent and direction of energy, of impact (i.e., baseball line drive, flyball, "bad hop," pitched ball).
B. **Topical anesthesia** may offer pain relief to obtain better exam. ***Do not use it to prolong play!***
C. Obtain visual acuity ***before*** any manipulation (hands or penlight) of the eye Exception: ***chemical injury*** (i.e., field markings or "turf dust"), which calls for immediate flushing of the eye for 15 to 30 min depend on amount and concentration.
D. Check eye movement (note limitation), pupillary response (in an afferent pupillary defect, the pupil dilates with light in injured eye)
E. Use appropriate first aid: crushed ice, shield, "moist chamber"

*Diplopia = two images of the same object with both eyes opened. When either eye is covered, one image disappears; monocular diplopia is rare, it is usually due to refractive error (i.e., astigmatism). It looks like television "ghost image"; when one eye is covered, the patient still sees "double."
†These individuals cannot obtain an unlimited driver's license in 80% of the United States.

F. Determine severity of injury; if in doubt ***refer*** *to ophthalmologist!*
   1. Determine need for further evaluation (i.e. imaging, more extensive treatment?)
   2. Determine if player may resume play now.

XI. Specifications of Sports Eye Protectors

A. Street-wear glasses or contact lenses ***provide no protection!***
B. Polycarbonate lenses with a 3-mm center thickness do offer protection.
   1. For low-eye-risk sports, polycarbonate lenses 2 mm thick and hinged frames are acceptable.
C. Sturdy frame with posterior retaining lip (so that lens cannot be dislodged back into eye).
   1. Polycarbonate frame with molded temple is strongest—hinges tend to be weak areas.
   2. Some have neon-colored cushions (nose and temple); kids love them!
D. Antifog lenses
E. Sports eye protectors should be fitted by an experienced optometrist or optician.
   1. Most complaints start with a ***poor fit.***
F. Face protectors attached to a helmet may be made of polycarbonate or wire.
   1. These are mandated in most collision sports (hockey, lacrosse, football)
   2. Helmet must fit properly and be secured with a strap for for maximum protection.
G. Children with narrow facial features may not be able to obtain sports goggles; a child's sturdy frame with polycarbonate lenses will suffice.

XII. Rehabilitation of the Athlete with an Injured Eye and Return to Play

A. **During the game:** immediate return to play depends on the complaint (i.e., blurred vision, pain) and team physician objective findings. Common sense medical judgment prevails.
B. **When ocular tissue has healed** sufficiently to sustain a blow to the head or body (producing a Valsalva maneuver and increasing the pressure inside the eye) and the injured eye is comfortable with adequate return of vision.
   1. **Appropriate, well fitting eye protection should be worn!**

XIII. Emergency Kit for Eye Injuries on Court or Field

A. Near-vision card
B. Penlight with blue filter
C. Fluroescein strips
D. Commercial eye wash (in plastic squeeze bottle)
E. Eye shields (plastic/metal)
F. Topical anesthesia (i.e., 0.5% proparacaine)
G. Lid retractor (or large paper clips)
H. Applicator sticks (Q-tips)
I. Eye medication (your physician's choice)
J. Plastic sandwich bags (ice/"moist chamber"*)
K. Tape (eye patches optional)

Suggested Reading

Jeffers JB. An on-going tragedy: pediatric sports related eye injuries. *Semin Ophthalmol.* 1990;5:216–223.

Larrison WI, Hersh PS, Kunzwerler T, Singleton BJ. Sports-related ocular trauma. *Ophthalmology* 1990;97:1265–1269.

Pashby TJ, Pashby RC,Chisholm LDL, Crawford JS. Eye injuries in Canadian hockey. *Can Med Assoc J* 1975;113:663–674.

PBA. *1994 Sports and recreational eye injuries fact sheet.* Chicago: Prevent Blindness America, formerly National Society to Prevent Blindness, 1995.

Vinger PF. The eye and sports medicine. In: Duane TD, Jaeger EA, eds. *Clinical ophthalmology,* rev ed, vol 45. Philadelphia: Lippincott, 1994; chap 45.

*One side of sandwich bag taped over orbital rim acts as "moist chamber" for exposed protruding conjunctiva.

60. DENTAL

John F. Wisniewski

I. Anatomy and Histology

Teeth are contained in the alveolar bone (alveolus) of the maxillary and mandibular arches. The alveolar socket is the location of each individual tooth, while the periodontal ligament retains the tooth in the alveolar socket. During displacement injuries (luxation, intrusion, avulsion), the gross relationship between the tooth and the alveolar socket is altered and the integrity of the periodontal ligament is violated at the cellular level.

The tooth contains four types of tissues: (1) enamel, (2) cementum, (3) dentin, and (4) pulp. The first three—enamel, cementum, and dentin—are hard tissues. The last, the pulp, is soft tissue. Each tooth has two main portions: (1) the crown, that portion of the tooth which is covered by enamel, and (2) the root, that portion of the tooth which is covered by cementum. The tip of the root is called the *apex*. The junction of enamel of the crown and the cementum of the root is known as the cementoenamel junction (CEJ) or cervical line. The main bulk of the tooth is made up of dentin. The innermost layer, which is solely soft tissue, is called the *pulp*. The pulpal tissue furnishes the arterial, venous, and nerve supply to the tooth. This tissue travels through the dentin via odontoblastic processes. Ultimately, these processes anastamose at the dentoenamel junction (DEJ) or end at the root surface.

II. Tooth Injuries

A practical system that describes tooth injuries simply divides them into two groups. Based upon which part of the tooth sustains the trauma, injuries of this nature are classified as involving the crown of the tooth or the root of the tooth.

A. **Class I fracture.** Fracture of the enamel portion only.
   1. **Symptoms**
      a. Athletes may express concern for appearance.
      b. Pain, if any, is minimal.
      c. The fractured edge may be sharp, rough. This may irritate soft tissue such as, the lips, cheeks, or tongue.
   2. **Treatment**
      a. If symptomatic to air or water stimuli, sealants or varnishes can be applied immediately to reduce sensitivity.
      b. Address the fractured edge for sharpness and/or roughness by either reshaping the tooth or restoring the tooth with a bonded tooth-colored restoration.
      c. Radiographs are taken to assess the possibility of root fracture and to serve as a baseline for future reference.
   3. **Return to play** Return to play can be immediate. Final determination in this matter can be made by the athlete. There is no immediate need for a dental consultation, but one should be scheduled at the earliest convenience.

B. **Class II fracture.** Fracture line includes dentin, but no pulp exposure.
   1. **Symptoms**
      a. Esthetic concerns, sharpness, and roughness are similar to that of the class I fracture.
      b. Pain or sensitivity to cold water or when breathing in air through the mouth is not uncommon.
      c. The yellowish color of dentin aids in the differentiating a class II fracture from a class I fracture.
   2. **Treatment**
      a. If symptomatic to cold water or breathing in air, sealants and varnishes can be applied immediately to reduce sensitivity.

b. The tooth can usually be restored with a bonded tooth-colored restoration.
c. Radiographs are taken to assess the possibility of root fracture and to serve as a baseline for future reference.

3. **Return to play.** Return to play can be immediate. The athlete's indication of sensitivity, to cold water or the intake of air while mouth breathing will ultimately determine his or her ability and/or willingness to compete. Irregardless of whether or not the athlete continues to compete, a dental consult should be attained immediately following the athletic event.

C. **Class III fracture.** Fracture of the crown with exposed pulp.

1. **Symptoms**
   a. An athlete exhibiting a class III fracture usually has significant pain in addition to any combination of the clinical symptoms which are associated with class I and class II fractures.
   b. Since the pulp is directly injured and exposed, the tooth may demonstrate a red spot or bleed. A pinkish hue in the dentin without bleeding is indication of a severe class II fracture.
2. **Treatment**
   a. Control pulpal bleeding by using sterile gauze or cotton pellets.
   b. In cases of moderate to severe bleeding, the physician can control the hemorrhage as well as the pain by utilizing a local anesthetic. Initially, preference is given to administering a periapical injection in lieu of an intracanal injection. If however, the later is required, added care need be exercised for this type of injection can cause or exacerbate a tooth fracture. Lidocaine with or without epinephrine is generally acceptable.
   c. In performing a ***periapical injection,*** reflect the lip or cheek so that the mucobuccal fold is clearly visible. Remove any debris, saliva or blood from the injection site. Use digital palpation to locate the apex of the root deep in the mucobuccal fold. Insert the 25- or 27-gauge syringe needle, with bevel toward the bone, at a 45 degree angle. Following aspiration, inject the anesthetic solution slowly.
   d. Prior to an intracanal injection, the physician should have administered a local anesthetic via a periapical injection and have identified the source of bleeding as pulpal and not from any of the surrounding soft tissue or periodontium.
   e. In performing an ***intracanal injection,*** the physician should administer the local anesthetic via a 27-gauge needle. The syringe should form a passive seal with the canal foramen and the anesthetic solution injected without force. The solution should be delivered intermittently, with short intervals, until the anesthetic flows out of the canal.
3. **Return to play.** Whether the anesthetic is used or not, the athlete should not be allowed to return to competition. To afford the best prognosis and reduce the risk of infection, an immediate dental consultation is required. Immediately, posttrauma, root canal therapy will be initiated.

D. **Class IV tooth fracture.** Fracture involving roots only (cementum, dentin, and pulp).

1. **Symptoms**
   a. Radiographs are essential for diagnosis.
   b. Clinically, the root may or may not have mobility in relation to untraumatized adjacent teeth.
   c. Clinical symptoms may range from none to a dull ache, to extreme pain, or even to numbness.
2. **Treatment**
   a. Root fractures can be horizontal or vertical. In regards to horizontal root fractures, the closer to the cervical line (gum line), the poorer is

the prognosis. Vertical root fractures may also involve enamel. Vertical root fractures originating in the center of the biting edge and extending down the middle, in either a labiolingual or mesiodistal direction, offer an extremely poor prognosis.

b. With horizontal or vertical root fractures, immediate treatment requires stabilizing the tooth.

3. **Return to play.** An athlete should not be allowed to resume play if a horizontal or vertical root fracture is suspected. A radiological and dental consultation should be performed by a dentist immediately post-trauma.

E. **Lip lacerations**

1. **Treatment**

a. Lip lacerations, in combination with tooth fractures, should be carefully inspected and debrided.

i. Irrigate the wound with sterile saline or anesthetic solution.

ii. Prior to suturing, take a radiograph to ensure that there are no tooth particles embedded in the soft tissue. These particles may serve as a nidus for infection.

iii. Evaluate for tetanus inoculation as well as antibiotic coverage.

III. Tooth-Bone Injuries

A second category of hard tissue injuries involves the violation of the tooth-to-bone relationship.

A. **Tooth luxation.** Loosening or displacement of the tooth in relationship to the existing arch form.

1. **Symptoms**

a. Athletes may experience no pain or a dull ache.

b. This trauma is often accompanied by fracture and/or fragmentation of the alveolar socket.

c. Usually caused by a blunt blow originating from the anterior toward a posterior direction.

d. An athlete's chief complaint is either "My tooth looks pushed in" or "My bite is off, I'm not biting right."

e. Bilateral digital palpation along the arch and alveolar socket and in the mucobuccal fold will help to determine the severity of the tooth/arch deformation.

2. **Treatment**

a. If the tooth is displaced in alignment (2 mm or less) or possesses mobility (2 mm or less in its socket), the health care provider should gently guide the tooth back into alignment. A soft diet, with no excessive biting to the injured area, is recommended. If the tooth is successfully repositioned, a dental consult need not be immediate but should be sought within 24 hr.

b. If the tooth exhibits extreme mobility—for instance, 3 mm or greater—the physician/trainer should attempt to gently reposition the tooth. Considerations for a soft diet and avoidance of excessive biting utilizing the traumatized dentition should be mandated. Passive splinting with acid-etch composite resin and orthodontic wire/dental floss is recommended. Depending on whether the tooth has been successfully realigned and/or the extent of mobility and arch deformation, a dental consult should be obtained either immediately or immediately following the athletic event.

c. In either of the above cases, repositioning of the tooth should be attempted only if the health care provider feels competent. Dental consultations will require radiographs and follow-up evaluation for possible endodontic therapy. Deciduous, primary or "baby" teeth should not be splinted.

3. **Return to play.** In either case of luxation, the athlete should not be allowed to return to competition until a dental consult has been obtained.

B. **Tooth intrusion.** Displacement of the tooth into the alveolar bone.
   1. **Symptoms**
      a. Athletes may experience severe pain.
      b. This trauma is usually accompanied by a direct fracture within the alveolar socket. Periodontal ligament cells are crushed, torn, and abraded. Bone marrow spaces are crushed or compressed.
      c. The blunt blow is usually received from an inferior direction toward a superior one.
   2. **Treatment**
      a. A clinical and radiographic examination by a dentist should be obtained immediately.
      b. Depending on the age of the patient and the size of the bone marrow spaces, intruded teeth are sometimes left alone to reerupt into proper position.
      c. In older individuals, teeth can be guided into reeruption via orthodontic care.
      d. Endodontic therapy is likely.
   3. **Return to play.** In the case of an intruded tooth, the athlete should not be allowed to return to competition. A dental consultation should be obtained immediately.

C. **Tooth extrusion,** or partial displacement of a tooth out of its socket.
   1. **Symptoms**
      a. Athletes may experience no pain to a dull ache.
      b. The periodontal ligaments, nerve, arterial and venous supplies of the tooth are torn.
      c. The blow usually entails a force originating from a superior toward an inferior reference point.
   2. **Treatment**
      a. Bilateral digital palpation is necessary in assessing and realigning the tooth.
      b. Instructing the athlete to bite down on a cotton gauze may be helpful in repositioning the tooth back into its socket. The health care provider should attempt this only if he or she feels competent to do so.
      c. Passive splinting and/or endodontic therapy are likely.
      d. Soft food diet and refrainment from utilizing excessive biting forces are recommended.
      e. A clinical and radiographic examination by a dentist should be obtained immediately.
   3. **Return to play.** In the case of an extruded tooth, the athlete should not be allowed to return to competition. A dental consultation should be obtained immediately.

D. **Tooth avulsion.** An exarticulation, or complete displacement, of the tooth out of its socket.
   1. **Symptoms**
      a. Athletes may experience various degrees of pain.
      b. Usually, the etiology is a blunt blow in a similar direction as that causing an extruded tooth.
   2. **Treatment**
      a. The amount of extraoral time is the critical factor in achieving a successful replantation. ***Time is of the essence.*** The rate of successful replantation is 90% at 15 min, 70% at 30 min, and 30% at 1 hr. There is a 95% failure rate after 2 hr of extraoral time.
      b. If the tooth is to be replanted on site, the following guidelines will help to ensure optimal results:
         i. Do not scrape or scrub the crown or root of the tooth. Do not clean the tooth with disinfectants or detergents. Avoid touching the root of the tooth.
         ii. Gently rinse off the tooth with milk, sterile saline, anesthetic, solution, or Hank's solution.

iii. Place the tooth into its socket; the socket should not be scraped clean. Guide the tooth back into its proper position by having the athlete gently bite down on a gauze.
iv. Deciduous, primary or "baby" teeth should not be replanted.

c. If the tooth is not replanted on site, transporting the tooth to the dentist should include the following considerations:
   i. The tooth should be kept in a liquid medium, such as cold milk, Hank's solution, saliva, or sterile saline. Avoid storage in tap water as it can cause damage to the periodontal ligament cells on the root of the tooth. Avoid transporting the tooth "dry."
   ii. The storage container should be break-resistant, nontoxic, and sterile; it should have a tight-fitting cap.
   iii. Occasionally, if the athlete is not bleeding intraorally, and is both coherent and of proper age, the tooth can be wrapped in a wet gauze and placed in the buccal vestibule or under the tongue.
   iv. The Save-A-Tooth System includes the ideal transporting medium in a scientifically designed container. Besides containing Hank's solution as the storage medium, the device is user-friendly for the attending health care provider as well as the recipient dentist.

d. Dental management will include:
   i. Radiological and dental examination.
   ii. Passive splinting with acid-etch composite resin and orthodontic wire for 7 to 10 days.
   iii. A tetanus booster.
   iv. Systemic antibiotics for 7 to 14 days.
   v. Soft diet.
   vi. Root canal therapy initiated within 7 days.
   vii. Follow-up radiological and dental examinations.

3. **Return to play.** In the case of an avulsed tooth, the athlete should not be allowed to return to competition. A dental consultation should be obtained immediately.

IV. Prevention

A. Dental screening examinations should be included as part of preseason or pre-participation physicals.

B. Mouth guards are recommended by the American Dental Association for ice hockey, field hockey, football, and lacrosse players. While not all sports require use of a mouth guard, physicians, dentists, and athletic trainers should advise athletes to use a mouth protector in any sport posing risk of an orafacial injury.
   1. Recommended mouth guards should be custom-made or "mouth-formed." Custom-made mouth guards are clinically ideal; "boil and bite" types are clinically acceptable.

C. Team physicians and athletic trainers should research these items prior to the beginning of the athletic season:
   1. Have a list of "on-call" dentists.
   2. Realize that the general dentists, pediatricians (children's dentists), endodontists (root canal dentists), and oral surgeons are capable of managing the avulsed tooth.
   3. Determine if the hospital of choice has a dentist or oral surgeon on call.
   4. Determine if the hospital of choice has a general practice residency program. If it does, are the dental residents on beeper call or are they in-house/hospital based?
   5. Keep a list of phone numbers for the appropriate dental professionals/hospitals and call ahead, especially in the case of an avulsed tooth.
   6. Keep the emergency kit up to date with the supplies needed to treat an avulsed tooth.

The author wishes to thank Ms. Betty Edgeworth for typing the manuscript of this chapter.

This chapter is dedicated to my wife, Annette, and daughter, Kristi, for their constant support of my professional work.

Suggested Reading

Castaldi CR. First aid for sports-related dental injuries. *Phys Sports Med* 1987:15(9):81–89.

Clark JW, ed. *Clinical dentistry,* vol 3. Hagerstown, MD: Harper & Row, 1978, chaps 33, 34, and 35.

Drasner P. The athletic trainer's role in saving avulsed teeth. *Athletic Training* 1989;24(2):139–142.

Kruger GO, ed. *Textbook of oral surgery,* 4th ed. St Louis: Mosby, 1974, chap 18.

Kumamoto DP, Jacob M, Nickelsen D, Howe WB. Oral trauma: on-field assessment. *Phys Sports Med* 1995;23(5):53–62.

PART XII. **OTHER INJURY**

61. THE THORAX

Harry L. Galanty and Douglas E. White

I. Anatomy of the Chest

The thorax extends from the clavicles to the diaphragm and contains the heart, major vessels, trachea, bronchi, lungs, and esophagus. The rib cage, sternum, and scapulae surround and protect these vital organs. The surface anatomy helps identify the underlying structures.

A. **Bony landmarks**
   1. **The suprasternal notch** forms the superior border of the sternum. It lies midline between the medial aspects of the clavicles. The trachea can be palpated in the notch and should also lie midline.
   2. **The sternum** is formed by the manubrium, sternal body, and xyphoid inferiorly. It extends from the suprasternal notch to the level of ninth thoracic vertebra. The manubriosternal junction lies at the second costal cartilage.
   3. **The ribs** provide shape, protection, and strength to the thorax.
      a. The ***first rib*** is not palpable and runs behind the clavicle.
      b. The ***second through seventh*** *ribs* articulate with the sternum via the costal cartilage.
      c. Ribs ***eight through ten*** form the inferior costal margin and are cartilaginous anteriorly.
      d. The ***eleventh and twelfth ribs,*** or floating ribs, remain without articulation.
   4. **The scapulae** lie over the second to seventh ribs, posteriorly.
   5. **The spinous processes of the thoracic vertebrae** are the prominent midline posterior landmarks.

B. **Viscera**
   1. **The heart** lies predominantly on the left side of the chest, spanning from the second left intercostal space to its apex in the fifth left intercostal space.
   2. **The aortic arch** lies behind the manubrium.
   3. **The lungs** surround the heart in the pleural cavities.
   4. **The diaphragm,** on inspiration, sits at the eighth or ninth costal cartilages rising as high as the fifth on expiration.

C. **Muscular anatomy** (see Fig. 61-1)
   1. **The pectoralis major and minor** are located in the anterosuperior chest wall.
   2. **The latissimus dorsi, serratus anterior, trapezius, rhomboids and levator scapulae** muscles sit laterally and posteriorly.
   3. **Internal and external intercostal muscles** assist the diaphragm in respiration.

II. Skin and Soft Tissue Injury

A. **Contusion.** Contusion of the chest, with or without associated hematoma is one of the most common sports injuries. The anterior chest has a relative paucity of overlying muscle; thus contusions here primarily involve the skin, breast, or underlying bone. In contrast, posterior chest contusion commonly affects the muscular layer.
   1. **Presentation.** The patient may complain of having his or her "wind knocked out" after a direct blow to the chest. Transient muscle spasm triggers this dyspnea. Localized pain is typically present. Exam reveals an area of tenderness, which may develop local swelling and ecchymosis.
   2. **Treatment** primarily consists of immediate ice packing. If pain persists, nonsteroidal antiinflammatory drugs (NSAIDs) may be appropriate.

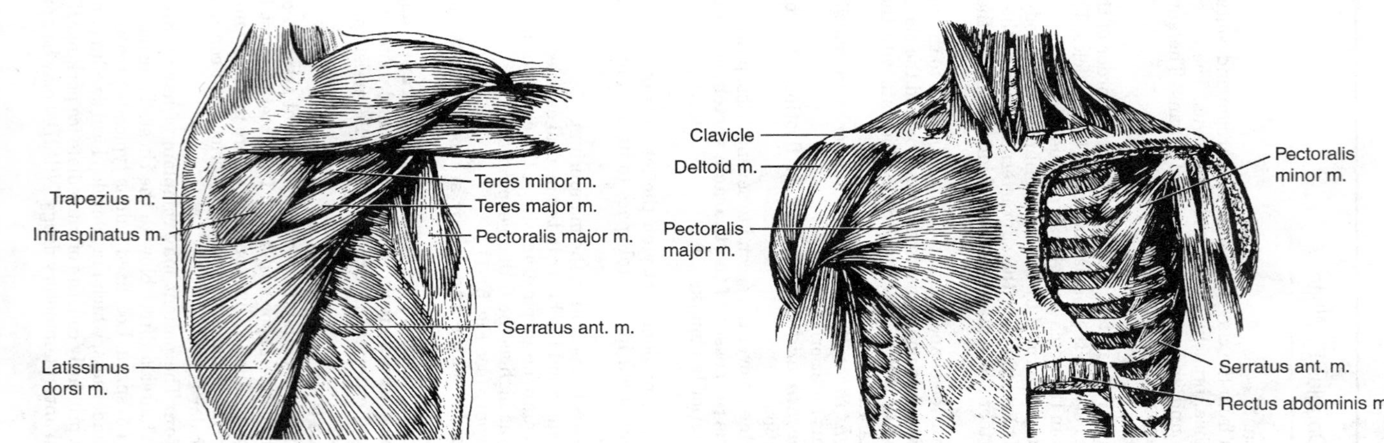

Fig. 61-1. Lateral and anterior views of the chest wall. The prominent bony landmarks and musculature are noted.

3. **Return to play** is based on symptoms. Local padding/protection is advisable.

B. **Muscle strain.** Muscle strains in the chest result from excessive tension, stretching, or overloading of a given muscle or muscle group. The pectoralis major and minor, and to some extent the intercostal muscles, are the most frequently injured. Pectoralis muscle strains most often occur when the athlete is performing bench presses or forceful internal rotation of the shoulder joint.

1. **Mechanism.** Because of the broad-based midline origin of the primary thoracic muscles, strains more often occur at a muscle's site of insertion. For example, pectoralis strain often involves its insertion at the proximal humerus; rhomboid strain damages fibers at its scapular insertion.
2. **Presentation.** Patients report an episode of pain or tearing, often during strenuous contraction or eccentric activity. Weakness, spasm, and local swelling may follow. On examination, there is local tenderness and increased pain with resisted muscle contraction. Marked tears may result in a palpable defect at the site of rupture.
3. **Treatment.** Analgesics and ice packing are used for the first 48 hr, with adjunctive therapy/modalities as needed. Severe pectoralis muscle tears may be treated with a sling for comfort, and elite athletes may require surgical repair.

C. **Breast Injury**

1. **Runner's nipple**
   a. **Mechanism.** This chafing condition results from friction of a runner's shirt, causing pain, irritation, and even bleeding in both women and men.
   b. **Treatment.** Coat the nipple with petrolatum, then bandage or tape it. Shirts made of synthetic material or silk can be preventive.
2. **Breast pain with running or activity**
   a. **Mechanism.** Athletic activity can generate as much as 70 ft-lb of force on the breast, which can lead to pain and local contusion, particularly in large-breasted women, those with fibrocystic changes, or those who are pregnant.
   b. **Treatment.** Ice or cold applications to painful, contused areas. A ***sports bra*** is recommended with further activity to provide comfortable support. Seams should not pass over the nipples. If needed, a 4-in. elastic bandage wrapped over the sports bra offers additional support and protection.

III. Bony Injury

A. **Rib fractures.** Rib fractures are very common chest injuries. They typically occur as a result of blunt trauma, but occasionally indirect forces or stress have been implicated. Contact sports such as football and hockey have a higher incidence of rib fractures, but they can occur with any inadvertent chest trauma (falls or collisions). The most commonly fractured ribs are the ***fourth through seventh,*** which comprise the longest, most prominent ribs.

1. **Single rib fractures.** Most often only a single rib is fractured. Typically, these are relatively minor injuries with few complications.
   a. **Presentation.** Pain is localized over the fractured rib. It will be exacerbated with inspiration, as the ends of the fracture will move and rub together. Physical examination reveals local bony pain on palpation and with anteroposterior compression of the chest wall.
   b. **Testing.** Radiographs are confirmatory but more importantly function to rule out complications such as pnuemothorax, hemothorax, or pulmonary contusion.
   c. **Treatment** is symptomatic. Since pain increases with respiration and motion, rest is the best initial plan. Analgesics will help keep the patient comfortable. Strapping, once common, is not recommended, as it can lead to complications from decreased lung volume, such as atelectasis.

d. **Return to play** is based on pain control. Pain will decrease with healing, but may be present for 6 to 8 weeks.
   i. After an initial 2 weeks of rest, pain control and healing should be such that the athlete may participate if comfortable.
   ii. Protection of the injury with padding and chest protectors will cushion blows to the chest.
   iii. If pain remains, even with clinical signs of healing, some suggest local anesthetic injections along the intracostal nerve to eliminate pain during activity.

2. **First-rib fracture.** The first rib is short, broad, and flat and lies in a position protected by the shoulder girdle. This rib can be fractured from severe direct trauma but more likely from repetitive forceful stresses.
   a. **Mechanism.** Forceful contraction of the scalenus anterior opposes the forces generated by the arm while throwing, weight lifting, or rowing. This action generates substantial torsional stress at the first rib attachment.
   b. **Presentation.** The athlete feels sharp pain and a snap. Pain is poorly localized, but shoulder and neck motion should remain intact.
   c. **Testing.** This fracture, which is minimally displaced, can be confirmed with an anteroposterior chest radiograph.
   d. **Treatment.** Sling and pain control are the treatments of choice, with healing evident by 4 weeks.
   e. **Return to play.** This is guided by pain; the patient can usually return in 4 to 6 weeks.

3. **Other stress fractures.** These are seen most often in rowers and beginning golfers. They are consistently found in the posterolateral segment of the ribs, where the highest bending stresses occur. These fractures develop from the forceful retraction and protraction of the scapula generated by the serratus anterior.
   a. **Presentation.** The athlete has tenderness over the affected rib, but radiation of pain along the costal margin may cause this injury to be mistaken for a muscle strain.
   b. **Testing.** Early in the course, radiographs are negative, but bone scans will confirm the diagnosis.
   c. **Treatment.** Treatment consists of rest from the offending activity.
   d. **Return to play** when pain resolves, usually about 6 weeks.

4. **Flail chest.** This complication of multiple rib fractures occurs when a segment of ribs is mechanically isolated from the rest of the chest wall.
   a. **Presentation.** There is local chest pain, and the affected portion of the chest wall will move paradoxically with respirations (inward with inspiration and outward with expiration). Concurrent sucking sound may be present.
   b. **Testing.** Chest and rib radiographs will confirm the diagnosis.
   c. **Treatment.** Prompt hospital transport with evaluation for intrathoracic injury are required. Supplemental oxygen or intubation may be required if respiratory status worsens. If the patient has little respiratory distress and no problems with oxygenation, management is primarily supportive, with close observation and pain control.

B. **Sternum fractures.** Sternum fractures are most commonly a result of direct trauma.

1. **Mechanism.** The lower part of the sternal body is relatively flexible, while the manubrium remains rigid. A posteriorly directed force to the sternum will usually be transmitted more cephalad to its stiffer segment just distal to the manubrium. The fracture can be incomplete, complete, or displaced.
2. **Presentation.** Transient dyspnea may accompany anterior chest wall pain. Symptoms are aggravated by inspiration. Localized tenderness is elicited at the level of injury. Deformity of the sternum is present with

displaced fractures. One may palpate crepitus at the fracture site with respiration. The examiner should auscultate for intrathoracic injury such as pneumothorax or pulmonary contusion and palpate for associated rib fractures. Injury to the great vessels must also be considered.

3. **Testing**
   a. **A lateral chest radiograph** is necessary for definitive diagnosis.
   b. **Anteroposterior films** should also be obtained to aid in fracture diagnosis and assess intrathoracic injury.
   c. **Pitfalls of X-ray diagnosis.** An unfused sternum can easily be mistaken for fracture. The second and third segments of the sternal body fuse near the age of 14 and the first and second fuse by about the age of 21.
4. **Treatment**
   a. **Nondisplaced sternal fractures** are treated conservatively. Rest and pain control are utilized until symptoms improve. These heal well between 6 to 8 weeks.
   b. **Displaced sternal fracture.** Reduction should be attempted. Place the patient in the supine position, with a roll behind and parallel with the thoracic spine, to expand the anterior chest wall. A posteriorly directed force can be applied to the anteriorly displaced part of the sternum. Reductions are typically stable.
5. **Return to play.** The athlete can return to play as symptoms abate, with padding specifically over the sternum to prevent further injury.

C. **Scapular fractures.** The scapula is infrequently injured, since it is protected by multiple layers of muscles. Most athletic fractures occur to the scapular body or the glenoid following a direct high-energy impact. Glenoid fractures can also result from the indirect trauma of shoulder dislocation. These injuries are discussed elsewhere.

1. **Presentation.** The athlete complains of diffuse shoulder pain, worsened with motion. The arm is kept in an adducted, protected position. Tenderness is present over the scapula itself. Palpate the acromion and coracoid, as these too can be fractured in athletes. Rotator cuff function is very weak and painful, mimicking a traumatic cuff tear.
2. **Testing.** The best views to visualize scapular fractures are a true anteroposterior and lateral of the scapula. A West Point view will evaluate glenoid fractures.
3. **Treatment.** The majority of scapular fractures are minimally displaced or not at all, requiring only supportive measures and a sling for protection. If a glenoid neck fracture appears unstable or moderately displaced, open reduction is advisable. Due to the significant force required to fracture the scapula, associated injuries like pneumothoraces, pulmonary contusions, and rib fractures should be considered.
4. **Return to play.** Athletes should be withheld from competition until the fracture is healed and full shoulder motion has returned, usually in 4 to 6 weeks. Protective padding can be applied for contact.

D. **Costochondral injuries.** The cartilaginous attachment of the ribs to the sternum is quite flexible to absorb force, but it can be torn or dislocated. The method of injury is similar to that of sternal fracture, usually by direct force.

1. **Presentation.** Pain can be severe and is localized over the injured costochondral junction. Deep inspiration is aggravating, as is coughing. A deformity may be palpable if dislocation is complete. A click can sometimes be elicited when the joint is stressed.
2. **Testing.** X-rays will not help define the injury, due to the radiolucency of the cartilage, but can help rule out sternal/rib fractures.
3. **Treatment.** Rest and analgesia are again the best treatment. Sometimes localized injections of anesthetic can be helpful in pain control. Healing of these injuries is slow, between 6 to 8 weeks.
4. **Return to play** after 6 to 8 weeks, as pain allows.

IV. Cardiovascular injury

A. Myocardial Contusion

1. **Definition.** Myocardial contusion (MC) is a force-related injury of cardiac muscle characterized by necrosis with or without hemorrhage into the myocardium. It is a serious complication of severe blunt trauma to the chest. The estimated incidence ranges from 8% to 71% of all cases, depending upon the diagnostic modality and criteria employed. The injury, similar to myocardial infarction (MI) in histopathologic appearance and can range from purely epicardial to full thickness in severity.
2. **Presentation.** Though not always present, the most common symptom noted in MC is nonspecific chest pain following severe blunt trauma. Physical examination often reveals sinus tachycardia. Other arrhythmias may be present. Severe cases may include pericardial friction rub, an S3 gallop, pulmonary rales, or an elevated central venous pressure.
3. **Testing.** Diagnostic testing for MC is problematic in that there is no gold standard.
   a. **Electrocardiographic (ECG)** changes—including conduction abnormalities, 1 mm ST elevation or depression, or T wave inversion in two contiguous leads—are highly suggestive of MC.
   b. **Creatine kinase MB (CK-MB)** isoenzyme level elevations to greater than 5% of the total creatine kinase lends further support for MC. ***Normal ECG and CK-MB*** *have a* ***reliable negative predictive value*** for further cardiac complications.
   c. **Echocardiography** is the most useful study for confirming diagnosis, evaluating wall motion abnormalities, and delineating the presence of pericardial fluid.
   d. **Radionuclide studies** add little to diagnosis or prognosis over the studies listed above.
   e. **Cardiac troponin I.** Recent studies have suggested that serial measurements of cardiac troponin I is more specific than CK-MB bands as a marker for cardiac injury and may become the diagnostic test of choice.
4. **Treatment.** Cardiac monitoring and supplemental oxygen should be instituted on all patients with suspected MC, given the tendency of injured myocardium to arrhythmia. Monitoring may be discontinued when rhythm is stable and acute symptoms have resolved. Treatment is otherwise expectant management. The course of MC is complete recovery in most cases, since patients are typically young and without concurrent coronary artery disease or other long-standing pathology. Complications of MC are rare but include arrhythmias, ventricular dysfunction, acute valvular or other intracardiac damage, ventricular aneurysm with thrombus, and free wall rupture.
5. **Preventive measures** for MC and other serious intrathoracic injury include proper use of chest protection in high-risk positions such as goalie, catcher, and quarterback.
6. **Return to play.** Guidelines are not well established, but return to contact sports should be delayed for several months to a year (if at all) after a significant episode of MC. Follow-up echocardiogram should be normal and appropriate protection should be used.

B. Cardiac concussion (commotio cordis)

1. **Definition.** Commotio cordis (CC) is cardiac arrest and sudden death following blunt trauma to the chest. It occurs primarily in otherwise healthy children and adolescents. Attempts to estimate its incidence are hampered by its rarity and by the absence of a formal registry for such cases. Precordial impact by a thrown or hit baseball account for two-thirds of the cases noted in a recent series.
2. **Etiology.** The cause of this dramatic event is uncertain. Ventricular fibrillation and acute bradycardia are considered the probable etiologies, since both arrhythmias have been induced experimentally by blunt chest trauma. Children and adolescents are thought to be at higher risk

because of their thin, compliant chest walls, which readily transmit the force of a precordial blow. Other theoretical mechanisms of injury include alteration of coronary blood flow and extreme vasovagal response or an undetected injury to the cardiac conduction system.

3. **Presentation.** Patients suffering CC collapse immediately or shortly after impact, becoming apneic and pulseless.
4. **Diagnosis and treatment.** Postmortem exam reveals no underlying cardiovascular damage. No intervention has been shown to benefit this situation, though prompt recognition, cardiopulmonary resuscitation, and electroshock treatment of ventricular fibrillation would theoretically be of value.
5. **Preventive measures.** Same interventions as discussed with myocardial contusion. Ideally, a person certified in cardiopulmonary resuscitation (CPR) should be available at all events involving solid, high-velocity projectiles. Debate over the practicality and efficacy of additional protective measures in organized sports, such as softer balls, is ongoing.

C. **Other cardiovascular injuries.** An appreciable number of case reports exist involving serious, sometimes fatal injury due to chest trauma sustained in sports. The incidence is rare but is understandably higher in collision sports such as downhill skiing, horse jumping, or climbing.

1. **Cardiac rupture and pericardial tamponade.** Severe blunt injury to the precordium may result in the disruption of a cardiac wall or, less commonly, the intraventricular septum or valves. Such injuries are rapidly fatal, particularly with rupture into the pericardium causing subsequent tamponade. With ruptures of the atria, however, as many as 10% to 30% of patients survive long enough to undergo surgery.
   a. **Presentation.** Classic features of tamponade are concurrent shock, distended neck veins, and narrowed pulse pressure, though these may be obscured in acute trauma. As a rule, any chest injury between the nipple lines, which results in unconsciousness and shock, must be suspected of causing cardiac rupture or other potentially lethal cardiac injury.
   b. **Testing.** With tamponade the electrocardiogram (ECG) shows low voltage and electrical alternans. Echocardiography is diagnostic.
   c. **Treatment** is initiated with pericardiocentesis, which can be temporizing as well as diagnostic. Definitive treatment is uniformly surgical.
2. **Great vessel rupture.** The great vessels lie in the superior mediastinum and include the thoracic aorta, its major branches, the superior vena cava, and the subclavian vein and tributaries. Injuries to these well-protected vessels range from contusion to disruption. Rupture of a great vessel is often rapidly fatal, but those patients surviving the initial injury may encounter a period of recovery during which signs and symptoms may be few. All patients who have withstood sufficient deceleration or compressive force injuries should be assumed to have a great vessel injury until proven otherwise.
   a. **Presentation.** Salient features include chest pain with or without hypotension and/or asymmetric pulses.
   b. **Testing**
      i. **The upright chest radiograph** should be examined for signs of ***mediastinal hematoma:***
         a. Loss of the normal aortic knob contour.
         b. Widening of the mediastinum to greater than eight centimeters.
         c. Tracheal shift to the right.
      ii. **An aortogram** confirms the diagnosis.
      iii. **Computed tomography (CT) with contrast** may be used in more stable patients.
   c. **Treatment** is prompt surgical repair.

V. Pulmonary Injury

A. **Airway injury.** Blunt trauma is the most common cause. Injury to the ***trachea*** and upper ***bronchi*** have been reported in boxing and other contact sports. The force can be severe enough to cause fracture to the tracheal or laryngeal cartilage.

1. **Presentation.** The athlete will appear with anterior neck and upper chest pain complaining of dyspnea. He/she may also have a hoarse voice or sonorous respirations. Hemoptysis may be present in severe cases.
2. **Testing.** Aids to physical exam include chest radiograph and CT scan.
3. **Treatment.** Most cases will require only supportive treatment, such as supplemental oxygen, topical ice packs, rest and analgesics. Frequent lung and airway evaluations are necessary to ensure the stability of respiratory status.
4. **Principal complication—airway obstruction**
   a. **Etiology.** Airway obstruction can result from laryngeal edema, hemorrhage, or physical obstruction secondary to tracheal derangement.
   b. **Presentation.** The patient will become dyspneic, agitated and cyanotic.
   c. **Treatment.** Emergency cricothyroidotomy will be necessary to maintain the airway with prompt transport to hospital thereafter.

B. **Pulmonary contusions** can occur following a forceful collision to the chest from another player or hard surface. Most will go undetected unless the athlete develops hemoptysis or respiratory difficulty. With improved imaging techniques, these injuries have been more accurately identified as pulmonary lacerations, surrounded by intraalveolar hemorrhage.

1. **Mechanism.** Two types of pulmonary laceration are found in athletes. Most commonly, injury results from compression of the air filled lung, with the glottis closed. This produces increased pressure in the parenchyma and subsequent tearing. Hematoma will typically develop around this air filled space. Lacerations may also occur from direct penetration of a fractured rib.
2. **Presentation.** Evaluation following blunt chest trauma should begin with attention to the ***airway, breathing,*** and ***circulation*** (the ABCs), with particular attention paid to respiratory ease. Auscultation will rarely reveal rales, but if these are present, further evaluation is necessary. Most athletes will be diagnosed when they complain of hemoptysis. However, the majority of sports-related lung lacerations go undiagnosed due to a paucity of symptoms. Athletic trauma results almost exclusively in the mildest or grade 1 injuries, with less than 18 % opacified lung parenchyma.
3. **Testing**
   a. **Chest x-ray.** A pulmonary laceration can be seen within hours of the trauma on x-ray as nodular densities or consolidation. These studies typically underestimate the severity of the lesion.
   b. **Chest CT** is more sensitive and can be used for diagnosis immediately after injury in otherwise stable patients.
4. **Treatment** for grade 1 injuries is supportive. Bed rest is best until the patient is stabilized, especially if hemoptysis is present. More severe injuries require hospitalization and may necessitate mechanical ventilation in hypoxemic or hemodynamically unstable conditions.
5. **Return to play.** These patients can resume routine activity within days and contact sports in 1 to 2 weeks if asymptomatic.

C. **Simple pneumothorax.** A pneumothorax occurs when the pleura is disrupted, allowing air to enter the pleural space. Penetrating trauma, such as a rib fracture, can cause this directly. Spontaneous pneumothoraces, usually seen in thin, tall males, can occur following rupture of a small bleb. Individuals with Marfan's syndrome are predisposed to these.

1. **Presentation.** The onset of symptoms may be insidious in spontaneous pneumothoraces. Pleuritic chest pain, dyspnea, and cough are common.

Physical examination reveals tachypnea and decreased breath sounds on the affected side. Percussion of the chest may reveal tympany. Subcutaneous emphysema is present when air travels outside the pleura into the tissues of the chest wall and neck. This can be detected by palpating crepitus over the areas involved.

2. **Testing.** Chest radiographs should include ***inspiratory*** and ***expiratory*** views to confirm the diagnosis and severity of lung collapse.
3. **Treatment.** In most athletes, these injuries are small and can be followed expectantly, with rest and serial radiographs to document improvement. The lung will reexpand as the free air is resorbed. If the lung is greater than 30% collapsed, serious consideration should be given to hospital observation, oxygenation, and thoracostomy.
4. **Return to play.** The athlete may return to play if he or she is asymptomatic after 2 to 3 weeks of rest (other injuries allowing). Recurrence is somewhat common in patients with spontaneous pneumothorax.

D. **Tension pneumothorax.** This condition occurs when inspired air accumulates into the pleural space without means of escape. As the amount of air increases, the lung is compressed, leading to progressive hypoxia and hemodynamic compromise.

1. **Presentation.** Absent breath sounds and hypertympany of the ipsilateral chest may be recognized, along with shift of the trachea to the opposite side.
2. **Treatment.** Immediate decompression should be performed by inserting a 16-gauge angiocatheter needle into the second intercostal space at the midclavicular line of the affected side of the chest. Eventually placement of a chest tube will be necessary.

E. **Pleuritic pain or stitches.** This describes the sudden sharp pain that occurs in the lower thoracic or upper abdominal region while playing.

1. **Mechanism.** The etiology is not known and has been postulated as colonic gas. It is most likely a spasm to the intercostal muscles.
2. **Presentation.** Pain is usually short-lived, lasting only 10 to 15 min and improves with rest. Physical examination is completely normal.
3. **Treatment.** Stretching of the thoracic muscles and arms or deep controlled breathing may relieve the pain. There are no known preventative measures.
4. **Return to play.** Return as symptoms allow—often after a brief rest.

Suggested Reading

DeLee JC, Drez D, eds. Orthopaedic sports medicine. Philadelphia: WB Saunders, 1994.

O'Donoghue DH. Treatment of injuries to athletes. Philadelphia: W.B. Saunders, 1984.

Turney SZ, Rodriguez A, Cowley RA, eds. Management of cardiothoracic trauma. Baltimore: Williams & Wilkins, 1990.

62. THE ABDOMEN

Jeffrey L. Tanji

I. Problem/etiology of Abdominal Injuries

A. **Sports-associated trauma** accounts for 10% of all injuries to the abdomen. Bicycling injuries represent the most common sports associated etiology, with collision and contact sports of all types strongly associated with abdominal trauma.

B. **Blunt abdominal trauma** is more likely than sharp trauma to result in abdominal injury. The spleen and the liver (less often) are the two viscera most commonly affected by blunt trauma. Much more rarely the colon, small intestine, kidneys, pancreas and bladder are affected. An enlarged spleen prior to trauma is the most significant risk factor for serious abdominal trauma in sport.

II. History Useful in Diagnosing Abdominal Injuries

A. **Abdominal/flank pain**
   1. Quality/character (sharp, dull, colicky)
   2. Onset (immediate or delayed)
   3. Frequency
   4. Duration (constant or intermittent)
   5. Radiation (Kehr's sign for splenic rupture if pain goes to shoulder)
   6. Location (what quadrant? Is it epgastric or suprapubic?)
   7. What makes it better/worse?

B. Mechanism of injury/how was the abdomen hit?
C. What sport was involved in the injury?
D. What position was the body in during the injury?
E. When was the last meal/last bowel movement/last urination?
F. Any risk factors for an enlarged spleen (such as mononucleosis)?
G. Previous history of abdominal injury or abdominal conditions
H. Medication use (prescription or over-the-counter)
I. History of allergies
J. Gastrointestinal/urological/gynecological review of systems
K. In young men, ask about scrotal masses (testicular cancer)

III. Physical Examination of the Abdomen

A. **Vital signs** in a young and healthy athlete are usually normal even with an intraabdominal bleed

B. **Inspection of abdomen**
   1. Scaphoid or distended abdomen
   2. Swelling or discoloration (Grey-Turner or Cullen's signs)

C. **Auscultation of bowel sounds** (prior to palpation and percussion)
   1. **Absent** (concern about pancreatic trauma or rupture)
   2. **Hyperactive** (concern about obstruction)
   3. **Hypoactive** (similar concerns as with absent sounds)

D. **Palpation of abdomen**
   1. **Perform light palpation** first to check for exquisite tenderness.
      a. Examine nontender area first, then move to area of tenderness
      b. Check for abdominal wall defect or hematoma
      c. Check for palpable herniation of abdominal wall
   2. **Deep palpation** examines the viscera
      a. **Liver** (enlargement or Murphy's sign)
      b. **Spleen** (knees up, palpate with both hands)
      c. **Kidneys** (costovertebral angle tenderness)
   3. **Rebound tenderness**
   4. **Peritoneal signs** (abdominal shake, percussion)

5. **Active resistance** against rectus and oblique muscles (sit-up position)
6. **Valsalva manuver** for dorsal hernia

E. **Percussion of abdomen**
1. General percussion for *masses*
2. Percussion for *liver size estimation*

F. **Digital rectal examination**
1. **Assess for masses** or tenderness
2. **Assess for bleeding** (grossly or with Hematest)

G. **Examination of hip flexors and abductors** against resistance
1. **Active and passive resistance against hip flexors**
2. **Active and passive resistance against hip abductors**

H. **Chest examination for related thoracic injury**
1. **Pneumothorax**
2. **Clinical rib fracture**
3. **Intercostal muscle strain**
4. **Costochondral injury**

I. **Scrotal examination** for masses
1. **Testicular cancer** possible in young men
2. **Check inguinal ring for hernias** with Valsalva manuver

IV. Diagnostic Tests Pertinent to an Abdominal Workup

A. **Laboratory tests**
1. **Serial complete blood count,** hemoglobin or hematocrit.
   a. If splenic rupture is suspected
   b. Frequency of blood draws every 4 to 6 hr
   c. Hospitalization should occur if splenic rupture is suspected
2. **Type and cross-match blood**
   a. May type and hold blood if index of suspicion is low
   b. Keep 2 to 4 units of packed red blood cells ahead
   c. Should have two large-bore intravenous access sites
3. **Urinalysis**
   a. Dipstick is a minimum to screen for hematuria
   b. Hematuria in the presence of flank pain—renal trauma
   c. A normal test does not rule out kidney laceration/contusion
4. **Diagnostic peritoneal lavage**
   a. Most sensitive and specific test for bleeding or visceral injury
   b. A positive test consists of the following
      i. 20,000 to 100,000 red blood cells red blood cells (RBCs)
      ii. 300 to 700 white blood cells white blood cells (WBCs)
      iii. Elevated amylase
      iv. Bile
      v. Bacteria by Gram's stain
5. **Serum amylase level** for blunt abdominal trauma
   a. Nonspecific
   b. Elevated in the following conditions
      i. Pancreatitis
      ii. Acute cholecystitis
      iii. Small bowel obstruction/laceration
      iv. Perforated peptic ulcer
      v. Colonic contusion
6. **Serum lipase** for suspected pancreatic rupture
   a. **Highly sensitive** and specific for pancreatic injury
   b. **Often drawn** in conjunction with the serum amylase level
7. **Preoperative laboratory panel if patient is unstable**
   a. **Prothrombin time/partial thromboplastin** time
   b. **Blood products** for transfusion
   c. **Complete blood count** and chemistry panel

B. **Imaging studies**
   1. **Upright abdominal series**—kidney, ureter, and bladder (KUB)—**and decubitus views**
      a. **Checks for free air** under the diaphragm (visceral rupture)
      b. **Check for obvious rib fractures**
      c. **Suspect injury to spleen**
         i. Depression of colonic flexure
         ii. Obliteration of splenic shadow of the colon
         iii. Elevation of left hemidiaphragm
      d. **Suspect renal injury**
         i. Loss of renal outline
         ii. Blurred psoas margin
         iii. Pulmonary atelectasis
         iv. Rib or vertebral fractures
   2. **Computed tomography** (intravenous and oral contrast of the abdomen)
      a. Visceral injuries
      b. Pancreatic injury
      c. Liver trauma
      d. Splenic injury
   3. **Intravenous pyelogram**
      a. Sensitive and specific for urinary tract trauma by dye leakage
      b. Images bladder rupture
      c. Renal injuries visualized
      d. Retrograde urethrogram if urethral tear is suspected
   4. **Liver/spleen scan**
      a. Can evaluate for rupture or bleeding
      b. Not an initial screening imaging test
   5. **Ultrasonography**
      a. Pancreatic visualization
      b. Testicular masses
   6. **Angiography** of the visceral vessels can isolate suspected bleeding
   7. **Testicular scan** for torsion of the testicles

V. Prevention of Abdominal Injuries

A. **Splenic rupture**
   1. Identification of players with splenic enlargement
   2. No clearance to participate in collision sport if spleen is enlarged
   3. Four weeks before clearance for collision sport after enlargement has clinically resolved

B. **Abdominal wall contusions**
   1. Strengthening exercises to the abdomen (to "corset" the viscera)
      a. Abdominal crunches
      b. Leg lifts
      c. Sit-ups
      d. Abdominal strengthening machines
         i. May not get as many angles as floor exercise sit-ups
         ii. Does protect the back and neck from strain
   2. Proper padded support can protect against blunt trauma
      a. Flak jacket
      b. Hip padding

C. **Bladder rupture**
   1. Contrary to conventional wisdom, a full bladder does not increase risk
   2. Lower abdominal strengthening exercises can corset the abdomen

D. **Testicular trauma** can be prevented by use of a jock strap and cup

E. **Incarcerated hernias** may be prevented by early detection on examination

VI. Treatment

A. All suspected visceral injuries require a surgical consultation
   1. **Immediate laparotomy** may be done diagnostically if unstable
   2. **Close observation** with serial exams may occur in house

B. **Ruptured spleen**
  1. Surgical splenectomy
  2. Hemostasis to bleeding sites
  3. Routine postoperative care

C. **Renal trauma** (urology consultation necessary)
  1. Most cases are nonoperative (intracapsular site of injury 85%)
    a. Do well with observation
    b. Bed rest, hydration
    c. Observe for postinjury hypertension
    d. Rebleeding is a risk at 15 to 20 days postinjury
  2. Operative cases (15%)
    a. Involve renal pedicle
    b. Lacerations across cortex or capsule
    c. Hemorrhage or extravasation of urine
    d. Intraperitoneal or retroperitoneal tears
    e. Bladder rupture associated with pelvic fracture
    f. Routine postoperative care

D. **Scrotal trauma**
  1. **Minor injuries** can be managed conservatively
    a. **Hematocoele** if blood accumulates in the tunica vaginalis
    b. **Hydrocoele**
    c. **Stable bleeding** can be managed conservatively
    d. **Contusion** can mask testicular trauma
  2. **Major injuries** require urological consultation
    a. **Rupture/dislocation** of the testes
    b. **Spermatic cord torsion**

E. **Pancreatic trauma**
  1. **Most treated conservatively**
    a. Follow lipase and amylase
    b. May need ultrasound to rule out
      i. Pseudocyst
      ii. Abscess
      iii. Hemorrhagic pancreas
  2. **Close follow-up** for recurrence of symptoms

F. **Abdominal wall injuries** generally do not require a surgical consultation
  1. **Mild hematomas, contusions, and strains**
    a. Avoid nonsteroidal antiinflammatory drugs (NSAIDs) early in the course to limit bleeding
    b. Ice
    c. Consider physical training (PT) modalities
    d. Judicious exercise
  2. Abdominal side stitch can be treated with observation, massage
  3. Solar plexus blows
    a. Observe for return to normal respiration
    b. Can be associated with temporary diaphragmatic paralysis
    c. Usually resolves immediately
  4. Ventral hernias
    a. Surgical consultation
    b. Education about symptoms of incarceration
  5. Severe abdominal muscle tears
    a. May appear like ventral hernias if complete substance
    b. Most often partial thickness tears
    c. Judicious PT

VII. Prognosis/Return to Competition

A. **Serious visceral injury** and rarely an abdominal muscle tear may take 4 weeks for a return to training and 4 to 6 months to return to collision sports
  1. Splenic rupture/splenectomy
  2. Renal laceration with surgical repair

3. Visceral perforation
4. Bladder rupture
5. Torsion of the testicle with surgical repair
6. Exploratory laparotomy
7. Severe abdominal muscle tear

B. **Moderate injury** may require 2 weeks for a return to training and 4 weeks to return to collision sports
1. Conservatively managed renal trauma
2. Scrotal trauma
3. Visceral contusion without hemorrhage

C. **Mild injury** may return to competition within days
1. Abdominal wall contusions
2. Abdominal hematomas
3. Abdominal muscle strains (mild)

Suggested Reading

Birrer RB. Abdominal injuries. In: Birrer RB, ed. *Sports Medicine for the primary care physician,* 2nd ed. Boca Raton, FL: CRC Press, 1994.

Bragg LE. Athletic injuries of the thorax and abdomen. In: Mellion MB, Walsh WM and Shelton GL eds. *The team physician's handbook.* Philadelphia: Hanley and Belfus, 1990.

Cianflocco AJ. Renal complications of exercise *Clin Sports Med* 1992;11: 437–451.

Green GA. Gastrointestinal disorders in the athlete. *Clin Sports Med.* 1992;11: 453–470.

Housner JA, Green GA. Gastrointestinal problems in the athlete. In: Sallis RE, Massimo F, eds. ACSM's *essentials of sports medicine.* St Louis: Mosby, 1996.

63. GENITOURINARY INJURIES

Brent S. E. Rich

Blunt trauma accounts for most athletically related injuries to the genitourinary tract. Life-threatening injuries are rare because of the anatomical protection of the genitourinary system. A thorough history regarding the mechanism of injury and onset of symptoms followed by a focused physical examination should guide the practitioner. Unstable vitals signs, pelvic fractures, or unremitting pain requires evaluation in the hospital setting.

I. Anatomy

The genitourinary system consists of the following structures: kidney, ureter, bladder, urethra, and external genitalia. Genital injuries are more common in the male even with the use of protective devices. Contact and collisions sports lead to the highest incidence of genitourinary injuries, though noncontact sports—such as bicycling, jogging and water skiing—also contribute to hematuria, pseuodonephritis, contusions, and lacerations.

II. Kidney

A. **Most commonly injured** organ in the genitourinary system.

B. **Well protected** due to anatomical location. Protected by retroperitoneal space, overlying ribs, abdominal musculature, perinephric fat, and thick renal capsule.

C. **Mobility** of kidney offers protection. Can move one to three vertebral levels without affecting function.

D. **Blunt trauma** leading to contusion or hematoma accounts for 80% to 85% of renal injuries. Renal lacerations or fractured kidneys account for 6% to 15% of injuries.

E. **Signs and symptoms** of renal injury include flank pain, hypotension, lower rib fracture, flank ecchymosis, flank mass, fracture of the lumbar vertebral transverse process, and hematuria.

F. **Classifications/stages of renal injuries**

1. **Renal contusions** with capsule intact, leading to subcapsular hematoma.
2. **Minor renal cortical lacerations** with the collecting system intact.
3. **Major renal parenchymal laceration** involving the collecting system.
4. **Renal pedicle injuries** resulting in laceration, avulsion, or thrombosis of the renal artery or vein leading to a devitalized kidney account for 1% to 2% of injuries and are life-threatening.

G. **Evaluation for renal injury.** Traditionally, all patients with hematuria, gross or microscopic, were evaluated with intravenous pyelography (IVP). One-third of patients with renal injury do not have hematuria.

1. **Workup indicated** for
   a. **Gross hematuria**
   b. **Microscopic hematuria** (greater than 5 RBCs per high-power field) with shock (systolic blood pressure less than 90 mm Hg).
2. **IVP or computed tomography (CT).** CT scanning depends on the institutions availability. Advantages include noninvasiveness, ability to assess other associated injuries, and ability to assess complete delineation of the injury.
3. **Treatment:** Stable patients are treated by expectant management, bed rest, hydration, and analgesics. Rest from strenuous activities for 2 to 3 weeks to prevent rebleeding from clot resolution. Hospital admission and operative exploration indicated for unstable patients.

III. Bladder

A. **Blunt trauma** is the most common cause of injury to the bladder. A pelvic fracture or direct blow to a full bladder may result in rupture.

B. **Signs and symptoms** of bladder injury include suprapubic pain, gross hematuria, urinary retention, pubic ecchymosis, and/or shock. Delayed diagnosis may present as peritonitis.
C. **Imaging.** Retrograde cystography is 100% accurate if properly performed. Evaluation of postevacuation film is very important to evaluate for extravasation.
D. **Treatment.** Extraperitoneal rupture with sterile urine managed with antibiotics and catheter drainage. Intraperitoneal rupture requires surgical exploration and closure.
E. **Runner's bladder** or "exercise-induced hematuria" may occur in athletes who exercise with an empty bladder. The posterior wall of the bladder may "slap" against the base of the prostate. Resolution of symptoms in asymptomatic patients may occur in a few days. Repeated episodes mandate evaluation with urography and cystoscopy to rule out more serious causes.

IV. Urethra

Urethral injuries in women are rare due to the short length (approximately 4 cm) of the urethra. Injuries are limited to lacerations when they occur. In the male, the injuries are described in relation to urogenital diaphragm.

A. **Anterior injuries** are distal to the urogenital diaphragm and affect the bulbous or pendulous urethra.
   1. **Mechanism of injury** is a straddle-type fall.
   2. **Signs and symptoms** include pain, perineal hematoma, urethral bleeding, and difficulty in voiding,
   3. **Imaging** is done by retrograde urethrography.
   4. **Types of injuries and treatment**
      a. **Contusion.** No extravasation of contrast. Catheterization until voiding possible.
      b. **Partial disruption.** Contrast flows proximal to injury with periuretheral extravasation. Treatment with catheterization or surgery, if indicated.
      c. **Complete disruption.** No retrograde flow of contrast proximal to the injury. Treatment with open resection and realignment.
B. **Posterior injuries** are proximal to the urogenital diaphragm and affect the membranous or prostatic urethras.
   1. **Mechanism of injury** is often significant trauma often with pelvic fracture.
   2. **Signs and symptoms** include urinary retention with inability to void, floating prostate, and blood at urethral meatus.
   3. **Imaging** by retrograde urethrography. Catheterization contraindicated because it may convert a partial tear into a complete tear.
   4. **Types of injuries and treatment**
      a. **Partial tear.** Consider surgical repair versus observation.
      b. **Complete tear.** Surgical repair with immediate or later urethral reconstruction.
   5. **Complications** include urethral strictures, impotence, and incontinence.

V. Genital Injuries in Males

Genital injuries in athletic events primarily occur from blunt trauma.

A. **Penile injuries** are unusual owing to the relative mobility of the penis.
   1. ***Contusions and lacerations*** are the most common injuries.
   2. ***Penile fracture*** or rupture of the tunica albuginea surrounding the corpora cavernosa may occur when the erect penis suffers a direct blow.
      a. ***Symptoms*** include pain, inability to void, and bending of the penis to one side. ***Treatment*** is initiated with ice followed by urologic surgery to evacuate the clot and repair the lesion.
   3. ***Cyclist's penis*** or "numb-crotch syndrome" occurs from pressure on the pudendal nerves between the bicycle seat and the pubic symphysis.
      a. ***Symptoms*** include tingling and numbness on the shaft of the penis or scrotum that resolve without treatment. Adjusting the height, angle, or width of the saddle seat resolves future problems.

B. **Testicular trauma** is most commonly due to a direct blow. Even with the use of protective devices (i.e., athletic supporters, plastic cups) the testicles are subject to injury.

1. **Contusion**
   a. **Signs and symptoms** include local pain, scrotal swelling, ecchymosis, nausea and vomiting.
   b. **Treatment** consists of observation, bed rest, ice application, elevation, scrotal support, and analgesia.
2. **Fracture**
   a. **Mechanism of injury** is rupture of the tunica albuginea.
   b. **Signs and symptoms** are similar to contusions with pain out of proportion to the injury.
   c. **Imaging** accomplished by testicular ultrasound to determine if the tunica is intact. Transillumination may aid the practitioner to evaluate the extent of an expanding mass and the need for ultrasound.
   d. **Treatment** is by surgical repair. If performed within 72 hr, 90% of ruptured testes can be salvaged, whereas success is 55% if surgery is delayed.
   e. **Complications** include ischemic atrophy, necrosis, secondary infection and prolonged discomfort.
3. **Testicular torsion**
   a. **The mechanism** of testicular torsion is a forceful contraction of the cremaster muscle. Trauma is not a direct cause of testicular torsion. The testicle may become malaligned in a horizontal rather than vertical arrangement, resulting in obstruction of venous return. The direction of torsion is usually counterclockwise in the left testicle and clockwise in the right.
   b. **Signs and symptoms** include unilateral scrotal pain, swelling, tenderness, and nausea and vomiting without voiding difficulties. The testicle may be "high-riding" or lying in a transverse direction. Pain may be alleviated by further elevating the testis.
   c. **Imaging** by ultrasonography, radionuclide scintigraphy or magnetic resonance imaging (MRI) scanning may assist in diagnosis. In technetium testicular scanning, decreased uptake indicates probable torsion, whereas increased uptake may indicated epididymitis with the contralateral testis as the control.
   d. **Torsion is a true urological emergency** leading to necrosis and infarction of the testicle if untreated. If repaired within 5 hr of pain, the salvage rate approaches 80%. With the delay of more than 6 hr, spermatogenesis may be lost; after more than 10 hr, necrosis of the Leydig cells occurs. Loss of the testicle necessitates orchiectomy.
4. **Testicular masses** should be thoroughly evaluated in the athlete. Testicular neoplasm is most prevalent between the ages of 20 and 40. Either testicular self-examination or physician examination should occur during the preparticipation physical examination. Suspicious lesions should be evaluated by a physician.

C. **Scrotum**

1. **Scrotal laceration** may be repaired by primary closure.
2. **Varicocele** are a common cause of scrotal swelling, occurring in approximately 15% of males.
   a. Dilation of the pampiniform plexus of veins (or "bag of worms") is the ***etiology.***
   b. Occurs on ***left side*** primarily.
   c. Association with ***infertility*** and testicular failure.
   d. **No contraindication to physical activity.**

VI. Genital Injuries in Females

Injuries to the female genital tract are uncommon but when they occur are a result of blunt trauma or straddle injuries. Labial hematomas or tears, vaginal lacerations, or clitoral tears may occur. Rarely, a laceration may result from the friction of a strong stream of water against the external genitalia, as in water skiing. Treatment with rest, ice, elevation and analgesic is usually adequate, but surgical consultation is necessary for significant injuries.

VII. "Athletic Pseudonephritis"

1. **Definition:** Strenuous exercise may cause benign and transient microscopic red and white cells, and protein with cellular and noncellular renal tubular casts to appear in the urine.
2. Urine generally clears with rest within 1 to 2 days.
3. **Degree of hydration and intensity of exercise** correlate with amount of urine sediment.
4. **Mechanism.** Exercise decreases renal blood flow and glomerular filtration rate, leading to an increase in glomerular permeability and decreased renal tubular reabsorption.

VIII. Preparticipation Physical Examination

1. **Routine urinalysis** during preparticipation physical exam is ***not indicated.***

Suggested Reading

Koch MO. Genitourinary trauma. *1992 Conn's current therapy.* Philadelphia: W.B. Saunders, 1992.

Schneider RE. Early strategies for genitourinary trauma. *Emerg Med* 1991; 30:27–36.

York JP. Sports and the male genitourinary system: kidneys and bladder. *Phys Sports Med* 1990; 18:116–130.

XIII. **REHABILITATION**

64. GENERAL PRINCIPLES OF REHABILITATION

W. Benjamin Kibler and Stanley A. Herring

Introduction

Goals of the Rehabilitation Process

The ultimate goal of rehabilitation of sports-specific injuries is maximal restoration of function for an anatomic area or a specific athletic activity. Contact and noncontact sports result in both macrotrauma and microtrauma injuries. Macrotraumatic injuries occur as an event with normal tissue becoming acutely abnormal with clinical symptoms. Microtraumatic injuries occur as a process over time, with a gradual transition from normal to abnormal tissues and resultant clinical symptoms. Both types of injuries require careful evaluation and specific rehabilitation to allow the athlete to return to normal function. To achieve maximum efficiency of the rehabilitation process, several goals should be met: (1) establishment of a complete and accurate diagnosis; (2) minimization of the deleterious local effects of the acute injury; (3) allowance for proper healing; (4) maintenance of other components of athletic fitness; (5) return to normal athletic function.

Establishment of a Complete and Accurate Diagnosis

Without a thorough diagnosis, adequate rehabilitation is not possible. The specific tissue damage must be identified, yet this may only partially define or even completely omit the tissues that were overloaded to cause the injury, especially in the microtrauma process. In long standing injuries, substitution patterns (compensation) develop as the athlete tries to maintain sports performance. A framework can be established around these findings to allow complete and accurate diagnosis. The specific tissue damage (*tissue injury complex*) and overloaded tissues (*tissue overload complex*) can be identified on physical examination. The clinical symptom complex comprises the presenting complaints. Specific inflexibilities, weaknesses, or imbalances (*functional biomechanical deficits*) and the substitution patterns (*subclinical adaptation complex*) can be identified if the patient and the athletic activity are considered in the context of the injury. Identification of the specific alterations and deficits associated with the clinical symptoms complex allows for the functional diagnosis to be made and for comprehensive rehabilitation to be planned.

Minimization of the Deleterious Local Effects of Acute Injury

Sports injury results in tissue damage, which is invariably accompanied by tissue inflammation. This initial inflammatory phase is followed by subsequent phases of tissue healing, repair, and remodeling. This process occurs with acute injury, acute exacerbation of chronic injury, or chronic injury and is the same regardless of injury site. There may be a difference in magnitude based on whether the injury is acute or chronic.

The amount of inflammation associated with the tissue injury can be controlled by measures which minimize its exuberance and promote recovery. Physical modalities such as ***therapeutic cold*** combined with ***compression*** and ***elevation*** are useful in acute pain and injury. ***High-frequency electrical stimulation*** also affords pain control while decreasing muscle spasm and increasing circulation. This helps to remove inflammatory waste products.

Medications such as ***nonsteroidal anti-inflammatory drugs (NSAIDs)*** may help to minimize the local effects of acute injury by limiting the extent of the inflammatory response and relieving pain. ***Corticosteroids*** are potent antiinflammatories but have no direct analgesic properties. If NSAIDs or corticosteroids are prescribed, dosage, timing and potential side effects should be considered. In addition, their role in inhibiting the beneficial effects of inflammation need to be considered.

The injured tissue may need to be ***rested, splinted,*** or occasionally kept nonweight bearing. However, treatment must be balanced with the known local side effects of immobilization. Local muscle may show a 20% strength loss after 1 week of immobilization and another 20% decline in residual strength every subsequent week of immobilization. Type I fibers are particularly effected by immobilization, with up to a 47% loss by the fifth week. The side effects from local immobilization extend beyond muscle. Significant biochemical and biomechanical alterations in the joint capsule, subchondral bone, bone-ligament complex, and cartilage also occur with immobilization. Prolonged rehabilitation is needed to regain strength and flexibility.

Pain is a potent inhibitor of muscle function and must be controlled early in the rehabilitation process to keep the muscle inhibition to a minimum and to decrease the chance of subclinical adaptation in the recovery process.

Allowance for Proper Healing

Injured tissue should be provided with the best environment for recovery. Proper healing is promoted by minimizing the deleterious local effects of injury, by appropriate medication, limiting the time of immobilization, and protection from shear forces as the tissue is healing. ***Mobilized injured muscle*** shows a more rapid and intense sprouting of new capillaries as compared to immobilized muscle. Collagen fiber growth and realignment are stimulated by early tensile loading of muscle in safe ranges. Hematomas, inflammatory cells, necrotic tissue, and degenerative changes disappear more quickly in injured muscle that is mobilized within mild ranges early in the process of healing. Early motion decreases the formation of adhesions between healing tissue and surrounding structures. Injured tissue may require rest in the early phases, but prolonged inactivity may not be the best way to allow proper healing. Anatomic repair and secure fixation of injured tissues, when indicated with surgery will allow more secure return to early ranges of motion and a more normal environment for healing.

Maintenance of Other Components of Athletic Fitness

In addition to managing the local effects of an injury, measures to maintain general fitness should be enacted as a part of the comprehensive treatment program. This will decrease the total rehabilitation time.

Cardiovascular fitness decreases relatively rapidly with inactivity. Maximum oxygen uptake ($\dot{V}O_2max$) decreases up to 25% after 3 weeks of bed rest. The positive effects of 7 weeks of endurance training are completely lost within 8 weeks of detraining and approximately half of the decrease occurs within the first 2 weeks. Cardiovascular changes are fairly quick to readapt, but it is obviously better not to have them occur at all.

Appropriate ***modified strength training*** contributes to maintenance of general fitness during rehabilitation. The injured site may initially tolerate little to no exercise and is relatively rested. However, strengthening can be designed for the rest of the body. Even when training is reduced to once per week, strength can be maintained over a 12-week period. This is especially important if other areas of the body were involved in the chronic overload process.

Cardiovascular and strength training should be combined with a continued ***flexibility*** program in order to maintain general athletic fitness. Cross training can be advised in order to avoid overloading previously undertrained muscles which are now being more regularly utilized. Inflexibility is a very common problem that occurs both as the result of inactivity or as an adaptation in the microtrauma process. Problems with inflexibility should be identified in the complete and accurate diagnosis and should be addressed as part of the rehabilitation process.

Maintaining fitness benefits the patient not only physiologically but ***psychologically*** as well. Injured athletes often feel frustrated and may develop self-defeating thoughts that can interfere with recovery. Regular exercise helps the patient maintain his or her previous fitness level and contributes to a sense of well-being that is very important for healing.

The training program should be coordinated so that the general athletic fitness and sports-specific activities are rehabilitated at the same pace. Thus, when the athlete is ready to return to sport as far as the injury is concerned, the rest of the body is also ready.

Return to Normal Athletic Function

It is essential to address the local and general effects of an injury to provide thorough treatment. However, one must understand the specific demands of the sport and prepare the athlete for them to assure total rehabilitation. Resolution of the anatomic and functional deficits associated with an injury include ***restoration of flexibility, strength, strength balance, power, aerobic fitness*** and ***proprioception*** that are specific for the sporting or athletic activity. These can be accomplished by completion of a ***sports-specific training*** and readiness program. Certain sports have certain demands and must be evaluated in terms of intensity, duration, and organization of the muscle firing patterns. The rehabilitation should be set up in the later phases of the program to closely resemble these activities so that the athlete is ready to return to the specific demands of the sport.

In summary, many methods can be used to accomplish the goals of rehabilitation. These include modalities, rest, medication, surgery, exercises for flexibility and strength, and sports-specific progressions. To be most efficacious, they must be used in a logical and scientifically based sequence in line with their benefit to tissue healing and function.

Methods of Rehabilitation

Initial Injury Management

Initial injury management should be based on the type, location, and severity of injury. Acute injuries with tissue damage and acute swelling should be treated with the goals of reducing swelling, reducing any deleterious local effects, and promoting healing as quickly as possible. In some instances, initial injury management includes surgery.

Rest

Rest should be used to relieve soreness and pain, prevent further injury, prevent the development of subclinical adaptations, and allow the body to start the healing process. In most instances this is actually relative rest. The rest of the body can still be exercised, aerobic endurance maintained, and some limited motion of the involved site allowed. Strict immobilization is kept to a minimum because of the deleterious neurologic and tissue effects. Periods of rest may also be necessary during the later stages of rehabilitation to allow recovery from exercise.

Medications

Medications should be used for specific purposes, mainly pain relief, in the early phases of rehabilitation. Pain, which is a potent inhibitor of muscle activation and coactivation, is especially deleterious around muscle-dependent joints. In acute overload situations, inflammation may contribute substantially to the pain or clinical symptoms. However, in chronic problems, such as tendinitis, the inflammatory process probably contributes a relatively small amount to the pain complex. In the acute phase of the pathologic problem, a case can be made for the short-term use of nonsteroidal antiinflammatory drugs (NSAIDs) or oral or injectable corticosteroids. NSAIDs should be used for their analgesic rather than their antiinflammatory properties in the more common chronic microtrauma injuries. Medications should be viewed as adjunctive rather than curative and should be prescribed with all the known risks to tendons, the gastrointestinal tract, and kidneys in mind. No specific NSAIDs appears to have an enhanced efficacy or better-benefit risk ratio. Long-acting crystalline corticosteroid suspensions provide the fastest relief and are preferred over aqueous preparations for injections. After injection, exercises should be avoided for 2 to 3 days. Injections should be placed *around* the injured area rather than directly into the area. Corticosteroids can also be used in phonophoresis or iontophoresis to allow delivery of the medication in this fashion.

Surgery

Surgery may be required to relieve clinical symptoms and heal the tissue injury complex. The surgical procedures should create conditions for optimal healing and optimal rehabilitation. Fixation of the injured tissue should be secure enough to start early protected motion and soft tissues should be tensioned after repair to allow a degree of mobility with stability. Overtightening of the tissues or immobilizing the tissues too long should be avoided as this creates undesirable biomechanics.

Ultrasound

Ultrasound (high-frequency mechanical vibrations) produces thermal and non-thermal physiologic effects for therapeutic purposes. Tissues with high protein content, such as muscle and nerve, absorb ultrasound more readily. An increased thermal response and possible tissue damage can occur at heterogeneous tissue interfaces such as the bone-muscle or tendon-bone interface. Ultrasound is the most effective deep-heating modality for muscles and deep-seated joints. Thermal effects result in increases peripheral blood flow, increased tissue metabolism, and greater tissue extensibility. Nonthermal effects of ultrasound on membrane stability have been advocated in the treatment of pain and inflammation; however, experimental studies have been contradictory. Ultrasound does have analgesic effects because of its action on membrane stability, presynaptic inhibition, and increased cortisol levels. Phonophoresis is a technique that uses mechanical energy to drive whole molecules of medication, usually corticosteroids, into tissue. Although some symptomatic relief is reported with phonophoresis as compared with placebo, there is incomplete evidence that the corticosteroid molecules can be driven into deep, symptomatic areas.

Electrical Stimulation

Electrical stimulation has been used in the treatment of both acute and chronic injuries. There is considerable support for its uses in modifying pain and inflammation but no scientific studies of its efficacy have been performed. High-voltage galvanic stimulation has been used to relax muscle spasm, reduce edema, increase blood flow, and maintain range of motion. Iontophoresis, which uses differences in electrical potential to deliver medication to deep tissues, allows medications to penetrate tissues with reduced vascularity, such as bursae and tendons.

Cryotherapy

Cryotherapy, the therapeutic use of cold, serves to decrease tissue temperature, inflammation, metabolic rate, circulation, and muscle spasm. In acute injury, all of these influences combine to reduce secondary hypoxic injury around the primary injury, decrease pain, and decrease swelling. In chronic injuries, the main effects are reduction in postinjury, postoperative, and postexercise pain or swelling. Cellular effects are to reduce swelling and hypoxia. Effects on pain and spasm are due to decreased nerve conduction and decreased spindle activity. Methods of delivery vary from ice bags to cold compression devices. The depth of penetration also varies. Cold must be used carefully to avoid skin damage due to overexposure.

In summary, the methods of rehabilitation described thus far have all been advocated to help treat pathologic problems in sports. Scientific studies showing their efficacy are lacking. Most appear to have a role early in the pathologic process in decreasing some of the symptoms of pain, muscle spasm, and inflammation. They appear to have less of a role in chronic problems that do not particularly involve pain or inflammation but mainly dysfunction. Rehabilitation beyond the resolution of symptoms requires achievement of proper flexibility and dynamic muscle stability in addition to anatomic healing. This flexibility and restoration of muscle strength must be both local and extend through the rest of the kinetic chain.

Flexibility

Flexibility exercises can be used to restore the mobility of joints and muscles. These areas may be tight as a result of repetitive microtrauma, disuse, or immobilization. Exercises can help improve flexibility in postoperative joints as well. The exercises appear to work by reducing connective tissue adhesions, reducing abnormal collagen cross links, and reducing tissue stiffness. Stretching also improves the viscoelastic properties of muscle. The net result is tissues that are pliable, pain free, balanced in flexibility, and not prone to abnormal translation.

Flexibility exercises may be ***passive,*** in which gravity or a therapist facilitates the stretching; ***assistive,*** in which the other extremity is used to move the injured limb;

or ***active,*** in which the involved joint is self-powered. The exercises are usually started in short arcs of motion and positions that do not put the injured tissues on tensile stress; they then progress by stages to full ranges of motion. The motions are controlled in regard to position, time, and speed, based on the degree of healing and the degree of motion required. Moderate tension should be developed, so that the viscoelastic properties of tension relaxation and creep are used to maximize tissue pliability. Flexibility exercises are usually started early in the rehabilitation program and should be continued throughout all of the phases of rehabilitation.

Flexibility is traditionally very slow to return to normal especially if the inflexibility is due to repetitive microtrauma. The key point in stretching is that the muscle or joint area that is tight must be isolated with a particular exercise so that this particular area is selectively stressed. Body mechanics can adapt to produce an integrated movement that masks a tight joint or muscle. ***Manual mobilization*** and manual capsular stretching as well as ***cross-friction massage*** can also be used to restore flexibility. These techniques must be done carefully in order not to disrupt internal repairs, create new damage, or reinjure the damaged tissue.

Muscle Strengthening

Muscle strengthening exercises are the key to complete functional rehabilitation of injured parts. Muscle is the most important tissue in terms of generating power, accepting load, and protecting joints. Full strength, balance, and force generation must be restored in the muscles before normal physical activity can be expected. Generation and summation of forces through all of the muscles will allow for the most effective and efficient athletic performance.

The mechanical properties of the muscle may be improved by loading a muscle so that it hypertrophies. This is usually done by isolating it and then progressively loading it ***isometrically, concentrically,*** and ***eccentrically*** as the muscle's ability to contract increases. The best ways to work isolated muscles are with rubber tubing or free weights. As the muscles get stronger, machine weights, which are less specific for individual muscles, may be added. However, the targeted muscles must have some strength to benefit from the machine weights. With the combined movement patterns created by the machines, strong muscles may compensate for weak ones and may retard development of weaker muscles. Rubber tubing and free weights may selectively strengthen certain muscles that can be identified on examination, thereby creating the possibility of normal force generation and force-coupled balance. They have disadvantages in that muscle hypertrophy is often a slow process, especially in chronic injuries, and isolated muscle activities are not functional around certain joints, such as the shoulder. This type of training becomes a prelude to normal joint muscle activity.

Neurologic control of muscle activity is a final element of muscle function and gain of muscle strength. Alterations in ***muscle firing patterns*** and neural drive as the result of fatigue, pain, altered proprioception, disuse, or injury are commonly seen in athletic problems. Most of the early strength gains seen in rehabilitating muscle are due to improvement in firing patterns, motor unit recruitment, and decreased threshold for firing. Therefore, early emphasis should be placed on making muscles contract safely and painlessly. This may be done through isometrics, very short arc isotonics, or mild co-contraction activities with the joint in a safe position. As more joint flexibility is achieved and tissue healing occurs, more positions for manual co-contraction in single planes of movement can be gained. More resistance can be added through the tubing, weights, or machines to allow for optimum strength gains. Emphasis does not have to be on maximal strength gains but on balance of agonist and antagonist in the early stages, with progression to maximal strength gains as the rehabilitation progresses.

Neurologic training can then progress to reestablishment of the motor patterns necessary for the fine control of joint movement in multiple planes. The major programs to promote this process are proprioceptive neuromuscular facilitation and other proprioceptive drills, closed chain exercises and open chain exercises. ***Proprioceptive neuromuscular facilitation*** activities are combined movement patterns that use specific sensory input from a therapist to the patient to bring about a specific activity or movement. Rhythmic stabilization techniques may be applied at various positions of flexion and abduction. The alternating stimulus requires a neurologic activation of stretch receptors and enhances the motor patterns that provide the dynamic stabilizing activity of the muscles around the joint.

Closed Kinetic Chain Exercises are defined as exercises in which the distal end of the extremity meets a considerable resistance. These exercises create a predictable sequential combination of joint positions and motions secondary to the distribution of the forces through this base of support. Closed chain exercises are very commonly used in lower extremity rehabilitation. These exercises are beneficial because they decrease strain and shear on ligaments around the joint by inducing coactivation of the quadriceps and hamstrings in the lower extremity, allow specificity of training in that most athletic activities are done with the foot on the ground, allow concurrent shift which is the pattern of agonist/antagonist muscle activity that occurs in locomotion, and may stimulate proprioception.

Closed chain activities can also be done for the upper extremity. The shoulder does fit most of the definition of a closed chain—it works as a funnel, transferring forces from the stable base of the trunk in a predictable manner to the joints of the arm. These exercises, by promoting coactivation force couples, enhance the dynamic joint stability that appears to be the primary role of the shoulder muscles. By fixing the hand, these exercises promote scapular stability, the base from which the shoulder and arm can function. Also, strengthening of the shoulder in a closed kinetic chain function will decrease tensile stress on the capsular ligaments, decrease tensile stress on the supraspinatus tendon and other structures that may be injured or repaired around the shoulder, and decrease the effect of the deltoid component of the abduction force couples. They may be done at loads safe enough to use early in rehabilitation. In the shoulder, they are best used early in the rehabilitation sequence, where neurological retraining is more important.

Open chain exercises are also necessary in rehabilitation to prepare for the fast ballistic movements that occur in sports activities such as kicking, throwing, or swimming. We use open chain activities after healing has progressed, after closed chain exercises have stabilized the joints and coordinated the muscle firing patterns, and when the range of motion is sufficient to allow for the rapid shifts in motion and position that occur with the open chain activities. All of the open chain activities require a preparation or cocking phase, an acceleration phase and a deceleration phase. In this situation, muscles are acting as agonist-antagonist force couples, and they need to reverse roles rapidly between acceleration and deceleration. Open chain exercises should emphasize large ranges of motion, rapid joint activity, and a prestretching followed by forceful agonist and antagonist force couple firing. The open chain exercises can be done with dumbbells, rubber tubing, or other types of exercises. We feel that plyometric exercises are the best type to achieve the goals of the open chain exercises. These exercises all involve a prestretch, which tensions the muscles and stores elastic energy, followed by a rapid explosive contraction.

Timing and Usage of Rehabilitation Methods

The methods of rehabilitation must be used in a logical, diagnosis-specific way to achieve maximum efficiency. The goal of rehabilitation of every pathologic problem is to restore normal function. However, the starting point for rehabilitation varies widely depending on the pathologic process, type of treatment, and complicating alterations in physiology or biomechanics either locally or distantly. This point varies widely and reinforces the need for a complete and accurate diagnosis as a starting place for rehabilitation.

Rehabilitation is divided into three phases, each based on the resolution of certain aspects of the tissue injuries or alterations noted and will use the basic methods outlined. There are specific goals, activity progressions, and criteria for movement from phase to phase. Within each phase, the specific activities will be classified by type, frequency, intensity, and duration. Since this is a function-based program, all of the protocols tend to progress to some common end points in later phases regardless of the starting point. Our framework includes three phases, the acute, the recovery, and the functional phase.

Acute Phase

The acute phase begins with the onset of clinical symptoms of injury or when the patient is seen for rehabilitation. Patient's injuries will vary widely from acute fracture or dislocation to postsurgical repair to overload tendinitis. However, in each instance attention is focused on resolving the clinical symptom complex and the tissue injury complex that have been identified in the evaluation. The ***goals*** of the acute phase of rehabilitation are to (1) create conditions for tissue healing; (2) reduce pain and inflammation; (3) reestablish nonpainful range of motion; (4) retard muscle atrophy, both locally and in the regional area around the injury; (5) establish neuromuscular control of the joint in neutral positions; and (6) maintain fitness of the rest of the kinetic chain.

Tissue healing will be promoted by a combination of rest, short-term immobilization, medication, injections, or surgery, based on the clinical findings. ***Pain*** symptoms should be aggressively addressed by the proper use of medications, modalities, and rest, because pain is such a potent inhibitor of normal muscle function, especially around the knee and shoulder. Early control of pain will decrease inhibition-based muscle atrophy and allow better control of the muscles by counteracting muscle weakness. ***Range-of-motion*** exercises should be started in pain-free arcs and may be passive or active assisted as tolerated. They may go on to larger arcs as healing progresses. ***Muscle strengthening*** may be started with isometric activity, which allows some strength gains without much joint motion.

Closed kinetic chain exercises begin with weight shifts with simple loading and will progress to increasing the amount of weight distributed through the arms or legs. For the shoulder, these exercises are usually done in glenohumeral positions with less than 60 degrees of flexion and less than 45 degrees of abduction. This allows minimal shear and evokes low-level muscle activity in the deltoid and rotator cuff. In the knee, these would be done with range of motion from extension to 45 degrees of flexion with support of crutches, a walker, or a wall.

Exercises for the rest of the ***kinetic chain*** should be emphasized in this phase. Aerobic exercises may be done in the legs for shoulder or elbow problems and in the arm and trunk for lower extremity problems. ***Flexibility*** exercises for all parts of the kinetic chain outside of the injured area should also be emphasized.

This phase of rehabilitation will be the most diverse because of the wide spectrum of clinical symptoms and tissue injuries and the variety of early treatments. The basic objective is the same—to create stable healing tissues that will allow tensile loading and improve joint health to allow for more advanced rehabilitation. ***Criteria for progression*** out of the acute phase include (1) progression of tissue healing where the tissue is healed or sufficiently stabilized for active motion; (2) passive range of motion to 75% of the opposite side; (3) minimal pain or tenderness, less than level II; (4) manual muscle test strength in nonpathologic areas 4+ to 5; (5) control of the periarticular regions; and (6) continued kinetic chain function.

Recovery Phase

The recovery phase will continue rehabilitation of the tissue injury complex but will also address the tissue overload and functional biomechanical deficit complexes. Entry into this phase assumes that the injured tissues may be loaded in tension and compression so that normal strength and flexibility may be reached. The ***goals*** of this phase are (1) to regain and improve extremity muscle flexibility, strength, balance, and endurance; (2) improve neuromuscular control in multiple planes of motion; (3) establish normal kinetic chain velocity in force generation patterns; and (4) establish normal range of motion of the joint.

Adequate joint ***range of motion*** is very important. Active assisted exercises should be done early in this phase and pushed toward normal motion. ***Strength, strength balance,*** and ***endurance*** gains in this phase are due to both muscle hypertrophy and improved neurologic firing patterns. Isotonic and isometric exercises should be done to facilitate the gains. Progressions can be achieved by increasing the speed of movement, changing the resistance, altering the number of repetitions, and increasing the frequency and duration of exercise sessions. Strength activities usually start with relatively light resistance and move slowly through relatively small arcs. As the muscles adapt, more resistance, more speed, and larger arcs are possible. Eventually muscles need to be trained for sport or activity-specific resistance, speeds, or motions. Machines are helpful to isolate and improve specific uniplanar motions but are also limited because most joint functions are multiplanar movements and are probably best for functional strengthening.

The strengthening program should move from proximal to distal and from large force generating muscles to smaller regulating muscles. Closed chain activities are a safe way to work without putting shear or tensile stresses on the joint structures.

As soon as shoulder flexibility to 90 degrees can be achieved, the arm can be placed at 90 degrees abduction either against the wall or against a movable object and scapular movement, and humeral rotation and humeral depression activities may be started. These exercises have the advantage of working the muscles at a low level of activity, eliminating excessive deltoid activity and rotator cuff inhibition, working the muscles in a co-contraction force couple and working them in positions more closely approximating the functional position of 90 degrees abduction. Scaption (scapular abduction) exercises have also been demonstrated to be effective in this stage.

Open chain strengthening can be built upon this base of strength and balance. Increased resistance, more repetitions, and work-rest ratios of 1:1 will increase muscle function. Generally, maximum strength can be achieved by lifting a maximum amount of resistance relatively slowly for four to six repetitions per set. Power is achieved by lifting 75% of the maximum quickly for five repetitions per set. Endurance is achieved by lifting 50% to 60% of the maximum rapidly for 8 to 15 repetitions per set. Many different exercises can be used, but it does not appear that one specific set or type of exercises is most beneficial.

Specific exercises for ***proprioception*** are also important in the recovery phase. Proprioceptive neuromuscular facilitation patterns, by stimulating the sensory receptors for stretch and enhancing coordinated firing patterns, are the major influences in establishing efficient motor control around a joint. Closed chain activities, by causing axial loading and joint compression, also simulate and facilitate the return of normal motor firing patterns. Proprioceptive exercises are based on putting the joint in a certain position that will allow muscle co-contraction and sensory feedback, then moving the joint through normal functional ranges to reestablish the normal motor feedback and motor control.

Recovery phase of rehabilitation is the longest and most complex because of the large amount of work required to restore all of the disordered components both locally and distantly. It is often ignored because there are very few symptoms in this phase. However, this is the phase that allows the creation of conditions for normal function. ***Criteria for progression*** out of the recovery phase include (1) full, non-painful active and passive range of motion of the joint; (2) no pain or tenderness; (3) strength at 80% of the opposite side with good force couple balance; and (4) a normal kinetic chain.

Functional Phase

The functional phase will address any of the remaining functional biomechanical deficits, correct any subclinical adaptations that may have developed, and use functional progressions to return to play. This is the final common pathway for the various protocols for the injuries that were first encountered. The ***goals*** of the functional phase are (1) to increase the power of the muscles around the joint to functional levels; (2) to increase neuromuscular control in multiple planes of motion; (3) to return to sport or activity-specific functions.

Power is the rate of doing work. Work must be done to move the joint or the extremity or to absorb a load and stabilize the joint. Power has a time component and, for most athletic activities, quick movements and quick reactions are the dominant ways of doing work. Methods to improve ***sports-specific power*** should include fast-speed isokinetic exercises, fast-speed isotonic exercises using light weights or tubing in multiple planes, plyometrics using tubing or medicine balls, and advanced open and closed chain activities.

Plyometric exercises are especially important in this phase of rehabilitation because they activate the stretch-shortening cycles of muscle activity that are common in most athletic activities. This prestretch improves the amount and efficiency of the muscle contraction.

Medicine balls are particularly effective plyometric tools. The weight of the ball as it is caught or handled creates a prestretch, creates a resistance, and demands a power contraction to be propelled forward. In the shoulder, progression is from two-handed chest passes to overhead throws to rotational passes. The ball may be initially held in the hands with progression to catching and returning the throw. Rotational movements of the hips and trunk are important of sports-specific activities of the shoulder and should be included in medicine ball drills. For the knees, catching the ball with knees flexed and going into a squat position and then coming up or rotating or actually moving the ball with the foot are similar types of progression.

Advanced closed chain activities play a role in functional phase especially in the lower extremity where loading, jumping, and sprinting activities are very important for return to play.

The functional phase is also the perfect time to instruct the athlete in preventative activities or ***"prehabilitation."*** A maintenance program of stretching, muscle-balance exercises, power exercises, and kinetic chain exercises is the best way to condition to prevent overload injuries and further problems in the sport. Most athletes who are injured in the sport will be going right back to the same activities. Therefore, the body should not only be healed from the symptoms but should also be prepared for resuming the stresses inherent in playing the sport. These exercises should be sports specific and should be based on the periodization principle of conditioning. ***Criteria for progression*** out of this phase into full competitions are (1) normal arthrokinetics and multiple-plane activities; (2) isokinetic strength balance and work at 90% of normal; and (3) completion of functional progressions and satisfactory clinical examination.

Summary

Rehabilitation in general and sports-specific rehabilitation are evolving in their techniques and in the amount of information that is available. At this point in time, there is no single best protocol because there has been little outcomes analysis of the results. Adherence to the basic principles that have been outlined in this chapter appear to be the best framework for constructing a good program. We have included specific rehabilitation programs for knee and shoulder in Appendix 5. In this period of emphasis on efficacious care, appropriate use of modalities based on understanding the pathophysiology of the injury will allow rehabilitation to be a part of the management and treatment of athletes.

Suggested Reading

Chandler TJ. Muscle Training in Injury Prevention. In: *Sports injuries: basic principles of prevention and care.* Boston: Blackwell, 1993:252–261.

Griffin L. *Rehabilitation of the injured knee. 2d ed.* St Louis: Mosby-Year Book, 1994.

Irrgang JJ. Rehabilitation. In: *Sports injuries: mechanisms, prevention, and treatment.* Baltimore: Williams & Wilkins, 1994:81–95.

Kibler WB. Current concepts in shoulder rehabilitation. In: *Advances in orthopaedics.* vol 3. St. Louis; Mosby-Year Book, 1995:249–300.

Kibler WB. *Functional rehabilitation of rotator cuff injuries.* Academy of Orthopaedic Surgeons, Rosemont, IL: American (video).

Wilk KE. Current concepts in the rehabilitation of the athlete's shoulder. *J South Orthop Assoc* 1994;3:216–231.

PART XIV. **SPECIFIC SPORTS**

65. BASEBALL AND SOFTBALL

Jan Fronek

Baseball and softball have traditionally emphasized skill and quickness. Recently, a variety of programs have focused on injury prevention and performance enhancement.

The epidemiology of these sports reflects the two types of injury patterns: (1) *acute macrotrauma* leading to injuries common to other running and pivoting activities where occasional contact or collision may occur and (2) *repetitive microtrauma*–induced injuries, particularly to the upper extremity and spine, specific to baseball and softball. For appropriate assessment and treatment, it is critical to understand the biomechanics of pitching, throwing, and batting.

The dominant side of most baseball players, especially pitchers, will demonstrate hypertrophy, especially of the proximal musculature. The shoulder will reveal approximately a 5° to 10° increase in external rotation (ER) and similar decrease of internal rotation (IR). Greater loss of IR usually indicates an injury and associated posterior capsular contracture.

In the past, the painful shoulder of the throwing athlete was considered to be due to impingement or external compression of the bursal surface of the rotator cuff, the vulnerable, relatively hypoperfused tendon. Recent basic science and clinical (motion analysis) research has been of critical importance in promoting further understanding of injuries to the throwing athlete.

During the late cocking and acceleration phases of throwing, the primary stresses to the shoulder involve the anterior aspect of the shoulder. The anterior structures include the glenohumeral (GH) capsule and specifically, the anteroinferior GH ligament in collaboration with the rotator cuff, especially the subscapularis, and pectoralis muscles. While the throwing athlete may present with the "external" bursal-side ***impingement syndrome,*** frequently, the presence of ***anterior instability*** or more commonly, ***multidirectional*** (anteroinferior) ***instability*** is responsible for the additional stresses to the rotator cuff. The rotator cuff trauma is due to direct injury to the tendon by the posterior glenoid labrum (***internal impingement***) as the arm is brought into maximal abduction and external rotation.

The deceleration phase places the arm into adduction and internal rotation, subsequently stressing the posterior GH capsule. With repetitive stress, ***posterior instability*** in enhanced, resulting in pain and posterior ***glenoid labrum tears.*** Associated rotator cuff trauma may occur due to the GH laxity or direct tensile forces applied to the tendon during deceleration of the arm.

The presence of a ***SLAP*** (superior labrum anterior posterior) lesion is due to repetitive stress or sudden tensile load on the biceps tendon. Importantly, it is frequently associated with increased shoulder joint laxity.

Neurovascular syndromes, arterial or venous thrombosis about the shoulder are uncommon; however, prompt diagnosis is critical for a successful clinical outcome. The Doppler study is valuable in the examination of the throwing athlete presenting with arm swelling, occasionally in association with exertional pain, paresthesias, or discoloration of the arm. This noninvasive study will evaluate the patency of the axillary and subclavian veins in order to diagnose this variant of thoracic outlet syndrome.

Suprascapular neuropathy is more commonly seen in volleyball players, yet this nerve is also vulnerable due to the repetitive stresses of pitching or pure compression at the suprascapular notch.

In skeletally mature players, bony injury is usually manifested as the rare ***rib stress fracture*** or spiral ***fracture of the humerus.*** Athletes with open growth plates are also at risk; however, they are more likely to develop ***stress-induced epiphysiolysis at the proximal humeral physis.***

During the acceleration phase of pitching, the marked valgus stress of the elbow is responsible for the most common injuries. The medial structures at risk are the ulnar collateral ligament (UCL), ulnar nerve, and the flexor muscle origin. The most disabling is a ***tear of the UCL,*** with the secondary osteophyte formation and calcium deposition within the substance of the ligament. Skeletally immature athletes are more likely to injure their growth plate as is discussed below.

The myotendinous strain of the flexor muscle results in ***medial epicondylitis*** and rare ***flexor muscle rupture.*** Bony injury resulting in medial ***epicondylar avulsion*** is more likely to occur in the player with open growth plates. ***Ulnar neuritis*** may also be present due to the increased valgus-induced stretch and/or local inflammation in the cubital tunnel. In distinction to the often injured medial tension side, the lateral compression side of the elbow joint is relatively spared. Occasionally, ***osteochondritis dissecans (OCD) of the capitellum*** is present. Rarely, one may see lateral epicondylitis and extremely rare is the posterolateral instability of the elbow joint. Posteriorly, ***triceps tendinitis*** represents the myotendinous injury and the olecranon will reveal the effects of the bony injury. The stress-induced ***posterior osteophyte formation*** and occasionally ***fracture of the tip of the olecranon*** and posterior fossa ***loose body*** are usually all sequelae of the chronic valgus overload.

During the later stages, progressive ***degenerative changes*** occur in both medial and lateral compartments of the elbow with the production of osteophytes, loose bodies, and ***adhesive capsulitis. Distal biceps tendinitis*** may be present due to repetitive overuse; however, with sudden high-stress, ***disruption of the biceps tendon*** generally results, producing significant disability. Therefore, surgical treatment for this problem should be considered.

Skeletally immature players, particularly pitchers, are at risk for ***medial apophyseal injury.*** The spectrum begins with stress-related widening of the physeal plate to actual avulsion and displacement of the medial elbow apophysis. On the lateral side of the elbow, the young child (less than 10 years of age) may develop osteochondrosis of the capitellum (Panner's disease) and the older child (typically in the second decade of life) may develop OCD of the capitellum.

Ulnar neuritis is most frequently seen in association with an UCL injury, though it may be the sole diagnosis especially in the presence of ulnar nerve instability (subluxation or dislocation). Other neuropathies (median and radial) are rare and not characteristic in this sport.

Baseball-related injuries to the hand and wrist occur due to direct trauma. Wrist dorsiflexion may result in the fracture of the distal radius or navicular. While all of the carpal bones are vulnerable, the ***navicular fracture*** is the most common and the ***fracture of the hook of the hamate*** may present as diffuse wrist pain. The most common ligamentous injury of the wrist results in ***scapholunate instability.*** Pain on the ulnar side of the wrist may represent an injury to the ***triangular fibrocartilage*** or ***subluxing extensor carpi ulnaris.***

Direct trauma (due to sliding or direct blow) to the fingers, may result in disruption of the UCL of the thumb metacarpophalangeal joint (***gamekeeper's thumb***), extensor tendon avulsion or fracture at the distal interphalangeal joint (***mallet finger***) and a variety of ***phalangeal fractures.*** Repetitive overuse results in soft tissue injuries including tendinitis, muscle strains and skin conditions (***fingertip blisters and calluses***).

Spine injuries in baseball may occur from direct trauma; however, they are more common from repetitive overuse. ***Neck injuries*** must be carefully assessed, especially in the presence of any cervical spinal stenosis. The pivoting and twisting motion necessary in pitching and hitting will stress the thoracolumbar spine. Most common are the ***myotendinous strains*** of the paraspinal, intercostal, and occasionally abdominal musculature. Rotational and axial stress to the ***intervertebral disc*** result in annular tears and occasional ***disc herniation.*** Repetitive loads, particularly in hyperextension, may result in ***spondylolysis*** and occasionally ***spondylolisthesis.***

Acute trauma to the lower extremities is less common in baseball; however, it accounts for a significant number of disabling injuries. ***Muscular injuries*** may involve the ***hamstrings, quadriceps,*** and, less commonly, the ***gastrocnemius-soleus*** complex.

Collision- or contact-induced bony trauma may affect the ***femur, patella, tibia,*** or ***fibula*** but usually results in ***ankle and foot fractures.*** The foot is particularly vulnerable to the errant ball fouled off the bat. Even without a fracture, the presence of a ***subungual hematoma*** is quite disabling. Other entities, such as ***calluses, corns,*** and ***blisters,*** are relatively uncommon.

In baseball and softball, ***ligamentous injuries to the knee*** represent the entire spectrum: from the grade I medial collateral ligament sprain to the dislocated knee with possible neurovascular compromise. Sliding-induced injuries result in a disproportionately higher incidence of injuries to the posterior cruciate ligament. Other injuries to the knee include ***meniscal and articular cartilage trauma,*** with secondary chondromalacia, intraarticular loose bodies, and early osteoarthritis.

Ligamentous injuries to the ankle are common, generally involving the anterior talofibular ligament and less frequently the calcaneofibular ligaments. In the presence of pain along the anterolateral aspect of the ankle and distal leg, it is important to consider the less common but more disabling ***injury to the syndesmosis*** membrane with possible widening of the ankle mortise. Rarely, the ligamentous injury will be associated with an ***osteochondral fracture of the talar dome*** and intraarticular loose bodies.

Chronic overuse of the lower extremities may result in ***stress fractures*** of the tibia, fibula, fifth metatarsal, and, extremely rarely, the patella. These injuries are less common but may occur due to high-impact loading activities: the running program (a component of the cardiovascular training) and landing on the lower extremity during the late cocking phase of pitching.

66. BASKETBALL

David N. M. Caborn and Michael J. Coen

Basketball has become one of the most popular team sports in the United States and the world. Participation in the sport requires a significant amount of running, jumping, and pivoting. As a game, it has developed into a high-speed, fast-paced, contact activity, with its share of traumatic injuries despite being considered a "noncollision" sport. Female participation has increased at all levels of the game, as have the number of acute injuries to the anterior cruciate ligament (ACL). Injury incidence has been reported at 3.5 injuries per 10,000 hr participation for males and 4.9 injuries per 10,000 hr participation for females. These injuries include those from conditioning, overuse, traumatic contact, and deceleration noncontact episodes. Basketball is enjoyed by athletes of all ages, but the adolescent player is at an additional risk for physeal, epiphyseal, and apophyseal injury, as an increased entry into participation often coincides with pubescent growth increases.

Lacerations and abrasions can occur from contact with the floor, another player, or the rim and backboard. ***Eye trauma*** accounted for 5% of the injuries incurred in the 1992 National Basketball Association (NBA) season. Approximately one of three were during rebounding with approximately two of three from fingers and one of three from elbows. Some 50% involved ***eyelid injury,*** 29% had ***periorbital contusions,*** 12% suffered ***corneal abrasions,*** and 5% had ***orbital fractures.*** The vast majority were not wearing eye protection. Additional facial injuries include nasal and other ***facial fractures*** and ***fractured or dislodged teeth.***

Closed-head injuries in the form of ***concussions*** do occasionally occur, and treatment, including exclusion from play, should be determined according to standard guidelines. ***Sudden cardiac death*** has received national attention even though it is a very rare event. It is usually caused by a congenital structural predisposition and must be emergently recognized and treated as an acute cardiac event.

Injuries to the proximal upper extremity are relatively rare in basketball. An occasional problem of overuse shoulder impingement or a traction-type injury due to "rim hanging" may occur. Other injuries may include ***acromioclavicular joint contusion*** or ***anterior glenohumeral subluxation*** due to acute trauma or repetitive microtraumatic stresses. ***Wrist*** complaints due to repetitive stress and minor traumatic events are usually from ***tendinitis or capsulitis. Hand*** metacarpal and ***phalangeal fractures*** and ***joint dislocations*** are seen owing to "jamming" by ball contact. A fall on an outstretched hand many result in a ***scaphoid fracture*** or an ulnar collateral ligament ***"gamekeeper's thumb"*** injury. Fingertip microtrauma in the form of a mechanical ***contact dermatitis*** from excessive ball handling on rough outdoor courts has recently been termed "pebble fingers."

The central axial skeleton is less commonly an area of significant problem, with lower back pain being an occasional complaint. The lower extremity takes most of the physical abuse induced by a vigorous basketball season. ***Muscle strains*** are common and include ***hamstring*** (usually midsubstance of medial), adductor ***(groin), iliopsoas*** (hip flexors), and rarely a ***calf muscle*** (medial head of gastrocnemius). Common knee problems during the conditioning phase of the season include ***iliotibial band inflammation, an inflamed medial plica, pes anserinus bursitis, lateral patellar syndrome, Osgood-Schlatter disease, Sinding-Larsen-Johansson disease (jumper's knee),*** quadriceps or ***patellar tendinitis*** (or occasionally rupture), and ***patellofemoral tracking problems*** with lesions in the area of the trochlear groove and the undersurface of the patella. Knee injuries accounted for 12% of the male injuries and 19% of the female injuries in one recent National Collegiate Athletic Association (NCAA) basketball study. Recent studies have shown female participants to be at a significantly higher risk than their male counterparts for acute ACL injuries. The majority of these are noncontact events in the form of landing, cutting, and sudden deceleration. ***Meniscal and collateral ligament injuries*** are commonly seen in a similar or concurrent pattern. There is approximately a three times increased risk for injury during a game versus practice. Last, insidious knee pain and swelling in an adolescent may herald an early ***osteochondritis dissecans*** lesion that is becoming symptomatic.

Lower leg injuries are also very common during a basketball season. ***Lateral ankle sprains*** are almost endemic in the sport. Prophylactic semirigid ankle stabilizers have been shown prospectively to decrease the rate of ankle injuries in military cadets. No difference in the incidence of ankle injury could be shown prospectively when the use of high-top was compared with that of low-top basketball shoes. Rehabilitation for ankle sprains has been advanced to include on expectation for a fairly rapid return to play, with an emphasis on strengthening, balance, and proprioception for prevention of recurrence. Occasionally ***anterior ankle impingement*** may cause chronic anterior pain at the ankle joint line. Other lower leg injuries include the overuse conditions of ***shin splints*** (periosteal inflammation); ***stress fractures,*** including tibial (34%), fibular (24%), metatarsals (18%), and the other bones of the foot including the navicular; ***plantar fasciitis, plantar nerve entrapment, heel pad syndrome; tendon overuse*** including ***Achilles, peroneal, anterior*** or ***posterior tibial,*** **or** ***long toe flexor; calcaneal apophysitis*** (Sever's disease), and the everyday ***blisters and calluses.*** Occasionally a traumatic base of the fifth metatarsal ***(Jones)*** fracture or a peroneus brevis avulsion fracture, a symptomatic accessory navicular, a ***"turf toe"*** (capsular injury, MTP joint of great toe), or ***hallux rigidus*** are also seen.

Overall, the sport of basketball provides an opportunity for participating in a safe, healthy athletic endeavor for a high percentage of the active population. The demands and contact of a high-speed, advanced, competitive level of play do place the athlete at risk for both overuse and traumatic injury. A healthy regard for prevention—including prior injury identification during preseason physical examination, regular surveillance during intensive preseason conditioning, and an astute comprehension of injuries as they occur during the season, along with timely, appropriate therapeutic intervention—will allow the continual enjoyment of basketball for player and spectator alike.

67. BOXING

Barry D. Jordan

I. General Concepts

A. **Amateur versus Professional.** Injury patterns in boxing are dependent upon the level of participation (i.e., amateur versus professional, sparring versus competition). Boxing, both amateur and professional, operates under distinct and separate rules and policies (Table 67-1). In general, amateur boxing tends to be safer than professional boxing. The use of protective headgear in amateur boxing results a relatively decreased frequency of facial lacerations, orbital hematomas, and nasal injuries.

B. **Practice versus competition.** Injury rates and patterns in boxing also vary according to whether they occur during practice (including sparring) or competition. Although the injury rates in competition are higher than those in sparring, the absolute number of injuries may be higher in sparring. This is probably a reflection of longer hours exposed to sparring compared to competition. Since practice also includes activities other than sparring (e.g., rope jumping, shadow boxing, heavy bag, speed bag, endurance running), the types of injury also differ. Injuries tend to be of the chronic overuse nature of injuries versus the acute injuries encountered during a boxing match.

II. Specific Injuries

A. **Neurological injuries**

1. **Acute brain injury.** The overwhelming majority of acute brain injuries (ABI) in boxing are concussions. More typically, these concussions are not associated with true loss of consciousness. Severe types of ABI (i.e., diffuse axonal injury, cerebral contusions, and intracranial hemorrhages) are extremely rare. The most common catastrophic ABI in boxing is the subdural hematoma, which accounts for approximately 75% of the deaths attributable to boxing.
2. **Chronic brain injury.** Chronic brain injury (CBI) is the cumulative, long-term consequence of repetitive head trauma. CBI is also referred to dementia pugilistica, the punch-drunk syndrome, or chronic traumatic encephalopathy. Typically, CBI occurs after retirement or late in the career of a boxer after a relatively long exposure. The clinical characteristic of CBI may include:
   a. Dementia, or psychiatric disturbances
   b. Extrapyramidal tract dysfunction presenting as parkinsonism
   c. Cerebellar impairment, as evidenced by dysarthria, impaired coordination, and/or ataxia
   d. Increased spasticity secondary to pyramidal tract involvement

B. **Head (Nonneurological) facial injuries**

1. **Facial injuries.** Facial lacerations and hematomas are common in boxing. However, these injuries are seldom severe enough to warrant termination of a bout. A profusely bleeding laceration that impedes vision represents an indication to end a bout. Other indications to terminate a fight include a full-thickness laceration of the eyelid or an orbital hematoma that totally occludes the eye.
2. **Eye injuries.** Ocular injuries are relatively common in boxing.
   a. **Conjunctival injuries.** Conjunctival hemorrhage secondary to direct trauma to the eye is relatively common in boxing.
   b. **Injuries of the iris and ciliary body.** Injury to the iris and ciliary body may result in traumatic iridocyclitis or abnormal pupillary reactivity. Other injuries to the iris and ciliary body encountered in boxing include iris sphincter tear and traumatic hyphema. Boxers with traumatic hyphema may experience angle recession. Angle

Table 67-1. Comparisons between amateur and professional boxing

Rounds	Amateur—three 3-min rounds or five 2-min rounds	Professional—four to twelve 3-min rounds
Headgear	Yes	No
Regulation	National level (USA Boxing)	State or local level
Gloves	10–12 oz	8–10 oz
Passport system	Yes	Variable
Physician can terminate fight	Yes	No (with exceptions)

recessions of greater than 180 degrees are more likely to result in glaucoma. Although angle recession can occur in boxers, elevated intraocular pressure is rare.

c. **Lens injuries.** Traumatic cataracts can occur in 10% of professional boxers and tend to be of the posterior subscapular type. Cataracts in boxers seldom result in uncorrected visual acuity of less than 20/40.

d. **Vitreoretinal injuries.** Vision-threatening retinal lesions may be encountered in 15% of professional boxers. The majority of these retinal injuries were retinal holes and tears. Retinal detachments and macular pathology are relatively uncommon, occurring in approximately 3% of professional boxers. Treatment of retinal tears and holes can prevent the progression of retinal pathology. Continued boxing after repair of a retinal detachment is controversial and should be determined on an individual basis, considering the size of the lesion, its proximity to macula, and the quality of the repair.

e. **Orbital fractures.** Fractures of the inferior and medial wall can be encountered in boxing. The boxer with an inferior wall (blowout) fracture will present with vertical diplopia that is accentuated with upgaze because of the entrapment of the inferior rectus muscle within the fracture site. Fracture of the medial orbit occurs with forceful blows to the nose, resulting in a fracture through the ethmoid sinus. There may also be an associated nasal fracture.

3. **Nasal injuries.** Nasal injuries are common in boxing. The frequency of nasal injuries may be reduced with the utilization of protective headgear with cheek padding.

   a. **Epistaxis.** Epistaxis represents the most common type of nasal injury. The majority of bleeds are benign, originate from the anterior nasal septum (Hesselbach's plexus), and are easily controlled by applying pressure.

   b. **Nasal fracture.** Nasal fractures are relatively common in boxing and an indication for the termination of a competitive bout.

   c. **Septal hematoma.** Although infrequent, the formation of a nasal septal hematoma is an important medical concern because of the risk of infection. Septal hematomas should be drained.

4. **Ear injuries.** Trauma to the external ear can result in a subchondral hematoma (a collection of fluid within the layers of cartilage of the ear). Subchondral hematomas should be drained to prevent cartilage necrosis and cosmetic deformity (i.e., cauliflower ear). The frequency of subchondral hematoma and cauliflower ear is significantly reduced with the use of protective head gear. Rupture of the tympanic membrane can also occur in boxing as the result of a slapping blow to the ear, forcing air into the external auditory canal. If rupture of the tympanic membrane is associated with inner-ear pathology, the boxer will experience vertigo and/or ataxia.

5. **Jaw injuries.** The jaw is particularly vulnerable to traumatic injury in boxing. The mandible is susceptible to fracture, especially when struck with the mouth open. Temporomandibular joint (TMJ) pain and dysfunction can also be encounted in boxing.
6. **Dental/oral injuries.** Dental Injuries in boxing include tooth luxation, avulsion, or fracture. Alveolar fractures may also be encountered. Lacerations of the lip, tongue, or buccal mucosa are also frequently observed in boxing.

C. **Musculoskeletal injuries.** The majority of musculoskeletal injuries in boxing involves the upper extremities, in particular the hands, wrists, and shoulders.

1. **Hand/wrist injuries.** Injury to the metacarpophalangeal (MP) joint is relatively common in boxing because this joint is vulnerable to direct forces when the fist is clenched. The differential diagnosis of MP joint pain (boxer's knuckle) includes contusion, synovitis, rupture of the collateral ligament, articular fracture, capsular tears, and rupture of the extensor mechanism. Axial forces delivered down the shaft of metacarpal can result into carpometacarpal (CMC) pathology such as carpal bossing or metacarpal fractures. Thumb injuries are also relatively common in boxing. Hyperextension forces to the thumb can result in disruption of the MP joint's collateral ligament. Other injuries to the thumb include dislocation of the CMC joint and Bennett's fracture-dislocation. The utilization of the thumbless or thumb-attached glove can reduce thumb injuries. Fractures of the scaphoid may also be encountered in boxing.
2. **Elbow injuries.** Repetitive overload of the elbow can injure the medial collateral ligament. Hyperextension injuries of the elbow may also be encountered.
3. **Shoulder injuries.** Rotator cuff syndrome can be readily anticipated in boxing. Other shoulder injuries include instability of the glenohumeral joint and acromioclavicular (AC) joint separation.
4. **Injuries of the lower extremity.** These injuries tend to be of the chronic overuse type and are typically associated with roadwork and rope jumping. Common injuries to the lower extremity include ankle sprains, meniscal injury in the knee, and chondromalacia patellae.

D. **Thoracic and abdominal injuries.** Rib contusions and fractures are frequently encountered in boxing and are typically associated with body blows.

E. **Genitourinary injuries.** Testicular contusion may be encountered in boxing; however this injury is largely prevented by prohibiting "low blows" and using the protective cup. Punches delivered to the flank may be associated with renal injury, as evidenced by hematuria and albuminuria.

68. **CRICKET**

Answorth A. Allen

Cricket is one of the most popular spectator sports in the world. The game is played extensively in England and former British colonies. The game is played in North America primarily by immigrants from the West Indies and Asia.

A typical team consists of 11 players: two to four ***bowlers*** (pitchers), four to five ***batsmen,*** a ***wicket keeper*** (catcher), and one or two ***all-around*** players. Although all the members of the team will go to bat, only the specialist bowlers or all-around players will bowl. A test series is a match that will usually last for 5 days. More recently, 1-day test matches have become quite popular. The wickets are two sets of three wooden stakes pounded into the ground, each set of wickets being located at the end of a specially prepared surface of soft clay bounded with grass. The distance between the set of wickets is 22 yd. The objective of the bowler is to hit the wicket with the ball or to bowl the ball in such a way that the batsman will hit the ball in the air, allowing the fielder to catch it. A *fast bowler* can pitch the ball at speeds exceeding 95 mph. A *spin bowler* pitches the ball at a significantly lower speed but depends on the changing direction of the ball to hit the wicket. Depending on the condition of the surface, the ball will change its speed and direction. The bowling action is different from that of pitching in baseball. The fast bowler will run 50 to 75 yd to gain momentum and deliver the ball in an overhead motion with the elbow extended. The spin bowler depends on twirling the ball with the fingers and internal rotation of the shoulder to achieve the correct turns and twists of the ball.

The objective of the batsman is to score points and defend the wickets. Points or *runs* are scored when the batsman hits the ball and run between the wickets or when the ball is hit over delineated boundaries.

Cricket is a noncontact sport. The athletes are primarily at risk from direct trauma from the ball and from chronic overuse injuries. The ball weighs approximately 5.5 oz; when it is thrown or hit, it is a potentially lethal projectile. Overuse injuries are common because the professional players will play all year round. Generally very little emphasis is placed on off-season conditioning. The repetitive motions of activities like bowling place tremendous stresses on the shoulder and back.

Protective gear includes helmet, gloves, and padding for the legs and thighs. More recently, pads have been added to protect the ribs. Most of the gear is worn by the batsman. The bowlers and fielders typically wear no protection. When the ball is hit, it travels at significant speeds, and players are expected to catch the ball on the fly and to stop it with their bare hands.

Most of the injuries that occur in cricket are position-specific. The bowlers will often develop back and shoulder problems, while the batsmen and fielders are more at risk for traumatic injuries. During fast bowling, there is hyperextension and rotation of the thoraco-lumbar spine, which stresses the pars interarticularis and the facet joints. Poor bowling technique will exacerbate this problem. Low back pain is a common complaint in the fast bowler, and the differential diagnosis includes ***paraspinal muscle strains, spondylolysis, degenerative spondylolisthesis,*** and ***degenerative disc disease*** of the lumbar spine. *Stress fractures of the* ***pedicle*** can develop on the contralateral side in a vertebra with a pars fracture.

One of the most characteristic findings in the fast bowlers is that, as the years progress, they will have difficulty throwing the ball in from the outfield, but they are still able to bowl. My personal impression is that this is due to ***anterior subluxation*** of the glenohumeral joint, secondary to repetitive microtrauma to the joint capsule from bowling. Unless the shoulder laxity affects their ability to bowl the ball, these patients are best treated with physical therapy to strengthen the rotator cuff and periscapular muscle.

I have personally seen two cases of atraumatic partial ***anterior deltoid detachment*** in professional fast bowlers. They presented with acute onset of shoulder pain and inability to bowl the ball at high speeds. They subsequently developed heterotopic bone around the anterolateral aspect of the acromion and were successfully treated conservatively. A ***stress fracture*** *of the* ***humerus*** in a fast bowler has been reported.

Spin bowlers are more vulnerable to shoulder problems, specifically ***impingement syndrome*** and ***rotator cuff tears.*** As the spin bowler ages, he will often have problems lifting and keeping his arm up above the horizontal to obtain the appropriate spin on the ball. This is usually secondary to ***partial-*** or ***full-thickness tears*** of the ***rotator cuff.*** The *spinning finger* will often develop a painful deformity from stretching of the collateral ligaments of the interphalangeal joints.

The batsmen and fielders are more susceptible to traumatic injuries from the ball. Although the batsmen wear helmets and face visors, the fielders do not. Direct trauma to the head can result in ***closed head injuries,*** which can be potentially fatal. When the ball hits the ground at high speeds, it can change its direction rapidly and bounce toward the player. The athlete must often move quickly to avoid getting hit by the ball. ***Orbitozygomatic fractures*** can result from a direct blow to the face. Potential ***ocular injuries*** include traumatic ***retinal detachment, choroidal tears, ruptured globes,*** and ***traumatic iritis.***

Traumatic wrist and hand injuries are the most common injuries among cricket players. The wicket keeper and fielders are predominantly at risk, because they are constantly catching the ball thrown or hit at high speeds. The fielders do not wear gloves. Soft tissue injuries include ***hand lacerations, web-space injuries, mallet fingers,*** and ***wrist sprains. Nail bed*** injuries and ***digital nerve*** injuries can also occur, while flexor tendon injuries are rare. Distal ***phalangeal fractures*** are common, while ***metacarpal fractures*** are more unusual.

Muscle strains and ***contusions*** are common in the lower extremities. There is a significant amount of running in cricket, and *pulled* ***groins, adductor strains,*** and *pulled* ***hamstrings*** are not unusual. Although knee injuries are relatively unusual in cricket players, ***meniscal*** and ***chondral*** injuries can occur in the fielders and bowlers. ***Cruciate ligament*** *injuries* are unusual. Chronic overuse injuries to the knee include ***patellofemoral chondromalacia, patellar tendinitis,*** and ***Osgood-Schlatter*** *disease* in adolescent patients. The wicket keeper is especially prone to ***anterior knee pain*** and ***meniscal tears*** because of the constant squatting the position demands.

Overuse injuries of the foot and ankle injuries are fairly prevalent because of all the running required in cricket. ***Achilles tendinitis, metatarsalgia,*** and ***sesamoiditis*** are common problems. ***Stress fractures*** of the metatarsals and sesamoids are more unusual. ***Subungual hematoma*** of the great toe, ***corns, calluses,*** and ***blisters*** are common in bowlers, because they pivot against the shoes repetitively as the ball is delivered. ***Ankle sprains*** will frequently occur from cutting while fielding the ball.

The game is usually played under hot or humid weather conditions and some of the matches can last for days. ***Heat cramps, heat exhaustion,*** and ***heat stroke*** are constant concerns. Athletes can present with fatigue, headache, dizziness, confusion, and unconsciousness. They are given scheduled water breaks to allow them to replace body fluid and electrolytes.

69. CYCLING: ROAD, VELODROME, AND MOUNTAIN BIKING

Robert E. Hunter

The modern bicycle dates back approximately two hundred years, although its most popular version (the mountain bike) had its inception as recently as the early 1970s. In the past 15 years, biking has seen an explosion in popularity, with an estimated 40 million Americans riding a bike at least once a year. It is estimated that over 27 million adults ride at least once a week, 4 million use a bike to commute, and approximately 250,000 compete. In fact, bike sales were felt to surpass auto sales in the United States in 1987, and they have continued to exceed auto sales ever since. The economic implications of this popularity are profound, with an estimated $4 billion in bike and related merchandise sold on an annual basis. However, with this increased interest in biking has come the inevitable increase in injury. In the United States, it is estimated that there are in excess of 750,000 emergency department visits annually due to bike trauma, with approximately 1,000 deaths. Of those deaths, approximately 80% are directly attributable to head trauma. The total number of injuries resulting from bicycling is unknown, but given the fact that a very small minority of the overall injuries sustained result in medical evaluation or management, the total number of injuries is clearly considerable.

Those injuries that are sustained can be divided into three large groups: acute trauma, overuse injuries, and injuries secondary to environmental conditions. Although acute injuries vary somewhat with age and gender, most of the acute pathology seen involves the upper extremity. This reflects the fact that the energy from a fall is generally dissipated through an outstretched arm. In evaluating an upper extremity for a bike fall, one should pay special attention to the areas at greatest risk for damage. The ***scaphoid*** is the most commonly fractured carpal bone. The distal radius is also frequently fractured ***(Colles fracture)***. Injuries sustained at the level of the elbow will frequently result in ***fractures to the radial head.*** The humerus, including the proximal humerus, is relatively spared from fracture. However, the shoulder region itself is frequently traumatized as the result of a fall on the outstretched arm or directly on the apex of the shoulder. Two clinical entities are most common. First, an acromioclavicular ***(AC) joint separation,*** and second, a mid-third ***clavicular fracture.***

Acute injuries involving the lower extremity are relatively uncommon. Spoke-related trauma caused by catching parts of the foot within moving spokes is a problem seen with young children and also with adolescents where more than one person is being transported.

The area of most concern in acute injuries secondary to biking is ***head and neck.*** The majority of hospitalizations caused by bike injuries and a large majority of resultant deaths are secondary to head and neck pathology. Therefore, any evidence of neurologic dysfunction or neck complaint should be associated with very careful transport to a medical facility where complete neurologic evaluation can be performed to rule out serious intracranial or cervical spine problems. Fortunately, most of the acute pathology is relatively minor, reflected in the high incidence of contusion, abrasion, and laceration. All wounds should be thoroughly cleaned in order to avoid infection or "tattooing" of the skin caused by the imbedding of foreign material.

Overuse injuries in biking are more common and problematic, with the primary areas of involvement being the knee, shoulder, neck, back, hands, buttocks, and groin. These overuse injuries can be attributed to improper bike fit, improper training, or training to excess. In the knee, the primary area of concern is the extensor mechanism, with ***quadriceps tendinitis*** being most common. Other problems to be considered are ***patellar tendinitis, chondromalacia patella,*** or ***patellar malalignment*** caused by abnormal tracking by the patellofemoral articulation. Medial knee pain is generally secondary to ***pes anserinus bursitis,*** or ***intraarticular medial bands*** (plica), which can snap over the femoral condyle after repetitive motion. On the lateral side of the knee, ***iliotibial band tendinitis*** is the principal cause of overuse pain.

In the shoulder, overuse injuries reflect the fact that weight is being borne through the shoulder joint with biking. This results in ***impingement-type symptoms*** resulting from ***subacromial bursitis*** and ***rotator cuff tendinitis.***

Neck pain is a very frequent overuse injury. It occurs because the head is held in a forward position, with chronic extension due to the position of the handlebars. This results in ***muscle strain*** and trigger-point pain, which is frequently in the area of the levator scapulae and trapezius. The left side is more often affected than the right. Likewise the ***low back*** is subject to chronic fatigue and pain because of the body's position on the bike. Because the upper extremity supports at least part of the body weight, the hand, and particularly the ***ulnar nerve,*** is vulnerable to repetitive trauma. The nerve is traumatized in Guyon's canal and can result in either motor and/or sensory deficits over the ulnar nerve distribution. The buttocks and groin are susceptible to repetitive trauma because of their position on the bicycle seat and the heat and perspiration associated with distance training. This can result in cutaneous changes as well as actual infection, both superficial and deep. Nerve dysfunction secondary to pressure can also occur, with resulting numbness, impotence, and other ***genitourinary*** complications. Management of overuse injuries includes correcting bike fit, with key areas being proper seat height, proper seat positioning in a fore-aft orientation, and correction for proper forward lean and forward reach onto the handlebars. Common training errors to be corrected include using too slow a cadence and too high a gear rather than maintaining a more energy-efficient cadence of approximately 80 rpm in lower gears that reduce loads to the knee extensor mechanism.

Common environmental conditions that can affect bikers include acute ***altitude sickness***—particularly if biking is done at an altitude of more than 1,500 m (5,000 ft), ***hypothermia,*** and ***heat illness*** in the form of heat syncope (light-headedness or fainting caused by transient hypovolemia), ***heat cramps*** (secondary to hyponatremia), ***heat exhaustion*** (either sodium-depletion heat exhaustion or water-depletion heat exhaustion), and ***heat stroke*** (a life-threatening form of hyperthermia requiring immediate medical management).

70. DANCE

Marie D. Schafle

Dancers make up a unique segment of the athletic population. Because of the artistic nature of their activity, dancers rarely interrupt a performance for injury, preferring to delay treatment until after the performance or even after the season. It is necessary for the physician covering dance events to understand and accept this attitude while continuing to deliver the best possible care.

In actuality there are few injuries in dance that would absolutely preclude participation. Most can be treated while the dancer remains active. Definitive treatment can often be delayed until the end of the tour or the season. In the interim, physical therapy, taping or strapping, felt padding, and specific stretching and strengthening exercises can be combined with relative rest to keep the discomfort and disability at a minimum.

Since most professional ballet companies have a "team physician," the primary care physician can expect to work with community dance companies and to be asked to cover local events and recitals. The family physician may also be called upon to treat injuries incurred by students of community dance schools, to determine readiness for pointe work, to evaluate scoliosis, and to advise the dancer and her or his parents regarding menstrual irregularities and weight-control practices (issues best dealt with in the privacy of the physician's office).

Most injuries occur in class and at rehearsal. For those that occur during performance, treatment is usually not sought until after the conclusion of the performance. Suddenly disabling injuries that may require on-the-spot treatment are rare but may include acute fractures, dislocations, sprains, strains, and ruptured discs.

Acute Injuries of Dancers

Ankle Sprain

The etiology and treatment of ankle sprain is essentially the same as for any athlete except that, during performance, visible bracing is difficult if not impossible to use. Taping is practical for a performing dancer and can be covered with body makeup if necessary. The dancer may complain about the ankle feeling stiff after taping, but he or she should be encouraged to warm up with the ankle taped and then to reassess the feeling of stiffness.

Lumbosacral Sprain / Strain

Acute low back pain may occur quite suddenly and be very severe. Trigger-point injection is sometimes very helpful just before a performance but should not be used as a substitute for a rehabilitation program and learning of proper body mechanics for nondancing activities. The dance instructor should also be consulted regarding the possible need for correction of alignment.

Cuboid Syndrome

This is an unusual problem that presents with sudden onset of severe lateral midfoot pain and inability to bear weight on the affected foot. Some podiatrists can successfully manipulate this joint and achieve relief. Postreduction and also failed reduction treatment consists of lo-dye taping with a small felt "bump" under the cubometatarsal joint. This may also be utilized as a first-line treatment. It is is very effective for pedestrian activities but may not be effective for dance. It is worth trying, however.

Ruptured Achilles Tendon

In discussing surgical versus nonsurgical treatment, it is important for the dancer to be aware that, postoperatively, he or she will almost certainly lose some of the depth of the plie on the affected side. This may be more important to an individual dancer than the height of the jump (which might be decreased by nonoperative treatment).

This is definitely a condition that should be recognized quickly and referred to specialist immediately.

Ruptured Plantar Fascia
This is immediately disabling. This problem should immediately be referred to a podiatric dance specialist or to a dance orthopedist.

Pelvic Epiphysial Avulsion Fractures in Adolescents
These fractures are usually not a cause for immediate intervention and rarely require immobilization or surgery. Such patients should be referred to an orthopedic surgeon prior to the initiation of any treatment other than acute care. If the specialist is not available immediately, the patient should be placed on crutches until he or she can ambulate without limping and without pain.

Hamstring Strain
This injury, even if seemingly minor, should be completely rehabilitated to prevent chronic hamstring pain and recurrent strains in the future. Both hamstring flexibility and strength are extremely important for many dance movements and should be restored to that particular patient's normal level of flexibility and strength.

Gastrocnemius Strain
The gastrocnemius is very important for power en pointe, in jumping, and for flexibility in the plie, which is the preparation for every jumping movement. It should be completely rehabilitated in the dancer.

Important Note.
All one-sided injuries in dancers should be completely rehabilitated—that is, strengthened until the dancer is completely symmetrical or "centered." Failure to follow through with this will be the cause of many future problems for the dancer.

Chronic and Overuse Injuries of Dancers

Patellofemoral Pain Syndrome
This is more difficult to treat in dancers owing to the lack of supportive footwear and to the dancer's inability to wear braces (etc.) during a performance. Lo-dye and McConnell taping techniques *can* be used and covered with body makeup during performances.

Hip Flexor Tendinitis
This is usually a result of forcing turnout or of repetitive flexion (the dancer will describe this as her or his *extension*) of the hip (e.g., repeated grand battement in a particular choreography or barre exercise).

Flexor Hallucis Longus Tendinitis
Dancers often vigorously attempt to improve foot "extension" (i.e., plantarflexion) or forcibly attempt to increase plantarflexion strength. Many draconian methods are used in the dance community to impose certain skeletal attributes upon dancers who have not been genetically gifted with the "perfect dance body." When problems arise, it is helpful to ask the dancer what he or she has been doing to improve turnout and foot flexibility. The answers are often surprising and occasionally entertaining as well.

Posterior Ankle Impingement
Passive methods of attempting to increase plantarflexion can be a cause of posterior impingement. Any activity or condition (e.g., lack of strength in the dorsiflexors or hypermobility in plantarflexion) that causes the dancer to increase pressure on the posterior tibia and talus or to impinge the os trigonum can cause posterior impingement syndrome. Such a condition might, for example, be a sudden increase in the number of hours en pointe or a sudden change to a much more flexible pointe shoe. Surgery should be considered only in dancers at the preprofessional and professional levels. It is not indicated for a child not yet seriously considered for entry into the pro-

fessional levels by her instructors. It is important to speak with instructors as well as parents before determining the status of such a dancer.

Stress Fracture (Metatarsal, Tibial, Fibular)
These fractures are most common in the second metatarsal in women dancing en pointe and in the tibia for all dancers. They may be indicators of more serious hidden problems like anorexia, bulemia, or other eating or menstrual disorders. They are not improved by nondance employment that requires long hours weight bearing (e.g., waitressing).

Plantar Fasciitis
This condition is more common in dancers with high, stiff arches; it can be treated with lo-dye taping, arch pads, physical therapy, and supportive footwear to be worn apart from dancing.

Sesamoiditis and Fracture of the Sesamoids
This is usually a problem of repetitive jumping and landing. The dancer will complain of pain over the sesamoid in the demipointe position, when rolling up onto the pointe, and when jumping and landing. It is treated with a dancer's pad (see appendix 2) and antiinflammatory measures. Occasionally fractures may require removal of the sesamoid. This surgery is not to be considered lightly in a dancer, since the sesamoids contribute greatly to the dancer's balance when on demipointe.

Sciatica
The usual tests, such as straight-leg raising, can appear to be perfectly normal in the dancer. The physician must rely upon the dancer to discover whether the affected side is painful or less flexible. Another cause of sciatica is *piriformis syndrome*. However, this diagnosis is not common and has been much overused.

Quadriceps and Patellar Tendinitis
These problems occur mostly in adolescent males who are learning grand leaps and older males who may be doing choreographies requiring a sudden increase in the number of leaps done over a short period of time. The severity of the condition will dictate whether the dancer must be asked to observe only, relative rest or complete rest.

Osgood-Schlatter Syndrome
This can greatly impede the artistic growth of the dancer by decreasing ability to take class, especially those classes devoted to learning the great leaps.

Bunions and Corns
These are usually the purview of the podiatrist, although protective padding, moleskin donuts, judicious paring, and antiinflammatory measures may be provided by the primary care physician. Consultation with the local podiatrist regarding early measures that can be begun by the primary care physician will, in many cases, preclude the need for specialty referral.

Instructor–Physician Interaction

It is very important for the physician to defer to the dance instructor when suggesting alterations in technique. The physician should explain the physical problem and suspected cause and suggest that there be a team effort to modify activity. It is psychologically and physiologically very advantageous for the dancer to remain active in class as much as possible. In the event that an injury absolutely precludes weight bearing, a floor or water barre or pilates-based exercises can be substituted. It is important for the dancer to take only those parts of class that she or he can do while remaining "centered." A dancer's centering is a proprioceptive skill that is learned over years of dance training and involves near-perfect symmetry of weight bearing and movement. In the long term, loss of center can be more destructive to the dancer than the original injury.

71. DIVING: PLATFORM AND SPRINGBOARD

Benjamin D. Rubin

Approximately 10,000 athletes are registered with U.S. Diving and there are many more divers in Young Men's Christian Association (YMCA), club, and high school programs who are not members. National team members in the United States average 24 years of age and train an average of 4.5 hr per day, 6 days per week. Diving competition for men and women includes 1- and 3-m springboard, 10-m platform, and recently introduced 3- and 10-m synchronized events. The diver must show proficiency in forward, back, reverse, inward, and twisting dives. In platform diving, men are required to do armstand dives and women occasionally elect to do them. Dives can be done in the straight, pike, tuck, or free (a combination) positions. The necessary intricate maneuvers require strength, agility, balance, timing, quickness, and courage. Although injuries can occur during any phase of the dive, more occur during the entry than during the takeoff (which includes the approach, hurdle, and press) or the flight or midair maneuver. Entrance velocities from the 10-m platform can exceed 35 mph, requiring enough strength to maintain a handstand position with the added demands created by deceleration forces on the water surface. Because of the increased forces upon entry from the 10-m platform, injuries there are more common than in springboard diving.

Injuries can be divided into those affecting the musculoskeletal system (spine and extremities) and those of a nonorthopaedic nature. No gender differences have been observed in the type or incidence of injury. More experienced and older divers have demonstrated higher injury rates.

Diving-related injuries to the ***cervical spine*** have received attention because of the catastrophic nature of the injuries to the spinal cord reported in recreational divers. These injuries are usually related to a lack of formal training in diving, inadequate water depth, inadequate supervision, and, often, alcohol ingestion. There has not been a single reported fracture or dislocation of the cervical spine in organized competitive diving. There is a potential for noncatastrophic injuries from repetitive axial loading; however, degenerative changes have not been observed. ***Cervical sprains and strains,*** infrequently associated with ***brachial plexus stretch injuries,*** have been observed; however, owing to the protection afforded by the hands and arms during entry, they are less frequent than would be expected. Strains and sprains of the cervical, thoracic, and lumbar regions are usually related to twisting and arching during the flight and/or entry of the dive.

The sport of diving requires mobility and stability in the lumbar spine. The anterior segments (vertebral body, vertebral end plate, and intervertebral disc) are particularly vulnerable to the compressive forces and increased load during the press of the board, at entry, and with trunk flexion during flight. The combination of a flexed or rotated spine during maximum loading is most likely to lead to disc injury. Springboard diving places more stress on the lumbar spine because of the upwardly directed force during the press and the decrease in axial stress absorbed by the hips and knees compared with platform diving.

The posterior elements (facet joints, pars interarticularis) are subjected to overload during maximum lumbar extension or extension combined with rotation. This can occur during the takeoff for back or reverse dives, on entry for a back rotating dive short of vertical, or a front rotating dive beyond vertical. ***Spondylolysis, spondylolisthesis, "kissing spines,"*** and ***lumbar facet arthropathy*** have been observed. Segmental hypermobility, occasionally in response to segmental hypomobility, is frequently the cause of middle and ***low back pain*** in divers.

Shoulder injuries are frequently precipitated by the multidirectional laxity required to perform the complex technical maneuvers and the weakness of the scapular stabilizers. Occasionally a single incident will disrupt the delicate balance of the musculature of the capsule-labral complex and shoulder girdle. More often, the repetitive microtrauma associated with overhead use, repetitive impact, "swimming" entries, and "saving" short dives leads to the progressive failure of the anterior ligaments. In both cases the result is the conversion of laxity to ***instability.*** Thus, problems related to instability are more common in more experienced divers. The diagnosis is made more difficult by the coexistence of ***traction tendinitis*** of the supraspinatus, infraspinatus, teres minor, and/or long head of biceps. Although true impingement syndrome is uncommon, ***subacromial bursitis*** and ***tears of the supraspinatus*** have been observed.

Elbow injuries occur upon impact with the water while the elbow is locked in extension. These include tears of the ***medial collateral ligament, strains or tears of the triceps*** mechanism (usually at the musculotendinous junction), and ***ulnar neuritis.*** Triceps injuries are more common in age-group divers because of their relative muscle weakness.

Wrist injuries occur from repetitive impact and forced dorsiflexion on entry utilizing the flat-hand technique, especially in platform divers. The most common injuries observed include ***dorsal impaction syndrome, volar subluxation of the lunate*** (occasionally associated with secondary subluxations), ***dorsal ganglion cyst, flexor carpi ulnaris tendinitis,*** and milder ***sprains. Hand injuries*** include sprains of the ***ulnar collateral ligament of the thumb*** as a result of "missing the grab" with the opposite hand before entry, ***contusions and fractures of the metacarpals and phalanges*** from striking the board, and contusion of the hand on the cranium seen in young divers with inadequate strength to lock the elbows on entry.

Most lower extremity injuries are associated with jumping. Patellofemoral problems include ***patellar tendinitis, quadriceps tendinitis, maltracking patella,*** and ***patellar compression syndrome.*** Also observed are ***posterior tibial and Achilles tendinitis, tibial periostitis, stress fractures of the tibia,*** and ***tendinitis in the foot*** and ankle. Ankle and foot sprains and ***fractures of the fifth metatarsal*** can occur when the foot lands in an awkward position during the approach or on landing from the hurdle on the springboard. ***Fractures of the metatarsals and phalanges*** may result from striking the board during flight.

Most nonorthopaedic injuries sustained by divers affect the eyes and ears and are related to the forces exerted upon entry into the water. ***Perforations of the tympanic membrane, vestibular abnormalities, retinal detachment,*** and ***ocular contusions*** have been observed. ***Otitis externa*** (swimmer's ear) is frequently related to retained moisture in the ear canal. ***Pulmonary contusion*** and ***hemoptysis*** can occur as a result of landing flat on the water surface from the 10-m platform. Pneumothorax has not been observed. All divers have returned to full workouts within 48 hr. ***Scalp lacerations*** occur on inward or reverse dives when the diver leans toward the board while spinning in that direction. There is usually significant bleeding and occasional loss of consciousness. Neurologic sequelae other than headaches are rare. Fatal head injuries have occurred in two cases in which divers struck their heads on the 10-m platform while attempting a reverse 3½ somersault in the tuck position.

72. ENDURANCE EVENTS: MARATHON, ULTRAMARATHON, TRIATHLON

Warren A. Scott

These three events (marathon, ultramarathon, and triathlon) share many common medical and musculoskeletal problems and present a number of hazards and environmental challenges. Specifically, problems related to high altitude, excessive heat and humidity, or extreme cold water pose threats to the competing athlete. Injuries, hypothermia, hyperthermia, near-drowning, dehydration, electrolyte imbalances, hypoglycemia, seizures, bowel ischemia, circulatory collapse, and death from combined systems failure can occur. Prevention is the key, with proper supervision by medical and safety personnel guiding the race through the lowest-risk scenarios. It is essential that these individuals have the authority to control portions of the race and carry out the medical disqualification if an athlete is in trouble. Proper education of the athletes via race promotion information is an important move toward safer events. For athletes participating in these sports, preparation for the specific challenges of each event is an important (and overlooked) component.

Many injuries can plague the enthusiastic endurance athlete. Of these, most are secondary to training errors. Increases in training volume or intensity can produce a variety of injuries from the low back to the big toe and everything in between.

Running causes many common injuries. ***Plantar fasciitis*** is an insidious problem that has a variety of direct and indirect causes. The pain is most commonly felt along the medial calcaneal tubercle but can vary anywhere along the entire plantar fascia. Improper shoe gear, training errors, or direct trauma received from walking barefoot on rough surfaces can precipitate an injury to the plantar fascia. Treatment is geared toward protecting the injury site, correcting biomechanical imbalances, and proper foot support. The most common ***stress fractures*** of the foot involve ***metatarsal shafts 3 and 4.*** Palpating pain directly over the metatarsal shafts reveals the diagnosis. X-rays can remain negative for up to 1 month in some cases and are not reliable in predicting return to running. ***Fifth metatarsal fractures*** occur at the tuberosity (usually not serious) or just distal to the tuberosity (Jones fracture, which is serious). ***Tarsal navicular*** and ***calcaneous stress fractures*** are less common and can be difficult to detect. A high index of suspicion would lead to diagnostic imaging. ***The first metatarsal phalangeal joint*** is subject to a variety of problems. The two ***sesamoid bones*** can become contused during the push-off phase of running. ***Hallux valgus*** (bunion) is a product of genetics, foot deformation from shoe pressure, and walking mechanics. Abnormal joint biomechanics can lead to progressive joint destruction and may set off a chain reaction of injuries further up the leg. ***Hallux rigidus*** is like hallux valgus, but the stiffness severely affects flexion and extension. This limits the the push-off phase during running, which can lead to problems affecting the foot, tibia, knee, or hip. ***Metatarsalgia*** describes a contusion to the second, third, and fourth metatarsal heads, usually from running on rough terrain. Proper selection of running shoes can be key here. ***Nerve injuries*** can occur with any nerve anywhere in the foot. The culprits are pressure and friction, either inside the foot or on its surface. Careful examination will reveal the diagnosis. ***Interdigital neuroma*** (Morton's) is commonly found in the third metatarsal interspace. The posterior tibial nerve is trapped in the ***tarsal tunnel,*** found just below the medial malleolus, producing the equivalent of the carpal tunnel syndrome in the wrist.

Running on trails can lead to an ***inversion sprain;*** however the vast majority of ankle injuries are overuse. Top on the list of injured structures is the ***gastrocnemius–Achilles tendon–calcaneous complex.*** The exact site of tissue breakdown and the specific injury pattern can vary depending upon the "sports-specific stress pattern." ***Achilles tendinitis*** is a runner's nightmare. The appearance of swelling at midportion of the tendon is an ominous sign. The newest terminology is ***tendinosis,*** and this condition can be seen on magnetic resonance imaging (MRI; mucoid degeneration). Healing time for mucoid degeneration is usually 9 to 18 months. The injury site can also manifest at the tendon-bone interface. The pre–and post–Achilles tendon ***bursae*** can become inflamed and further complicate the problem. The ***posterior tibial*** and ***peroneal tendons*** are also subject to injuries. The peroneal tendon becomes injured during an inversion sprain, which can produce partial or complete tears. ***Ganglion cysts*** can develop at any site around the ankle; they may reach 2 cm in size and be painless.

The lower leg is susceptible to a injuries that occur along a continuum from ***muscle strain to tendinitis to periostitis to tibia stress fractures.*** The exact point of tissue failure may be identified with a careful physical exam and any combination of x-rays, bone scan, and MRI. The diagnosis must include a biomechanical analysis of the problem in order to construct a definitive treatment plan. Additional problems of the shin include ***exertional compartment syndromes*** of the lower leg. The history and the physical examination can differentiate compartment syndrome from tibial stress fractures/tendinitis. If conservative treatment fails (trial period up to 4 months) then compartment pressures should be measured for the possible consideration of surgical release.

The term ***runner's knee*** or ***patellofemoral syndrome*** is self-explanatory. Hard downhill running, especially on uneven terrain, is one of the fastest methods for precipitating an injury. One race 10 to 20 km in length run hard by an ill-prepared athlete can damage the patellofemoral joint so severely that healing may require 4 to 12 months. Careful examination will differentiate three distinct entities: (1) tenderness under the medial patellar facet, (2) tenderness along the side of the patella, and (3) tenderness on the patellar tendon. Diagnostic arthroscopy would reveal ***chondromalacia patella, synovitis*** or ***plica band.*** Pain along the patellar tendon, is called different names depending on age. The juvenile form is called ***Osgood-Schlatter*** syndrome (tibial tubercle apophysis) and ***Sinding-Larsen-Johanson*** (distal patellar apophysis) syndrome. The adult form of ***patellar tendinitis*** may present with pain anywhere along the tendon; however, beware of the chronic condition at the medial, distal pole of the patella-tendon interface. This point can undergo mucoid degeneration and can take 12 to 24 months to rehabilitate. Pain along the lateral aspect of the knee can be an enigma. The lateral side of the knee is a convergence of many structures, including the ***lateral collateral ligament, the popliteal tendon, the iliotibial tendon,*** and the ***lateral meniscus.*** Very careful history and physical examination is required. For this area an MRI is a helpful imaging study. Sometimes arthroscopy is the only way to make the final diagnosis. The ***iliotibial band friction syndrome*** is frequent in runners and infrequent in cyclists. Supinated feet, tight buttocks/thigh/calf muscles, lateral bowing of the leg, wider pelvis, downhill running, and canted road surfaces are contributory factors. ***Bursitis*** and ***synovitis*** presents as ***Baker's cyst*** in the popliteal fossa, or ***pes anserine bursitis*** along the medial tibial plateau, at the termination of the medial hamstring tendons. Middle aged and older athletes can develop ***degenerative meniscal tears*** by sprinting and trail running.

Thigh injuries are less frequent in occurrence but can be more devastating to the athlete. Acute muscle pulls of the ***rectus femoris*** and ***semimembranosus*** are the more common types. These can be graded mild (muscle knot), medium (knot plus mild hemorrhage), and severe (large hemorrhage). These pulls occur during faster-paced training runs or late in the marathon/ultramarathon/triathlon, when dehydration, fatigued legs, and muscle glycogen depletion occur. Immediate management with ice, compression, massage, and stretching can significantly decrease tissue damage. Keeping the muscle in slight tension as much as possible significantly speeds healing. ***Chronic low-grade muscle strains*** can occur in the calf, hamstring, or quadriceps. A combined therapy approach of stretching, deep tissue massage, tension-producing night splints, progressive strengthening, and counterforce bracing can produce a cure. ***Stress fractures*** of the femoral shaft are rare and present with vague symptoms. X-rays are not accurate and bone scan should be an early consideration.

The most common hip problems are ***gluteal/iliotibial strain/tendinitis,*** and ***greater trochanteric bursitis.*** Etiologic factors include overtraining, fast downhill running, or running on uneven terrain. Not stretching after running can lead to progressive muscle tension buildup in the low back and buttocks, rendering these muscles susceptible to strain. The ***femoral neck stress fracture*** is a serious condition. Diagnosis may be elusive but can usually be revealed via the medical history, high index of suspicion, and a confirmatory bone scan. Thin female athletes, high mileage (more than 60 km per/week), and poor biomechanics (heavy-footed runner) will contribute to the problem. A vague ache in the groin is the first symptom. Full fracture with displacement can occur if the problem goes untreated. ***Osteoarthritis*** of the hip (and knee) is seen in runners who are over age 50. Pain, time off from running, medication usage, and long-term prognosis tend to vary from individual to individual. "Remissions" from arthritis whereby the patient/athlete can return to running without pain (and without medications) may sometimes occur.

The pelvis is susceptible to a number of different problems. ***Stress fractures*** of the ***pubic rami*** can develop and present with vague symptoms. Juveniles suffer from ***apophysitis*** along the iliac crest, anterior superior iliac spine, and ischium. ***Osteitis pubis*** is an injury to the pubic symphysis, resulting from shear overload and asymmetrical running postures. Several different tendinopathies can also affect the pelvis. The ***rectus abdominis, adductors, gluteals, piriformis,*** and ***proximal hamstring tendons*** can all exert a traction overload on the pelvis, provoking a periostitis or tendinitis. Chronic problems in this area can be secondary to injuries in the sacroiliac joint and the lumbar spine. Biomechanical neutral running posture is an essential part of the treatment plan.

Low back pain is a frequent complaint in modern society. It is important to differentiate whether the problem is secondary to running. ***Degenerative disc disease*** of the lumbar spine is a common progressive problem that is probably caused by poor posture, prolonged sitting, and poor physical conditioning. Leg asymmetry, weak abdominals, tight hamstrings, bent-over running posture, and uneven running surfaces are additional risk factors. Many back experts recommend physical exercise as treatment, and most runners with this condition will verify that they feel fine while running. Treatment plans must be individualized, since no specific pattern will reliably predict a runner's outcome. Regardless of the problem, most runners can be successfully rehabilitated and return to running.

All runners are subject to the above problems; however, due to the length of the ultramarathon event (6 to 30 hr), several seemingly benign problems can grow to large proportions. ***Runner's nipples, corns, calluses,*** and ***blisters*** are common among "ultra runners." Early recognition of "hot spots" is essential during these long events. The skin receives much abuse and may break down and bleed during the course of one race. The tricks of the trade include lubricants on the skin, "corn pads" to protect the nipples, synthetic socks that wick away moisture, and changes of running shoes during a race. Profound dehydration and energy depletion can occur in the novice ultramarathon runner. These races are frequently held on trails and at higher elevations, where additional hazards include slips, falls, sprained ankles, sunburn, and bee stings. Preparation must include altitude acclimatization and training oneself to eat and drink on the run.

The triathlete is susceptible to all of the aforementioned problems, plus the additional insults from swimming and bicycling. Swim training is associated with a variety of overuse injury patterns to the shoulder. Repetitive interval training and the use of hand paddles can overload the shoulders of swimmers in search of improved performance. ***Supraspinatus tendinitis*** is very common and results from overtraining, strength and flexibility imbalances, shoulder instability, and improper technique. ***Biceps tendinitis*** is another frequent problem in swimmers and is usually experienced only in the long head of the tendon. Both of these tendinopathies can be short-lived and mild or longstanding and severe, with progressive tendon deterioration and possible rupture. Open-water swimming requires lifting the head out of the water to sight position, which can produce ***cervicothoracic strain.*** Cold-water swims (55° to 65°F, 12° to 18°C) can place the swimmer at risk for ***muscle cramps*** and ***hypothermia,*** thus increasing the risk of drowning. Warm-water (over 80°F, 26.6°C) hazards include ***hyperthermia*** and ***venomous stings.***

Bicycle-related problems are either traumatic falls (85% to the head, neck, and shoulders) or overuse. Common overuse injuries include ***compression*** of the ***ulnar*** and ***median nerves*** in the wrist, ***pudendal nerve*** in the perineum, and ***interdigital nerves*** of the foot (***Morton's neuroma***). The aerodynamic racing posture used in the triathlon produces excessive strain on the ***cervicothoracic spine. Cervical disc disease*** is a common complaint among many mature cyclists. The ***patellofemoral joint, patellar*** and ***iliotibial tendons*** can become injured; however, this is more frequent in runners. Proper equipment selection and bike fit are essential precautionary measures. Long bike rides can produce skin irritation at pressure points along the saddle, causing ***perineal abscesses.*** Preventive lubrication and hygiene of the skin of this area is an important first aid step.

During triathlon races (2 to 17 hr), additional problems occur during the transition from one event to the other. The swim-bike transition promotes orthostatic changes as blood shifts from the upper body to the legs. Cramping may occur in the legs with the first few steps out of the water. The excitement of the race can cause an unsuspecting athlete to pull a calf, hamstring, or quadriceps muscle. During the bike ride, it may be necessary to consume large volumes of fluid and carbohydrates in order to maintain fluid homeostasis, body cooling, and blood sugar levels. The bike-run transition is the most difficult phase. At this point in the race, the athlete is often suffering from fatigue and dehydration, possibly hyperthermia, electrolyte imbalances, muscle cramping, and confusion. Proper race preparation and pacing strategies are the best prevention. The medical team must remain vigilant for compromised athletes and institute a medical disqualification if the safety of the competitor is in jeopardy.

73. EQUESTRIAN ACTIVITIES

Anastasios V. Korompilias and Anthony V. Seaber

Each year in the United States an estimated 30 million people ride horses, and half of these ride on a regular basis. Equestrian activities are diverse in character and include fox hunting, polo, point-to-point races, dressage, calf roping, trail riding, jumping, and showing, while professionals are involved in all types of showing, jumping, and racing as well as harness racing and rodeos. These activities offer excitement and vigorous exercise demanding a high degree of athletic skill, but they also carry a measure of risk. Horseback riding is the only sport in which the two partners are members of two different species and the athlete is not always in control of his or her destiny.

The mechanism of the injury influences the injury sustained and is of some importance in the management of the patient. Most equestrian injuries occur in falls from the ridden horse (63% to 99%) and mainly involve the upper part of the body. The unpredictability of the accident and the capacity of the horse to travel at speeds up to 30 mi (50 km) per hour with the rider's head approximately 3 m from the ground creates an opportunity for serious injury. Injuries to the upper half of the body occur if the rider lands on the outstretched arms, the shoulder, or the back or the head, while injuries to the thoracolumbar spine occur if the rider lands on the buttocks. A variety of minor and serious injuries can be produced: soft tissue injuries; ***fractures of the clavicle; fracture of the humerus; fractures and dislocations around the elbow; fractures of the forearm, wrist, and the hand; multiple fractures of the ribs with internal chest injuries and complications; blunt abdominal injuries; closed head injuries; skull fractures; spinal fractures or dislocations;*** and finally, but not rarely, ***lethal craniocerebral injuries.*** Another hazard arising from a fall is that the rider may be kicked by the horse as it tries to regain its feet or the horse may step on the rider. Sometimes, having survived falling from the horse the rider may be injured when another horse kicks or treads on him or her. Kick injuries usually occur at a point of contact 1 m above the ground and thus involve the lower part of the back, the buttocks, groin and thigh, or the patient's chest, abdomen, head, or face if the rider was bending forward at the time of injury. Stepping or trampling injuries vary from mild ***contusions and fractures of the foot and toes*** to more severe ones such as ***cerebral contusions, comminuted fractures of the lower leg,*** or damage to the trunk. Horses can weigh 1,000 lb (450 kg), so that compression injuries—including ***fractures of the pelvic ring, ribs, and injuries of the lower extremity***—may be inflicted if the horse rolls over or falls backward on its rider after rearing. If the rider's leg is trapped beneath the horse as it lands, major ***ligamentous injuries of the knee, tibial fractures,*** and ***injuries of the ankle and foot*** are common. Being dragged by the reins after falling may cause relatively mild injuries, while being dragged by a foot caught in the stirrup generally results in severe injuries or lethal events from repeated blows against the ground or objects (e.g., walls, tree branches) as the rider is dashed against them. Serious injuries including ***fractures of the facial bone, nose, and teeth*** as well as, ***head injury*** may result from the rider's face striking on the horse's neck when the horse rears or throws its head backward. Although ***rope burns and fractures of the fingers*** are the most common injuries following entanglement of the hand and fingers with the reins, inappropriate grip of the reins or halter rope while leading a horse may result in ***avulsion injury to a finger or thumb. Flexor tendinitis*** can be caused by prolonged gripping of the reins. ***Myositis ossificans*** of the hip adductor muscles has been seen in horseback riders.

Undoubtedly the majority of accidents occur when the patient falls from a horse. However, a significant number of injuries occur while handling horses (1% to 27%), the most serious injury related to being kicked. Horse bites also occur and tend to consist of severe crushing injury of soft tissues. If ***lacerations*** occur, they should be treated in the same manner as other animal bites. In addition to *Staphylococcus* and *Streptococcus* infections, horse bites may involve *Bacteroides* spp., *Clostridium tetani,* and rabies.

Although medical studies concerning equestrian activities sometimes present conflicting data, sufficient information is available to define the demographics and injury patterns of equestrian injuries. The most common location of horse-related injuries is the upper extremity (24% to 61%), with injuries to the lower extremity second in frequency, comprising nearly 25% of injuries in all equestrian activities according to the reports of the National Electronic Injury Surveillance System (NEISS). Approximately 20% of horse-related injuries occur to the head and the face, with a 10% incidence of spinal injuries. An estimated 22.4% of horse-related accidents comprise injuries to the upper and lower trunk.

Soft tissue injury (e.g., laceration, contusion, or abrasion) is the most common type of injury (45.7%), followed by fracture or dislocation (27.6%). ***Concussion*** is the third most common type of injury (10% to 15%). Of the injured persons, 5% to 10% required hospitalization, with the most common diagnosis being concussion and fracture. Furthermore, 2% of the riders with ***head and spinal injuries*** had persistent posttraumatic disabilities attributed to damage of the central nervous system trauma (posttraumatic epilepsy).

Higher rates of injuries occur in 5- to 24-year-olds because persons in this group are more likely to ride horses. More women than men engage in equestrian sports from age 5 to 24 years, and more women have equestrian accidents than men. From 24 to 44 years of age, men and women have similar injury numbers, while over 44 years, men have an increasing incidence. Most of the accidents occur during recreational riding or riding lessons rather than at competition. A different pattern of injuries can be identified with professional jockeys. Most jockeys sustain injuries to the limbs, whereas amateur riders sustain lesions to the head and face. Head and spinal injuries in jockeys are infrequent, which may be attributed to better head protection or more rigid safety standards.

The risks for severe injury related to equestrian activities are well defined, and it is not an exaggeration that horse riding carries high participant morbidity and mortality. The severity of riding injuries has been compared with that of injuries sustained by motorcyclists and automobile racers. Although mortality in equestrian activities is less than 1%, lethal accidents have been reported in numerous studies from neurosurgical sources. Craniocerebral injuries caused over 70% of deaths, followed by chest and abdominal injuries. Accidents in females before the age of 25 and in males over this age are more common. Although more women have horse-related accidents than men, this probably is because more women ride horses than men, yet men have almost 1.5 the total number of deaths in equestrian accidents.

Horse-related injuries in comparison with those from other sports activities are fewer in number but are considerable in severity. Head injuries constitute the major etiology of more serious injuries and, unfortunately, most of the reported accidents occurred without the use of protective headgear. Head protection by appropriate helmet use is of great importance in reducing the incidence and severity of equestrian-related injuries. Helmets meeting the requirements of the American Society for Testing and Materials (ASTM) provide excellent protection when appropriately secured. In addition to protective headgear, proper riding clothing, boots, and adequate training in the handling and care of the horse and falling techniques could also decrease the incidence and severity of equestrian accidents. There is no doubt that safety practices among horseback riders improve when the riders are trained by certified instructors with teaching experience who have successfully completed a horse safety course from an accredited organization that emphasizes safe riding techniques.

74. FENCING

Rebecca Jaffe and Julie Moyer Knowles

Fencing is a sport in which two people attempt to score touches or points by making their weapon contact their opponent. In international competitions their are three weapons with different scoring rules. The ***foil*** is scored when the tip of the weapon touchs the torso. The entire body is a legal target for the tip of the ***epee.*** The ***sabre*** can be scored when the tip or the cutting edge makes contact, but the legal areas are only the torso, head, and arms. Unique to this sport is the playing field, called a ***piste.*** It is a linear strip approximately 5 ft wide and 47 ft long.

Improper training and conditioning can lead to problems related to fatigue and balance and thus a higher incidence of injury. By nature of the sport there is a predominance of one side of the body, with the weapon arm and the lead leg; however, it is important to stress bilateral strengthening for injury prevention. The type of weapon used does not seem to relate to injury distribution, but more contact injuries occur with the epee because the legal target area is the entire body.

Injuries most commonly seen in this sport are ***sprains*** (muscle), followed by ***strains*** (ligaments). ***Contusions*** are also a common consequence of fencing from the strike of the weapon. The most common area affected is the lower extremity. This is because the piste may be concrete, thus making ***heel bruises*** and ***joint trauma*** possible. The piste can be an elevated platform from which the athlete may fall; thus ***ankle sprains*** are commonly seen. In addition, ***tendon ruptures*** and frank ***fractures*** may also occur. Ankle sprains are the most common significant injury in the sport.

The equipment and facilities account for about one-fourth of all injuries. Personal factors including poor technique, inadequate warmup, fatigue, and dangerous tactics may factor into about half of all injuries.

The stance of the fencer's trail leg is a planted, flexed, and externally rotated valgus stressed position. This makes the leg prone to acute injuries such as ***medial collateral ligament sprains, medial meniscal tears, lateral subluxating patella, groin strains, ruptured Achilles tendons,*** and ***eversion ankle sprains.*** The front leg is prone to ***quadriceps strains, blisters,*** and ***nail contusions*** including ***subungual hematomas.***

The weapon itself can cause ***contusions*** as well as ***lacerations.*** These lacerations can occur anywhere on the body but are most commonly seen about the target areas—the torso, arm, and head. There are rare reports of ***penetrating wounds*** despite careful checking of equipment. Weapons are known to break. There have been reports of punctures of the lung, creating a pneumothorax. Case reports include two immediate deaths due to penetrating wounds to the brain. Survival from penetrating lesions to the brain has also been reported. These injuries occurred despite vigorous checking of equipment, including a spring-loaded point to the mask at 12 kg of force. At events the physician is responsible for providing emergency treatment as necessary and as referred from the athletic trainer.

Overuse injuries are very common in these athletes. They must maintain a balanced position with weapon poised in a correct stance for prolonged periods of time. ***Tendinitis of the wrist and hand*** are seen. Many fencers suffer from ***lumbosacral strains*** mostly involving the trunk extensor musculature. ***Iliotibial band syndrome*** due to the stance is also seen. The hyperpronated stance and poorly supportive footwear lead to an increase in ***plantar fasciitis, posterior tibialis tendinitis, shin splints, stress fractures,*** and possibly ***periostitis of the navicular.***

Heat injury/illness is frequently seen. The venues are warm and the clothing is restrictive. The lack of hydration may cause ***muscle cramps*** as well. Intravenous fluids are sometimes used between bouts for quick and reliable rehydration.

Foreign bodies about the eye are another frequently seen problem during practice and competition.

The maximum time allowed for treatment of an injury is 10 min during a bout. The injury must be confirmed by a Federation Internationale de Escrime (FIE) medical representative or a physician or trainer on duty. If a player cannot be cleared in that time by the qualified medical person, he or she must withdraw from the event. If the player returns to competition that day and suffers from the same injury, the fencers immediately forfeit that event. In team competitions, in order to return to competition, the fencer must be cleared by the appropriate medical representative. There are no time outs allowed for muscle or heat cramps.

After adjusting for exposure time, there does not appear to be a gender difference when it comes to injuries in fencing.

75. FIELD HOCKEY

Cato T. Laurencin and W. Jay Gorum II

More than 100,000 athletes currently participate in field hockey in the United States, and the popularity of the sport has grown steadily throughout the decade. Field hockey athletes range in age from 9 to 60 years, and 80% are females. Individuals compete at both the club and team level and skills range from beginner to Olympian. Little has been written regarding injuries among field hockey athletes, but with the tremendous growth this sport is experiencing it is important for those in sports medicine to be aware of the patterns of injuries that can be found.

The lower extremity is the *most common* region for injury in field hockey, with ankle ligamentous problems and overuse type injuries predominating. This region accounts for approximately 60% of serious injuries that are encountered. The *second most common* region for injuries is the upper extremity, particularly the hands and fingers. This is followed by face and head injuries as the *third most common* site, with less than 20% of injuries seen in this region.

Field hockey requires skills in running, dribbling, accelerating/decelerating quickly, and the ability to change direction abruptly on grass and/or Astroturf surfaces. Loss of balance can happen while executing these maneuvers, and often this occurs in association with incidental contact with an opposing players stick. The ***ankle sprain*** is the *most common* acute injury seen. The ankle is also vulnerable to ***traction-compression spur*** phenomena at the ***medial and lateral malleoli*** and to ***malleolar fractures. Overuse injuries*** are quite common and must be continually watched for by the sports medicine practitioner. The overuse injuries seen include ***shin splints, medial tibial stress syndrome, chronic compartment syndrome, iliotibial tendinitis, stress fractures of the tibia,*** and ***hamstring/groin strains.*** The ***patellofemoral stress syndrome*** is very common among teenage female athletes who play field hockey. ***Achilles tendinitis*** can occur in an overuse setting and/or with inadequate warm-up. This condition can predispose athletes to Achilles tendon tears.

Acute trauma about the knee can lead to such injuries as ***meniscus tears, soft tissue contusions, abrasions, lacerations, various types of bursitis, ligamentous sprains,*** and frank ***ruptures,*** particularly involving the ***ACL (anterior cruciate ligament),*** and the ***MCL (medial collateral ligament).***

Injury rates in field hockey are greater (in general) on Astroturf than on grass. In the middle-aged female athlete with unilateral burning pain of the foot, the most likely diagnosis is ***Morton's neuroma.*** Shin guards prevent much of the direct acute trauma seen from the ball and stick, but the knees, quadriceps, and feet are still vulnerable.

About 80% of all athletes experience ***back injury/pain*** at some point while playing field hockey. This rate is much higher than that in most other field sports. The mechanisms of injury include trunk/spinal flexion over a stick, high-velocity rotational movements when hitting or pushing the ball, overuse, and running in a flexed position (thus increasing spinal loading). Axial rotation and lateral bending forces may also produce ***intervertebral disc herniation.*** Injury to the back reduces with trunk extension stretching and strengthening (isotonic and endurance) exercises.

Acute traumatic injury of the upper extremity *most commonly* occurs to the ***dorsal side of the hand/finger.*** Contact from the ball or stick is the *most common* mechanism of acute trauma. ***Contusions and fractures*** are very common, most often affecting the ***first digit,*** causing ***mallet fingers*** and ***dislocations*** of the ***proximal interphalangeal joint*** with tearing of the ***collateral ligaments.***

Other mechanisms of upper extremity injury include ***overuse, falls,*** and ***collisions. Dorsal ganglions, De Quervain's tenosynovitis (abductor pollicis longus and extensor pollicis brevis tendinitis),*** and ***ulnar/median nerve inflammation*** can develop secondarily to ***overuse. Tennis elbow (lateral epi-***

condylitis) is seen with supination on the elite level after multiple stick saves in goalie drills. After a fall or collision, ***subluxation*** of the ***glenohumeral joint*** or ***fractures of the clavicle*** or ***scaphoid*** may occur.

More than half of all acute traumatic injuries to the face and head are caused by direct impact from either the ball or the stick in field hockey. ***Ocular trauma*** occurs after the ball/stick rises abruptly after a pass or the ball ricochets from a divot in the grass field. This can result in ***hyphema, corneal abrasion, perioral lacerations/contusions*** or ***hematomas.***

A defensive player occasionally runs into an offensive player's moving stick from behind while trying to steal the ball. Resulting injuries include ***fractures, contusions,*** and ***lacerations*** of the defensive player's ***nose, cheeks,*** and ***lips. Lacerations of the face*** often require sutures. ***Cerebral contusions*** and ***concussions*** secondary to collision are relatively common. When athletes play on Astroturf, there is an increased incidence of acute traumatic injuries to the ***face and head*** because the balls attain greater velocities and the reaction times to them are shorter.

In general, patterns of injuries found in female field hockey athletes are essentially the same as for male athletes. However, a few injuries have been found to occur at a higher frequency in the female athlete. For example, ***"runner's nipple"*** can occur secondarily to irritation from rubbing clothing and ***breast tenderness*** occurs after exercise without a sports bra. ***Loss of menses*** can arise in some athletes, requiring thorough evaluation to rule out ***amenorrhea, pregnancy,*** and/or ***hypothalamic dysfunction.***

The most dangerous setting in which injuries occur in field hockey is in the awarding of a penalty corner. The goalkeeper's position is associated with an injury rate about three times higher than that of an outfield player. The risk of injury during a match exceeds the risk of injury at practice by a factor of 20 to 1. It is hoped that with a better understanding of patterns and levels of sports injuries in field hockey, there will be improved treatment of the injuries outlined above.

76. FOOTBALL

James P. Bradley and Michael J. Rytel

Football is a violent sport requiring explosive strength as well as exceptional speed and endurance. While epidemiologic studies have reported an incidence of injury between 11% and 81%, to those who care for these athletes, injuries in football are so common that the phrase "football injury" seems redundant. For example, in the National Football League (NFL) the rate of injury has been reported to be 1.5 injuries per athlete per season. Many factors influence the rate of injury, including weather conditions and playing surfaces, with wet, slippery fields producing the fewest injuries. Offensive and defensive players suffer equal numbers of injuries, but the relative risk of injury is highest for running backs, followed by quarterbacks, tackles, and centers. Tackling is the most dangerous maneuver, leading to 32% of injuries, followed by blocking (29%), carrying the ball (19%), and being blocked (10%). Passing, running, and receiving are relatively safe activities, resulting in less than 3% of injuries. Players are much more likely to be injured during a game than during practice, and teams that limit the number of contact practices have fewer injuries. The impact of artificial surfaces on injury rates has not been clearly determined. The NFL is currently conducting a leaguewide study to address this concern. The nature of the game makes certain injuries prevalent.

Approximately 250,000 head injuries occur during football annually. More head injuries occur in football than any other sport, and these injuries are twice as frequent as cervical spine injuries. Some 90% of head injuries are ***concussions,*** with the incidence of concussion in high school varsity and college football being approximately 20%. Concussions occur when making a tackle (43%), being tackled (23%), blocking (20%), or being blocked (10%). Any player who loses consciousness should be considered to have a concomitant neck injury and be treated accordingly. Many players who reach the professional level have sustained multiple concussions during their careers, resulting in the possibility of permanent neurologic impairment. These athletes need to consider this when contemplating return to play. ***Facial lacerations, ocular injuries, nasal fractures,*** and ***injuries to the teeth*** and ***oral cavity*** make up the remaining 10% of head trauma. Prevention of head injuries relies upon a number of factors. Advanced helmet design, including proper fit and an appropriate face mask and mouth guard, is crucial. Adequate conditioning and correct tackling techniques are valuable measures which aid in the prevention of head injuries as well. Furthermore, rule changes can decrease injury rates by eliminating dangerous tactics. For example, a rule change in 1976 to outlaw spearing resulted in a 50% decline in head and neck injuries.

Cervical strains (overload of the musculotendinous units) and ***cervical sprains*** (injury to the ligamentous structures) are the most common neck injuries in football. Less common but certainly of greater consequence are ***fractures, dislocations, subluxations,*** and herniated discs. These potentially catastrophic events can damage the spinal cord, resulting in temporary or permanent paralysis. Studies have shown that the most devastating neck injuries stem from an axial compression applied to the top of the head. In 1976, the National Football Head and Neck Injury Registry was established to compile data concerning such injuries. The initial data showed that advances in helmet design during the 1960s led to an increase in the number and severity of cervical spine injuries because players were able to use the helmet as a weapon when tackling and blocking. Subsequent rule changes prohibiting the use of the top of the helmet to "spear" an opponent have led to a decrease in the incidence of fractures, dislocations, and subluxations from 7.72 to 2.31 per 100,000 among high school players and from 30.6 to 10.66 per 100,000 for college level athletes. In short, avoiding the use of the top of the head in tackling is the most important factor in decreasing the incidence of severe neck injury. Coaches should emphasize this fact to their players and teach proper techniques to avoid such injury.

"Stingers" are caused by traction to the brachial plexus when the shoulder is depressed while the neck is flexed laterally to the opposite side. They represent the most common neurologic injury in football. Studies have shown that between 50% and 65% of college football players experience a stinger during their careers. Repeated or prolonged stingers may lead to permanent loss of neurologic function.

Up to 30% of college football players and approximately 12% of players in the NFL will lose playing time because of injury to the lumbar spine. The most common injury to the ***lumbar spine*** involves ***strains*** and ***contusions*** following a direct blow to the back. Moreover, a blow to the flank may also result in ***injury to the ribs*** or underlying ***kidney.*** Repetitive microtrauma to the pars interarticularis from hyperextension and heavy weight lifting may lead to a stress fracture known as ***spondylolysis.*** Displacement of the fracture is referred to as ***spondylolisthesis.*** Linemen are most susceptible to these injuries with studies showing that approximately 50% of college linemen are affected. The heavy weight lifting required of linemen and not football itself may be the direct cause of spondylolysis. The incidence of spondylolysis among high school and college players is between 15% and 21%, many of whom are asymptomatic. Furthermore, the incidence does not increase during college, suggesting that this is a condition that arises during adolescence.

The shoulder is subject to a wide variety of trauma during football. The term *separated shoulder* refers to an ***injury to the acromioclavicular (AC) joint,*** which results when a player strikes the ground with the "point" of the shoulder. This is a very common injury in football, which accounts for approximately 41% of these injuries in athletics. ***Contusions*** involving the shoulder are common in linebackers and may lead to ***"tacklers' exostosis,"*** which is new bone formation in the region of the deltoid insertion. ***Shoulder dislocations*** most commonly occur anteriorly. Typically, the arm is forced into excessive abduction and external rotation when attempting an arm tackle. Offensive linemen are at risk for ***posterior instability*** because of the repetitive posterior loads placed on the arm when it is elevated and adducted during blocking. Quarterbacks are predisposed to the same overuse injuries as other throwers. These include ***anterior instability, internal impingement, subacromial impingement,*** and ***partial or full-thickness rotator cuff tears.*** Proper conditioning and throwing mechanics help prevent these conditions.

Quarterbacks are also subject to ***instability problems at the elbow*** similar to those seen in baseball pitchers. This is the result of repetitive ***valgus overload*** during the early acceleration phase of throwing, which leads to attenuation or rupture of the ulnar collateral ligament. Offensive linemen may experience recurrent ***hyperextension episodes*** resulting in ***extension overload*** or ***posterior impingement*** syndrome. This is frequently complicated by flexion contracture and ***loose body formation.*** Traumatic ***olecranon bursitis*** can be seen in players of any position following a fall onto a flexed elbow. The use of elbow pads, especially on artificial surfaces, may help to prevent this injury.

Hand and wrist injuries are common and affect the player according to his position. Offensive linemen frequently suffer ***contusions, sprains,*** and ***interphalangeal joint dislocations,*** but they may often continue to participate with modifications to protective equipment or taping. Athletes who handle the ball may have more difficulty playing after a similar injury. ***Scaphoid fractures*** occur during a fall onto an outstretched hand and are fairly common football injuries. Studies have shown that college football players with nondisplaced scaphoid fractures may use a playing cast may for practice and games with a union rate of 92%. Asymptomatic nonunion of the scaphoid was reported in 28 NFL players in 1982. These players performed at this high level of competition despite a 20% to 30% loss of grip strength. A ***"gamekeeper's thumb"*** is a sprain of the ulnar collateral ligament of the first metacarpophalyngeal joint. This can occur with a fall onto an outstretched hand or when grasping an opponent to make a tackle. ***"Jersey finger,"*** an avulsion of the deep flexor tendon, is more common in defensive players and occurs when a flexed finger is forcibly extended while clinging to another player's jersey. A direct blow to the finger tip as when a receiver "jams" his finger on the ball can cause avulsion of the extensor tendon resulting in a mallet finger.

A ***"hip pointer"*** is a contusion over the iliac crest. In the United States, football is the most common cause of hip pointers. ***Periostitis*** and the formation of ***exostoses*** occasionally develop secondarily. ***Hamstring*** and ***adductor muscle strains*** can be disabling and are common in players at positions requiring speed. Kickers and punters are prone to ***rectus femoris strains. Quadriceps contusion*** is caused by a direct blow to the anterior thigh. Severe intramuscular bleeding can significantly limit knee flexion. ***Myositis ossificans*** (bone formation in the muscle) is a relatively common complication of thigh contusions occurring 4% to 18% of the time. The use of thigh pads to prevent contusions is encouraged.

The knee is the most commonly injured joint in football, representing approximately one-third of all injuries. Football players are 5.8 times more likely to sustain a knee injury than the general population. The ***medial collateral ligament (MCL)*** is the most frequently injured structure, with ***meniscal injury*** ranking as the second most common site. MCL tears typically occur in linemen when a valgus force is applied to the lateral aspect of the knee with the foot planted. Receivers, defensive backs, and running backs injure the ***anterior cruciate ligament (ACL)*** when planting the foot to make a sudden change of direction. Some athletes, mostly linemen, may be able to return to football with a torn ACL following rehabilitation and with the use of a functional brace. The ***posterior cruciate ligament (PCL)*** is typically torn when a player is tackled causing his flexed knee to strike the ground. If symptoms of pain and instability are negligible, athletes with isolated posterior laxity can return to football without surgery after completing a rehabilitation program emphasizing quadriceps strengthening. Of note, 2% of the athletes at an NFL predraft physical exam were noted to have asymptomatic isolated PCL laxity. ***Knee dislocation*** is a potentially catastrophic injury that may end in amputation in players who suffer concomitant vascular injury. Patellofemoral pain syndrome (***chondromalacia patella***), ***patellar tendonitis*** (jumper's knee), and ***patellar dislocations*** are other common maladies affecting the knees of football players. Numerous studies have examined the effect of prophylactic braces in preventing knee injuries. One study showed a definite decrease in MCL injuries in defensive players only. Two others studies demonstrated an increase in knee injuries among both high school and college players. Because data are conflicting, the use of prophylactic braces remains controversial.

The ankle is the second most commonly injured joint in football, accounting for 18% of all injuries. ***Lateral ankle sprains*** occur most frequently and are the result of pronation and internal rotation mechanisms. The ***syndesmosis*** is injured with external rotation of the talus in the mortise. These "high" ankle sprains can lead to heterotopic ossification of the syndesmosis secondarily. Chronic instability may follow severe sprains, occasionally necessitating reconstruction. Ankle taping decreases ankle and subtalar motion while increasing proprioception. Unfortunately, its effect is diminished after a short period of exercise, hence it may not provide continued protection. Ankle braces are more effective, but many athletes feel encumbered by these devices.

"Turf toe" is a sprain of the plantar capsular ligament of the first metatarsophalyngeal (MTP) joint. The injury occurs when the MTP joint is forcibly hyperextended. Lightweight, flexible shoes and artificial playing surfaces have been implicated in increasing the incidence of turf toe. Running backs, offensive linemen, tight ends, and wide receivers have a higher incidence of turf toe. ***Midfoot sprains*** are caused by a variety of mechanisms including axial load to a plantarflexed foot, axial load applied to the heel of a dorsiflexed foot, and rotation of the forefoot with the heel fixed. Orthotics to support the midfoot may be necessary upon return to football.

Football is likely to continue as the most popular collision sport in the United States. Improved injury prevention will rely upon further modifications of equipment, rule changes to eliminate hazardous play, and awareness and experience among coaches to teach safe and effective techniques.

77. GOLF

William J. Mallon

Introduction

It is well known that golfers play in spite of numerous ailments. Over 50% of touring professionals have sustained some injury that required them to stop playing competitively. As in all professional sports, the demands placed on the touring professional to remain competitive require pushing the body to the edge of overuse.

The benign appearance of golf causes many health care providers not to expect significant injuries among recreational or weekend golfers. Yet they do occur in the amateur golfer. Weekend golfers do not place the same demands upon their bodies while playing golf, yet these lesser demands are placed upon less well conditioned bodies. In addition, their swing techniques are less refined and efficient.

Epidemiology of Golf Injuries

Among professional and amateur golfers, the left wrist is the most common site of injury, followed by the lower back, the left elbow, and the left shoulder. The lead or target-side arm is injured much more frequently. It is interesting to note the rarity of lower extremity golf problems, which represent less than 10% of injuries.

The lateral elbow is much more frequently a source of injury (by nearly 5 to 1), than the medial elbow. *"Tennis elbow,"* the common name for *lateral epicondylitis,* is the most frequent elbow problem in athletics. *"Golfer's elbow"* has also been described and usually refers to *medial epicondylitis.* But it appears that tennis elbow, or lateral epicondylitis, is more common among golfers than golfer's elbow, and occurs mostly in the lead arm.

Prevention of Golf Injuries

Warm-up before playing is critical to prevent injuries. Most professionals begin their day by practicing on the range, starting out with short or half-strength shots. Few amateurs follow this routine, yet they should, especially those who are attempting to overcome injuries.

One of the causes of injury in sports is poor technique. Studies have shown that professionals generate less stress in the lumbar spine than amateurs, despite the fact that professionals generate a higher velocity of the body segments and more clubhead speed. This efficiency is due to the professional's use of better technique. Development of proper golf technique is best done with lessons from a qualified Professional Golfers' Association (PGA) golf professional.

Low Back Injuries

Chronic back injuries may necessitate some changes in technique and equipment to allow the golfer to "play around the injury." Golfers with back pain will benefit from using one of the newer extralong putters. These prevent the player from having to bend over from the waist, a position that stresses the lumbosacral muscles and articulations.

Three swing modifications may help a player with back pain: (1) The player may have to learn to swing with less torque in the back muscles. This is more of a "classic" swing as opposed to the modern swing, espoused by today's touring professionals, with a large shoulder turn and minimal hip turn. The classic swing uses virtually equal amounts of hip and shoulder turn, with the player often rising up on the left toe. (2) Golfers with back pain will often benefit from a more upright stance, using more knee flex to reach the ball. This takes stress off the lumbosacral area but will necessitate a slightly flatter swing plane. (3) Players with back pain should learn to shorten their swings.

Shoulder Injuries

Shoulder pain in golfers usually results from impingement, which generally occurs in the left shoulder in right-handed golfers. Golfers with impingement syndrome may benefit from shortening their swing and flattening their swing plane so as to minimize left arm elevation.

Golfers with instability symptoms will benefit from a shorter swing, as this places less stress on the shoulder capsule. Instability at the top of the backswing may be due to posterior subluxation of the shoulder.

Recent studies have shown that professionals and low-handicap amateurs often develop acromioclavicular joint problems in the lead shoulder. Treatment with distal clavicular excision has allowed these athletes to return to their former levels of competition.

Elbow Injuries

The most common elbow problem in golfers is lateral epicondylitis. Golfers with elbow pain present a difficult challenge to the physician. This is because impact and the act of taking a divot places a great deal of stress on the wrist and forearm musculature. If the elbow or wrist pain is chronic, the player may need to change his or her swing to "sweep" the ball off the turf without taking a divot. The golfer with left elbow pain should forget the old axiom to keep the "left arm straight." Also, more flexible shafts, possibly including graphite shafts, may take stress off the forearm and elbow by absorbing more of the shock of impact.

Wrist Injuries

Among people who play or practice golf often and complain of wrist or hand pain near the hypothenar eminence, a stress fracture of the hook of the hamate bone must be ruled out. Standard radiographs will not usually reveal this injury, and special imaging techniques, such as magnetic resonance imaging (MRI) or computed tomography (CT), are required if the diagnosis is suspected. The important point is that one must suspect this injury to make the diagnosis. The treatment is excision of the hook of the hamate, which has allowed many professionals to return to competitive golf.

Wrist ganglia are quite common in golfers, possibly due to repetitive trauma from taking divots. Other common hand and wrist injuries, such as carpal tunnel syndrome and DeQuervain's tenosynovitis, are actually relatively rare among active golfers.

Environmental Concerns

Golfers are often exposed to the environment for 4 to 6 hr at a time. Sunburn and heat exposure are concerns, but appropriate precautions can be taken to prevent both from occurring. Dressing properly helps, with light cotton clothing and a wide-brimmed hat. Adequate fluid replacement is important on very hot days. Golfers may wish to use a sunscreen lotion.

Snakebites do occur to golfers, especially those straying frequently from the fairway in high-risk geographical areas. Treatment of a poisonous snakebite is to transport the victim off the course quickly and seek appropriate medical help. Golf shops should have available kits that provide immediate aid to golfers who are allergic to toxic venoms, such as those of poisonous snakes and bee stings.

Lightning kills several golfers each year. Caution will prevent this if golfers leave the course immediately when lightning or thunder are seen or heard in the area.

78. GYMNASTICS

Bert R. Mandelbaum and Aurelia Nattiv

I. Introduction

Globally, gymnastics has evolved into an extremely popular and competitive sport. The long hours of disciplined training during childhood required to master the risky and complex maneuvers of gymnastics produce a variety of characteristic medical and orthopedic problems. The health care team responsible for the young gymnast must prevent injuries, minimize morbidity after injuries occur, and help maximize performance and personal development. Girls' and boys' gymnastics are distinctly different sports whose participants differ significantly in the ages of initiation, peak level of performance, and retirement. Men's gymnastics includes six different exercises: pommel horse, vault, floor exercise, parallel bar, high bar, and rings. Women's gymnastics includes uneven parallel bars, floor exercise, the balance beam, and the vault. These different events make different biomechanical technical demands on the gymnast. The problems attendant on each of these sports are decidedly different.

II. General Medical Concerns

A. **Nutritional problems.** Historically, the trend among the young female gymnast is toward thinness. Severe caloric restrictions can result in deficient nutrition, decreased metabolic rate, and disordered eating. In addition, this constant pressure to minimize weight can lead to calcium and iron deficiencies. Specifically, the young female gymnast who is euestrogenic requires 1200 mg of calcium per day.

B. **Disordered eating.** Disordered eating represents a spectrum of disease including anorexia nervosa, bulemia, and milder patterns. Most athletes fall, somewhere in the middle. It is important to recognize these individuals, since prevention and minimization is the key goal. At times, this can be complex. The health care team must work in concert.

C. **Menarcheal status.** Delayed menarche among young female gymnasts is common, and the prevalence of secondary amenorrhea in gymnasts can be as high as 66%. In this population, amenorrhea is secondary to low body fat, inadequate calories, poor nutrition, disordered eating patterns, stress, frequency of high-intensity exercise as well as other variables. The most serious complication associated with this is premature osteoporosis and an increased risk of stress fracture and other fractures. Some athletes may require hormonal intervention with estrogens.

D. **Growth problems.** The gymnast population has demonstrated that puberty and high-intensity gymnastics can alter the growth rate, so that full adult height may not be attained. The mechanisms of this growth inhibition remain obscure.

III. Orthopaedic Issues

The young gymnast's growing and developing body is susceptible to acute and chronic repetitive injury. Epidemiologically, the most common injuries affect the lower extremity. Specifically, ankle sprains are the most common of all traumatic or overuse injuries.

A. **Wrist injuries.** Wrist pain has been an increasingly common problem in young, avid gymnasts. This may be debilitating in gymnastics in an upper extremity weight-bearing sport. The debilitating symptom seemingly comes from adaptive changes that cause positive ulnar variance and tears of the triangular fibrocartilaqe. Other problems may include ganglion cysts, extensor tendinitis, or overuse injuries to the distal radial physis.

B. **Elbow injuries.** Elbow dislocation is most likely to occur in the female gymnast on uneven bars. Medial epicondylitis and tendinitis of the flexor tendon origin is common with upper extremity weight bearing.

C. **Shoulder injuries.** Gymnasts, by virtue of flexibility requirements, tend to have a spectrum of glenohumeral instability problems. In addition, painful impingement syndromes may be caused by instability, supraspinatus tendinitis, and/or bicipital tendinitis.

D. **Ankle injuries.** Sprained ankle is the most common problem, as the gymnast lands with the foot not flat, subjecting the knee-ankle to torsional loads and resulting in complex ligamentous injuries. Ankle sprains and/or impingement syndromes cause pain, functional instability, and weakness. It is imperative to differentiate ankles that are unstable because of lax ligaments from those that are functionally unstable.

E. **Knee injuries.** Knee trauma is a significant problem during dismounts and floor exercise. High-energy trauma can lead to complex ligamentous injuries, meniscus tears, physeal fractures, and other fractures. Most knee injuries can be attributed to premature attempts to practice new skills, poor mental and physical conditioning, and inadequate athletic or coaching preparation. The key in these situations is prevention.

F. **Spinal injuries.** Acute injuries to the cervical, thoracic, and lumbar spine may have catastrophic consequences if they involve neurologic compromise. These may be true emergencies. The key elements in the prevention of these injuries include details such as level of participation, skill, fitness, adequate spotting, and coaching. These techniques will ensure safe participation with minimal risk to the spine. Chronic spinal overuse injuries may from repetitive flexion, rotation, and extension be pose a difficult problem. Common problems include discogenic pathology, vertebral end-plate abnormalities, and damage to the pars interarticularis with resultant spondylolysis or spondylolisthesis. The health care team must clearly understand the potential of spondylolysis and the need to prevent it from progressing to spondylolisthesis in the 9- to 13-year-old.

IV. Prevention

The concept of the dose of gymnastics and the stress response of the gymnastic body should be understood by the health care team. Age of initiation, sports activity, progression of advancement, and technique should be individualized and reevaluated at various intervals. Adherence to these specific recommendations is essential to ensure safe, enjoyable, and successful participation.

79. **ICE HOCKEY**

Arthur R. Bartolozzi III, Michael Palmeri, and Peter F. DeLuca

Ice hockey is one of the fastest and most physical team sports in which violence and injuries are quite frequent. In recent years, ice hockey has grown tremendously in popularity, and this expanding interest has led to an increase in the number and severity of injuries.

Several studies of the epidemiology of injuries in hockey confirm that more than two-thirds of the injuries occur during the game. This is most likely related to the aggressive intensity of the games. While most of the injuries recorded were new, approximately 25% were recurrences or complications of prior injuries. Almost 70% of injuries were the direct result of contact, with the majority of these occurring due to contact with another player. Forwards were found to have a greater injury rate than defensemen and goal tenders.

The most frequently injured body parts were the ***knee, shoulder,*** and ***groin,*** where sprains, strains and contusions predominated. Injuries to the ***head, face, and neck*** were also common. Surgery was seldomly necessary.

Lacerations are common about the ***head*** and ***face,*** but studies have shown that face shields will prevent many of them. It is important to realize that behind every facial laceration is a potential fracture; lacerations over the cheek may overlie ***malar, zygomatic,*** or even ***orbital fractures. Mandibular fractures*** are not infrequent and can be diagnosed in the player who presents with pain and a sense of malocclusion; these injuries often require operative reduction with internal fixation.

Aside from lacerations, ***concussions*** are the next most common injuries to the head. Any player found unconscious from a head injury should be presumed to have a ***cervical spine injury*** and the appropriate precautions should be undertaken when transporting the player. Fractures and head injuries resulting in sudden death have virtually ceased in the era of the helmet. Although serious spine fractures are a rare occurrence, they do occur with axial loading of the cervical spine with the neck in a neutral or slightly flexed position. There is some fear that the helmet and face mask apparatus may be associated with the increased frequency of cervical spine injuries. Probably the best preventative measures against neck injury are to be involved in a comprehensive neck strengthening program and to avoid lowering the head.

Cervical fractures are not the only serious neck injuries. ***Laryngeal fractures*** have been reported to occur and are potentially life-threatening. Stridor, hemoptysis, subcutaneous crepitus, and loss of the Adam's apple promontory are the most flagrant signs, with emergency tracheostomy sometimes being necessary. These fractures occur from a cross-check over the neck or garroting from behind with the stick across the front of the neck.

Eye injuries are not infrequent, but visual loss or compromise has been greatly reduced by proper use of the face mask or visor and the introduction of high-sticking rules. Currently, the incidence of eye injuries is more common among older players who choose not to wear a mask or visor.

Injuries to the upper extremity occur quite frequently, with the ***shoulder*** most commonly affected. ***Acromioclavicular* (AC) *separations*** are the most common type of injury to the shoulder sustained by adult players, whereas ***clavicular fractures*** are more common among preadolescent and teenage players. Injury to the AC joint is often caused by the transmission of force due to the impact of the outstretched, abducted arm, which drives the clavicle forward and away from the acromion. The AC joint may also be disrupted from a direct blow to the acromion where it is struck against the boards or ice. Regardless of the cause of injury, operative intervention as a primary treatment is rarely needed and the athlete is usually able to return to play once adequate strength is regained. Of note, strength in horizontal abduction is usually the last to be restored to normal and is of extreme importance in pushing opponents away in struggles against the boards.

Rotator cuff strains and tears are also common due to the repetitive shooting drills, but they also occur from collisions into the boards or ice. ***Shoulder dislocations*** also occur from encounters with other players, sticks, and the boards but are an infrequent cause of missed games.

The ***sternoclavicular joints*** can be injured by hitting the boards chest first while experiencing a sudden retraction of the shoulders from a hit in the back. These injuries as well as injuries to the ***costochondral junctions and ribs*** usually respond well to abstinence from play.

Injuries to the ***elbow*** commonly present as ***olecranon bursitis and hyperextension*** or ***valgus injuries to the capsule.*** These may occur through direct falls on the ice, through collisions into the boards, or through forces leveraged through the player's stick by an opponent.

The ***wrist and hand*** are often afflicted with a variety of injuries. ***Fracture of the first metacarpal*** is often seen as a result of slashing, whereas other metacarpal fractures may be seen with fisticuffs. ***Scaphoid fractures*** as well as other carpal fractures may be encountered from falls on the flexed or extended wrist. ***Gamekeeper's thumb*** is seen from a fall with the stick in the hand, whereby the stick imparts a radially directed force that causes rupture of the ulnar collateral ligament of the metacarpophalangeal joint of the thumb. ***Jersey finger,*** or rupture of the flexor digitorum profundus tendon, commonly affects the ring finger and occurs in a fight when the finger slips off the opponent's jersey. ***Mallet fingers*** or disruption of the extensor tendon to the distal interphalangeal joint, either through tearing or avulsion fracture, also occur. Many of these hand problems require surgical intervention for correction.

The lower extremities are the most frequently injured areas, with the ***groin and knee*** being responsible for the majority. The ***groin or adductor pull*** is the predominant soft tissue injury and usually involves strains of the musculotendinous origin of the hip adductors. The groin muscles are critical in the force generation required for the quick and powerful starts of ice hockey. The occurrence of a groin strain is thought to be related to factors that include tight muscles, lack of adequate warm-up, weakness or fatigue, and muscle imbalances. This problem can be recalcitrant in nature; symptoms may progress more proximally toward the pubis, resulting in ***osteitis pubis,*** and further proximally to ***the lower abdominal wall,*** necessitating herniorrhaphy for resolution. This progression is an apparent recruitment of the more proximal musculature to perform the tasks normally thrust upon the adductors.

Contusions of the thigh (charley horse) are frequent injuries resulting from a direct hit into the boards, goal post, or an opponent's knee or hip. The ***hip pointer*** or ***contusion along the iliac crest*** also occurs frequently and can be quite disabling. Both can lead to prolonged myositis and eventual ***myositis ossificans,*** which will appear on a soft tissue x-ray as calcification at approximately 3 weeks, with new bone formation apparent at approximately 6 to 8 weeks.

The ***knee*** is the most frequently injured area in hockey, almost exclusively as a result of contact. The player is often hit from the lateral side to a flexed knee, resulting in a valgus and internal rotation strain that often sprains the ***medial collateral ligament (MCL)*** and may tear the ***anterior cruciate ligament (ACL) and medial capsule. Hyperextension injuries*** from a direct blow to the anterior aspect of the knee are also fairly common, but ligamentous disruption is rare. Magnetic resonance imaging (MRI) will often show bruising of the anterior aspects of the femoral condyles. A hyperextension-blocking brace and physical therapy are the usual treatments.

Despite the knee-shin protective apparatus, ***patellar fractures*** do occur and usually result from pucks, falls against the ice, and hitting the boards with the knee first. Traumatic ***patellar tendinitis*** can also result from a direct blow from the puck.

Ankle sprains are infrequent due to the rigidity of the skate boot. However, entrapment of the skate blade by the ice or the boards can cause a low-grade ***syndesmosis rupture*** as the pronated ankle is abducted and externally rotated by the player's inertia. Fractures of the ankle are also relatively uncommon, but ***bursal enlargements*** over the malleoli are common due to repetitive impact from pucks. ***Tenosynovitis of the extensor tendons*** has been attributed to the tight lacing of the skates.

Fractures of the feet are relatively common and are usually the result of being struck by the puck. The ***navicular*** is the most commonly fractured bone; if it is not displaced, the player can often play through the pain.

Back injuries are very common but are most likely to be in the realm of the muscle spasm or strain and usually respond to a preventative rehabilitation program of stretching and strengthening.

Injuries to the viscera do occur in ice hockey; the ***spleen*** is the most vulnerable. It is relatively unprotected in the left upper quadrant and injuries range from subcapsular hematomata to rupture, a surgical emergency. Preexisting splenomegaly, as from mononucleosis, predisposes the spleen to rupture. Less often, the ***kidney*** can be injured as the player presents with frank hematuria and back pain after being cross-checked from behind. ***Testicular hematomata*** also have been reported as a result of the direct contact from the puck or stick.

Last, ***contact dermatitis*** is a common entity among hockey players and is commonly referred to as the "creeping crud" or "gonk." It is due to the excessive sweating beneath the protective equipment.

80. LACROSSE

Stephen J. O'Brien, Eva M. Anisko, and Answorth A. Allen

Lacrosse is an aggressive sport that demands strength, endurance, and agility. The game is played on grass or turf. Athletes are at risk for sustaining injuries from body checking, falls to the ground, the ball, and the stick. The lacrosse equipment includes helmets, face visors, shoulder pads, and chest pads. Female players are not required to wear protective equipment and hence are more susceptible to head and facial injuries. The most common injuries reported by the National Collegiate Athletic Association (NCAA) Men's Lacrosse Injury Surveillance System for the 1994–95 season were sprains (26%), strains (20%), and contusions (18%). However, most of the significant injuries involved the ***hands,*** the ***shoulder girdle,*** the ***knee,*** and the ***foot*** and ***ankle.*** For purposes of this discussion, these injuries are classified according to anatomic region.

Head and Neck Injuries

The headgear used in lacrosse is essentially a plastic shell with or without a face visor. There is no air in the helmet and it is relatively light, so as to allow the athlete to move quickly. Potential head injuries include mild or moderate ***concussions,*** which occur relatively infrequently. Serious closed head injuries are rare. ***Facial lacerations*** are often caused by the stick or falls to the ground. The lacrosse ball is a hard, fast-moving projectile that can cause ***ocular injuries*** and ***facial fractures.*** Because of the lack of headgear in women's lacrosse, the head has the second highest rate of injury, after the ankle, among female players. ***Tooth avulsions*** and ***lip lacerations*** can result from direct trauma from the ball or body-to-body contact. For this reason mouth guards should be used routinely. Although ***neck sprains and strains*** are not unusual in lacrosse players, the most significant injury to the neck is a ***laryngeal fracture.*** This can happen from a cross-check with the lacrosse stick, fracturing the thyroid cartilage and placing the athlete at risk for respiratory compromise. Goalkeepers are especially susceptible to this injury and are required to wear throat protectors.

Injuries of the Upper Extremity

Clavicular fractures and ***acromioclavicular separations*** occur frequently in lacrosse players. The former is usually secondary to a direct blow to the clavicle from the stick. The latter is usually the result of a fall onto the point of the shoulder. The shoulder padding is light to emphasize speed and provides less than optimal protection. Potential associated injuries include ***rotator cuff contusions, labral tears,*** and ***osteolysis*** of the distal clavicle from repeated microtrauma. ***Shoulder dislocations*** are possible but occur infrequently unless the athlete has some predisposing risk factors.

Elbow injuries are relatively uncommon in lacrosse. Skin ***abrasions*** and ***olecranon bursitis*** can result from repeated falls to the ground on the point of the elbow. Athletes who play on hard surfaces, like Astroturf, tend to have this injury more frequently. Secondary ***infection*** of the olecranon bursa is a potential complication that should be managed aggressively. Elbow overuse symptoms include ***triceps tendinitis, lateral epicondylitis,*** and ***apophyseal*** injury in young players. Forearm ***contusions*** can result from a direct blow with the lacrosse stick. If the stick is swung hard enough, this can result in a forearm fracture. The classic ***night-stick fracture*** is more common than an isolated ***radial shaft fracture*** or ***both-bone fracture*** of the forearm.

Hand injuries are especially common in lacrosse players and include both ligamentous injuries and hand fractures. The lacrosse glove does not provide enough protection from slashing with the stick, hence most injuries occur from direct trauma. Common soft tissue injuries include rupture of the ***ulnar collateral ligament*** of the thumb metacarpophalangeal (MP) joint and ***collateral ligament*** injuries of the interphalangeal joints. ***Hand abrasions, lacerations,*** and ***nail bed injuries*** are also relatively common. ***Flexor tendon*** avulsions occur infrequently. Impaction injuries to the distal phalanx can result in jammed fingers or ***distal phalangeal fractures. Metacarpal*** and ***phalangeal fractures*** are usually the result of direct contact with the lacrosse stick. Hand injuries are especially common in women because they do not often wear gloves.

Torso Injuries

Injuries to the torso primarily involve the chest and rib cage and usually result from illegal picks and falls to the ground. Chest ***contusions*** and ***multiple rib fractures*** are fairly common. In the setting of multiple rib fractures, there is always the potential for a ***pneumothorax*** or ***hemothorax.*** It has been reported that a direct blow to the chest can cause ***cardiac arrhythmia*** in athletes without any previous history of cardiac disease. Conceivably in lacrosse, this could occur from a direct blow to the chest with the lacrosse ball. Abdominal injuries are relatively rare in lacrosse; however, athletes with blunt trauma to the abdominal region should be evaluated for ***splenic injuries.***

Injuries to the Lower Extremity

Most of the injuries to the lower extremity will occur from either a noncontact or contact mechanism. ***Groin strains, hamstring pulls,*** and ***calf muscle strains*** occur frequently. Direct trauma to the thigh muscles can cause ***quadriceps contusions*** and subsequent development of ***myositis ossificans.*** Knee injuries are extremely common in both female and male lacrosse players. They usually result from some kind of a twisting or pivoting mechanism. ***Meniscal tears, collateral ligament sprains,*** and ***anterior cruciate ligament ruptures*** are relatively common. As in a number of other sports, females have a higher incidence of anterior cruciate ligament injuries than males. Posterior cruciate ligament and multiple ligament injuries are uncommon. ***Prepatellar bursitis*** can result from repeated falls onto the patella. Chronic overuse injuries include ***patellofemoral chondromalacia, patellar tendinitis,*** and ***Osgood-Schlatter*** disease in the adolescent. The incidence of these injuries can be reduced with a good off-season conditioning program, appropriate shoe wear, and by changing the playing surface (grass is preferred to Astroturf). Injuries to the leg include ***pretibial hematomas, tibial stress syndrome, stress fractures,*** and ***exertional compartment syndrome.*** Hard playing surfaces appear to increase the risk of these injuries.

FOOT AND ANKLE INJURIES

Ankle injuries are the most common injury in women's lacrosse and the second most common injury in men's lacrosse. ***Ankle sprains*** occur routinely as a result of the frequent cutting and twisting motions required by the sport. ***Peroneal tendon subluxation or dislocation*** can be confused with an ankle sprain and must be considered when the patient is examined. Although ankle fractures are uncommon, ***syndesmosis sprains*** can occur. Overuse syndromes include ***Achilles tendinitis, posterior tibialis tendinitis,*** and, rarely, ***anterior tibialis tendinitis.*** Foot injuries include ***plantar fascitis, heel pain, metatarsalgia,*** and ***turf toe.***

Although a number of injuries can occur in lacrosse, fewer than 15% will require operative management. According to the NCAA Men's Lacrosse Injury Surveillance System, less than 30% of the injuries sustained during the season prevented the athletes from participating in practices and games for more than a 7-day period. The medical staff and coaches have become more aware of the potential for injury in lacrosse, and more emphasis is being placed on safety. The NCAA regulations limit the protective equipment for women's lacrosse in an attempt to prevent contact; however, this often compromises protection. The padding in men's lacrosse is light to emphasize speed and is often not used by the athletes. The gloves do not protect the hands adequately to prevent injuries from slashing. Injury rates can be reduced by changes in the rules and coaching techniques and in the equipment designed to protect the athlete.

81. MARTIAL ARTS

Answorth A. Allen

The martial arts, which originated in China, can be traced back to approximately A.D. 500. They were originally developed with potentially lethal intent and make use of the extremities to attack and disable an opponent. The use of weapons, such as knives, swords, and sticks, may be incorporated. The various styles include karate, tae kwon do, kung fu, akido, and kendo. Although the martial arts have been introduced as a sport in the western hemisphere relatively recently, there is tremendous interest and it is one of the fastest growing sports in the U.S.A.

The popularity of the sport has spawned a multimillion dollar industry incorporating schools, clothing and equipment. There are a number of local, national, and international competitions. Tae kwon do is one of the more popular forms practiced in this part of the world and was introduced as an Olympic event in 1988.

Competition includes both contact and noncontact drills. In the latter, the participants are judged in terms of their ability to perform exact forms with style and grace. Contact sparring is a sophisticated game of tag, where the competitor scores point by hitting the opponent while avoiding getting hit.

It is important that the physician covering a marital arts competition be cognizant of the way the medical team is organized and have an appreciation of the basic rules of the sport. The athletes usually compete on a flat mat or pad on a wooden or carpeted floor. Concrete flooring is usually not allowed because of the potential for injury. The *center referee* is in charge of the match and has the ability to give warnings, disqualify competitors, and award points. He is also responsible for the safety of the athletes. If there is an injury, it is the referee who will determine whether or not a physician is needed and the physician can enter the ring only if summoned by the referee.

Protective equipment includes head protector, chest protector, breast protector for female athletes, forearm guard, a mouthpiece, and shin/instep guard. Athletes usually compete with bare hands and feet with a maximum of two layers of tape. In most national and international tournaments, the match consists of three 3-min rounds with a one 1-min rest period between rounds. In junior competitions, the rounds usually last for 2 min. The rules state that eight counts are mandatory for all knockdowns. If the injured competitor does not respond to the eighth count, the count continues to 10 and the attacker is declared a winner. If an illegal attack caused the injury, the competitor must be immediately evaluated by the physician and has 1 min to get the appropriate medical care and to determine whether the match should continue. If the competitor is unable to continue, the referee must decide whether this illegal blow was intentional. If the attack is judged to have been intentional, the injured competitor wins; if it is judged to have been accidental, the attacker wins. It is imperative that the physician be close to the ring because of the time constraints before the competitor is disqualified. It is recommended that the physician wear appropriate clothing or labels so that he can easily be identified and he the physician should also stay close to the ring to facilitate immediate assessment of an injured participant.

How many injuries occur during organized martial arts competition is a controversial issue. Some authors have suggested that serious, potentially lethal injuries never occur. However, one cannot ignore the fact that the techniques were initially developed to inflict potentially lethal force, and even with the use of protective gear, serious injuries can occur. The majority of injuries involve the extremities and include contusions, abrasions, lacerations, sprains, and strains. Most of the serious injuries are traumatic in nature and are due to the tremendous forces that can be transferred from kicks and blows from the hands and feet. For the purpose of this discussion, these injuries are classified into different anatomic regions.

Head and Neck Injuries

Even with the use of the appropriate headgear, serious injuries to the head can occur. A ***concussion*** can result from a direct blow to the head or can be secondary to a fall. If there is an head injury with loss of consciousness, the match is usually stopped and the injured athlete is evaluated using standard criteria. ***Epidural*** and ***subdural hematomas*** are potentially lethal complications of head trauma. There is one report of a patient who sustained a spinning hook kick to the face, fell to the floor, and died within 24 hr in a local hospital. ***Fractures*** of the maxillofacial bones, the nasal bones, the orbits, and the mandible can also occur. ***Dislocations*** of the temporomandibular joint, though rare, are also possible. Potential eye injuries include ***corneal abrasions, diplopia, periorbital hematoma,*** and ***retinal detachments.***

Neck strains, though relatively common, should raise the index of suspicion for a possible fracture/dislocation of the ***cervical spine.*** Other potential injuries include ***epistaxis, teeth avulsion,*** and ***lacerations of the tongue and face.***

Injuries to the Torso and Groin

The torso presents a large surface area for contact during fighting, hence injuries to it are fairly common. The ribs are relatively subcutaneous and ***rib fractures*** can occur quite easily from a blow to the chest. Potential complications include ***pneumothorax*** and ***hemothorax.*** The ***sternoclavicular joint*** can dislocate anteriorly or posteriorly; the latter is potentially life-threatening and requires immediate reduction to prevent respiratory failure. ***Sternal fractures*** can occur but are highly unusual. Direct trauma to the upper back can cause ***scapular fractures,*** which can often go unrecognized initially. It has recently been reported that direct blows to the chest can lead to ***cardiac arrhythmia*** and possible sudden death in the absence of any congenital or acquired cardiovascular disease.

Blunt abdominal trauma can cause ***hepatic, renal,*** and ***splenic*** injuries. The athlete can bleed into the abdomen or retroperitoneal space, creating a potentially life-threatening situation. More common injuries include ***solar plexus*** and ***abdominal concussions.*** Injuries to the back include ***paraspinal*** and ***thoracolumbar muscle*** strains, sprains and spasms. Blunt trauma to the lumbosacral region can cause ***contusions.*** Direct blows to the groin region can result in injuries to the testes, including ***testicular hematomas*** and ***contusions. Strains*** of the ***hip musculature,*** specifically the ***rectus femoris*** and ***adductors,*** occur frequently.

Injuries to the Upper Extremity

The extremities are used as the main offensive and defensive weapons in the martial arts and hence are prone to injury. In the upper extremity, from proximal to distal, the most common injuries include ***acromioclavicular separations,*** usually from a fall to the mat, and ***clavicular fractures,*** from direct blows. ***Forearm contusions*** are common as the athlete blocks punches and kicks. Long bone ***fractures of the forearm*** are distinctly uncommon but can occur. Hand injuries occur frequently. ***Phalangeal*** and ***metacarpal fractures*** usually result from a direct blow. ***Dislocations of the interphalangeal joint*** can often be reduced to allow the athlete to continue competing. Other injuries to the hand include lacerations and ***nail avulsions.*** The ***"boxer's knuckle"*** is unique to martial artists and boxers. Direct impact to the flexed second or third metacarpophalangeal (MP) joint can cause a rupture of the joint capsule, resulting in a painful deformity over the knuckle.

Injuries to the Lower Extremity

The lower extremity can be used as an effective weapon in the martial arts. More power is usually generated and transferred from kicks than from punches because of the weight of the extremity and the relatively long lever arm. Kicks to the head, torso, and groin region are potentially lethal and can inflict serious harm to the opponent. Poor technique and lack of conditioning are risk factors for injuries to the hip, thigh, knee, and leg. The most common injuries are ***contusions, muscle strains,*** and ***sprains. Quadriceps contusions*** and ***pretibial hematomas*** are usually secondary to direct trauma.

Knee injuries can result from both noncontact and contact injuries. Athletes will frequently jump and land in positions that stress the knee ligaments. Women athletes are at significant risk for noncontact knee ligament injuries. Potential problems include ***patella subluxation*** and ***dislocation, meniscal tear, rupture of the anterior cruciate ligament,*** and ***collateral ligament sprain,*** primarily the ***medial collateral ligament. Osteochondral fractures*** are more unusual and can present with recurrent knee effusions and mechanical symptoms. Although femoral and tibia fractures are distinctly unusual, they can also occur.

Injuries to the Foot and Ankle

Significant foot and ankle injuries from the martial arts are relatively uncommon; although ***ankle sprains, phalangeal fractures, nail bed*** injuries, and ***foot contusions*** are not unusual. ***Midfoot sprains*** can occur but are relatively rare.

82. MOUNTAINEERING AND CLIMBING

Allan Bach

Mountaineering and climbing are activities that intrinsically involve an element of risk. These activities have been increasingly popular over the last 20 years and deaths and injuries from mountaineering in North America have increased tenfold from the early 1950s to 1992. As the great modern alpinists Reinhold Messner and Walter Bonatti have pointed out, extreme preparation and training are necessary for survival in the mountains. These lessons can be applied to leisurely 1-day scrambles as well as to extreme Alpine adventures. Environmental extremes, risk of foreign travel, psychological stresses, and the significant chance of physical injury make many aspects of medicine important in mountaineering. Over the last 15 years the interest in sport climbing has exploded, with once isolated mountain crags being literally covered with vertical gymnasts during good weather. The advent of rock climbing gyms have allowed people to train year 'round for climbing; as a result, training injuries and overuse problems, particularly in the upper extremity, have become much more common.

High-altitude medicine involves the mountaineer almost exclusively. We consider high altitude to be anywhere from 1,500 to 3,500 m (5,000 to 11,500 ft) above sea level, where there can be some physical effects due to the decreased arterial oxygen content. Above 2,500 m (8,200 ft), ***acute mountain sickness*** is common, especially when ascent has been rapid and the mountaineer may be ***dehydrated*** or otherwise physically stressed. Very high altitude is defined as 3,500 to 5,500 m (11,500 to 18,000 ft). Rapid ascents at this altitude can lead to acute mountain sickness, ***high-altitude pulmonary edema,*** and ***high-altitude cerebral edema.*** The upper slopes of many commonly climbed peaks are at these altitudes. Ascent rates greater than 300 m (1,000 ft) per day and dehydration are probably the two most important factors contributing to mountain illnesses. Extreme high altitude is defined as over 5,500 m (18,000 ft). It is in general considered impossible to live for long periods above this altitude, where physiologic deterioration is inevitable. Acute mountain sickness incorporates numerous symptoms and can be considered mild when a climber suffers only from anorexia, nausea, malaise, and headache. When these symptoms become more severe or unrelenting and the patient shows signs of respiratory or central nervous system compromise, the illness is severe and can be life-threatening. High-altitude pulmonary and cerebral edema also run a variable course, with a classification made on the severity of symptoms. Primary treatment for these problems is descent. Several drugs have been used as adjuncts to altitude illness including acetazolamide, nifidipine, furosemide, and dexamethasone. Other serious problems common at altitude are ***venous thrombosis*** and ***polycythemia, peripheral edema, retinopathy,*** and ***immune system suppression.*** Diseases that can be aggravated by high altitude include chronic lung disease, arthrosclerotic heart disease, and hypertension. Any disease aggravated by oxygen desaturation of hemoglobin can contraindicate travel to extremely high altitudes. High-altitude environments are, as a rule, dry, and dehydration is extremely common. Fluid intakes of 6 L or more per day, depending on activity levels, are necessary to maintain fluid homeostasis. The drier environment can also contribute to a very common chronic cough and bronchitis at high altitude. Exposure to solar ultraviolet radiation increases 4% with every 300 m (1,000 ft) of increased elevation. Thus, at high altitudes, the risk of problematic ***sunburn*** increases significantly and sunscreen protection is necessary.

Foreign travel may expose the climber to ***viral*** and ***bacterial gastroenteritis*** and ***protozoan diseases*** due to poor water and food quality or improper food handling. Immunizations are often necessary against infectious diseases, including gamma globulin shots for ***hepatitis A.*** At low altitudes or approaches in many mountainous areas, prophylaxis for ***malaria*** is mandatory. Traffic safety in foreign mountain environments is often marginal at best, therefore rescue and accident insurance are strongly recommended.

Cold weather may precipitate ***hypothermia*** and ***frostbite.*** Hypothermia can be caused by obvious situations, as when a climber is caught by an avalanche or is forced to spend an unprotected night out in an extremely cold environment. More commonly it occurs in mountaineers who are stressed, dehydrated, and in a catabolic state while in a cold environment. Early symptoms include lassitude and increased respiratory rate. Frostbite, of course, involves actual freezing of tissue, which is usually limited to exposed skin areas on the hands, face, or feet. Contributing factors are improper gloves or footwear, including poorly waterproofed boots or wet socks or glove liners. External pressure from boots or tight gloves is also a contributing factor. The most effective way of treating frostbite is rapid rewarming, but this should be done only if the injured part can remain warm after treatment. Refreezing causes severe soft tissue injuries.

The mountaineer should have at least some training in basic first aid before going on a trip into the wilderness, and a plan for rescue should be in place. It is customary to give a description of the planned route and expected date of return when venturing into mountain environments. The long hike in for a mountain adventure may precipitate many foot problems, including ***blisters, Achilles tendinitis,*** and ***ankle sprains.*** Prevention of these problems by use of proper footwear and foot preparation is much more effective than trying to treat them in the field. Many underlying knee problems can worsen during hikes on steep ground, particularly ***patellofemoral problems*** during descent. With individuals carrying heavy packs, ***lumbar strain*** and ***overuse*** of the ***hip abductors*** is frequent. Use of ski poles or properly adjusted walking sticks is very helpful in relieving these symptoms.

At low altitude, ***insect bites*** and ***bee stings*** are common. In the western United States, pit viper bites are a concern, particularly in rocky areas. Skin irritation from toxic plants, such as poison oak, can be extremely uncomfortable and debilitating. Although rare, attacks by large animals do occur in some remote areas of the United States and Canada. The suggested local precautionary rules should be heeded.

Upon reaching steep terrain, climbers are faced with the threat of falling or having something fall on them. Some 60% of injuries in the mountains occur on rock and the remainder on ice and snow. The immediate causes of injury are most frequently a fall or slip on rock, a slip or fall on snow and ice, or being struck by a rock or other object. Hypothermia with concomitant impaired judgment is an important causative factor of injury. Thunderstorms, of course, can occur daily in mountain environments and lightning injury is reported every year. The most common contributing causes of injury are unroped climbing and exceeding one's ability. Inadequate equipment, weather, and inadequate protection are also associated with many climbing injuries. Virtually ***any fracture or joint injury*** can be sustained by a fall from a height, and head injuries are a significant cause of death during falls, particularly if a climber fails to use a hard hat. Rock fall may also cause ***severe head or extremity injuries*** including amputation. Basic first-aid skills, including cardiopulmonary resuscitation (CPR), can be lifesaving in many of these situations.

In winter environments, extreme or steep ice climbing involves the use of crampons and sharp ice axes. Penetrating injuries can occur from these devices. Shards of extremely hard ice can be broken off while inserting the axes, and eye protection is strongly recommended.

Sport climbing has allowed many people to participate in climbing adventures without an increased threat of severe bodily injury. Sport climbing often involves short routes and bolted protection, where the threat of severe injury from a fall is low or with the use of top ropes, which can completely prevent a serious fall if used properly.

The upper extremities are put to an extreme test during high-level sport climbing. The ***shoulder*** can be ***dislocated*** or ***strained,*** often with associated ***shoulder instability.*** At the level of the elbow, underlying arthritic conditions can be worsened by sport climbing. The development of ***medial epicondylitis*** and—less commonly—***lateral epicondylitis*** is seen in sport climbers. ***Brachialis tendinitis*** or ***anterior capsular injury*** is common and often referred to as ***"climber's elbow." Tenosynovitis of wrist extensors*** and ***finger flexors*** is often seen. Compression neuropathies of the upper extremity—including ***cubital tunnel syndrome, radial tunnel syndrome,*** and ***carpal tunnel syndrome***—are often seen. Skin injuries of the hands are frequent, particularly during crack climbing with improper technique or protection. Virtually all climbers sustain ***abrasions to the fingertips. Ligamentous strains*** or ***ruptures of the metacarpophalangeal joints*** are seen, as well as acute ***capsulitis of the interphalangeal joints. Partial ruptures of the sublimis tendons*** can occur during extreme use, particularly with one-finger pulls or other extreme climbing techniques. Almost all high-level climbers experience pain or ***capsulitis of the distal interphalangeal joints. Annular pulley rupture,*** particularly along the proximal phalanx of the finger, is seen almost exclusively in sport or high-angle climbers. Prevention of these overuse injuries is highly important since treatment almost always involves some curtailment of climbing activities. Gradual training to increase strength and maintain flexibility is extremely important, while sport climbing and can help prevent many of these problems. It takes years for ligaments and tendons to adapt to the strains of high-level rock or sport climbing. It is the injuries to these structures that most often limit the aspiring climber's progress.

83. POWER LIFTING, WEIGHT LIFTING, AND BODY BUILDING

William F. Luetzow and David Hackley

Weight training is increasingly popular in a broad spectrum of the population as a means of conditioning, strengthening, and altering esthetic appearance. Therefore it is essential for the sports medicine physician to be familiar with common training practices and typical injuries associated with weight training, competitive lifting, and body building.

Definitions

Weight training refers to the use of a variety of resistance methods, including free weights and weight machines, to increase ***muscular strength, endurance,*** and/or ***power*** for sports-specific goals or for general conditioning.

Power lifting is a competitive sport in which an athlete attempts to lift a maximal amount of free weight in the defined lifts (squat lift, dead lift, and bench press).

Weight lifting is a competitive sport in which an athlete attempts to lift a maximal amount of free weight in clean-and-jerk and snatch lifts.

Body building is a competitive sport in which the participant uses resistance training methods to maximize muscle size, symmetry, and definition.

Dietary Issues

Perhaps no other area of athletics is as inundated with homeopathic folklore, fad diets, and the use of ***unproven dietary supplements*** as recreational and competitive weight training. Popular high-protein powdered supplements are highly concentrated. The resultant high osmotic load can cause ***cramping*** and ***diarrhea.*** Extremely high protein supplementation can lead to ***renal tubular overload.*** A widespread form of ***polypharmacy*** has evolved promoting various vitamins, minerals, enzymes, and even growth factors—all popularized to enhance the anabolic process.

Creatinine monohydrate, chromium picolinate, phosphates, inosine, and l-carnitine are currently popular. (Yet, for example, less than 2% of an oral dose of l-carnitine is actually absorbed.) More concerning is the use of ***stimulants*** (often with beta blockers). Clearly troublesome, the use of ***growth hormone, insulin,*** and ***insulin-like growth factor (IGF-1)*** is on the rise, with an ample supply apparently available through the black market.

Abuse of anabolic steroids is prevalent despite well-publicized adverse effects on health. Essentially all body builders restrict their fluid and caloric intake before competition. ***Diuretic abuse*** combined with restricted fluid intake has caused severe dehydration and electrolyte disturbance. ***Metabolic disturbances, hemoconcentration, myoglobinuria,*** and ***renal failure*** have been reported. Multiple ***deaths*** have occurred.

Cardiovascular Effects of Weight Training

The ***"athlete's heart"*** is well-documented in weight lifters and is characterized by an ***increase in both left ventricular cavity size and wall thickness.*** Recent studies suggest that the ***dimensions of the typical weight lifter's heart still lie within normal limits*** (less than 13 mm left ventricular thickness). Therefore a diagnosis of pathologic cardiomyopathy should be considered when abnormal values are encountered. Resistance-trained young males have been shown to have ***cardiovascular disease risk profiles comparable*** to those of aerobically trained young males. Both groups have favorable profiles compared with those of untrained cohorts. Low body fat and low fat intake in trained groups appear to be important factors.

Training Techniques

The sports medicine physician must maintain familiarity with commonly utilized training methods. Fad methods are subject to unsubstantiated popularity in the lay

Table 83-1. Common injuries: their prevention and treatment

Location	Type	Prevention	Treatment
Neck	Cervical strain, disc herniation	Neck positioning and support. Caution with neck exercise machines.	Rest, stretching (strain), traction (disk).
Shoulder	Acromioclavicular joint	So common as to appear unpreventable.	Stretching and warm-up. Wider grip on bench press. Avoid painful exercises, Steroid injection, surgery.
	Rotator cuff	Avoid lateral raise above 90 degrees, abduction, stretching, external rotator training.	Avoid overhead lifting. Subacromial steroid injection, physical therapy.
	Pectoralis major rupture	Rare in absence of anabolic steroid abuse.	Surgery generally recommended.
	Instability	Avoid "at risk" positions, such as hyperextension with butterfly machine.	Condition Rotator Cuff and scapular stabilizers. Bankart repair as indicated for anterior instability. Multidirectional instability typically treated nonoperatively.
Elbow	Lateral epicondylitis	Wrist supports to avoid extensor overload.	Rest, strap, occasional injection, rarely surgery.
Wrist	Tendinitis, most commonly flexor carpi radialis and De Quervain's	Use straps and techniques to avoid excess loads while training larger muscles.	Wrist supports, taping, rest, conditioning.
Lumbar	Strain, disc herniation, pars defect, instability	Maintain lordotic posture, feet off floor for bench press, spotting, belt.	Rest, "back school," dominal and spinal stabilizer muscle strengthening, epidural injection (disc). Surgery generally reserved for neurologic symptoms or severe slip.
Knee	Patellofemoral	Gradual progression with squats and lunges. Avoid leg-extension machine. Closed chain training.	Avoidance, low-load cross training. Alter stance during squats.
	Meniscal	Avoid twist or bounce with squats. Keep knee aligned with toes.	Rest, arthroscopic surgery
	Patellar tendinitis	Avoid squat and lunge past parallel with floor (90 degrees).	Rest, strap/brace

press. The ***Weider principles*** comprise the most common training techniques. The basic weight lifting "set" involves performing repetitions to exhaustion, followed by assisted and/or forced concentric repetitions. "Negatives" or eccentric muscle loading is a well-proven method for improving muscular size and strength; however, ***muscular strains are more common with eccentric loading.***

Weight Training and the Prepubescent or Adolescent Athlete

The reported incidence of injury by weight training in junior and senior high school football players, which caused more than 7 days of missed participation is 7.6%. 74% were classified as strain injuries. Several reports indicate that few injuries occur in carefully supervised programs.

Common Injuries (Table 83-1)

The vast majority of weight training–related injuries fall into the category of ***musculotendinous strains*** from acute or chronic overload. Nearly any region of the body may be involved. Strains of the ***lumbar spine*** are consistently the most highly reported (50% of reported power-lifting injuries). However, neck, shoulder, wrist, and knee injuries are all quite common. These injuries are more easily ***prevented*** than cured. Preventative measures include a ***stretching*** regimen before and after each workout. Wrist wraps and lifting gloves are used for comfort and safety and to reduce wrist and forearm strains. ***Weight belts*** are felt to decrease the load on the lumbar spine. One study documented loss of disc space after heavy lifting in all participants but significantly less with the use of a weight belt.

Most acute injuries are felt to occur due to ***loss of form*** during excessive loading without adequate supervision or assistance. Emphasis on ***appropriate training techniques, spotting,*** as well as ***commonsense progression of load and repetitions*** are likely to limit such injuries. When they occur, most strain injuries will respond to relative rest, ice, and nonsteroidal antiinflamatory medication.

84. RODEO

Jack Harvey

Rodeo is one of the original sporting events of North America. This high-risk sport frequently presents the medical team with acute trauma, often occurring in remote and rustic settings. This places a premium on trauma first aid skills and the establishment of communications, transport, and medical backup to care for injured cowboys and cowgirls adequately. Recently the competitors have realized the importance of athletic training skills to provide preevent preparation of stretching, taping, and bracing as well as the rehabilitation of chronic injuries.

The injury rate in rodeo surpasses that of the more traditional collision sports of football, wrestling and hockey. The variety of events that make up a rodeo each have their own particular injury patterns as well as the acute trauma that accompanies competing with or against 1,200- to 2400-lb animals. There is no "injured reserve," and tradition promotes competing with existing injuries. Further, the competitor's schedule often may require participation in three or four rodeos in a weekend, each separated by hundreds of miles of driving or air travel.

The events are classified as **rough stock,** which includes bareback, saddle bronc and bull riding, and **timed events,** consisting of calf and team roping, steer wrestling, goat tying, and barrel racing. Competitors often participate in more than one event, and injuries received early in the bareback riding may require treatment and taping to allow participation in the bull riding an hour later. Bull riding is the most injury-prone of the events, leading to 37% of the total injuries. It is followed by bareback riding and saddle bronc, at 23% and 16%, respectively. However, timed events do also produce many acute traumatic injuries, with goat-tying producing an epidemic of anterior cruciate tears.

Preparations for providing medical care to a rodeo should start at least 6–8 weeks prior to the rodeo with communication with the rodeo committee. During this meeting, times of competition, facilities, and provision of ambulance and medical transport should be confirmed. The ideal location for the sports medicine area is in back of the chutes, to allow easy access by the cowboys for preevent preparation as well as convenience for transporting injured competitors from the arena. Arena protocols as to who will attend to the injured competitor can also be established. Communication and cooperation with the paramedics prior to the rodeo is important to ensure optimal care for the injured cowboys. Sports medicine personnel will note that a traditional uniform of cowboy hat, long-sleeved western shirt, and jeans is required to enter the arena. Tradition in rodeo is that, if possible, the injured competitor will ambulate from the arena without assistance. If the injury is obviously serious, the sports medicine team should first enter the arena and assist with ambulation after initially assessing the injury. The paramedics, with appropriate equipment, can be summoned with prearranged signals if further on-site care is required prior to transport to the sports medicine facility or ambulance. If the bull is still in the area, careful consideration needs to be given prior to entering the arena to help a downed cowboy. Bullfighters (clowns) and the pick-up riders can usually clear the bull from the area rapidly, but if this is not the case, proceed with caution!

The sports medicine facility can be a room, tent, or mobile trailer located in an area convenient to the arena. Availability of electricity, lighting, water, and ice cannot be taken for granted and must be arranged prior to the event. The general equipment and supplies found in a training room should be available. This would include ice, modalities, tape, and bracing supplies as well as treatment tables. The medical supplies would be similar to those for sideline attendance and would also include casting, splinting, and suturing materials. Since many competitors are leaving after the rodeo instructional materials on icing, wound care and head injury are a convenience.

The medical team usually consists of an athletic trainer and/or physical therapist with sports experience in combination with a physician. Prior to the rodeo, all members of the team are available to help cowboys prepare for the upcoming events as well as evaluate and treat injuries received in the days or weeks prior to the present event. When the rodeo starts, one or more members of the team must constantly monitor the arena events in case of injury. One member can remain in the facility to continue taping and treatments as the rodeo progresses. If a serious injury occurs and the competitor is transported from the arena to the sports medicine facility, one member of the team must return to the arena monitoring as quickly as possible while other members of the team care for or transport the patient.

Upon completion of the performance, the team finishes with treatments and provides for follow-up care for the injured. This follow-up care may include regular visits to the sports medicine facility during the weekend of the rodeo or consultation with other personnel at the rodeo to which the competitor is traveling. Further care can also be arranged with doctors or therapists when the competitor finally returns home. The final task is to prepare the facility for the next performance, which may start within a few hours or the next day.

Bareback riding is the most punishing of the events to the rider, causing many chronic problems as well as acute traumatic injuries. As with all rough stock events, ***lacerations, contusions,*** and ***fractures*** can occur if the rider collides with the chutes, fences, or hard arena ground. The most injury-prone times are at the beginning of the ride while the rider is mounting the horse, upon exit from the chutes, or during dismount, especially if the rider is thrown from the horse or if the rider's hand gets hung up in the bareback rigging. Getting a hand hung up in the handle of the bareback rigging usually happens because of too tight a fit with the glove and rigging or being bucked off on the side opposite the riding hand. In the latter case, the rider is often dragged around the arena by one arm and may be seriously injured if flung against the fence or pulled under the animal's hooves.

Chronic pain in the ***cervical spine*** and radiculopathy ("***burners***") are common in this event. The use of a protective neck collar (made of a rolled towel or foam and stockinette) to limit ballistic neck extension during the ride is helpful in prevention and treatment. ***Shoulder strains*** and ***rotator cuff problems*** as well as ***glenohumoral dislocation*** occur from being hung up or upon landing when bucked off. ***Elbow hyperextension*** and chronic ***arthritis*** are the result of the tremendous eccentric forces the riding arm experiences during the ride. Treatment is with ice, modalities, and antiinflammatories. However, prevention with elbow hyperextension, taping, or bracing is most important. A unique arm pain, like "shin splints," along the edge of the ulna occurs in this event and in bull riding. The usual training-room techniques are helpful in controlling the pain, but taping the arm or the use of an orthoplast hard brace taped along the middle of the forearm along the ulna helps tremendously. The ***wrist*** also receives a lot of abuse and is protected by taping, but the tape must be applied so as not to interfere with the fit of the glove or placement of the hand into the rigging. The placement of several single layers of circumferential tape starting at the base of the thumb and continuing proximally up the forearm for 3 to 5 in. is usually successful.

Saddle bronc riding is notable for the high-flying buck-offs that produce the whole spectrum of ***lower extremity sprains, strains,*** and ***fractures.*** The cowboys in this event hold on with a single thick buck rein and thus avoid the chance of getting a hand hung up. However the stirrups can catch a foot, and if the loosely fitting boot does not come off, the cowboy can be dragged around the arena—most dangerously under the horse—receiving serious ***head injuries.*** If this occurs, it is the job of the pickup riders to stop the bronc and extricate the rider. Knee sprains of the ***medial collateral*** and ***anterior cruciate ligaments*** are caused by upright landings in the soft but uneven turf of the arena. Many riders wish to return to competition early, and bracing or taping is an important consideration. The most popular braces are those with no medial hinge or a small, thin medial component so as to allow close contact between the rider's leg and the animal. ***Ankle sprains*** usually do not keep the cowboys from participation and are supported with taping or a lace-up style of brace that allows for the boot to come off easily if the rider's foot gets caught in the stirrup. ***Fracture of the lower leg*** is the result of a twisting while landing or getting stepped on by the still bucking animal. ***Serious head and neck injury*** may result if the rider is thrown over the front of the horse onto his head or gets run over and kicked in the head. Neurological assessment, stabilization with a cervical collar and backboard, and rapid transport to a facility with neurosurgical backup should be expedited for serious cases. Less serious ***concussions*** and ***neck sprains*** will test the diagnostic acumen of the sports medicine team as the now conscious cowboy will usually insist on leaving shortly for the next rodeo or perhaps compete in the bull riding in an hour. Dealing with these problems can be assisted by recruiting the cowboys' traveling partners, girlfriends, or wives to allow for adequate recovery time from the more minor head and neck injuries. An authoritarian approach is usually doomed to failure.

Bull riding is the most dangerous of the rough stock events. Again the most dangerous times for the rider are while getting on the bull and exiting the chute and upon getting off at the end of the ride. During the ride the danger is in hitting heads with the bull as it snaps the rider down and forward or in ***tearing an adductor muscle*** while trying to hold on with his legs while the bull spins. The bull rope and grip also present the opportunity to get hung up. Once off the bull, scrambling for the safety of the fence is paramount; many injuries occur from being thrown under the bull during a spin or upon being caught by the bull catching before the rider can make the safety of the fence. The bullfighters (rodeo clowns) are very important in that they can often save a rider from injury by distracting the bull and drawing it off, allowing the rider to reach safety or the sports medicine team to reach the downed rider. Bull riders suffer the same ***chronic arm injuries*** as bareback riders. The other major chronic problem is repeated ***adductor strains.*** These are treated by the usual sports medicine techniques, and the use of taping, sports girdles, a structured stretching and concentric and eccentric adductor strength program.

The timed events produce less than 15% of the injuries. **Goat tying,** which requires the cowgirls to dismount at speed produces many ankle sprains as well as tears of the ***medial and anterior cruciate ligaments.*** **Steer wrestling** produces these same injuries as well as ***shoulder dislocations*** and ***pectoralis strains.*** Contusions and lacerations to the face accompany an ill-timed dismount onto the steer. Both **team ropers** and **calf ropers** may suffer the ***loss of a thumb*** if a coil of rope encircles the thumb during a catch. Calf ropers also get ***lower extremity sprains*** during their dismounts to quickly tie the calves. Lifting the calf prior to throwing and tying ("flanking") produces ***acute and chronic low back pain.*** Barrel racers usually have very few injuries except for hitting the barrel with a knee or if a horse falls during the run.

Injury prevention in rodeo events centers around good sports technique, matching the skill and age of the cowboys and cowgirls with the ranking of the stock, and the use of protective equipment. Protective vests are required in high school and collegiate rough stock rides. Mouthpieces are also required and must be remembered in clearing the airway of an unconscious rider. Use of a helmet is controversial among the cowboys for a variety of reasons but would prevent many serious head and facial injuries if the helmet were equipped with a mask and were required during bull riding. Use of helmets should be strongly encouraged among riders with a recent history of concussion. Stretching programs and well-designed sports specific strength programs are starting to be recognized by the cowboys as an important part of injury prevention. Proper and complete rehabilitation of recent or chronic injuries is also an important aspect of keeping the competitor going in the long run.

85. RAFTING/ROWING/KAYAKING/CANOEING

David M. Jenkinson

For thousands of years, human-powered crafts have been the major means of local transportation. For the early Native Americans and later the French trappers, the "Indian" canoe was the prime means of transport for great distances. This art of simple transportation has developed into a widely diverse field of paddlesport. Around the turn of this century, rowing was challenging baseball as America's most popular sport; since then, crew has been well established in the college ranks. Currently the American Canoe Association estimates that over 24 million people are involved with the sport of canoeing or kayaking. Paddlesport includes everything from extreme whitewater canoe, kayak, and rafting; Olympic rowing, canoeing, and kayaking; to ultra–long distance wilderness tripping or sea kayaking. Paddlesport is broken down by the type of paddle, body position, and environment in which the boat will be used. Competitions have occurred in every possible environment at every imaginable distance. The one constant to this diverse and rapidly advancing group of sports is that a person uses a paddle to propel the boat through the water.

When physicians think about the epidemiology of paddlesport they primarily concentrate on injuries of the upper extremity. However, one of the most common injuries in commercial rafting is the ***ankle injury;*** physicians forget about the walk to the river. The outdoor, wilderness nature of paddlesport yields a diversity of injury patterns.

Dermatologically, canoers, kayakers, and rowers (boaters) are exposed to a wide variety of skin pathologies. These range from simple overuse ***blisters*** on the hands, heels, and buttocks to ***allergic dermatitis*** from exposure to the fiberglass, kevlar, and other complex materials and resins that make up the boats. Dependent ***dermal breakdown*** is a very real threat to long-distance paddlers. ***Lacerations*** are common occurrences while scouting or portaging. The on-water conditions warrant special attention to sun protection; ***sunburn/sun poisoning*** and the prevention of ***skin cancer*** are important to long-time boaters. In addition, overgrowth of ***calluses*** on the hands can be a serious problem, especially for rowers. Occasional paring can easily keep this under control.

Foreign wilderness travel can also expose boaters to an assortment of ***fungal and parasitic infections*** of the skin and gastrointestinal tract. Numerous infections have been reported in the literature, from ***schistosomiasis*** and ***pulmonary blastomycosis*** to simple multisite ***Staphylococcus aureus.*** Boaters should not drink untreated water. Other simple steps of infection prevention are frequently overlooked, from simple laceration and blister care to current ***tetanus immunization.*** Some wilderness organizations are currently debating whether guides and instructors need to have ***hepatitis immunization.***

Head and neck injuries, while relatively uncommon in flatwater canoeing and rowing, are a significant consideration in whitewater boating. The combination of gradient, water volume, and rocky river channels makes ***blunt head trauma, loss of consciousness,*** and/or ***neck hyperextension injury*** possible in the case of an upset (or roll); hence it is recommended that all whitewater canoers, kayakers, and rafters wear helmets. Any ***loss of consciousness*** on the water always mandates immediate cervical spinal precautions and physician evaluation.

Ocular trauma is common during associated waterside travel in whitewater and wilderness boating. Frequently ***corneal abrasion*** occurs from surrounding vegetation during scouting and/or portaging. Occasionally ***lid laceration*** or ***corneal hemorrhage*** can occur during scouting, falls or rolls. Contact lenses can be worn during whitewater and wilderness boating; however, the risk of loss during upset and recovery requires one or two backup devices.

Exostosis formation is a unique threat to extended-season whitewater boaters and sea kayakers. This condition, while known to physicians, has recently gained recognition among the boating community itself. If the condition is recognized early enough, watertight ear plugs can frequently slow the progression of the disease. ***Perforation of the tympanic membrane*** has been reported in whitewater boaters after forcible submersion events.

Blunt trauma to the face and teeth is always a concern in rafting. ***Dental trauma*** usually occurs when a boater lets go of the end of the paddle (or oar) during an upset. Proper control of the handle easily minimizes this possible injury; "hold it, don't eat it" is a guide's common admonishment. Rarely, more severe facial trauma / fracture can occur during upsets in kayaking or canoeing.

The introduction of high-tech dry suits and synthetic clothing has extended the paddlesport season well into the late fall and early spring. In southern states, rowing and whitewater boating are year-round sports. In the north, sea kayakers and recreational rowers frequently "break ice" to start their season. ***Hypothermia*** is always a threat. Most cases of hypothermia occur in rainy weather (40° to 60°F; 4.5 to 15.5°C) in the unprepared commercial customer/paddlers and usually not in the well-prepared, experienced boater.

One of the most devastating injuries a boater can suffer is ***anterior-inferior shoulder dislocation*** or ***subluxation.*** Unlike most sports, an improperly performed whitewater kayaking/canoe roll and static turning stroke puts the paddler in the classic externally rotated, abducted position. Quick identification and field reduction of anterior dislocation by properly trained medical personnel is a key to minimizing sequelae. There are also anecdotal reports of ***posterior dislocation*** suffered by whitewater kayakers who reach forward for the next stroke only to plant the paddle into a fixed position, thus forcing the humeral head into the posterior medial capsule.

Other common shoulder injuries are either of ***glenohumeral capsular instability*** or, more commonly, ***impingement/bursitis/overuse*** variety. One interesting abnormality that has been seen in "non-side-switching" canoeist (freestyle, whitewater) is an ***asymmetrical development*** of the large motor units around the shoulder (increased latissimus dorsi and trapezius size on the "shaft hand" side, while the contralateral or "control hand" side shows marked underdevelopment of the serratus/rhomboid complex). All boaters can benefit from muscle rebalancing exercise, scapular stabilization, and postural work.

Elbow and wrist injuries present another problem for the boaters. While ***medial/lateral epicondylitis*** is relatively rare in whitewater sports, flatwater athletes commonly suffer from this condition. A common injury in beginning boaters is overuse of the "control side," or rotating grip wrist. This repetitive flexion and extension of the wrist can cause ***median nerve palsy*** and general ***extension tendinitis.*** A lesser problem is that of ***De Quervain's tendinitis.*** One possible solution to this is decrease the "feather" or offset of kayak paddle blade from the traditional 80- or 90-degree angle to the newer 45-degree offset.

Rowers can also be subject to ***blunt trauma*** from a missed stroke of the oar, known as "catching a crab." It can result in ***contusions or broken ribs,*** even ***puncture wounds of the abdomen or legs.*** In addition, several reports of a rare overuse injury, ***rib stress fracture,*** have been reported in college rowers.

A common complaint of new boaters is ***lumbar back pain.*** Numerous studies of rowers have reinforced the value of preevent stretching for all boaters. In most cases the athlete can benefit from increasing hamstring flexibility and abdominal strengthening. In kayaking, transient back pain can be helped with added lumbar support, or a "back band." Biomechanically, attention should be paid to improving trunk rotation on the catch phase of the forward stroke, rather than leaning forward from the waist. In the rower, attention should be paid the back position during the stroke-glide, and to use of the quadriceps instead of pulling, arching with the back. For back pain that does not resolve, ***herniations and spondylopathologies*** should be ruled out.

Overuse injuries to the lower extremities are, by nature of the sport, relatively minor. Rowers occasionally suffer from ***ischial tuberosity bursitis, quadriceps strains, hamstring pulls, IT band syndrome, patellofemoral syndrome,*** and ***patellar tendintious.*** A whitewater boater in an improperly fitted boat can sometimes suffer from transient numbness and tingling. This lower extremity pain is usually due to vascular insufficiency/occlusion from extreme flexion of the foot and knee in combination with a general decrease flexibility and improper outfitting. Modifying the outfitting of the boat and a general program of stretching can usually resolve this problem quickly. ***Fractures of femur, lower leg, ankle, and foot*** have all been reported during whitewater entrapment situation or after a fall during scouting.

Finally, a word about one of the obvious complications of paddlesport, ***accidental death and drowning.*** In reviewing the medical, U.S. Coast Guard, and American Whitewater Association literature, most accidental deaths can be broken down into two categories: (1) Inexperienced boaters without proper training and not wearing a personal floatation device (PFD) or (2) experienced boaters in a boat and/or body entrapment situation. Some simple rules are important in preventing serious consequences: (1) never boat alone; (2) make sure your boat is in good repair with the appropriate safety equipment; (3) Wear your PFD; (4) never use alcohol before or during boating; (5) good swimming skills and good physical condition are important; (6) If you are new to the sport, get some training in the basic techniques and rescue skills; and (7) for the experienced boater, know your skills and limits. Many local YMCAs, local paddling/rowing clubs, or university clubs will provide the basic training at low or no cost.

Paddlesport comprises a diverse group of athletic events. They can range from high-risk whitewater kayaking in remote river canyons to a rowing workout on the local river. The risk involved in these sports, while relatively minor, requires respect for the water and the environment. Physicians involved with these athletes should familiarize themselves with the biomechanical subtleties of each branch. The physician should not forget that up to 50% of all injuries occur not on the water but rather during dry-land training, scouting or other boat-related chores.

86. RUGBY

Peter Brukner

Rugby is a body-contact type of football played in two forms. Rugby union, a traditionally amateur 15-a-side game, is popular in New Zealand, South Africa, Great Britain, Australia, and France. Rugby league is a professional, 13-a-side game played primarily in Australia and the North of England as well as New Zealand, France, and Papua New Guinea. In most of the surveys conducted, rugby league has a higher injury incidence than rugby union, but the distribution of injuries between the two sports is relatively similar with one or two exceptions to be described further on. Because of the heavy body contact in rugby, the overall incidence of injuries is relatively high. Injuries are distributed fairly evenly among the positions in rugby league; however, rugby union centers and flank forwards tend to have a higher injury rate, as they tend to be more involved in tackling. Front-row forwards in rugby union also have a higher incidence of neck injuries.

Despite the high incidence of injuries, the number of serious injuries in rugby is relatively low. Until relatively recently, the most common serious injuries were cervical spinal injuries occasionally leading to quadriplegia. These tended to occur in rugby union front-row forwards involved in the scrum. Changes to the scrummaging rules in the 1980s have dramatically reduced the incidence of these injuries. The number of serious injuries of the head and face has also been reduced as a result of stricter policing of head-high tackles.

The head and face are still the most common sites of injury in rugby. ***Lacerations*** are relatively common but are usually of a minor nature and in many cases the player is able to continue playing after appropriate treatment is carried out during the game. Minor forms of ***concussion*** are common in rugby either due to direct contact with an opponent or as a result of the head hitting the ground after a tackle. The majority of rugby players with concussions appear to suffer mild forms and, on average, miss only 1 week as a result. There has been no evidence of the second concussion syndrome or of any chronic brain damage resulting from repetitive episodes of concussions. Protective headgear is not used widely in rugby, although some players, particularly those who have had previous episodes of concussion, choose to wear soft padded helmets. Further research in to the effectiveness of these helmets in reducing the incidence of concussion is needed.

Facial fractures are also seen relatively commonly in rugby. The most common site of facial fracture is the ***nose,*** followed by the ***zygoma. Blowout fractures of the orbit*** are occasionally seen. ***Eye injuries*** occur, usually as a result of an accidental finger poke in the eye. These are almost invariably minor injuries.

The most common upper limb injury seen in rugby is ***acute sprain of acromioclavicular joint.*** This injury occurs when the shoulder is struck by an opposing player or, more commonly, by contact with the ground when falling. Most injuries of the acromioclavicular joint are first-or second-degree injuries. ***Glenohumeral joint subluxations or dislocations*** usually occur as a result of landing on an outstretched arm. "***Burners,***" injuries involving traction of the brachial plexus, are seen occasionally in rugby, as are ***fractures to the clavicle*** and ***injuries to the rotator cuff tendons.***

Fractures of the metacarpals and finger bones are relatively common. Fractures and dislocations of the fingers occur when, in attempting to catch the ball, contact is made at the end of the finger. Fractures of the metacarpals usually occur because of direct contact with an opponent, either accidental or deliberate.

The most common trunk injury is an ***injury to the ribs or rib cartilages.*** This is usually ***bruising,*** but occasionally ***rib fractures*** may occur. Complications of rib fractures such as a ***pneumothorax*** or ***pneumohemothorax*** are occasionally seen. ***Low back strains*** and ***disc prolapses*** are also seen.

As with other sports that involve sudden changes in direction, ***groin strains*** are seen frequently in rugby. These are usually ***adductor muscle tears. Chronic groin***

pain is not as common in rugby as in other forms of football that involve more kicking, such as soccer and Australian football. The ***hip "pointer" or subperiosteal hematoma of the iliac crest*** is also seen occasionally as a result of direct contact.

Contusions to the quadriceps muscle are extremely common in rugby, but they are almost invariably relatively minor injuries and seldom cause a player to miss a subsequent match. Occasionally ***myositis ossificans*** may develop, and this usually results in a lengthy absence from the game. ***Quadriceps and hamstring strains*** are the most common acute muscle injuries seen in rugby. These strains still occur frequently despite increased attention to warm-up and stretching. The role of the lumbar spine in the development of these strains is still a matter of some controversy.

In any sport that involves high-speed changes of direction and the likelihood of an opponent falling across the player's knee, knee ligament injuries are common. The ***medial collateral ligament (MCL)*** is the most commonly injured ligament in rugby. The usual mechanism is the application of a valgus force to the knee as a result of a direct contact with an opponent while the foot is fixed on the ground. ***Anterior cruciate ligament (ACL)*** injuries may be seen in isolation or in association with an MCL tear. ACL injuries may result from direct body contact or from hyperextension or sudden pivoting movements. ***Meniscal tears, posterior cruciate ligament (PCL) tears,*** and ***dislocation to the patella*** are other knee injuries seen occasionally in rugby.

Contusions to the calf muscles and ***calf strains*** are also seen occasionally. ***Achilles tendon injuries*** and ***fractures to the fibula*** are even less common.

The ***ankle*** is the most commonly injured joint in rugby. The majority of these are inversion injuries and result in ***partial or complete tears of the lateral ligament complex. Fractures of the ankle*** are relatively rare. ***Medial ankle ligament strains*** are much less common.

Stress fractures have been recorded occasionally in recent years and are probably due to the increased amount of training performed by more serious rugby players.

Preventive equipment has not been used widely in rugby. The majority of players wear mouth guards to protect their teeth and possibly to decrease the likelihood of a concussive episode. As mentioned previously, soft helmets are worn occasionally. Ankle strapping is performed uniformly at the elite level as well in those who have previously had ankle injuries at club level. Coach education is generally well organized in rugby football and most coaches have at least a basic qualification. Coaching courses usually have a small component dedicated to injury prevention.

In conclusion, rugby football has a relatively high injury incidence due to the contact nature of the game. However the vast majority of injuries are relatively minor and the incidence of serious injuries has decreased in recent years due to rule changes and stricter refereeing.

87. SPEED SKATING, IN-LINE SKATING, FIGURE SKATING

Wade Smith

Speed Skating

Ice speed skating encompasses short- and long-track styles. Short-track racing is performed on a 111-m oval, pack style, within a hockey rink. Competitors generally race all events including the 500- 1,000-, 1,500-, and 3,000-m races. Team relay races are 5,000 or 3,000 m. Races include five to eight skaters traveling at speeds up to 35 mph, drafting within inches of one another. Passing is done at high speed, often in the corners, and no overt physical contact is allowed. Safety padding is placed along the boards around the ice rink to protect skaters during falls. Mandatory safety equipment includes solid-shell helmets, knee padding, and gloves. Optional equipment such as kevlar neck guards, shatterproof eye protection, and soccer-style shins guards are recommended but not uniformly worn.

The majority of serious injuries are impact injuries occurring after high-speed falls in short-track speedskating. ***Extremity fractures***—including ***ankle, tibia, distal radius,*** and ***femur***—may result when skaters fall at the apex of the turn and collide at speed with the boards or the padding. Despite adequate padding at the point of impact, torsional forces generated when a skater's extremity is twisted underneath him or her while sliding may result in spiral or oblique extremity fractures. ***Cervical spinal injuries,*** including fractures and sprains, may be caused after pad or board collisions. The mechanism is usually axial loading with the neck in flexion. ***Head injuries*** may also occur, the most common being ***concussions*** without amnesia. ***Brachial plexus traction injuries*** are seen in less experienced skaters who attempt to protect their heads during a fall with outstretched arms. All skaters who remain down after a fall and board collision need immediate medical attention and should be initially treated as having potentially ***unstable cervical spinal injuries.*** While waiting for medical evaluation or transport, skaters lying on the ice should be kept warm to prevent ***hypothermia.***

Skate blades are another source of serious injury in short track. When skaters fall, they are often close together and may either be stepped on by other skaters or knock other skaters down as they slide toward the boards. ***Laceration*** of an exposed area occurs with even minor contact because of the skate blades' sharp edges. Lacerations of upper and lower extremity vessels or of the carotid artery require immediate direct pressure and emergency transport. Of ***peripheral nerve injuries,*** the most common is the ***superficial peroneal.*** With nerve lacerations, there is often concomitant vessel and muscle disruption.

Long track is skated as a time-trial event on a 400-m oval. Distances range from 500 to 10,000 m. Two skaters race simultaneously in separate lanes "against the clock." The basic body position for all types of speed skating requires approximately 90 degrees of knee flexion and 60 to 70 degrees of hip flexion. The explosive stroking performed in the bent over "down position" requires powerful hip abductors, adductors, and extensors as well as quadriceps and hamstrings. Non-impact injuries in short and long track are primarily due to overuse or sustained during high-intensity training sessions. ***Low back pain*** is common in both groups, especially in distance skaters. ***Minor lumbar strain*** is common early in the skating season when training consists of a relatively high load of off-ice sessions combined with an increasing length of time spent on the ice in the down position. Off-ice sessions consisting of heavy weight training, hill sprinting, and explosive jumping (plyometrics) contribute to low back pain. Individual athletes with predisposing conditions such as ***spondylolisthesis*** need to be monitored, particularly during periods of increasing volume or intensity, for development of ***lumbar spasm, radiculopathy,*** and ***disc injury.*** Moderate to severe back pain may also occur after falls. Because of the high volume and large amount of cross training required in advanced skating programs, ***muscle strains*** and ***overuse injuries*** are frequent and often difficult to treat. ***Hip adduc-***

tor, hip flexor, and ***hamstring injuries*** are common in the off season training period and during on-ice sprint training. Tired athletes attempting explosive sprint runs, jumps, or starts appear to be at increased risk. Season-long stretching programs combined with thorough warm-up periods decrease the overall incidence of muscle strains. Other overuse syndromes include ***patellar tendonitis, anterior knee pain, achilles tendonitis*** and ***exertional compartment syndrome.*** Distance running, sprinting, plyometrics and heavy squatting, particularly in athletes with lower extremity malalignment or predisposing histories should be carefully monitored. ***Chronic bursitis of the foot and ankle*** is frequently caused by improper skate fit, but may also occur with large skating volumes in well-fitting skates. Symptomatic treatment is by boot adjustment or padding of affected areas.

In-Line Skating

In-line skating has become one of the fastest growing recreational pasttimes in recent years. Along with this increasing popularity has come an increase in in-line skating injuries. The majority occur in recreational use. Novices are at increased risk. Many injuries occur in the first month of skating and often while standing still or skating at very low speeds. Frequent injuries include ***distal radius, ankle, elbow, clavicular, and patellar fractures, ulnar collateral ligament tears of the thumb, acromioclavicular separations,*** and ***wrist sprains. Head injuries, spine fractures,*** and ***multiple long bone fractures*** have been reported, especially in children skating on city streets without head protection. Available protective gear includes hard-shell helmets, gloves, wrist protectors, knee pads, and elbow pads. Safety gear, especially helmets, decrease injury rates, as do proper instructions in skating, braking, and falling technique. Skating terrain plays an important role as well, with gravel, uneven surfaces, automobile traffic, and hills contributing to an increased risk of falling.

Competitive in-line skating comprises speed skating either on a hard wood oval track or outdoors, usually on a road. Distances may be from 300-m (984-ft) to 95 mi. (59-m) marathon races. Traumatic injuries are much less common than among novice recreational skaters because of the technical expertise of competitive skaters. Speeds on downhill road courses may exceed 60 mph. Five-wheel skates with custom leather boots provide increased glide and stability at high speed but decreased maneuverability and braking. All participants wear helmets, but few wear any additional padding. The most frequent injury is ***skin abrasions*** ("road rash") from sliding falls at speed on cement. These may be quite extensive and painful and are best treated with frequent cleaning and silver sulfadiazine (Silvadene) dressings. Overuse injuries similar to those in ice speed skating are common, as is ***overtraining syndrome*** because of the large number or races throughout the year, especially in the warmer climates.

Figure Skating

Figure skaters sustain high-impact and torsional loads to their lower extremities, especially during the landing and takeoff phases of jumping. In addition, for each particular jump, many practice attempts are required, often resulting in a fall, before the jump can be landed successfully. Consequently, ***ligamentous injuries to the knee and wrist, hematomas of the hip and buttocks,*** and ***meniscal injuries of the knee*** are common. The injury severity is often dictated by the velocity and height of the jump. With the advent of triple and quadruple revolution jumps, these injuries are increasing in severity. ***Repetitive hyperextension*** of the lumbar spine in the landing position can contribute to ***low back strain*** and ***spondylolisthesis*** in younger skaters. ***Ankle sprains*** are uncommon with custom-molded boots but are more frequent with poorly reinforced skates. ***Acute muscle strains*** commonly occur in the ***hip flexor, adductor, and hamstrings,*** particularly when the skater is learning high-velocity jumps. Skeletally immature skaters are at risk for ***tibial tubercle apophysitis*** and ***physeal fractures at the knee.*** Pairs and ice-dance skaters may sustain ***blade lacerations*** from their partners. They are also at risk for ***lumbar strain, impingement syndrome of the shoulder,*** and ***rotator cuff tendinitis*** resulting from repetitive lifting of their partners. Foot problems include recurrent ***perimalleolar bursitis, Achilles tendinitis, Haglund's syndrome, hammertoes,*** and ***hard and soft corns*** occuring from poor skate fit or high-volume training. Children spending large amounts of time on the ice may complain of ***arch and plantar fascia pain, bunions,*** and ***bunionettes.*** Because of esthetic demands and rigorous training schedules begun at an early age, some skaters are at risk for eating disorders such as ***anorexia nervosa*** and ***bulemia.***

88. ALPINE SKIING

J. Richard Steadman and Mark T. Dean

Skiing continues to increase in popularity and, accordingly, the number of skiing injuries treated, continues to rise. The incidence of ski injuries, however, has decreased over the past 20 years. The injury rate in recreational skiers has decreased from approximately 7.6 per 1,000 ski days to 2.6 per 1,000 ski days, with an approximately 60% decrease in lower extremity injury rate. Much of the decreased injury rate can be accounted for by improvements in equipment. Improved ski bindings and changes in boot height and construction have affected injury patterns. The incidence of ankle injuries and "boot top" tibial fractures has decreased with the advent of higher, stiffer boots. However, along with this decreased incidence of tibial fractures has come an increase in ***knee ligament injuries.*** Snow conditions also contribute to injury occurrence and improved trail grooming and maintenance may play a role in decreasing injuries in the recreational skier. The competitive skier has a much higher incidence of injury and, in fact, virtually all competitive ski racers sustain an injury at some point in their careers. Particularly, competitive skiers' bindings must be tightened a great deal more than those of recreational skiers to prevent prelease; therefore, an increase in knee ligament injuries is noted. Speed also is a determining factor in the severity of injuries as downhill skiers often reach speeds of up to 100 km/hr.

Preparations for the medical coverage of ski races is far different from that for the coverage of other sporting events. Medical professionals who provide coverage for ski events must be proficient skiers to be able to navigate the course safely if a "downed" skier needs assistance. The medical team must also be positioned carefully along the race course so as to provide expedient care. This is particularly important in longer races with more vertical drop, such as the downhill. Radio communications with trainers and coaches positioned along the course is critical.

The team physician covering ski racing as well as the local physician treating recreational ski injuries must be trained to evaluate and initiate treatment for a wide variety of traumatic injuries. Although the elite ski racer is required to wear a helmet, ***head injuries*** may still occur. Recreational skiers may also incur head injuries; most of these are due to high-velocity falls or impact with stationary objects such as rocks or trees. A careful neurological assessment should be performed as well as evaluation for ***orbital or facial fractures.*** The "downed" skier should never be moved until palpation of the entire spinal column and a careful neurological examination is performed as ***cervical, thoracic, and lumbar spine injuries*** may occur. A skier with a suspected spinal cord injury should be carefully immobilized before transport down the mountain to medical facilities. Thoracic injuries such as ***pneumothorax*** and ***intraabdominal injuries*** such as ***splenic ruptures*** and ***liver lacerations*** also occur with some frequency in recreational skiers and may precipitate surgical emergencies.

One of the most common injuries of the upper extremity is the ***ulnar collateral ligament tear of the thumb,*** or "skier's thumb," which may occur secondary to jamming the thumb into the ski strap or into the snow during a fall. Other upper extremity injuries that may occur are ***acromioclavicular joint separations, anterior shoulder dislocations,*** and ***proximal humerus fractures*** as well as ***humeral shaft, olecranon,*** and ***scaphoid fractures. Rotator cuff tears*** are common in mature athletes with shoulder dislocations and careful, early evaluation and follow-up should be ensured.

Knee ligament injuries are the predominant lower extremity injuries due to skiing. Tears of the ***anterior cruciate ligament (ACL)*** have been reported to occur in up to 66% of all knee injuries during skiing in some studies. Three common mechanisms of injuries can account for the majority of ACL injuries. The most common is a valgus and external rotation mechanism to the knee. This commonly result in injuries to the

medial collateral ligament as well as ***meniscal injuries.*** Hyperextension and internal rotation can also occur, especially novice skiers when the ski tips cross and the skier's weight falls backwards. This injury can occur at low speeds and, in fact, the skier may be surprised that such a severe injury could occur in this way. Fatigue, poor conditioning, and difficult terrain or snow conditions increase the risk of "sitting back" and therefore increase the rate of ACL injury. More advanced skiers often injure the ACL by direct anterior translation of the tibia on the femur, or the "boot-top drawer." This injury may occur as the skier lands from a jump or a mogul (bump) as the skis hit the snow with a combination of anterior pull from the quadriceps and an anterior force produced by the boot top in this hyperflexed position. This mechanism of ACL injury is unusual in other sports and explains the higher incidence of isolated ACL tears in downhill skiers. Sprains of the medial collateral ligament (MCL) are also quite common and may result from an external rotation force with or without binding release. ***Knee dislocations*** may occasionally occur, and if there is any evidence of multiple ligament injuries or knee dislocation, careful vascular examination should be performed both on the hill as well as by the emergency department physician. ***Hip fractures*** are relatively common at recreational ski areas, particularly in mature skiers. ***Hip dislocations*** may occur and should be treated and reduced at an appropriate facility on an emergency basis. ***Femoral fractures*** may occur and should be splinted on site before transport down the mountain is allowed. Although decreasing in frequency, ***tibial shaft fractures*** may occur and may result from rotational forces or a direct blow to the tibia. Other injuries commonly seen are ***tibial plateau fractures*** and ***patellar dislocations.***

Weather-related injuries such as ***hypothermia, frostbite,*** and ***sunburn*** are extremely common. ***Altitude sickness*** is an ever-present danger, particularly among recreational skiers traveling from low altitude levels for ski vacations. Symptoms of altitude sickness include fatigue, nausea, dizziness, and confusion; they should be treated aggressively by return of the skier to a lower altitude and by oxygen therapy.

Snowboarding, Cross-Country Skiing, and Telemark

Snowboarding is increasing in popularity at an extremely rapid rate. It accounts for most of the growth of ski areas at the present time. Organized snowboarding competitions are now commonplace and are becoming more popular as well. Snowboarders may, of course, experience any of the injuries previously listed for Alpine skiers, but the general trend for snowboarders is for fewer lower extremity injuries and particularly less injuries to the knee ligaments. There are, however, significantly increased rates of upper extremity injuries, as snowboard falls tend to occur on an outstretched hand. ***Scaphoid fractures*** and ***forearm fractures*** are particularly common.

Cross-country skiers are less prone to traumatic injuries but may experience overuse injuries as well as weather- and exposure-related injuries. Upper extremity overuse injuries such as ***lateral and medial epicondylitis*** and ***De Quervain's tenosynovitis*** may be seen. Also, lower extremity muscular strains are not uncommon. Although traumatic injuries may occur during a fall; however, the rates are dramatically lower than that with Alpine skiing and snowboarding.

Telemark skiing is a variation of downhill skiing and, as such, similar injury patterns may occur. However, telemark skiers may experience increased ***patellofemoral pain syndromes*** secondary to the constantly flexed position of the knees required for the technique of telemark.

89. SOCCER: FUTSAL AND INDOOR

Jonathan B. Ticker

Futsal, which is abbreviated from *futbal salon,* or indoor football, is played internationally. In 1962, the Federation Internationale de Football Association approved this sport as the internationally sanctioned version of indoor soccer, and in 1981 the United States Futsal Federation was established. World Cup competition began in 1989, with the United States winning medals in each of the first two tournaments.

The United States, however, has had leagues from the amateur to the professional levels playing indoor soccer, with rules different from those of futsal but with similar injury patterns. Futsal uses five players, including one goalkeeper, on a court that measures approximately 20 by 40 m (65 by 131 ft), with boundary lines, not boards. The surface is usually a parquet floor or synthetic surface and the ball is smaller, with much less bounce. In addition, penalties are called as in outdoor soccer. Indoor soccer, on the other hand, is usually played in an ice-hockey rink on Astroturf, with the boards maintained to keep the ball in play. There are six players on each team, including one goalkeeper. The ball is similar to that used in outdoor soccer, and penalties are served as in ice hockey. Although these two sports have other differences, both allow frequent substitutions and emphasize individual ball-handling skills, speed, and a quick release of the ball.

The frequency of injuries during futsal appears to be no greater than in outdoor soccer, based on small studies for futsal injuries. The incidence of injuries during indoor soccer has been reported to be less than for outdoor soccer at the professional level but greater at the youth level. There are more injuries during games than practices in both sports. For indoor soccer, injuries increase with age and are highest in players over 25 years of age. Furthermore, while women have a similar incidence of injuries overall, they have a greater incidence of serious injuries, especially of the knee.

Injuries most commonly encountered in these sports, as in most sports, are ligament sprains, muscle strains, and contusions (bruises). These injuries are often associated with contact between players as well as contact with the ball. The lower extremity is most often injured, with ***ankle sprains*** being the most common injury in both sports. In one study of indoor soccer, the distribution of injuries by body parts was as follows: ankle (23%, with 84% of these being sprains), knee (23%, with 48% ligamentous), head (12.5%), leg (9.5%), foot (8%), torso (6%), fingers (5%), and other (13.5%). While ankle and knee injuries may account for almost half of the injuries, the third most commonly injured area was the head. The players are in close proximity because of the relatively small size of the field. Also, particularly in futsal, where a smaller ball is used, the ***face and eyes*** are at risk for injury. ***Retinal detachment*** has been observed in futsal competition.

By far, the majority of injuries are considered minor. As a result, return to play is often not affected. A severe injury—such as a fracture, dislocation, laceration requiring sutures, eye injury, or ligament injury compromising joint stability—is much less frequent. ***Tears of the anterior cruciate ligament*** appear to account for a majority of the ligamentous knee injuries in indoor soccer, particularly in females. Serious injuries, such as a displaced ***ankle fracture*** or an ***elbow dislocation,*** have been reported during futsal competition. By position, goalkeepers are more likely than other players to sustain an upper extremity injury, such as an ***interphalangeal joint dislocation,*** in both futsal and indoor soccer.

An additional risk for these sports is the hard playing surface. Therefore, injuries can occur to the body as a result of a direct blow or by breaking a fall with the upper extremity. Thus ***wrist sprains*** are seen in futsal as well as ***abrasions*** from the Astroturf of indoor soccer and futsal. For indoor soccer, collision with the boards accounts for additional injuries. Furthermore, poorly maintained playing fields (e.g., irregularities in the surface, such as a defect or edge in the carpet of the Astroturf, or moisture on the floor) can account for some injuries. Specifically designed shoes for both futsal and indoor soccer are recommended. Fluid management and ***heat exhaustion*** pose fewer problems than in outdoor soccer, unless the venue is constructed outdoors or the arena or gymnasium is poorly ventilated.

Suggested Reading

Albert M: Descriptive three year data study of outdoor and indoor professional soccer injuries. *Athletic Training* 18:218–220, 1983.

Lindenfeld TN, Schmitt DJ, Hendy MP, Mangine RE, Noyes FR: Incidence of injury in indoor soccer. *American Journal of Sports Medicine* 22:364–371, 1994.

Putukian M, Knowles WK, Swere S, Castle NG: Injuries in Indoor Soccer: The Lake Placid Dawn to Dark Soccer Tournament. *American Journal of Sports Medicine* 24:317–322, 1996.

Ticker JB, Para AJC, Galpert A, Fu FH: Futsal: A preliminary report on injuries in a growing sport. *Pittsburgh Orthopaedic Journal* 6:73–75, 1995.

United States Futsal Federation Injury Registry, USFF, Berkeley, CA.

90. SOCCER: OUTDOOR

Darren L. Johnson and Ray L. Neef

Soccer is the world's most popular team sport and is the fastest-growing team sport in the country with over 2 million league players in the United States. Soccer is often regarded as a relatively safe sport; however, it is estimated that 50% to 60% of all European sports injuries and 3.5% of all hospital-treated injuries are related to soccer. With the advent of indoor soccer and the increasing participation of women at every level of play, the incidence of injury continues to climb and is currently similar to that observed in lacrosse or hockey.

Injury rates among strikers, midfielders, and goalkeepers appear to be the highest, with ***ligamentous sprains*** and ***muscle strains*** accounting for approximately one-third of injuries at all levels of play. Tackling is the mechanism by which most injuries commonly occur. The incidence of injury increases as the average age of the participants rises, peaking with the 20- to 24- year-old group, with women sustaining nearly twice the number of injuries as men. The severity of injuries involved in soccer is relatively low, with only 10% to 23% of occurrences resulting in time lost from practice or play, representing less than 0.1% of injuries at all levels.

The ***lower extremity*** is the most often injured body part in soccer, representing from 60% to 88% of all injuries. ***Muscle strains (adductors, hamstrings,*** and ***quadriceps***), as well as ***contusions to the thigh and calf*** are common acute injuries. Strains of the quadriceps, hamstrings, gastrocsoleus, and adductors are extremely common in soccer players and may result in extended periods of limited or lost playing time if not appropriately recognized and treated. Deep muscle contusions can be quite disabling and may lead to complications such as acute ***muscle compartment syndrome*** or ***myositis ossificans.*** The use of shinguards greatly reduces the frequency of ***leg contusions*** and is now required in many leagues. ***Chronic exertional compartment syndrome*** may frequently be seen in soccer players and must be differentiated from ***tibial periostitis, stress fractures,*** or ***local nerve compression.***

Knee injuries in soccer are less frequent than expected representing 16% of all injuries in men and 19% in women; however, these injuries account for the greatest amount of lost playing time. ***Collateral ligaments*** have the highest rates of injury, representing 0.51 per 1,000 athlete exposures in men and 0.62 per 1,000 exposures in women. Other structures that may be injured include the ***meniscal cartilage, patella*** or ***patellar tendon, posterior cruciate ligament,*** and the ***anterior cruciate ligament.*** Tears of the anterior cruciate ligament (ACL) have been shown to be significantly more common in female players than in their male counterparts (0.31 per 1000 versus 0.13 per 1000 athletic exposures) and are frequently the result of non-contact mechanisms. Many theories exist concerning this increased injury rate among women. Contributing factors may be divided into extrinsic (muscle strength and coordination, body movement in sport, shoe-surface interface, and level of conditioning/skill) and intrinsic (limb alignment, joint laxity, notch dimensions, and ligament size) factors. Tears of the ACL are generally the most disabling of knee injuries for the soccer player and account for most of the time lost to knee injury. Few players are able to return to their previous level of play with an ACL-deficient knee, despite strengthening and bracing. Surgical reconstruction is often recommended for those who wish to remain competitive. ***Illiotibial band friction syndrome, popliteus tendinitis, patellar tendinitis, pes anserine bursitis,*** and irritation of the synovial plicae are common overuse syndromes observed in the knees of soccer players.

Ankle sprains are the most common soccer injuries, accounting for lost playing time at all ages and levels of competition and representing 17% to 20% of all injuries. As in other sports, the typical ankle injury involves a plantarflexion inversion stress, with injury to the ***lateral ligamentous complex.*** An external rotation/eversion injury may result in a ***high ankle sprain,*** which may tear the anterior and posteroinferior tibiofibular ligament, the inferior transverse ligament, and/or the ***syndesmotic ligament.*** Prophylactic taping is expensive and time-consuming and has not been shown to reduce the incidence of sprains in previously uninjured players. However, if a player has a history of repeated ankle sprains, particularly within the same season, taping and/or bracing has been shown to reduce the incidence of recurrent injury. Tears of the lateral ligament complex should be differentiated from ***peroneal tendon subluxation, dislocation,*** or ***rupture. Achilles tendinopathy*** and ***acute partial*** and ***complete ruptures*** are occasionally seen in soccer, with gross rupture more commonly occurring in the older player. Inflammations of the ***peroneal tendons, posterior tibial tendon,*** or ***FHL*** are common overuse syndromes observed in competitive players. ***Anterior ankle impingement syndrome*** stemming from chronic tibiotalar osteophytes is very common in veteran players and has been termed "footballer's ankle."

Because of the active use of the foot in soccer, it is not surprising that injuries of the midfoot and toes are common. Acute injuries include ***midfoot sprains, fifth-metatarsal fractures,*** and the rare ***tarsalmetatarsal dislocations (Lisfranc injury***), usually as a result of hyperextension overload during tackling. ***Subungual toe hematomas*** and ***digital fractures*** are quite common, with studies showing greater than 30% incidence of phalangeal fractures and osteophytes in elite soccer players. With the repetitive stresses of soccer in the forefoot, overuse injuries such as ***metatarsal stress fractures, sesamoid injuries, turf toe, reverse turf toe (soccer toe***), and ***hallux rigidus*** are frequently encountered.

Upper extremity injuries represent 5% to 15% of soccer injuries occurring primarily in goalkeepers involving the hand. ***Phalangeal fractures*** are the most common—usually the result of catching the ball on the end of the finger. ***Shoulder acromioclavicular separations*** are also seen in all players, relating to falls on the shoulder or outstretched arm.

Injuries to the ***trunk, back,*** and ***pelvis*** are relatively uncommon, accounting for less than 10% of injuries resulting in lost playing time. ***Chronic groin pain*** or ***pubalgia*** is often encountered, relating to the chronic stresses on the lower abdominal wall, hip flexors, and adductors as a result of the biomechanics of repetitive forcible kicking motions.

Head, neck, and face injuries account for 5% to 15% of soccer injuries and usually represent ***minor lacerations*** or ***contusions.*** Both ***dental*** and ***eye injuries*** are relatively uncommon despite the infrequent use of protective headgear, eye wear, and dental guards. The dental mouthpiece can reduce dental injuries and is recommended for goalkeepers and players with orthodontic devices.

Soccer is unique in its use of the head in advancing the ball, and this poses special injury concerns. In the upper levels of the sport, a player will strike the ball with the head an average of six times per match, subjecting the head, cervical spine, and neck musculature to potential injury. ***Concussion*** and ***cervical injury*** can both result from contacting the ball with the head, especially in a lateral impact as opposed to a more frontal strike. Studies in children have shown that strikes at a relatively slow ball speed can exceed head injury tolerance levels. Even with proper technique, impact forces involved in soccer heading approach the upper limits of safety and significant injury can potentially result from any combination of poor technique, accidental contact, or mismatch of ball-to-head weight.

The most important preventative measure for avoiding acute head and neck injuries as a result of heading is to establish proper technique, using the head actively to counteract the force of the oncoming ball, and striking with the forehead rather than passively absorbing the shock with the top or side of the head. Also, the use of smaller balls for young players can significantly reduce the risks inherent in heading.

91. SURFING

Marvin Bergsneider and Ronald A. Navarro

An accurate enumeration of the incidence of surfing-related injuries has not been determined, in part owing to the heterogenous and evolving nature of this sport. Most injuries or afflictions are related to the surfer's interaction with the ocean and/or the surfboard. Certain conditions, such as surfing over shallow rocks or coral reefs or utilization of a shore break, increase the risk of injury. Particular forms or preferences of surfing, such as body surfing or riding large waves, expose the surfer to more serious risks. Surfers are vulnerable to injury, largely because of the inherent power of an ocean wave. Wave energy is proportional to the square of the height of the wave. For example, a 4-ft-high wave delivers approximately 300 ft-lb of energy per foot of wave crest, whereas that number increases to 300 ft-*tons* for a 12-ft wave. In the impact zone (whitewater area), the downward and turbulent forces can easily turn the buoyant surfboard into a missile or hold a surfer under water for prolonged periods of time (more than 2 min in large surf). Among professional surfers, a injury incidence of four moderate to severe injuries per 1,000 surfing days (3.5 hr surfing per day) has been estimated.

Minor lacerations account for over 40% of all surfing injuries, with the surfer's own board being responsible for most. The skull, chin, foot, leg, and eyebrow are most commonly affected. Lacerations and abrasions are common in surf areas characterized by tubular wave breaks over shallow coral reefs. These abrasions frequently contain small pieces of animal protein and skeletal material that act as foreign bodies and may lead to ***chronic suppurative wound infections*** if not promptly and adequately debrided. Near industrial cities, sewage spillage near surf breaks greatly increases the ocean water's bacterial count, thereby requiring thorough irrigation of wounds prior to closure. Some advocate delayed closure if the wound had prolonged exposure to the aquatic environment before definitive irrigation. Lacerations have a higher propensity to develop into infected or chronic ulcers, since many surfers will attempt to "get back into the water" before adequate epithelialization can occur. Skin lacerations may occur despite no apparent break in the overlying wet suit.

Surfer's ear is the presence of ***exostoses in the external ear canal*** in response to the irritation of water and wind. Symptomatic surfer's ear can be treated with antibiotic drops, with cortisone to reduce inflammation. Use three to four drops per ear, three to four times per day for a week. ***Tympanic membrane rupture*** has been reported. Application of topical antibiotics and avoidance of the ocean is required. Occasionally surgical myringoplasty may be required to close a large perforation. ***Pingueculae*** and ***pterygia*** are hyaline nodules of the conjunctiva, usually found on the nasal side of the cornea. They are also thought to be caused by the irritation of sun, water, and wind. While pingueculae can be treated symptomatically, pterygia can encroach on the pupillary area and interfere with vision. Those that do can be removed with a simple operative procedure. ***Blunt eye trauma*** has decreased with the introduction of padded nose guards, which eliminate the sharp point of surfboards. ***"Surfer's sinus"*** is a ***chronic rhinitis*** seen commonly in individuals who frequent the ocean.

Dermatologic conditions are common, especially among avid and fair-skinned surfers. A ***rash*** of the nipple and/or axilla is normally due to wet-suit irritation. Treatment is preventive by encouraging the use of a rash-guard nylon shirt under the wet suit. ***"Surfer's chest knots"*** are innocuous subcutaneous masses over the lower rib cage found more commonly in veteran surfers. ***"Surfer's knots*** or ***knobbies"*** are overgrowths of connective tissue at the tibial tubercle and dorsal foot seen in surfers who paddle long boards in the kneeling position. As in the case of most water-related activities, severe and/or repeated ***sunburn*** can be problematic. Surfers should be screened routinely for signs of ***skin cancer,*** especially on top of the ears, the scalp, and the back. "New moles" and previously badly sunburned areas should be especially scrutinized, with referral to a dermatologist if the area looks questionable. Surfing is becoming increasingly popular in tropical countries, with the associated risks of ***stings*** from various ***sea organisms.*** Most produce a burning discomfort and are benign. Contact with certain toxic jellyfish and sea urchin species can produce severe localized dermatitis, generalized muscular cramps, pulmonary edema, and, rarely, death. Treatment of man-of-war stings consists of bathing the wound in salt water and then with vinegar or isopropyl alcohol before scraping off clinging tentacles.

Musculoligamentous sprains and ***strains*** are relatively common, accounting for 35% of injuries. Most muscle sprains involve the ***cervical and lumbar spine.*** Overuse and stress from vigorous surfing maneuvers are the leading causes of injury. The shoulder is frequently injured due to ***rotator cuff impingement*** during the act of prone paddling (excessive hyperextension and internal rotation), a condition commonly referred to as ***"surfer's shoulder" syndrome. Acromioclavicular, glenohumeral,*** and ***knee dislocations*** have been reported. ***"Surfer's elbow"*** has been described as a form of ***lateral epicondylitis.*** Rest, functional rehabilitation, and antiinflammatory medications usually treat most of these injuries adequately. Stretching and warm-up activities prior to surfing should be emphasized to reduce the incidence of these injuries.

Skeletal fractures represent 15% of surfing-related injuries. These most commonly involve the nose, arms, hands, tibiae, feet, and teeth. An exacerbation of ***spondylolisthesis*** has been described, as have ***wrist and humerus fractures*** in body surfers. A rare injury is ***"surfer's rib,"*** an isolated ***fracture of the first rib*** secondary to performing a "layback" maneuver, in which the surfer is in a hyperextended position while making a left turn. A ***talar osteochondral lesion*** has been described following a penetrating injury of the surfboard's fin. Basic splinting techniques are employed before the surfer obtains definitive fracture care.

Injuries of the cervical spine occur most commonly with body surfing, although they may occur with any type of surfing in shallow water. Typically, the surfer either falls off the surfboard head first or is caught in the lip of the breaking wave. Therefore the mechanism of injury is often a vertical compression, hyperflexion, or extension. A cervical fracture not associated with a neurologic deficit should be suspected in a surfer who strikes his or her head and complains of neck pain. The cervical spine should be immobilized until cleared by neuroimaging studies. Injuries associated with neurologic impairment may require immediate ocean rescue and resuscitation. Quadriplegia may be accompanied by ***neurogenic shock,*** manifest by hypotension, bradycardia, and possibly hypothermia. The ***central cord syndrome*** has been reported in older surfers who sustain even mild flexion injuries. ***Fractures of the thoracolumbar spine*** are rarely encountered.

The incidence of traumatic brain injury is unknown. Undoubtedly, some surfing-related drownings are due to ***concussive head injuries*** with the associated loss of consciousness. A closed head injury may occur following a collision with the surfboard, a rock, or a coral reef. ***"Surfer's neuropathy"*** is a ***peroneal compression neuropathy*** due to prolonged sitting on a surfboard. ***Brachial plexus injuries*** have been reported, although the etiologic mechanism is not clear.

The risk of ***near-drowning*** (and drowning) increases with the size of the surf. The most common scenarios include a closed head injury, being held under water in large surf for a prolonged period, or becoming trapped under water by either the leash or the board snagged in a coral reef. Surfers with ***seizure disorders*** involving loss of consciousness are clearly at increased risk of drowning. Rescue of the drowning surfer can be delayed because of the lack of recognition of the incident or the severity of the surf conditions.

A variety of surfing-related injuries of the internal organs have been reported, including ***splenic rupture*** and ***axillary artery injury. Scrotal sac rupture*** with testicular expulsion has occurred despite no obvious break in the wetsuit. ***Shark attacks*** occur more commonly in certain coastal waters, notably those of Australia, South Africa, and northern California. Most attacks are nonfatal, although significant blood loss may occur. Sting-ray attacks may result in loss of flesh from the leg or foot.

Prevention of surfing-related injuries is mainly educational. The use of protective headgear should be recommended for surfing in shallow coral reef breaks. Rubber nose guards for surfboards decrease the incidence of lacerations and ocular injuries. Liberal use of sunscreens should be encouraged. Surfing should be postponed for several days following a significant rainstorm in areas known to have city sewage runoff. Surfers who intend to travel to tropical countries should be counseled with regard to vaccinations, antimalarial prophylaxis, and recognition and treatment of stings by sea organisms.

92. SWIMMING

Allen B. Richardson

Competitive swimming is one of the largest participation sports in the United States, claiming some 210,000 athletes registered with the National Governing Body, United States Swimming, Inc. A large number of swimming athletes are registered with other programs, such as the Young Men's Christian Association (YMCA) and local country club leagues. Further, there are a growing number of athletes who continue to compete on the master's level and who participate in events of which swimming is a part, such as triathlalons and biathalons. Open-water and marathon swimming are also gaining in popularity.

There are four primary events in competitive swimming, freestyle, butterfly, backstroke, and breaststroke. A fifth event combines all four strokes and is called the individual medley. International competition usually takes place in a pool 50 m in length, while the American winter season takes place in a 25-yd pool. Freestyle, or Australian crawl, has individual events ranging from 50 m (or 55 yd) to 1,500 meters, while the other strokes have events at 100 and 200 m. Individual medley is swum over 200 and 400 m. There are different skills and body types are associated with the different strokes and events.

As opposed to many other sports, competitive swimming does not give rise to a wide variety of traumatic or disabling musculoskeletal problems. Success in competitive swimming favors those athletes with upper extremity strength and flexibility, which allows them to "flow" through the water, thereby incurring less drag. Almost all problems of an orthopaedic nature fall into the category of overuse syndrome, in which prolonged and intense use of a body part leads to "wear and tear" of that part and therefore painful symptoms.

Shoulder pain, commonly known ***"swimmer's shoulder,"*** is the most common orthopaedic ailment to affect the competitive swimmer. It is reported to affect some 60% of athletes, usually after approximately 6 to 8 years of participation in the sport and more often among those swimming freestyle, butterfly, and backstroke, because of the overhead use of the shoulders. Sprinters tend to be more susceptible to symptoms, and training aids, such as hand paddles and drag swimsuits, are known to aggravate symptoms.

The underlying cause of shoulder pain in swimmers is a ***"sub-clinical multi-directional instability"*** of the shoulder. The pain is located about the acromion, although it is also commonly located over the posterior capsule; it is usually associated with overhead activities, especially at hand entry into the water. In this regard, the symptoms are the same of those of an impingement syndrome.

Physical examination will demonstrate tenderness to palpation about the acromion, a positive impingement test, and instability to anterior and posterior stress of the glenohumeral joint, with a reproduction of symptoms.

Radiographic examination is usually normal except if one finds an abnormally shaped acromion on the outlet view. Arthrography or magnetic resonance imaging (MRI) might reveal a tear of the glenoid labrum but will rarely show any abnormality of the rotator cuff.

The nonsurgical treatment of swimmer's shoulder is directed at strengthening the rotator cuff muscles and thereby increasing the stability of the glenohumeral joint and decreasing the inflammation caused by its overuse ice packing, nonsteroidal anti-inflammatory drugs, and judicious rest periods from training.

Surgical treatment of swimmer's shoulder is arthroscopic debridement of the torn or redundant glenoid labrum. If the tear is well defined, repair may be possible with one of the newer arthroscopic stapling techniques. An acromioplasty is usually done at the same time to relieve those symptoms related to impingement of the humeral head against the acromion.

Low back pain is quite common among competitive swimmers, especially butterfly swimmers. Freestyle and backstroke also require considerable rotational movement during the swimming stroke, and starts and turns require repeated rapid flexion and extension of the lumbar vertebrae, leading to pain and disability. While the diagnosis is usually a ***chronic strain of the paraspinous muscles*** of the lumbar spine, the treating physician should evaluate the swimmer for ***spondylolysis, spondylolisthesis,*** and ***Scheuermann's kyphosis*** with routine x-rays.

Chronic knee pain is seen in some 25% of swimmers and is usually related to ***chondromalacia*** or patellofemoral pain. Once again, the underlying cause of this discomfort is probably excessive movement between the patella and the femoral trochlea. Breaststroke swimmers are also susceptible to ***chronic strain of the medial collateral ligament.*** Ligamentous or meniscal tears are distinctly rare as a result of competitive swimming.

Over recent years, ***exercise-induced bronchospasm (EIB),*** which occurs with remarkable frequency among competitive swimmers, has become better recognized and treated. Because the treatment of asthmas requires the use of central nervous system stimulants, which are banned for use by the International Olympic Committee, only aerosol bronchodilators (beta $_2$ agonists) are allowed for routine use (albuterol, salbutamol, Brethaire Inhaler, Ventolin, etc.). Athletes and their families should be aware that the use of these medications must be declared to the International Federation to prevent disqualification from competition.

93. TENNIS AND OTHER RACKET SPORTS

Marc R. Safran and David A. Stone

At present, tennis is a game in transition from a sport requiring coordination, agility, and tennis-specific skills to one that also demands power and places a premium on conditioning. However, this evolution has not apparently altered the epidemiology of tennis injuries. The lower extremity and the spine represent 50% to 75% of all tennis injuries. The majority are sprains or repetitive-trauma overload injuries.

Acute traumatic injuries that are relatively uncommon include ***strains of the thigh adductors, rectus femoris,*** and ***hamstrings, ankle sprains,*** and occasionally ***meniscal injuries. Muscle strain*** injuries are more common on slick grass surfaces. ***Tennis leg*** is a partial rupture of the medial head of the gastrocnemius muscle during foot push off of the affected leg, while ***tennis toe*** is a subungual hematoma caused by jamming of the toes within the shoes and occurs more commonly on hard courts. ***Shin splints*** and ***medial tibial stress syndrome*** can occur in tennis players who change their training habits. Symptoms from these entities are worse when they result from playing on a hard court. Tennis players may also complain of ***turf toe, plantar fascitis, calluses, corns,*** and ***blisters. Blisters*** are more common during hot or humid times, with new footwear, or slippage of the foot in the shoe on a high-friction playing surface (hard courts).

Tennis elbow (lateral epicondylitis) has been related to stroke mechanics, age, frequency of play, and racquet vibration. As many as 30% to 40% of tennis players develop elbow pain at some time in their careers. Lateral epicondylitis tends to afflict the 30- to 50-year-old recreational (three to four times a week) or inexperienced player who has poor form, particularly the backhand, and inadequate conditioning. Heavier, stiffer, more tightly strung rackets with incorrect grip sizes are also contributing factors. ***Medial epicondylitis*** is less common than lateral epicondylitis but may be seen in players who try to hit with excessive top spin on the forehand side or maximal pronation on the serve by incorporating a wrist snap. ***Valgus extension overload*** injuries may occur when players lack leg drive or open up their body stance too early on the serve. ***Stress fractures of the ulna*** have been reported in tennis players who use a two-handed backhand.

Shoulder problems are common in older athletes and in elite tennis players, among whom over 50% note shoulder pain. The majority of shoulder problems are similar to those of other throwing athletes: ***impingement*** and ***instability.*** The dominant shoulders of elite players have been found to have increased shoulder flexibility in external rotation and decreased flexibility in internal rotation. Further, their sit and reach flexibility and hip rotation is also reduced. These flexibility adaptations may play a role in injury production.

Wrist injuries in tennis players can occur from direct trauma or, more commonly, from overuse. ***De Quervain's syndrome, extensor carpi radialis brevis and longus tendinitis,*** and ***flexor carpi ulnaris tendinitis*** may result from overstretching the muscles during serving, excessive eccentric contraction of muscles to stabilize the wrist during off-center shots, or using incorrect form. ***Recurrent dislocation of the extensor carpi ulnaris*** may occur when players hit the forehand with the wrist in ulnar deviation and supination, imparting excessive slice. ***Ulnar carpal impingement*** and ***triangular fibrocartilage tear*** may also occur in tennis players with ulnar-sided wrist pain. ***Fractures of the hook of the hamate*** occur less frequently than in golf and baseball. ***Kienbock's disease*** due to repeated impact has been reported in tennis players. Compression of the index finger metacarpal head against the racket handle may injure the ***radial digital nerve.*** Rarely reported is ***ulnar artery thrombosis*** at the hamate due to repetitive injury from hyperflexion of the wrist or contact with the grip.

The stroke most commonly associated with injury in tennis is the serve, generally also considered the most important stroke in the game. It is the most strenuous of all strokes and requires integrated movement of the legs, trunk, and arms to minimize risk of injury and maximize performance. Particular serves, such as the top-spin serve, require a significant increase in lumbar lordosis (extension) to be hit effectively. Ground reactional forces are transmitted to the spine by the hips and knees, forcing lordosis and rotation in the spine and external rotation of the shoulder. Muscles such as the rectus abdominis and internal and external obliques flex and rotate the spine for serving. The thoracolumbar fascia act as the attachment site for multiple paraspinal muscles that contract eccentrically to decelerate spinal flexion. As a result, ***rectus abdominis strains, paraspinal muscle strains,*** and ***thoracolumbar myofascial injuries*** are common among tennis players. The axial rotation and lateral bending forces may also produce ***intervertebral disc herniation. Spondylolysis*** occurs occasionally in tennis players, presumably due to repetitive hyperextension. ***Sacroiliac joint dysfunction*** is relatively common in tennis, with the most likely mechanism being repeated jumping during the serve. Landing from the jump may induce ipsilateral pelvic translation and contralateral side bending/rotation of the spine on an internally rotated femur. The end result may be a unilateral upward shear. ***Sacroiliac stress fractures*** have also been reported in these athletes. Up to 40% of male professional tennis players miss at least one tournament a year due to low back pain.

The evolution of the racket to composite oversized frames and wider bodies continues at present with the introduction of the "extra-long" racket, introduced in 1995 by several companies. The effect that extra-long rackets will have on tennis injuries is not clear. Much work has gone into the study of racket vibration and the risk of injury to the upper extremity. Racquet vibration at impact is higher when the player grips the racket more tightly and vibration is prolonged with off center hits. Racquet vibration dampening systems are effective, but the effect on injury is not clear.

Tennis shoes have also evolved over the past decade, both in materials and construction, to prevent injury. A notch for the Achilles tendon provides better rear-foot fitting and a reinforced toe guard prevents injury in players who drag their toes. Special shoes, with multiple small spikes to reduce slippage, are made for play on grass. For play on hard courts, shoes with midsoles made of ethylene vinyl acetate improve shock absorption. Shoes made from polyurethane are more durable but heavier. Environmental concerns during tennis play including ***heat illness, muscle cramps,*** and ***bee stings.***

Badminton, Squash, and Racketball

In badminton, squash, and racketball, the rackets are lighter than in tennis; as a result, it is less likely to cause ***strain*** to the upper extremity's musculature. The same upper extremity injuries listed in tennis occur in these sports as well. Since the serve in these sports is more like a forehand stroke, low back injuries are less frequent. ***Strains of the thoracolumbar musculature*** are still quite prevalent because of the rotational forces involved in hitting the ball, but disc herniation, spondylolysis, and sacroiliac dysfunction do not occur as commonly. In racketball and squash, collisions with other players and the wall can result in a variety of acute injuries, such as ***sprains and fractures of the wrist, contusions of the thoracoabdominal region and extremities,*** and ***skin abrasions.*** Since these sports are played within a small enclosed space, there is a high risk of being hit by either the ball or racket, causing a ***contusion*** and ***laceration*** anywhere on the body. ***Hyphemas*** and ***orbital fracture*** are risks in the racketball or squash players not wearing appropriate protective eye wear. Appropriate eye wear involves wrap-around configuration, fully enclosed glasses or goggles with polycarbonate lenses, antifog coating, and secure stabilization to the back of the head. Lower extremity injuries, such as ***meniscal tears, anterior cruciate ligament disruptions, ankle sprains,*** and ***ankle fractures*** are more common in these sports, as with badminton, since the surface produces more friction with the shoes, making noncontact twisting injuries more likely. With the better traction and the need for short, quick bursts of movement, acute musculotendinous injuries are more common than in tennis. These include ***Achilles tendinitis and rupture*** (in the 30- to 50-year-old athlete), ***tennis leg, plantar fascia rupture,*** and ***hamstring strains.***

94. TRACK AND FIELD

R. Douglas Shaw

In the average track-and-field competition, there will be relatively few injuries. These will generally consist of acute ***lower extremity muscle strains*** in sprinters and jumpers or acute ***ankle or knee ligamentous sprains*** from improper jump landings or falls during running races, hurdling, or pole vaulting. Most injuries in inexperienced athletes result from inadequate early-season training or improper technique. The average competitive runner or jogger may encounter the common conditions of ***Achilles tendinitis, chondromalacia, iliotibial band syndrome, plantar fasciitis, or shin splints*** at some time during his or her running career. A variety of other conditions vary between running, jumping, or throwing events.

In sprinters—distances up through 400 m (440 yd)—***acute hamstring strains*** are by far the most common injury. Often these injuries represent a recurrence of a prior strain that has not been allowed to heal fully and has been inadequately rehabilitated. They may also relate to poor flexibility or inadequate warm-up in cold weather. ***Plantar fasciitis*** and ***Achilles/gastrocnemius strains or ruptures*** are not uncommon in the short sprints and explosive jumping events.

Middle- and long-distance runners—800 m (880 yd) and longer—are most susceptible to overtraining problems due to ***repetitive overload trauma*** to the lower extremity. ***Achilles tendinitis/tendinosis, peripatellar overuse problems, iliotibial band syndrome, plantar fasciitis,*** and ***shin splints*** are all common. At the mass start of a race, one may occasionally see lower extremity ***puncture wounds*** or ***lacerations*** from ***spike injuries,*** as well as ***abrasions*** and ***contusions*** from falls. ***Stress fractures*** are not infrequent in the metatarsals, tarsals, and tibia. A young runner with hip pain may suggest a ***proximal femur stress fracture.***

Hurdlers are subject to the same problems as sprinters; in addition they may suffer injuries from collisions with or falls from a hurdle. ***Medial ankle and foot abrasions and contusions*** are frequently seen in the athlete's trail leg. A fall from a hurdle may sometimes cause a ***sprain*** or ***fracture to the wrist.*** Assorted ***abrasions and contusions*** to the knees, arms, and back often occur from falls on unforgiving track surfaces. ***Achilles and plantar fascial strains*** are also common.

Steeplechase competitors are susceptible to the same problems as middle- and long-distance runners. In addition, they may suffer significant ***contusions or ankle and knee sprains*** from hitting or falling from the immobile steeplechase hurdles and water-jump hurdle.

Javelin throwing puts the athlete at risk for multiple injury sites. Elbow injuries are frequent, the majority related to overuse, such as ***medial epicondylitis.*** Less common are ***muscular strains*** of the shoulder. Rare but reported arm injuries include ***avulsion fractures of the medial epicondyle, olecranon stress fractures, and a humeral spiral stress fracture.*** Back pain is a common complaint due to the rotation and compressive forces of the throw compounded by an abrupt deceleration with the plant of the blocking foot. ***Lumbosacral muscular strains*** are common. Less commonly, ***spondylolysis*** or ***disc herniation*** may occur. An aggressive footplant of the blocking leg may cause a ***hyperextension type of ligament injury*** to the knee, possible ***meniscus tears*** to the knee joint, ***patellar and quadriceps tendon strains,*** as well as ***groin strains*** to the rear leg. Potentially life-threatening ***penetrating injuries*** to the head, neck, and thorax have occurred when athletes were struck with a thrown javelin or have accidentally fallen onto a javelin stuck in the ground.

Shot-putters often develop pain in their throwing hands due to ***hyperextension injuries*** to the wrist or fingers. ***Muscular groin strains*** may occur. ***Patellar tendon strain or tendinosis*** is often seen and is likely more related to heavy leg presses during weight lifting than to throwing.

Discus throwers have relatively few serious injuries but often complain of ***blister*** and ***callous*** formation on the fingers of their throwing hand. ***Groin strains*** are also common.

Hammer throwers are also plagued by ***blister*** and ***callus*** formation on their fingers. A rarely reported injury is ***brachial plexus neuritis*** in elite hammer throwers.

"Jumper's knee" refers to ***patellar tendinitis*** or ***quadriceps tendinitis*** related to repetitive trauma overload and can occur in any of the jumping events. ***Heel bruises*** are commonly seen in the long jump and triple jump. The term "***stone bruise***" refers to a chronic heel bruise that is best prevented by the use of plastic heel cups. ***Achilles tendon ruptures*** occasionally occur in the mature jumper at takeoff, and ***hamstring strains*** may occur in the landing phase of the jump. In the triple jump, if the jumper lands on the edge of the landing pit at the end of the step phase of the jump landing, a serious ***knee strain, meniscus tear,*** or ***cruciate ligament rupture*** may occur. ***Lumbar muscle strains*** may also be seen from repetitive landings on the runway in all phases of the triple jump.

High jumpers often develop ***heel bruises*** and "***jumper's knee.***" A faulty foot plant on takeoff may cause ***acute ligamentous sprains or repetitive overload stress to the medial structures of the foot and ankle. Acute strain or tendinitis of the posterior tibialis tendon*** may occur below the medial malleolus. Flop-style jumpers landing on their necks rather than their upper backs may suffer a ***cervical muscle or ligament strain*** or potentially catastrophic ***cervical spinal cord injury,*** especially if they should land off the pit entirely. ***Shoulder dislocations*** have occurred from falls related to slippage of the takeoff foot on a wet jumping surface.

In the pole vault, an improper pole plant may cause a ***lumbar or shoulder muscle strain.*** The most severe injuries while vaulting are usually the result of landing off of the landing pit from heights up to 20 ft (6m). These could be ***ligamentous joint strains or fractures of the extremities or spine,*** depending on the landing. Pole vaulters are also vulnerable to the same lower extremity problems as sprinters.

Decathlon and heptathlon athletes, because of the extended hours of preparation for diverse events, are susceptible to overtraining and may present with any of the problems of the individual events. Often they will have more than one ongoing condition. Although uncommon, ***osteitis pubis*** has occured in several decathletes.

Environmental concerns relate mainly to ***heat illness.*** On warm and especially humid days, distance athletes as well as multievent competitors and athletes running in multiple heats may suffer from ***dehydration, heat cramps, heat exhaustion,*** and possibly ***heat stroke.***

95. VOLLEYBALL

H. Paul Hirshman

Volleyball is among the most popular sports in the world, with an estimated 150 million players. Most injuries are relatively mild. In Schafle's study, conducted in the 1987 Amateur Volleyball Tournament, the overall injury rate was 1.97 per 100 hr of play, but the rate of injuries causing a player to lose 5 or more days of play was only 0.10 per 100 hr of play. Overuse injuries are common, as well as acute injuries. Front-row players are at much higher risk of injury than back-row players.

Inversion ankle sprains are the most common acute volleyball injuries. Since players can step over the center line as long as at least part of the foot is in contact with the line, there is considerable risk of contact with the opposing players. Most sprains occur when a player lands on the foot of an opposing player (50%) or when the blocking player lands on the foot of a blocking teammate (25%). Most injuries occur while blocking (60%) or attacking (30%), as one would expect, since blockers do jump after the attackers, so the attackers usually land first. Bracing or taping is sometimes utilized to try to lower the incidence of ankle sprains, which may be recurrent. ***Knee injuries*** are much less frequent in volleyball.

Isolated ***meniscal injuries*** occur when players twist, especially from the defensive position with the knee flexed 90 degrees or more. Significant ***ligamentous injuries*** can occur, especially when the player lands off balance from a jump. The ***contusions*** are rare when players wear knee guards. Elbow pads are used in a similar fashion to prevent injuries that may occur—for example, as commonly happens when diving in the back row.

Traumatic finger injuries, especially ***sprains of the interphalangeal joints*** of the ring and little fingers, are fairly common in blocking in volleyball. ***Lacerations of the web space*** due to abduction injuries, ***fractures,*** or true ***dislocations*** occur less frequently. ***Avulsion of the extensor tendon*** from the dorsum of the distal phalanx, with or without bony injury, may also occur during blocking and is analogous to baseball's ***mallet finger*** injury. ***Muscle sprains and strains*** in volleyball most commonly involve the ***hamstrings, rectus femoris, medial gastrocnemius,*** and occasionally the ***anterior deltoid.***

Overuse problems are common in volleyball, especially in the knee extensor mechanism. ***Patellofemoral pain*** and ***patellar tendinitis*** are most common, as would be expected in a sport that involves so much jumping. The type of playing surface affects the incidence of these problems, with concrete floors being among the worst and wood floors among the best.

Conditioning and proper warm-up may decrease the frequency of these problems. ***Achilles tendinitis*** also occurs, although it is less frequent.

Overuse problems in the ***shoulder*** include ***rotator cuff injuries, instabilities,*** and ***suprascapular neuropathy.*** Spiking and serving are biomechanically similar to throwing in baseball and serving in tennis, so the pathophysiology of the rotator cuff and atraumatic instability problems in volleyball are thought to be analogous to shoulder problems in other sports. Traumatic ***shoulder dislocation*** in volleyball is rare. Suprascapular neuropathy with marked atrophy, especially of the infraspinatus, seems to be much more common in volleyball than in other overhand sports but is usually not symptomatic.

Back problems are, unfortunately, common in volleyball. Repetitive jumping is implicated, as well as the hyperlordosis and twisting of the jump serve. ***Stress fractures*** in volleyball are uncommon and usually involve the ***fibula, metatarsals,*** or occasionally the ***tibia.***

96. WATER POLO

John A. Gansel

European countries have historically dominated the sport of water polo. Legendary match-ups have mirrored political events in the area. Shortly after the Soviet Union's occupation of Hungary in 1956, the two water polo teams met. The water in the pool following the game was said to have been red-tinged from the fights that occurred. Water polo was introduced into the United States in the late 1940s. Inspired by the U.S. Navy's success using yellow rubber life-raft materials, the original leather ball—which became slippery and tripled in weight during the course of play—was replaced by a yellow rubber ball. The popularity of the sport in the United States continued to grow. Improved continuity of national team coaching, development programs, and financial support have allowed the United States to evolve into an international power in water polo. Growth at home led water polo to become a men's and women's collegiate sport, supported by hundreds of age-group and high school programs with thousands of participants.

The game has been described as a combination of soccer, basketball, and wrestling in the water. The regulation pool is 30 m (33 ft) long, 20 m (22 ft) wide, and 2 1/2 m (8 ft) deep. Six field players work to score a goal by throwing the ball past the defending goalie into the opposing team's "cage." Players cannot use the sides or bottom of the pool to their advantage. They sprint from end to end of the pool, with changes in direction dictated by turnovers and fouls. Quarters are 6 min long, with the game clock stopped for fouls and when the ball is out of play. Unlike the case in many sports, when the game clock stops, players continue to work for position advantage. Because of this unique feature, 6-min quarters translate to 15- to 20-min quarters of sprints, treading water, and wrestling for position, with few breaks in play. This requires a level of conditioning matched by few other sports. The flurry of shots, physical contact, referee whistles, and counterattacks can be confusing to the uninitiated observer. The water polo player is susceptible to injury from throwing and swimming as well as from direct contact. Owing to the great amount of time spent in the pool training and playing, these participants often develop ***otitis externa*** (swimmer's ear).

A ball thrown by an elite water polo player can approach 50 mph with a shot on goal. This requires a vertical position with an eggbeater kick to stabilize the lower body while elevating the shoulders and upper body from the water. The legs are relatively anchored and the rotation of the body to throw the ball, from windup to follow through, occurs at the hips and above. This significantly strains the elbow, shoulder, and back. ***Medial epicondylitis, subacromial bursitis, and rotator cuff tendinitis*** (both from ***overuse tendinitis*** and ***subtle shoulder instability***), and ***musculoskeletal back problems*** are common causes of pain. Laxity of the ***elbow's ulnar collateral ligament*** and exacerbation of subtle shoulder instability as seen with swimmers can occur when a player's upper extremity is forcibly externally rotated from behind by an opponent during the early phase of throwing. Frank ***shoulder dislocation*** is rare.

The eggbeater kick is a modified breaststroke kick with the legs alternating. The knees are stressed in valgus, flexion, and external rotation as they are extended. Players must overcome the resistance of the water and often the body weight of their opponent. Stress is to the medial knee structures, including the medial capsule, medial collateral ligament and pes tendons. ***Pes aneserinus bursitis, tendinitis,*** and ***medial collateral ligament strain*** are common. ***Patellofemoral problems*** are less common.

Water polo is a contact sport. Physical contact is required to maintain and improve a player's position in relation to an opponent. A defender can initiate contact if the opponent holds up the ball to shoot or pass. Rules prohibit acts of "brutality" such as kicking, scratching, and striking an opponent with a closed fist. Referees check fingernails and toenails before players enter the water to ensure that ***gouging,*** accidental or intentional, will be minimized. The body is somewhat protected from blunt trauma by the resistance of the water, but a player's head and neck are vulnerable to injury. Various contact injuries do occur, causing ***contusions*** to the ***lower extremity*** and ***low back*** as well as the ***groin.*** Cheap shots outside of the referees' field of vision occur and are, unfortunately, an acknowledged way to gain advantage over one's opponent.

The head is most vulnerable to injury during the opponent's shot follow through or from being kicked during the transition game. Ears are protected from ***perforation of the eardrum*** by the plastic ear guard attached to the water polo cap. Many players wear mouthguards to protect against ***chipped or lost teeth. Facial lacerations*** are common. ***Periorbital contusion, nasal fracture,*** and ***concussion*** are less common. ***Finger fractures and dislocations*** as well as ***lacerations of the intermetacarpal web space*** with rupture of the intermetacarpal ligament can occur during the follow-through phase of throwing if an opponent is struck or by the goalie trying to block a shot on goal.

Most players are aware of the potential for injury, and intentional infliction of injury is rare. Water polo is generally considered a safe sport, with the most common injuries being ***contusions*** or ***abrasions*** that are usually not limiting and heal before the next competition.

97. WATERSKIING: STANDARD AND WAKEBOARDING

George L. Caldwell, Jr.

Waterskiing has become a popular sporting activity that appeals to a diverse group of athletes, encompassing all age ranges and levels of ability. Over 15 million Americans participate annually and injuries range from minor muscle strains to the sensational accidents that are occasionally reported in the news. The various forms of water skiing include two-skiing or slalom, barefoot skiing, trick skiing, ski jumping, and wakeboards. The four components that differentiate waterskiing significantly from other recreational sports are the high velocity with which a participant can hit the water or collide with a fixed object, the danger posed by the boat's propeller, potential contamination of wounds, and possible drowning of a disabled or unconscious patient. Fortunately, the fatality rate is estimated to be less than 1 per 30,000 participants. The epidemiology of injuries is similar to that seen in contact sports. The majority are secondary to single traumatic episodes, not repetitive overuse, as in many recreational sports. It is the recreational skier who is much more apt to incur major injuries, while the competitive athletes are generally disciplined and safety-conscious.

Injuries of the lower extremity predominate at all levels of competition. ***Hamstring and quadriceps strains*** frequently result from the stress of acceleration during start or eccentric loading suffered during attempted deceleration during a fall or the landing from a jump. The vast majority of strains are at the musculotendinous junction, although ***avulsion of the tendinous origin of the hamstrings*** has been reported. ***Strain of the hip adductors*** may occur when the two skis of a novice skier are forced apart or from the slack and "catch" during landing with toehold maneuvers by a trick skier. ***Spiral femoral fractures*** are rare but are generally ascribed to novice ski jumpers who land with all the force directed to one leg at an awkward angle of impact.

Common knee problems include meniscal tears and ligamentous strains/ruptures. The length of the ski can transmit tremendous torque to the lower extremity during "normal falls." ***Strain of the medial collateral ligament*** often results from valgus stress during a fall. Both ***medial and lateral meniscal tears*** result from sudden falls or twists. A concomitant or isolated injury to the ***anterior cruciate ligament*** (ACL) also follows falls. Ski jumpers hit both the ramp and then the water with a great deal of force, risking injury to the menisci or the ACL. ***Rupture of the posterior cruciate ligament*** (PCL) most commonly occurs in trick skiers during "toehold turns," which inflict a rotational injury to the knee if the foothold fails to release during excessive force. The PCL is less commonly injured secondary to hyperflexion during a ski-jump landing. Prepatellar bursae develop in wakeboarders secondary to overuse.

The trick skier may suffer an ***ankle sprain*** from an uncontrolled twist or a late binding release during a fall. ***Talus fractures*** have been reported in slalom skiers. ***Ankle fracture/dislocations*** have been reported secondary to tow-rope entanglements during a beach start. ***Bruised heels*** result from landing a jump with the body weight positioned posteriorly and are common among competitive jumpers.

Forearm and hand injuries are relatively uncommon. Painful, torn ***calluses*** across the palmar aspect of the metacarpal heads are seen in skiers competing in warm water. ***Degloving and digit avulsion*** have been observed during entanglement with a tow line during acceleration. The ***flexor/pronator strains*** of the forearm generally result from overuse in competitive slalom skiers.

Shoulder problems include overuse injuries as well as traumatic dislocations. Slalom skiers forcefully raise their arms upward as their bodies lean more horizontally when turning buoys and then move to lessen the slack in the tow line. The subsequent rapid acceleration, as the slack is taken up, subjects the rotator cuff to tremendous forces, resulting in ***subacromial bursitis*** and occasional ***rotator cuff***

tears. Anterior shoulder dislocations may follow uncontrolled falls, especially when the skier fails to release the tow line quickly.

Spinal injury is commonly associated with a strain, although catastrophic injuries have been reported. ***Strain of the cervical and thoracic paraspinal muscle*** occurs in slalom as skiiers forcefully extend and twist while accelerating in turns, these injuries also occur in trick skiers who rotate in the air as they jump over the wake. As a ski jumper hits the ramp, he or she experience upwards of 10 to 20 g's of upward force, straining the lumbar spine. ***Herniated lumbar discs*** may occur during the takeoff or landing of a jump.

As stated, "routine" falls during skiing can result in a multitude of extremity twisting and shearing injuries as well as other miscellaneous injuries secondary to the impact. These include ***costochondral separation*** of the ribs secondary to falls at high speed. Direct trauma due to impact with a loose ski includes ***laceration of skin, muscle, and/or neurovascular*** structures. ***Splenic rupture*** or ***renal contusion*** results from blunt trauma to the abdomen. ***Rope burns*** occur when a skiier does not release the rope handle properly as he or she falls backward. The handle is eventually forcefully extracted from the skiier's grip, allowing the line to be dragged across the thighs skiier's at considerable speed and friction.

Douche injuries are caused by a high-pressure stream of water that is forced into a body orifice. Rectal ***enemas*** and less commonly ***rectal lacerations*** have been reported. High-pressure vaginal douches can result in ***vaginal or cervical laceration*** as well as ***tuboovarian abscesses, infertility,*** or even ***miscarriage*** during pregnancy. Water forced into the ear or nasal passage may lead to ***otitis externa, tympanic rupture,*** or ***sinus infection.***

Major head and neck injuries occur in both the novice and professional groups. ***Fractures and dislocations of the cervical spine*** have been reported following awkward falls into the water or collision with a fixed object, such as a ski ramp, pylon, or dock. Also, neck fractures with resultant ***paraplegia*** have been reported when skiers were hurled forward by rapid deceleration and then striking the shore during a "beach landing." ***Concussions*** and major ***closed head injuries*** often result from impact during collision. Competitive ski jumpers now routinely wear helmets to minimize this risk.

Fatal injuries may occur. Collisions with fixed objects often lead to injuries resembling those seen in pedestrians struck by motor vehicles. These injuries are quite variable in location and magnitude, depending upon the momentum of the athlete and the nature of the object struck. Entanglement in the tow rope can result in forceful acceleration injuries to the upper limbs or fatality if drowning results. Properly approved ski vests are essential equipment. Propeller injuries can be devastating. They result in massive, contaminated soft tissue and osseous injuries that resemble battlefield wounds. Recognition of these potentially serious injuries must be a paramount concern for the skier, observer, and boat operator.

98. WRESTLING

Edward M. Wojtys and John E. Kuhn

Wrestling is the fifth most popular sport for high school boys and the fourth most common college sport where participants are likely to require surgical treatment for injuries. ***Overall injury rates*** for wrestling range from 4% to 12% in preadolescent boys and 12% to 31% in high school and college participants. While most of these injuries are minor, approximately 25% fall in the moderate to severe range and 5% require withdrawal from participation. In general, injuries seem to occur more commonly in practice than during competition; however, the injury rate per tournament match is as high as 22.3%.

An association between weight class and injury rate has not been established for high school or college wrestlers. The majority of injuries occur on the mat, either with both wrestlers in the down position or, more commonly, during the takedown. Fatigue and inadequate conditioning may be responsible for an increase in injuries during successive periods of a match. Most often, the injured wrestler is behind in the scoring. The most commonly injured areas are the head and neck (36%), the knee (20%), and the shoulder (13%).

The most common head injury is the ***auricular hematoma,*** with almost 40% of wrestlers reporting some form of permanent auricular deformity. With auricular trauma, blood collects between the perichondrium and the cartilage. New cartilage is formed by the tightly encasing perichondrium, leading to deformity of the auricle or a ***cauliflower ear.*** The use of headgear, although not completely effective, can reduce the occurrence of this deforming condition. This injury most often occurs during the takedown maneuver.

Eye injuries are usually not severe and are usually ***periorbital contusions*** or ***lacerations;*** however, ***corneal abrasions*** and ***lacerations*** can occur. ***Herpes gladiatorum,*** a common infectious skin condition in wrestlers, may affect the eyes as well, causing ***follicular conjunctivitis, blepharitis,*** and phlyctenular disease.

Injuries to the face and nose, particularly ***epistaxis*** and ***nasal fractures,*** may also occur during wrestling. ***Concussions*** are rare, and appropriate headgear may decrease their occurrence.

Approximately 10% of all reported wrestling injuries involve the neck. Most are neurogenic pain syndromes such as ***stingers,*** cervical sprains, or strain-type injuries. All wrestlers with neck injuries must be evaluated cautiously; catastrophic neck injuries should be assumed unless proven otherwise.

Acute cervical strains can involve the trapezius, sternocleidomastoid, erector spinae, scalene, levator scapulae, and rhomboid muscles. These occur under a variety of conditions where mechanical loading exceeds the ability of the muscle to generate force. Wrestlers may return to competition when a near-normal pain-free range of motion is achieved. ***Acute cervical sprains*** involve the articular capsular structures and ligaments of the cervical spine. There should be no discomfort with axial neck compression prior to returning to wrestling. A positive compression test would require further evaluation.

Neurogenic pain syndromes, such as ***stingers,*** occur by stretching or compressing the nerve roots or brachial plexus. These are usually mild, neuropraxic (grade I) injuries in wrestling. Wrestlers with this type of injury may be predisposed to recurrence. Some may progress to permanent neurologic loss and cervical radiographic changes such as osteophyte formation and foraminal narrowing. ***Acute disk herniations*** which present with radicular symptoms may also occur with wrestling.

The greatest number of cervical injuries seems to be related to "bulling" the neck into a hyperextended position while attempting, or blocking a takedown. While rare, ***catastrophic injuries of the cervical spine*** have been attributed to being thrown and landing in a twisted position on the head or to illegal holds such as a full nelson. These can result in partial or complete paralysis.

Low back injuries are less common, representing 5% of all injuries reported. These almost always represent ***paraspinous muscle strains.*** These injuries can occur during takedowns or during sparring, where the wrestlers pull, push, and twist against each other while standing with the lumbar spine in mild extension. Many injuries are a result of repeated episodes of microtrauma or overuse. ***Facet syndromes,*** though uncommon, present with back and leg pain, morning stiffness, and relief of pain with ambulation. Prevention of low back injuries through proper wrestling technique, conditioning, and a stretching program that includes the hamstrings and hip musculature is essential. Overuse injuries to the low back may have far-reaching effects later in life. Unfortunately, low back pain is seen more commonly in retired wrestlers than age-matched controls.

Injuries to the trunk and ribs may also occur in wrestling, including ***rib fractures*** and ***costochondral separations.*** These can be caused by the wrestler's own exertion during a "bear hug" or by a fall on an opponent's leg or arm. Wrestlers should withdraw from participation until movement is painless.

Knee injuries are common in wrestling and account for up to one-third of all serious wrestling injuries. ***Prepatellar bursitis,*** both infectious and noninfectious, is common and results from mat friction. This may be prevented with well-fitting knee pads. ***Ligamentous sprains, meniscal tears,*** and ***patellar dislocations*** seem to involve the lateral side of the knee more often than expected and usually affect the lead leg, which is twisted during a takedown maneuver. Wrestlers on the defensive seem to be more at risk. Sprains of the ***anterior and posterior cruciate ligaments,*** although possible, occur much less frequently than in other sports.

Foot and ankle injures are infrequent, and generally involve ***sprains of the lateral ankle ligaments.*** Unfortunately, the high wrestling shoe has been designed to grip the mat, not support the ankle. Tripping or stepping on the edge of the mat or twisting over a foot fixed on the mat are common causes of this injury.

Upper extremity injuries are most common at the shoulder, with ***acromioclavicular sprains*** most frequent, especially during a takedown. Good technique and proper mats may reduce the frequency of these injuries. ***Shoulder dislocations*** are rare when legal holds are used but may occur during a sudden pull on the opponent's arm in a switch or drag maneuver.

Elbow injuries, including sprains and dislocations, typically result from falls while landing on the extended arm or from aggressive holds. Like prepatellar bursitis, friction on the mat may induce ***olecranon bursitis;*** elbow pads may offer some protection.

Fractures or ***dislocations of the fingers*** as well as ***sprains of the wrist*** may occur in wrestling. These occur as a result of twisting injuries when wrestlers are using the hands to grab or obtain a hold or position. Alternatively, finger injuries may occur when a wrestler tries to unlock an opponent's grip. This can produce ***phalanx and metacarpal fractures, scaphoid fractures, and sprains, including the ulnar collateral ligament of the thumb.*** Fracture of the finger is the most common fracture in the sport of wrestling.

Dermatologic problems are particularly difficult for wrestlers. The close contact of the sport provides ample opportunity for the transmission of infectious agents. Viral agents include ***herpes gladiatorum,*** a skin infection caused by the herpes simplex virus 1, which affects up to 2.6% of high school wrestlers and 7.6% of collegiate wrestlers in a given year. Contact with opponents having active infections is the greatest risk factor for spread, particularly if the infected wrestler has a cold sore or active skin infection. Skin-to-skin contact through abrasions or breaks in the skin is thought to be the pathway of infection in susceptible hosts; abrasive clothing may be a contributing factor. By prohibiting infected wrestlers from competing, prevention remains the mainstay of control. Other viral infections seen in wrestlers include ***molluscum contagiosum*** and ***verrucae,*** or the common wart virus.

Fungal infections in wrestlers, called ***tinea corporis gladiatorum,*** are caused by *Trichophyton* species and other dermatophytes. These lesions are thought to occur through skin-to-skin contact and not through fomites, such as the wrestling mat. Control by prohibiting infected individuals from participation may prevent spread. Wrestlers can return to competition if lesions have been shown to respond to treatment after 10 days of topical treatment or 15 days of oral treatment.

Bacterial skin infections include ***impetigo,*** a staphylococcal or streptococcal infection characterized by bullae or sharply demarcated erosions covered with a heavy yellow crust.

Of particular importance in wrestling is the problem of ***weight control.*** Most wrestlers will lose 3% to 20% of their preseason body weight in order to participate in a lower weight class, despite having preseason body fat averaging less than 8%. Most of this weight reduction occurs in the final days before each match, causing the wrestler's body weight to fluctuate 15 to 30 times in a season.

This rapid weight loss is usually guided by wrestling peers and is rarely under the supervision of a coach or physician. Methods for this weight loss include restricting food, induced vomiting, fluid deprivation, and dehydration by sweating through exercise and/or thermal methods. These practices have been shown to reduce strength and endurance, deplete liver glycogen stores, decrease work performance times, lower oxygen consumption, impair the thermoregulatory process, possibly increase susceptibility to infection, lower plasma and blood volumes, reduce cardiac function, decrease renal blood flow and filtration fractions, and increase loss of electrolytes from the body, with a profile in some similar to that of anorexia nervosa.

Guidelines to reduce this dangerous practice proposed by the American College of Sports Medicine include (1) Assess body fat content, and require medical clearance for those under 5%. (2) Observe daily caloric requirements with a balanced diet and discourage wrestlers from adopting diets that provide less than their minimal nutritional needs without prior medical approval. (3) Discourage the practice of fluid deprivation and dehydration through education; prohibiting the use of rubber suits, steam rooms, saunas, laxatives, and diuretics; scheduling weigh-ins just prior to competition; and scheduling weigh-ins throughout the season. (4) Permit more participants per team to compete in the more common weight classes (119 to 145 lb). (5) Regulate tournaments so that wrestlers can compete only in those weight classes that they competed in most frequently during the regular season. (6) Encourage the collection of data on hydration state and its relation to growth and development.

APPENDICES

Appendix 1. INJECTIONS

Marc R. Safran

I. Intraarticular Injection

Joint injection is primarily used to deliver intraarticular corticosteroids to treat inflamed joints, bursae, or tendons. They can also be used selectively as a diagnostic tool. ***Contraindications*** are (1) coagulopathy and (2) infection in the overlying skin or soft tissue. Corticosteroid should not be injected into a joint until infection (including that caused by atypical bacteria or fungi) has been excluded. There is some evidence that repeated injection into the small joints of the hand may cause deformity. Similarly, injections into tendon insertions may result in rupture. Injection with corticosteroid into the Achilles or patellar tendons is absolutely contraindicated. Large joints should not be injected more than three or four times a year or ten times cumulatively. Small joints should be injected less often, not more than two or three times per year or four times cumulatively.

II. Supplies

A. **Aseptic skin preparation materials**
   1. Sterile gloves
   2. Iodine (Betadine or Iodophor) solution
   3. Alcohol solution
   4. Sterile gauze pads

B. **Local anethesia materials**
   1. 1% Lidocaine for skin, subcutaneous tissues, and joint structure
   2. Ethyl chloride spray for skin
   3. 0.25% to 0.5% bupivacaine HCl (Marcaine) for joint structure

C. **Sterile needles** from size 18- to 25-gauge, depending on the where injections are to be given.

D. **Syringes** from size 3 to 60 cc depending on the size of the joint and if injection is to be preceded by aspiration.

III. Cortisone

Cortisone usually takes 24 to 36 hr to begin working. The duration of benefit depends on the corticosteroid preparation utilized.

A. **Risks**
   1. Steroid flare (crystal synovitis)
      a. Resolves spontaneously within 24 to 36 hr
      b. Treat with rest, ice, and a nonsteroidal antiinflammatory drug (NSAID) such as ibuprofen
   2. Subcutaneous fat atrophy
   3. Skin depigmentation
   4. Rupture of soft tissue and tendons
      a. Particularly with repeated injections.
      b. Reduce risk by not injecting same area more than 3 times in a year.
   5. Infection

IV. Technique

The most important maneuver before injecting a joint is to locate the appropriate ***landmarks*** (usually bony) and mark the proposed injection site with indelible ink. While ethyl chloride will usually reduce most of the pain of the injection itself, some physicians recommend generous injection of the skin and subcutaneous tissues with local anesthesia prior to joint injection/aspiration. If one is to only inject a joint, thus making only one pass with a needle, and feels comfortable with the technique and anatomy, then injecting with local anesthesia prior to joint injection is unnecessary. The patient is going to feel one shot either way, so the second injection (local anesthesia) is unnecessary. The patient should note that the pain may be ***exacerbated*** by the injection, either by steroid flare, distention of the joint or soft tissues by the injected solution, or just from the added traumatization to the area by the needle. Thus the patient should be warned of the possible short-term aggravation of symptoms in the injected joint or soft tissue region and receive the appropriate analgesia instructions. If corticosteroid solution is given with lidocaine and/or bupivacaine, the patient should be made aware that the immediate relief obtained with the anesthetic medications will likely wear off before the corticosteroid preparation begins to provide relief. When injecting into a large joint, a larger-bore needle (18 to 20 gauge) is helpful. The injected solution should ***flow in easily*** (without resistance) if the needle is truly into the joint. If a large amount of resistance is encountered, either the joint has a tense effusion or the needle is in the soft tissues.

After discussing the risks with the patient and identifying the landmarks ***prior to injection,*** clean the region with iodine prep (if the patient is not allergic to iodine), then wipe with an alcohol swab. The area is then sprayed with ethyl chloride to provide skin anesthesia, and finally the joint or soft tissue region is injected. After removal of the needle and syringe, apply pressure to the injection site with a sterile gauze pad.

The type of medication and dosage, syringe size, and needle size are based upon the joint to be injected. Generally do not give more than 1 mL of a corticosteroid preparation. The rest of the injection includes a combination of lidocaine and bupivacaine (for longer duration of anesthetic benefit). When injecting large joints intraarticularly, if there are no health contraindications, use of bupivacaine or lidocaine with epinephrine for an even more prolonged benefit. Do not use lidocaine or bupivacaine with epinephrine when injecting digits or smaller joints.

A. **The shoulder.** The glenohumeral joint may be injected either anteriorly or posteriorly. The subacromial space can be injected separately to isolate the subacromial bursa and rotator cuff.
    1. **Anterior approach (Fig. 1).** With the patient seated, hand resting in lap and shoulder muscles relaxed, the glenohumeral joint can be palpated by placing one's fingers between the coracoid process and the humeral head. As the shoulder is internally rotated, the humeral head can be felt turning inward and the joint space can be felt as a groove just lateral to the coracoid. A 1.5-in. 20- or 22-gauge needle is inserted lateral to the coracoid. The needle is directed dorsally, laterally into the joint space, and slightly superiorly. This avoids risk of injury to the neurovascular structures about the shoulder and provides anterior exposure to the shoulder. No more than 10 mL of solution needs to be injected.
    2. **Posterior approach (Fig. 2).** The posterior aspect of the shoulder is identified with the patient seated, hand resting across the abdomen and shoulder muscles relaxed. The posterolateral corner of the acromion can be palpated easily in most patients, regardless of size or body habitus. A 1.5-in. 20- to 22-gauge needle is inserted 2 cm distal and 2 cm medial to the posterolateral corner of the acromion and advanced anteriorly and medially toward the coracoid process. Passing through the musculature of the external rotators, occasionally a pop will be felt as the needle penetrates the posterior shoulder capsule. No more than 10 mL of solution needs to be injected.
    3. **Subacromial Space (Fig. 3).** The patient is seated with hand resting lap and shoulder muscles relaxed. Traction may be applied to the lower arm to open the subacromial space, though this is rarely necessary. The lateral approach to the subacromial space is the most accessible and safest. Injection of the rotator cuff tendon itself or to the glenohumeral joint is nearly impossible with this approach. If the injectable solution flows in easily, the only place your needle can be is in the subacromial space. The tip of the acromion is identified. The needle is entered 2 to 3 cm below the midpoint of the acromion and angled up

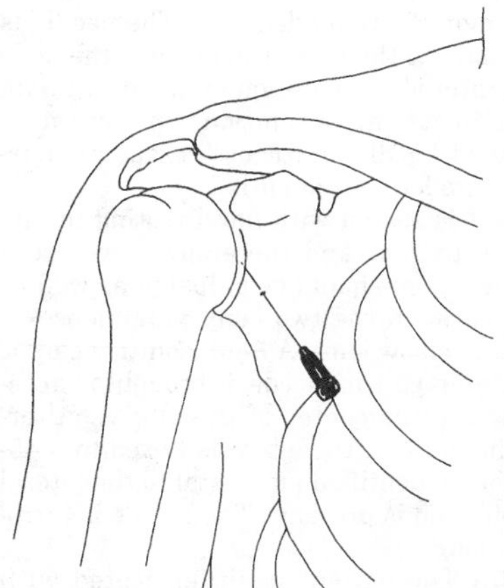

Fig. 1. Anterior approach to the shoulder. Reprinted with permission from Paget S, Pellicci P, Beary JF III, eds. *Manual of rheumatology and outpatient orthopaedic disorders,* 3rd ed. Boston: Little, Brown, 1993, fig. 4-1.

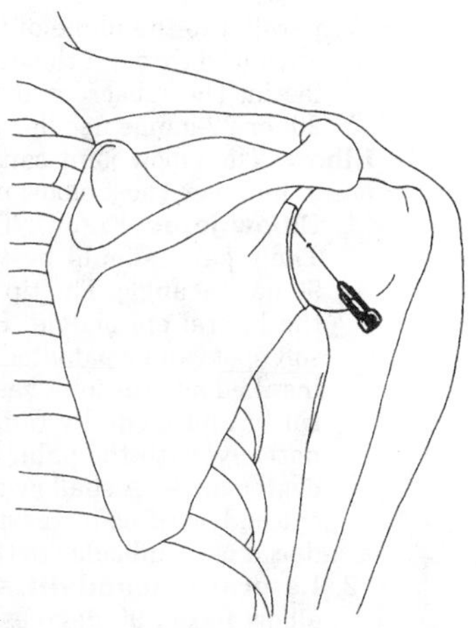

Fig. 2. Posterior approach to the shoulder. Reprinted with permission from Paget S, Pellicci P, Beary JF III, eds. *Manual of rheumatology and outpatient orthopaedic disorders,* 3rd ed. Boston: Little, Brown, 1993, fig. 4-2.

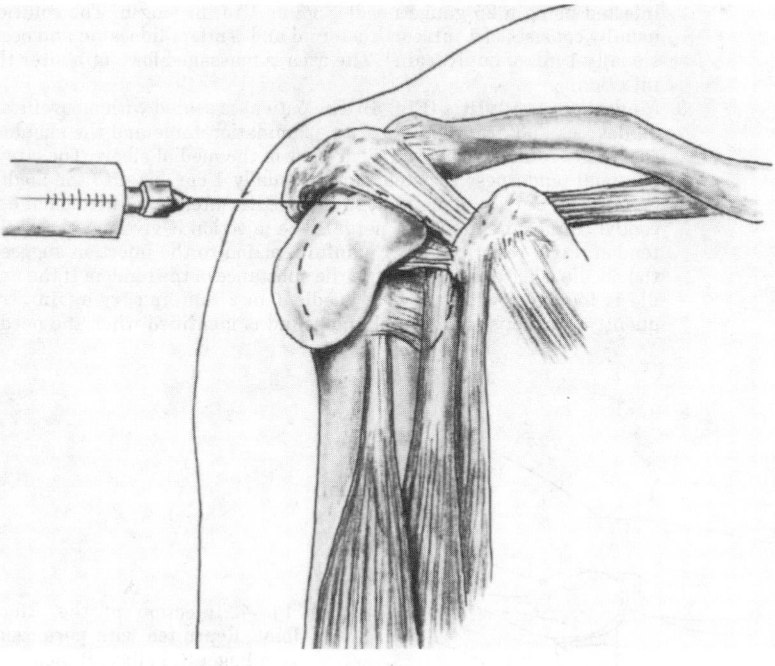

Fig. 3. Subacromial Injection of the shoulder. Reprinted with permission from Brems JJ. Degenerative joint disease of the shoulder. In: Nicholas JA, Hershmann EB, (eds). *The upper extremity in sports medicine,* 2nd ed. St. Louis: Mosby–Year Book, 1995, fig. 10-4.

parallel to the plane of the acromion (30 to 60 degrees). The needle is advanced through the deltoid muscle to the firm resistance of the deep fascia. The subacromial bursa is entered and solution instilled. A 1.5 in. 20- or 22-gauge needle, and injecting 10 mL of solution is preferred.

B. **Elbow.** The elbow joint can be injected for diagnostic or therapeutic purposes; however, most elbow injections are for epicondylitis.

1. **Elbow joint (Fig. 4).** The patient is seated with hand resting in lap. Their palm should be facing the patient and the elbow flexed to a 90 degree angle. The tip of the olecranon should be palpated as well as the lateral epicondyle. Halfway between the two bony prominences a soft spot can be palpated; this is the elbow joint. A 5-mL solution can be instilled into the joint easily if a 22-gauge 1-in. needle is brought in anteriorly and medially (angling toward the center of the elbow). Alternatively, with the palm facing the patient, the elbow is flexed to a 45-degree angle. A shallow depression is identified just distal to the lateral epicondyle (if no intraarticular effusion is present). The needle is introduced perpendicular to the elbow joint.
2. **Lateral epicondylitis (Fig. 5).** The patient is either seated with elbow flexed 90 degrees and arm resting on an examination table or lying supine with elbow flexed 90 degrees and hand resting on the ipsilateral buttock. This injection is given at the site of maximal tenderness, usually 1 to 2 cm distal to the lateral epicondyle and just over the tendon. Firm resistance or a painful reaction to the injection suggests that the needle is too deep and within the substance of the tendon. If the needle is too deep, withdraw the needle 1 to 2 mm and try again. Frequently, a sandpaper-like feel and sound is identified when the needle enters the inflamed tissue region. Then 2 to 3 mL of solution is injected using a 25 gauge needle, 5/8 or 1 in. in length. The solution usually consists of 1 mL corticosteroid and 1 mL of lidocaine and occasionally 1 mL of bupivacaine. The area is massaged for 5 min after the injection.
3. **Medial epicondylitis (Fig. 6).** The patient is seated with elbow flexed 90 degrees and arm resting on an examination table and the shoulder externally rotated to allow a clear view of the medial elbow. The site of maximal tenderness is noted; this is usually 1 cm distal to the medial epicondyle. Care is taken to keep the needle anterior to the medial epicondyle (and thus the ulnar nerve). The injection is given just over the tendon. Firm resistance or a painful reaction to the injection suggests the needle is too deep and within the substance of the tendon. If the needle is too deep, withdraw the needle 1 to 2 mm and try again. Frequently, a sandpaper-like feel and sound is identified when the needle

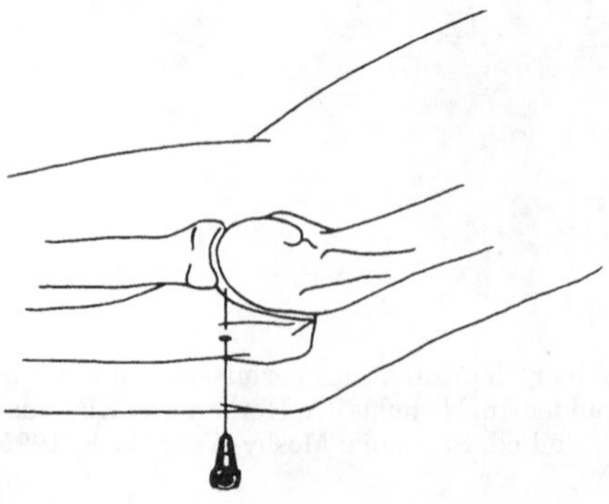

Fig. 4. Injection of the Elbow Joint. Reprinted with permission from Paget S, Pellicci P, Beary JF III, eds. *Manual of rheumatology and outpatient orthopaedic disorders,* 3rd ed. Boston: Little, Brown, 1993, fig. 4-3.

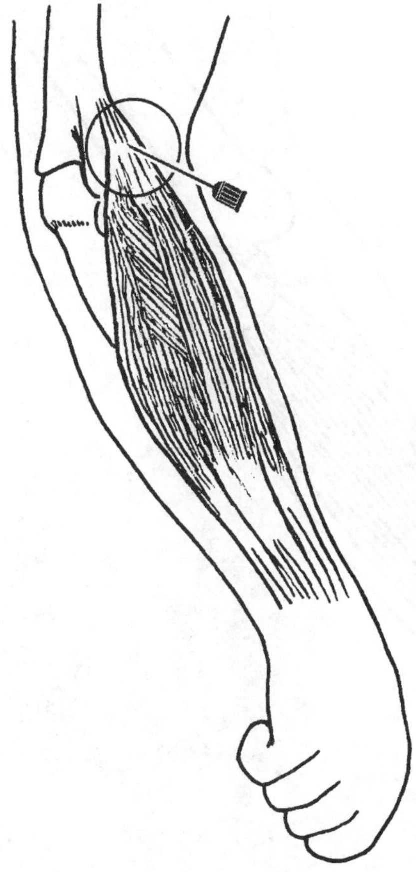

Fig. 5. Injection for lateral epicondylitis.

enters the inflamed tissue region. Paresthesias in the distribution of the ulnar nerve (medial forearm and ring and little fingers) upon passage of the needle or during injection of the solution indicates this may be in the ulnar nerve. Stop immediately, as injection into the nerve can damage it. Remove the needle, exchange it, and redirect more anteriorly and superficially. Then inject 2 to 3 mL of solution using a 25-gauge needle, 5/8 or 1 in. in length. The solution usually consists of 1 mL corticosteroid and 1 mL of lidocaine and occasionally 1 mL of bupivacaine. The area is massaged for 5 min after the injection.

C. **Wrist.** Wrist injection is performed from the dorsal aspect of the wrist just distal to the radius or ulna, as indicated by clinical examination.

1. **Radial entry (Fig. 7).** The patient is seated and the hand and wrist are relaxed in a slightly flexed position on an examination table. The joint space can be located by palpating the edge of the distal radius just medial to the extensor tendon of the thumb. A 1-in. 22-gauge needle should be directed into the joint from the dorsal aspect. All that is needed to inject this joint is 5 mL of solution.
2. **Ulnar entry (Fig. 7).** The patient is seated and the hand and wrist are relaxed in a slightly flexed position on an examination table. The joint space can be located by palpating just distal to the distal ulna.

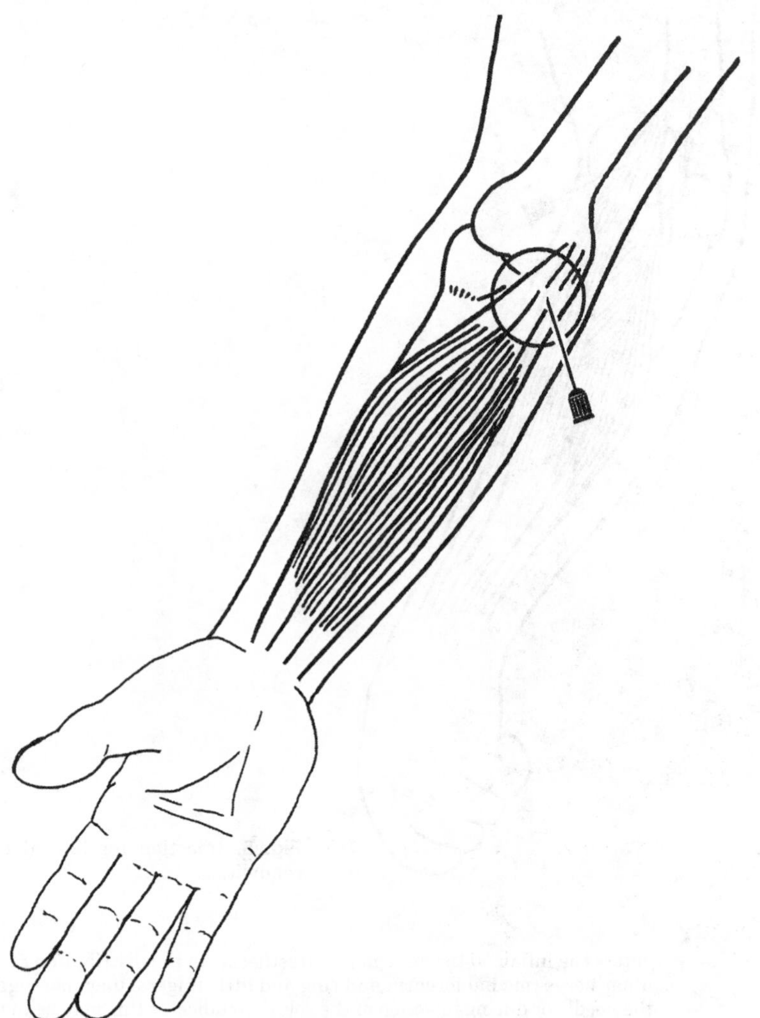

Fig. 6. Injection for medial epicondylitis.

A 22 gauge needle should be directed in a volar and radial direction into the joint from the dorsal aspect. All that is needed to inject this joint is 5 mL of solution.

D. **Knee.** The knee is the largest and easiest joint to enter. The knee can be injected with the knee extended or flexed, from medial or lateral. I find that aspiration of a knee with a large effusion is best performed with the knee extended. However, when no effusion is present, the knee is easily injected with the patient sitting up and knee flexed.

1. **Knee extended (Fig. 8).** With the patient lying supine, the knee should be comfortably extended and quadriceps relaxed. Relaxation is adequate if the patella can be moved medially and laterally between the

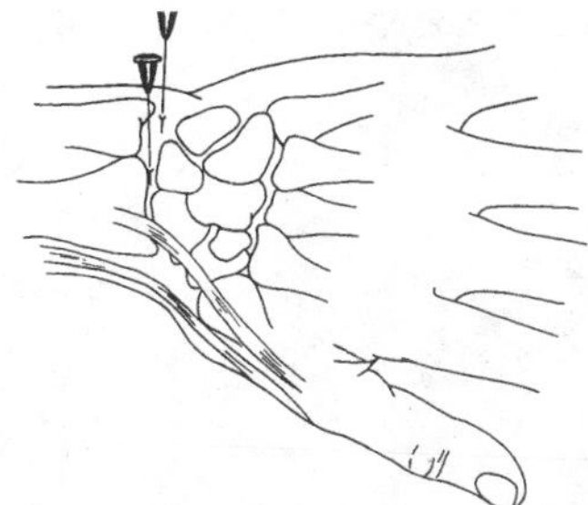

Fig. 7. Injection of the wrist joint. Reprinted with permission from Paget S, Pellicci P, Beary JF III, eds. *Manual of rheumatology and outpatient orthopaedic disorders,* 3rd ed. Boston: Little, Brown, 1993, fig. 4-4.

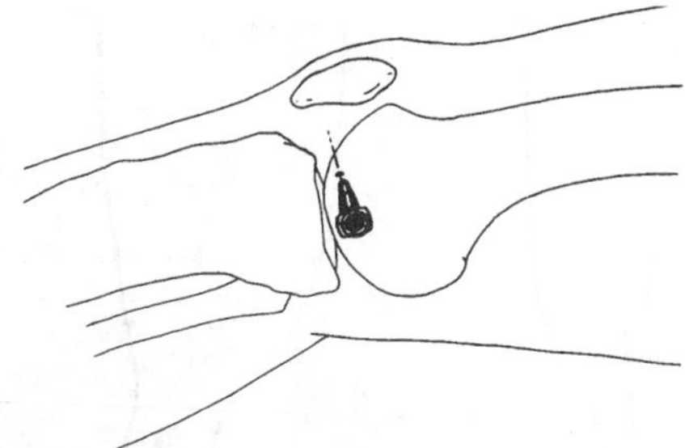

Fig. 8. Injection of the knee joint (with knee extended). Reprinted with permission from Paget S, Pellicci P, Beary JF III, eds. *Manual of rheumatology and outpatient orthopaedic disorders,* 3rd ed. Boston: Little, Brown, 1993, fig. 4-6.

examiner's fingers. Grasping the medial and lateral margins of the patella, a skin mark is made that corresponds with the posterior aspect of the patella (when looking from the side of the patient, the margin of the patella closest to the table). An 18-to 20-gauge 1.5-in. needle is introduced from the lateral or medial side of the knee, in a direction parallel to the plane of the posterior aspect of the patella. With very large effusions, the needle may be introduced at the level of the suprapatellar pole, while with little or no effusion, the needle should be introduced just distal to midpatellar height. Larger needles are occasionally necessary to drain the knee. Most commonly 10 mL of solution is used to inject this joint.

2. **Knee flexed.** With the patient sitting or lying supine comfortably and the knee at the edge of the examination table, the patient's leg, foot, and ankle are hanging over the edge of the table. The patellar tendon at the level of the joint is palpated. The joint may be entered from either the medial or the lateral aspect; however, with the tendon being more lateral, it is easier to inject from the medial parapatellar side. A soft spot just medial to the patellar tendon is palpated. This is bordered by the medial femoral condyle, medial tibial plateau, and patellar tendon. The 20-gauge 1.5-in. needle is introduced through this soft spot, directing the needle posteriorly, 30 degrees laterally, and slightly superiorly. This brings the needle into the intercondylar notch region. There should be no resistance when injecting. If there is resistance, the injection may be going into bone or the cruciate ligaments. Most commonly, 10 mL of solution is used to inject this joint.
3. **Pes anserine bursa (Fig. 9).** With the patient sitting or lying supine comfortably and the knee at the edge of the examination table, the patient's leg, foot, and ankle are hanging over the edge of the table. The point of maximal tenderness is palpated over the per anserine bursa. The pes anserine bursa lies between the aponeurosis of the co-joined tendons of the sartorius, gracilis, and semitendinosis and the medial collateral ligament approximately 5 to 6 cm below the anteromedial joint line. This is approximately 2 in. below the joint line, 1 to 2 in. medial to the tibial tubercle. The 20-gauge 1 in. needle is inserted at this site and advanced down to bone, then withdrawn 2 to 4 mm. Withdrawing the needle assures placement superficial to the periosteum and in the bursa.

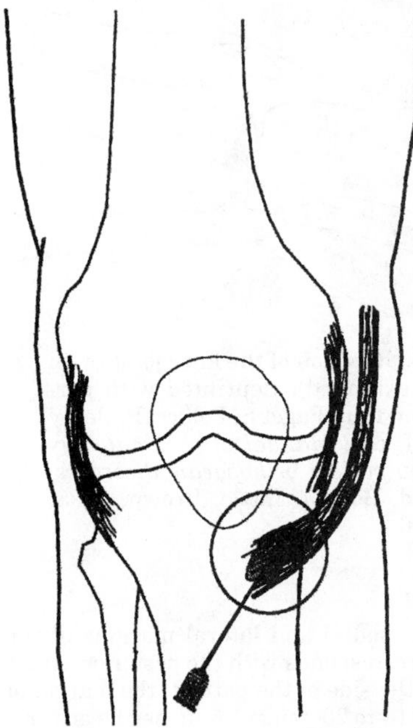

Fig. 9. Injection of the pes anserine bursa.

There should be no resistance to the injection. Resistance indicates injection into bone or the tendon. Most commonly, 5 mL of solution is utilized to inject this bursa.

E. **Ankle.** The ankle may be difficult to enter, but it can be entered from the anteromedial or anterolateral direction. For both approaches, the foot is first placed at about a 45-degree angle of plantarflexion. It is important for the leg, foot, and ankle to be completely relaxed. This may be achieved by having the patient sit on an examination table with the knee at the edge of the table and the leg, foot, and ankle hanging over the edge.

1. **Medial approach (Fig. 10).** A 22-gauge 1-in. needle is placed about 2 to 3 cm proximal and lateral to the distal end of the medial malleolus.

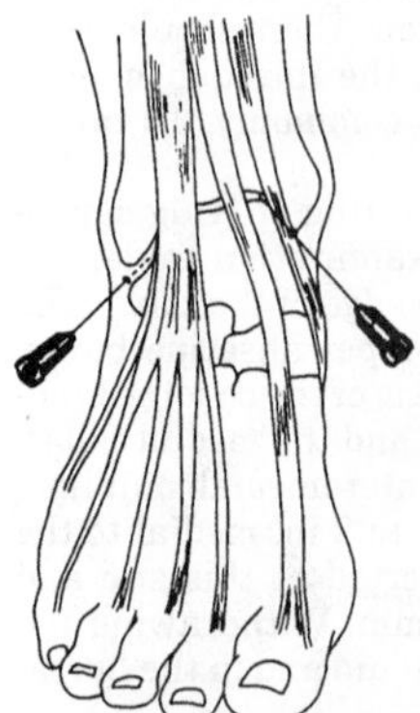

Fig. 10. Injection of the ankle joint (medial and lateral approaches). Reprinted with permission from Paget S, Pellicci P, Beary JF III, eds. *Manual of rheumatology and outpatient orthopaedic disorders,* 3rd ed. Boston: Little, Brown, 1993, fig. 4-4.

The extensor hallucis longus is just lateral to the needle at this point. The needle is directed 45 degrees posteriorly, slightly superiorly, and laterally.

2. **Lateral approach (Fig. 10).** The lateral approach is preferred because the joint space is larger and fewer obstructing soft tissue structures may be encountered with this approach. A 1-in. 22-gauge needle is placed about 2 cm proximal and 1 cm medial to the distal end of the lateral malleolus. The extensor digiti minimi is just lateral to the insertion site of the needle. The needle should be directed 45 degrees posteriorly, slightly superiorly and 30 degrees medially. No more than 5 to 7 mL is used to inject this joint.
3. **Posterior tibial tenosynovium (Fig. 11).** It is important for the leg, foot and ankle to be completely relaxed. This may be achieved by having the patient sit on an examination table with their knee at the edge of the table and the leg, foot and ankle hanging over the edge. The tip of the medial malleolus is palpated. The 20-gauge 1 in. needle enters just behind the posteroinferior edge of the medial malleolus and advanced proximally and superficially. The bevel of the needle is kept parallel to the course of the tendon fibers. Once the bone of the medial talus is touched, the needle is withdrawn 1 to 2 mm, and the 3 to 5 mL of solution is injected. Minimal pressure is necessary if the needle is within the tenosynovial sheath. Do not inject if resistance is encountered.

F. **Plantar fascia (Fig. 12).** The patient is placed prone with the foot hanging just off the edge of the examination table. The origin of the plantar fascia is identified approximately 3 to 4 cm from the back of the heel. This is usually the point of maximal tenderness. A 1.5-in. 22-gauge needle enters the heel 2 cm distal to the origin and is advanced at a 45-degree angle down to the firm resistance of the fascia. The needle is passed through the fascia onto the shelf of the calcaneus. The solution is injected between the fascia and the bone. Never inject the corticosteroid on the fat-pad side of the fascia due to the risk of heel fat-pad atrophy. No more than 3 mL is used to inject the plantar fascia region.

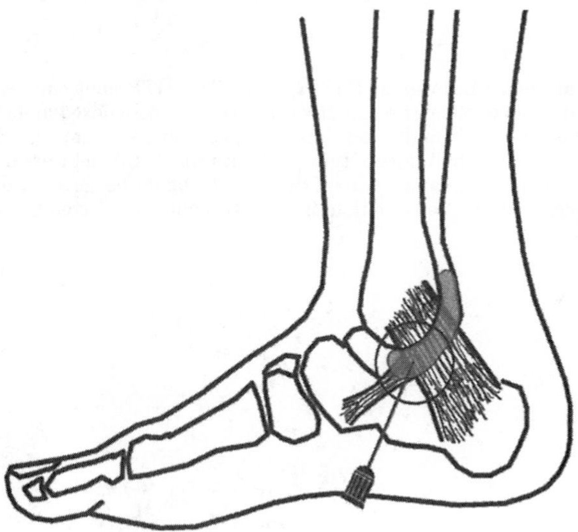

Fig. 11. Injection of the posterior tibial tenosynovium.

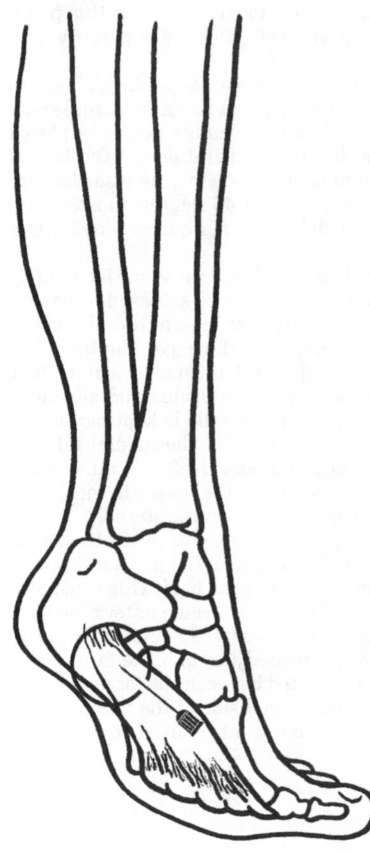

Fig. 12. Injection of the plantar fascia.

G. **Metatarsal phalangeal (MTP) joint.** The MTP joint can easily be palpated on its dorsolateral aspect with the toe slightly flexed and relaxed. The joint is entered from the dorsolateral aspect using a 22-gauge, 5/8 in. needle. Because it is a "ball-in-cup" type joint with the distal metatarsal convex and the proximal phalanx concave, the needle should be directed distally at a 60 degree angle. No more than 2 to 3 mL should be injected into the joint.

Appendix 2. **ATHLETIC TAPING AND BANDAGING**

Gary B. Johnson

Athletic trainers have developed many skills to help an athlete return to practice and/or competition as safely and as quickly as possible. Among those skills is the knowledge of appropriate bandaging and taping. When bandaging or applying tape, you should have a goal. The following are some general purposes for the use athletic tape.

1. Protect a body part against injury
2. Protect a body part against further injury
3. Limit abnormal or excessive range of motion
4. Enhance proprioceptive feedback
5. Allow an athlete to participate with as little restriction as possible

Preparation of Body Part for Taping

The skin should be clean and dry prior to taping. This includes removing any body oils or lotion. Perspiration and dirt will prevent the tape from properly sticking to the skin. Better tape adherence can also be obtained by having the body part clean-shaven. Sensitive areas of friction like the Achilles tendon or the front crease of the ankle may be covered with a thin piece of foam and lubricated to prevent blisters or cuts. All minor cuts and blisters should be cleaned and covered prior to taping. The area can be lightly sprayed with a quick-drying adherent to prevent the tape from loosening. In most tape applications, prewrap or underwrap is used prior to taping to protect the skin against irritation. This is especially true during two-a-day practice sessions.

Tape Application Techniques

1. Body part placement is important in getting an effective tape application. When attempting to limit excessive or abnormal range of motion, the joint should be placed near a neutral position.
2. Anchor strips of tape can often be placed over large muscular areas. When applying strips of tape, it is important to allow for contraction or expansion of the muscle. Tight tape over a muscular area can restrict blood flow and be very uncomfortable. Use of elastic and/or stretch tape and having the athlete contract the muscle while the tape is being applied will allow adequate blood flow.
3. To give maximum support and assure that the tape does not separate with activity, overlap the tape by at least half the width. Every area should have at least a double thickness of tape.
4. Avoid applying too much thickness (greater than four times) of tape over an area. Excessive tape can cause bunching and constriction, leading to skin irritation and discomfort.
5. Try to avoid wrinkles, especially over crease areas. Go at a pace where you can smooth and mold the tape to the skin. Getting the correct angle is important in decreasing wrinkles. Inappropriate angles and trying to force the tape in a certain direction will lead to excessive wrinkles.
6. For a novice taper, tearing the tape with your fingers can be challenging. With practice and patience, tearing can become quite easy. Place the tape between the thumb and finger of both hands. Your hands should be placed close together. With a quick snapping type of motion in the opposite direction, tear the tape. If the tape becomes folded over or crimped, tearing it will be very difficult. Pick a new spot at which to tear the tape.
7. When applying tape to a body area, consistent tension is important. A loosely applied strip followed by a tightly applied strip can cause bunching of the skin. Even tension is also important along both the upper and lower edges of the tape. Uneven tension can lead to tape cuts and skin blistering.

8. Make sure all spots within the area of application are covered. Leaving uncovered areas make the application less effective and can lead to skin irritation and discomfort.

Tape Selection

It is important to select the correct type and width of tape. The width is directly proportional to the size of the body area.

Fingers, thumbs, and toes—1/2 to 1 in.
Hands, wrists, and feet—1 to 1 1/2 in.
Ankles—1 1/2 or 2 in.
Elbows, shoulders, and knees—1 1/2 to 2 in.

Use of Elastic "Ace" Bandages

Ace bandages can be used for several reasons when treating athletic-related injuries. They are most commonly used for:

1. Restricting joint movement
2. To provide support to large muscle groups
3. Provide compression to reduce swelling
4. Secure wound dressing
5. Secure ice bags over an injured area.

Ace wraps are available in widths of 2, 3, 4, and 6 in. They also come in different lengths: regular (approximately 5 yd) and double width (approximately 10 yd). It is important to select the appropriate length and width for the body part you are treating. The small-size wraps (2 and 3 in.) are best used on hands, wrists, feet, and ankles. The larger wraps are best for hips, groins, thighs, knees, and shoulders. Double-sized wraps are used when going around the waist, especially for wrapping the hip and groin or going around the shoulder.

Ace wrap application is similar to that of tape. Tape adherent can be used to prevent slipping of the wrap. Wraps are usually applied in a distal-to-proximal direction. The wrap should overlap by least half the width. Apply even tension with no unexposed areas. To get the greatest support and compression, remove most of the elasticity from the wrap as it is being applied. Make sure the wrap is not too tight, because it can restrict blood flow and be very uncomfortable. The wrap can be secured by using stretch tape or small clips.

Common Taping Procedures

Ankle Technique (Fig. 1)

Materials: 1 1/2- or 2-in. white tape
prewrap
tape adherent
heel and lace pads (optional)

Position: Athlete should be seated with the knee straight and the ankle at a 90 degree angle.

Step 1: Apply two anchor strips about one-third of the way up the lower leg. Starting on the inside part of the leg, apply a stirrup strip coming down the leg, under the heel, and up the outside of the ankle. Next, apply a strip (horseshoe) around the Achilles tendon in either direction (Fig. 1A).

Step 2: Repeat the stirrup and horseshoe strips two more times. Overlap the strips by at least half the width of the tape. Next, apply closure strips, starting at the ankle and moving up the leg. (Fig. 1B).

Step 3: Starting on the inside of the ankle, apply a strip of tape around the foot, crossing over the top of the ankle and then around the leg and finishing at the starting spot. This should resemble a figure eight when finished (Fig. 1C).

Step 4: The next strip (heel lock) starts along the inside of the foot, crosses through the bottom and the outside of the heel/Achilles tendon and progresses around the back of the lower leg, returning to the side of the ankle (Fig. 1D). Repeat this with a similar strip going in the opposite direction or around the bottom and inside part of the heel (Fig. 1E).

Step 5: Apply circular closure strips around the foot and up the lower leg. Make sure there are no uncovered areas (Fig. 1F).

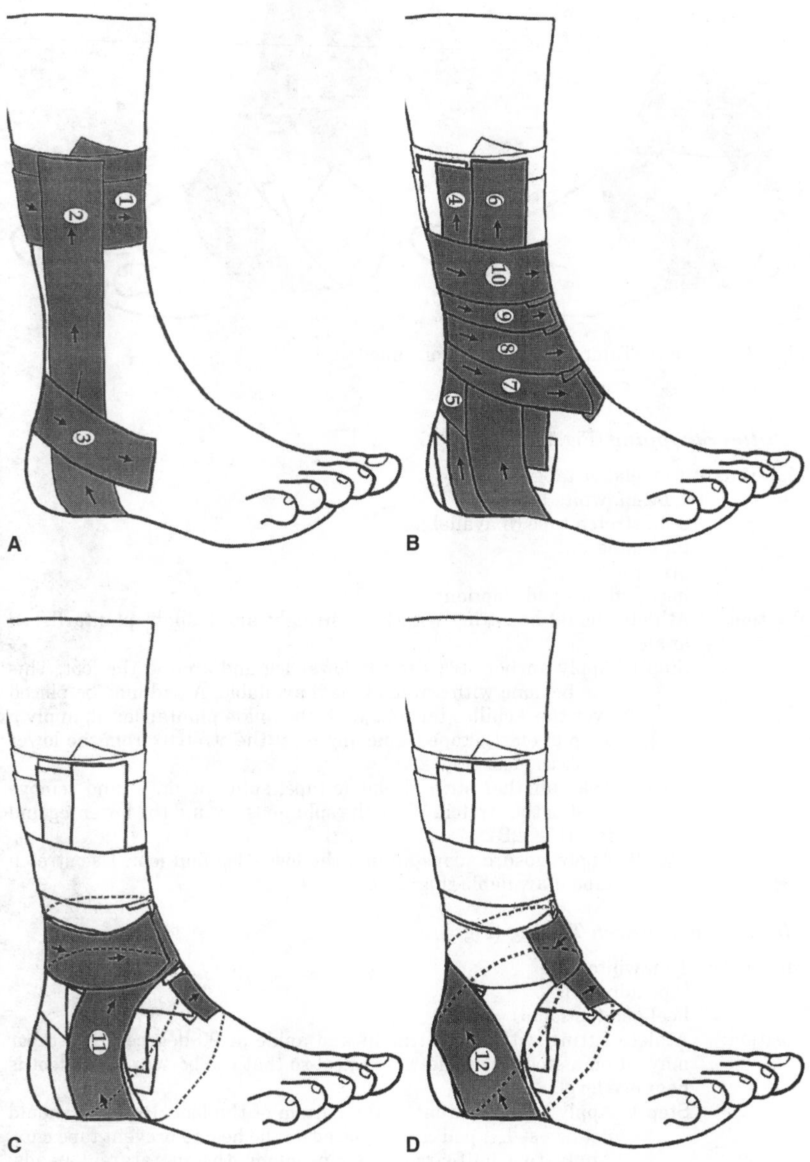

Fig. 1(A-D) Ankle Taping Technique.

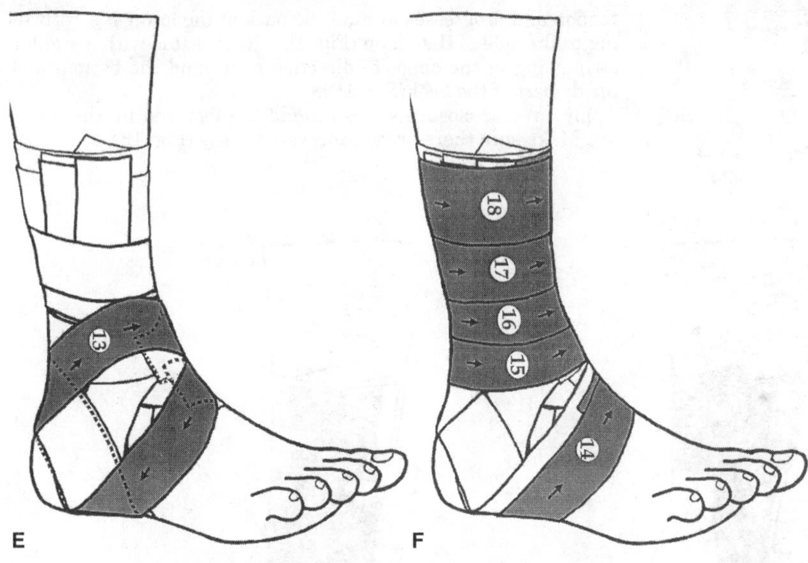

Fig. 1(E-F) Ankle Taping Technique (continued).

Achilles Strapping (Fig. 2)

Materials: 3-in. elastic tape
1 1/2-in. white tape
2-in. stretch tape (if available)
tape adherent
prewrap
heel and lace pads (optional)

Position: Athlete should be sitting with knee straight and a slight plantarflexed ankle.

Step 1: Apply anchor strips to the lower leg and around the foot. This can be done with stretch tape if available. A pad may be placed over the Achilles tendon. With the ankle plantarflexed, apply a strip of elastic tape (removing most the stretch) from the lower leg to the foot (Fig. 2A).

Step 2: Take another strip of elastic tape, split the ends, and remove most of the stretch. Wrap the split ends around the lower leg and foot (Fig. 2B).

Step 3: Apply closure strips around the lower leg and foot. Use stretch tape if available (Fig. 2C).

Plantar Fascia/Arch Taping (Fig. 3)

Materials: 1-in. white tape
tape adherent
heel pad (optional)

Position: Athlete sitting with knee straight and ankle at 90 degrees. The taper may sit on a stool or will have to kneel so that the bottom of the foot is near eye level.

Step 1: Apply tape adherent to the bottom of the foot. Prewrap should not be used. A pad can be placed on the heel to prevent tape cuts. Apply two half-circular strips along the metatarsal heads. Starting along the medial side of the foot, run a strip down the

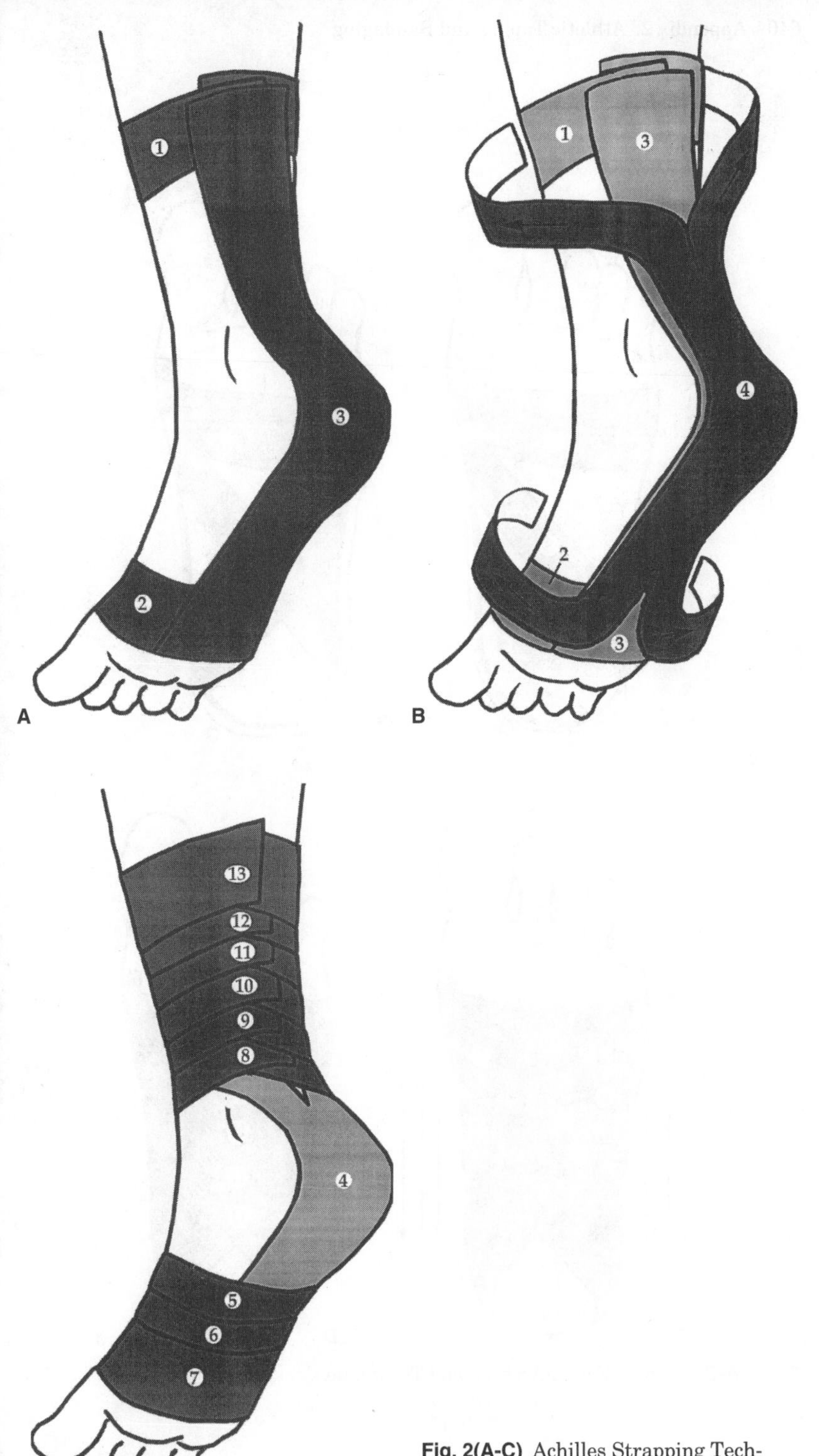

Fig. 2(A-C) Achilles Strapping Technique.

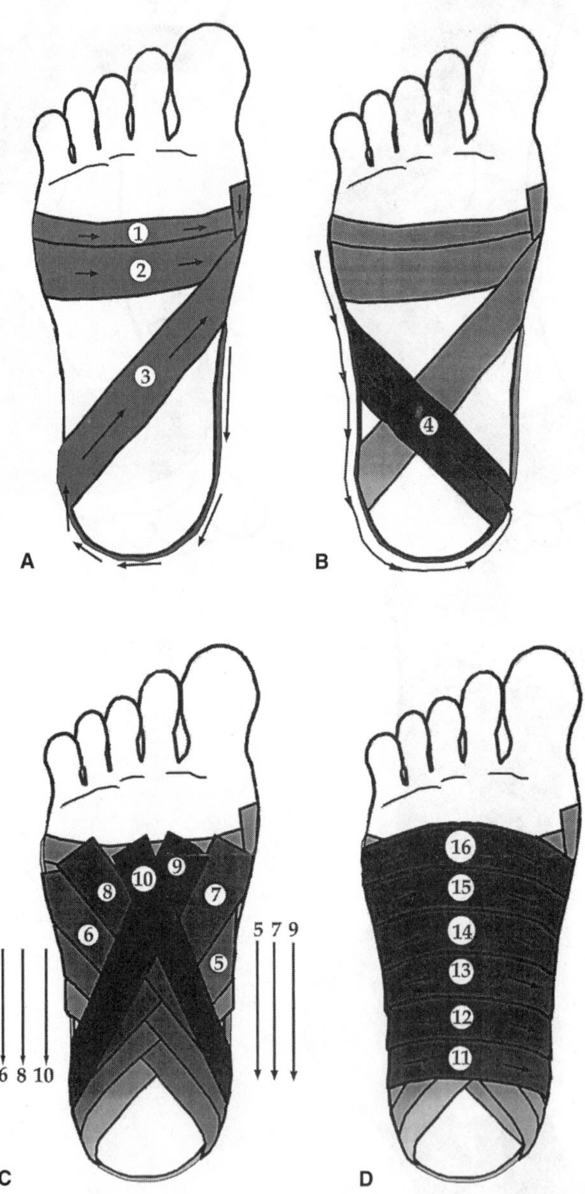

Fig. 3(A-D) Plantar Fascia/Arch Taping Technique.

foot and around the heel. At the lateral aspect of the heel, cross the tape across the bottom of the foot. As you cross the bottom of the foot, apply a slight tug as you return back to the starting position (Fig. 3A).

Step 2: Start a strip of tape along the lateral part of the foot and around the heel returning to the starting point. Again as you come across the foot, apply a slight tug (Fig. 3B).

Step 3: In an alternating fashion, apply three additional medial and lateral strips (Fig. 3C).

Step 4: Apply half-circular strips with a lateral to medial pull. The half-circular strips should extend from the heel to the head of the metatarsals (Fig. 3D).

"Turf Toe" Technique (Figure 4)

Materials: tape adherent
1-in. white tape

Position: Athlete should be sitting with the knee straight. The big toe should be slight plantarflexed.

Step 1: Apply tape adherent to the bottom of the great toe and foot. Apply two anchor strips around the great toe. Along the medial surface of the great toe, apply strips of tape from the distal aspect of the great toe to the arch (Fig. 4A).

Step 2: Continue with strips of tape as you move to the plantar surface of the foot (Fig. 4B).

Step 3: Start along the dorsum of the foot and angle the tape to make a circular pattern around the great toe. As you come around the toe, apply a slight tug on the tape as you come across the joint. End the tape along the plantar surface of the foot (Fig. 4C).

Step 4: Apply half circular strips from the arch to the head of the metatarsals (Fig. 4D).

Dancer's Pad (Figure 5)
For sesamoiditis and fractures of the sesamoid.

Materials: 1/8 or 1/4-in. felt pad
tape adherent
white tape (width depends on size of foot)

Position: The dancer should be prone with the ankle in neutral flexion and foot relaxed.

Technique: The felt pad is fashioned with scissors as shown (Fig. 5). It is fitted to the plantar aspect of the forefoot proximal to the metatarsal heads and extending the proximal skin creases of the toes, with the area of the first metatarsophalangeal joint (ball of foot) left uncovered. It is secured to the foot either by using an adhesive felt pad with tape adherent or affixing with the widest tape as comfortable for the athlete. This relieves the stress on the sesamoids.

Hyperextension Wrist Technique (Figure 6)

Materials: 1-in. white tape
prewrap

Position: The forearm should be fully supinated and the wrist should be in a neutral position to slightly flexed position. The fingers should be spread.

Note: For athletes who need to catch a ball and/or need full function of the hand, this taping technique may not be practical. Some athletes will not tolerate tape on the palm.

Step 1: Apply two circular strips around the wrist and to the area just proximal to the metacarpal heads. Apply crossing strips of tape from the metacarpals to the wrist (Fig. 6A).

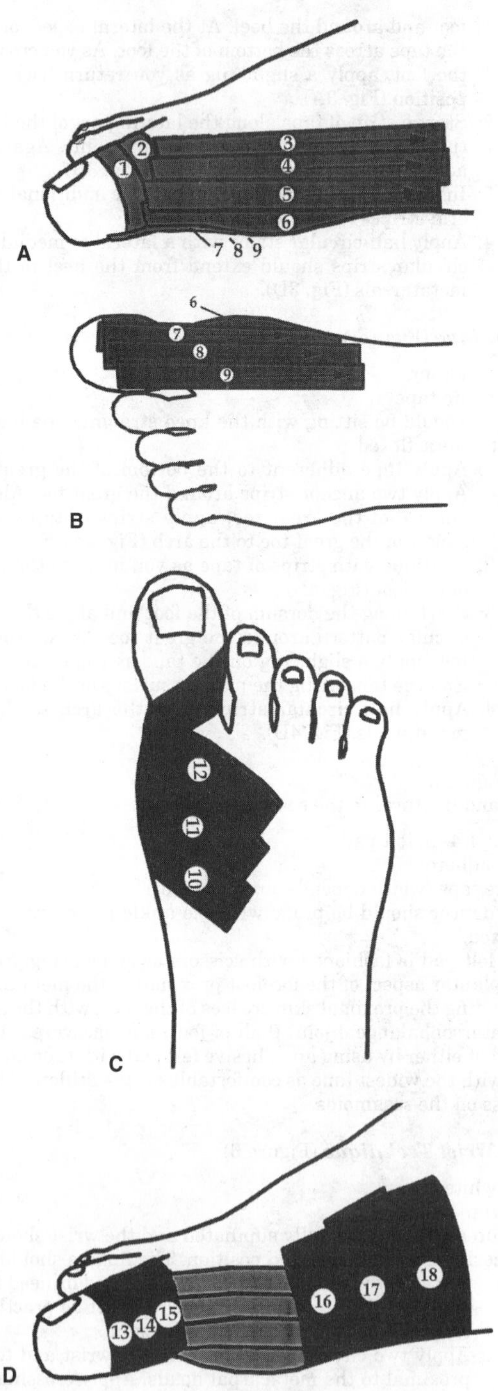

Fig. 4(A-D) "Turf-Toe" Taping Technique.

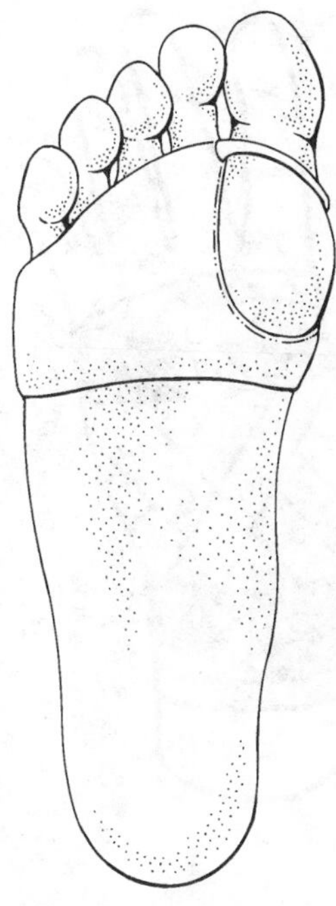

Fig. 5 Dancer's Pad Technique

Repeat crossing strips two or three times, covering the entire hand area. Optional circular strips can be applied in a figure-eight fashion starting at the wrist, crossing the palm and circling the metacarpophalangeal joints.

Step 2: Apply two to three closure strips around the hand and the wrist (Fig. 6B).

Thumb Technique (Fig. 7)

Materials: 1-in. white tape
Prewrap

Position: Athlete should have the hand in a normal resting position with the thumb slightly spread. The forearm should be in a pronated position.

Step 1: The tape should be started on the lateral aspect of the hand. Apply a couple of circular anchors around the wrist and with a continuous motion, move up the outside aspect palm of the thumb, through the web space, around the thumb, and over the back of the hand (Fig. 7A). Apply increased tension in the tape, pulling the thumb slightly toward the hand as you go around the thumb.

Step 2: In a continuous motion, apply two more strips around the thumb. If you cannot get the correct angle, then tear the tape to start a new strip (Fig. 7B).

Step 3: Finish with one or two closures around the wrist (Fig. 7C).

Finger Buddy Tape (Fig. 8)

Materials: 1/2-in. white cloth tape
cotton or prewrap (optional; use if taping must last longer than just for game or practice)

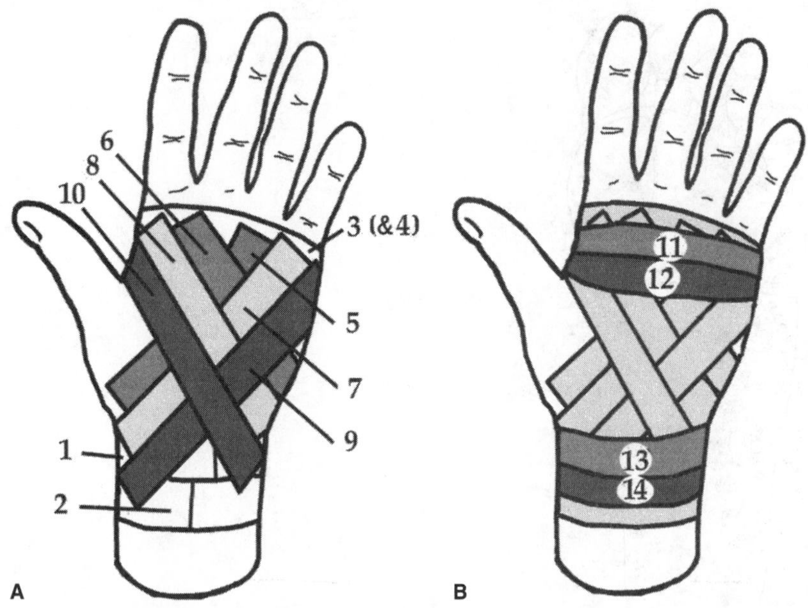

Fig. 6(A-B) Hypertension Wrist Taping Technique.

Position: Athlete should be sitting with the hand and fingers in the normal resting position. The injured finger and adjacent finger should be slightly spread apart.

Step 1: Apply tape adherent to the injured and adjacent fingers at the level of the proximal phalanx and the middle phalanx, between the interphalangeal joints. Place cotton or prewrap between the injured and adjacent finger to prevent maceration (if taping longer than just practice or event). The cotton or pre-wrap are not necessary if taping only for practice or play (using splint at other times). Wrap the 1/2-in. tape one to two times around the proximal phalanges of the two fingers snugly, but not too tightly to affect circulation (Fig. 8A).

Step 2: Wrap tape one to two times around the middle phalanges of the two fingers. (Fig. 8B).

Velpeau Bandage (Fig. 9)
For immobilization of acute shoulder fractures and dislocations, humeral fractures, and certain elbow fractures.

Materials: long Ace wrap or bias stockinette
pad or towel

Position: Athlete should be sitting or standing with the hand of the injured arm holding the opposite shoulder as shown. An ABD pad or towel is placed in both axillae and between the affected and arm/shoulder.

Step 1: The wrap is started under the affected arm in front of the chest and brought under the opposite axilla, up the back, and over the top of the affected shoulder (Fig. 9A). This is then brought in front of the affected arm and wrapped under the arm in front of the chest and then under the opposite axilla again. It is then brought around the back of the athlete.

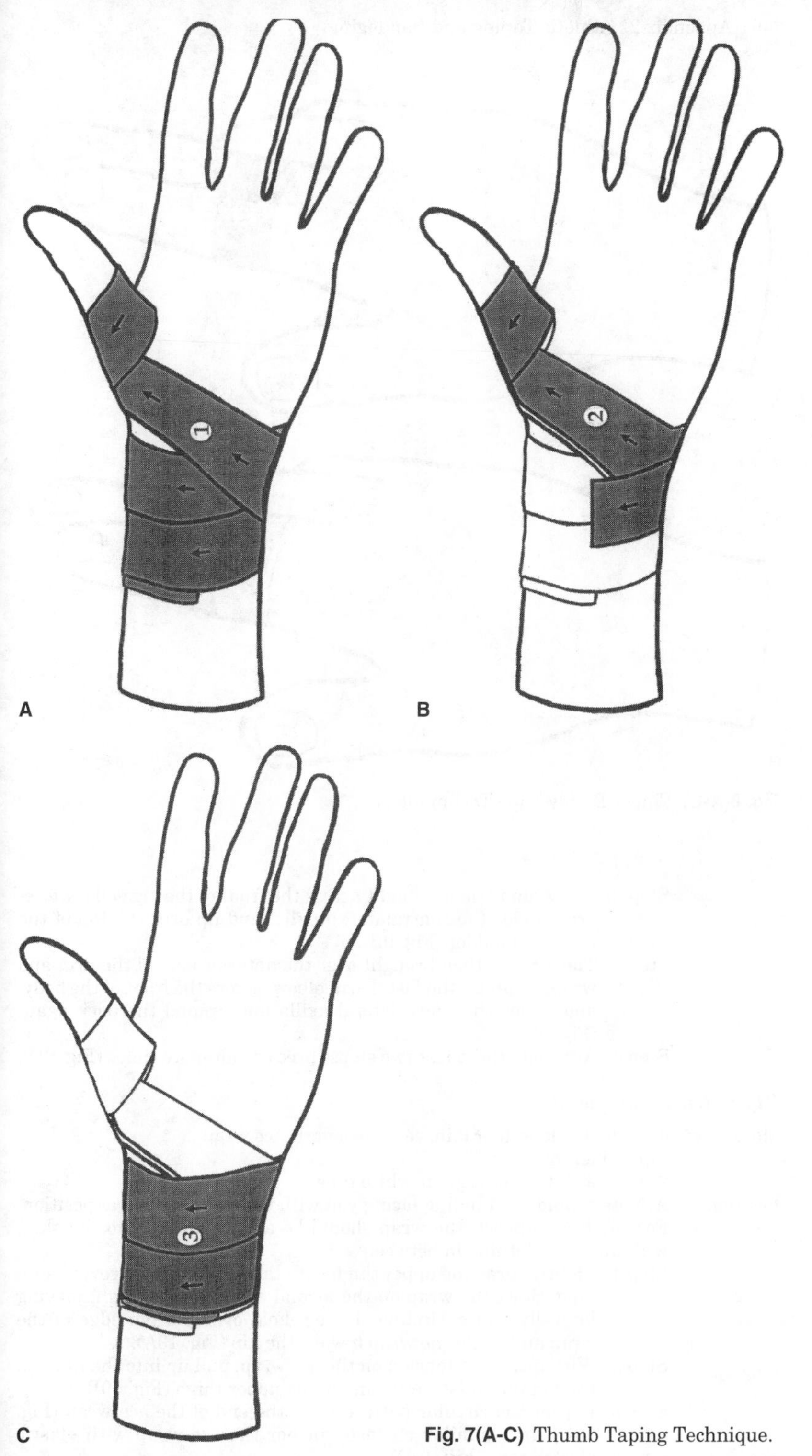

Fig. 7(A-C) Thumb Taping Technique.

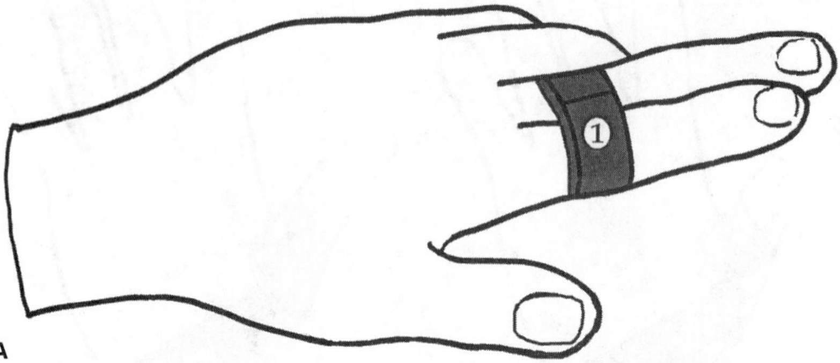

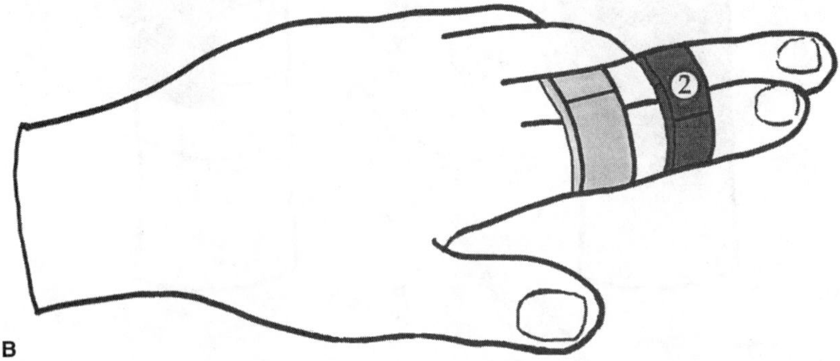

A

B

Fig. 8(A-B) Finger Buddy Tape Technique.

Step 2: The wrap is then brought across the front of the arm/elbow/forearm, under the contralateral axilla, and up over the top of the injured shoulder (Fig. 9B).

Step 3: The wrap is then brought over the anterior part of the arm and wrapped under the distal arm/elbow, across the front of the body, and under the contralateral axilla and around the back again (Fig. 9C).

Step 4: Alternate these last two steps three or four more times (Fig. 9D).

Hip Spica Wrap (Fig. 10)

Materials: 4-in. double-length or 6 in. regular-length Ace wrap
tape adherent spray
2-in. stretch tape or regular white tape

Position: Athlete should be standing facing you with the leg in a neutral position. For the best support, the wrap should be applied directly to the skin, with minimal clothing in between.

Step 1: Lightly spray the upper thigh with tape adherent to prevent slipping. Start the wrap on the medial aspect of the thigh, moving laterally and encircling the leg. Fold over the top edge of the wrap and angle the wrap toward the hip (Fig. 10A).

Step 2: With increased tension on the ace wrap, pull up into the hip and around the waist, returning to the upper thigh (Fig. 10B).

Step 3: Repeat the circular pattern until the end of the ace wrap (Fig. 10C). In a similar pattern, anchor the ace wrap with elastic stretch tape (Fig. 10D).

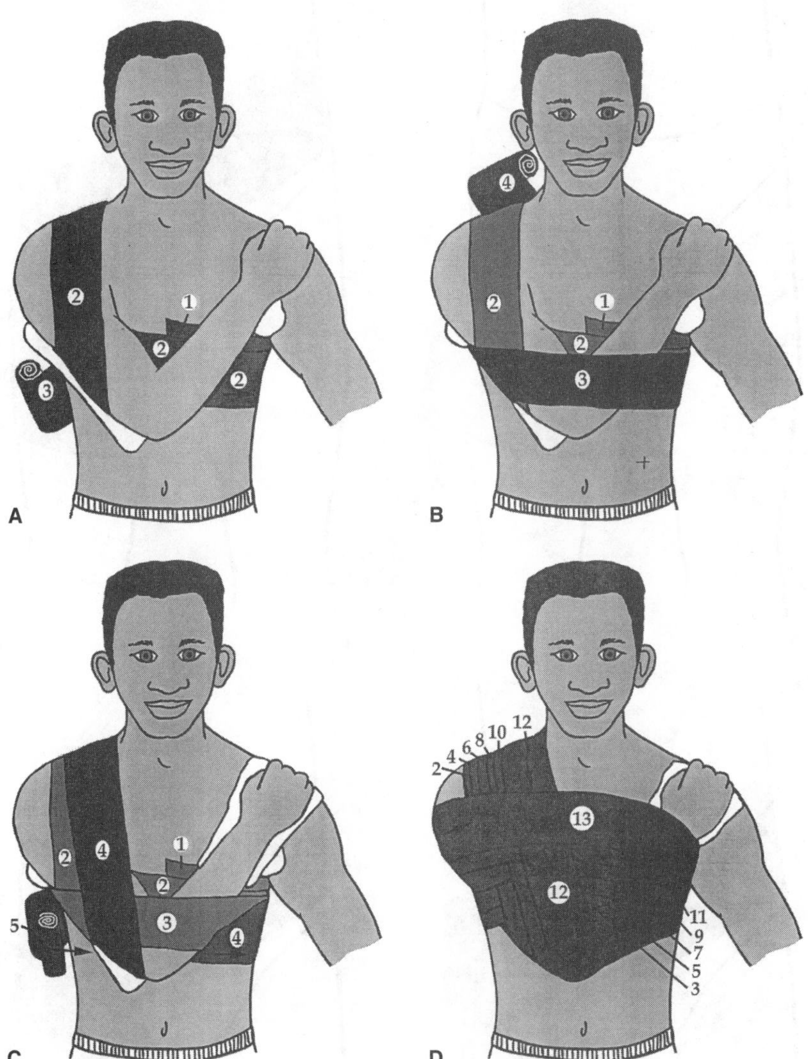

Fig. 9(A-D) Velpeau Bandage Technique.

Groin Spica Wrap (Fig. 11)

Materials: 4-in. double length or 6-in. regular Ace wrap
tape adherent
2-in. stretch tape or regular white tape

Position: Athlete should be standing facing you with the leg internally rotated. For best support, the wrap should be applied directly to the skin, with minimal clothing in between.

Step 1: Lightly spray the upper thigh with tape adherent to prevent slipping. Start the wrap on the lateral aspect of the thigh, moving

(*Text continues on page 652*)

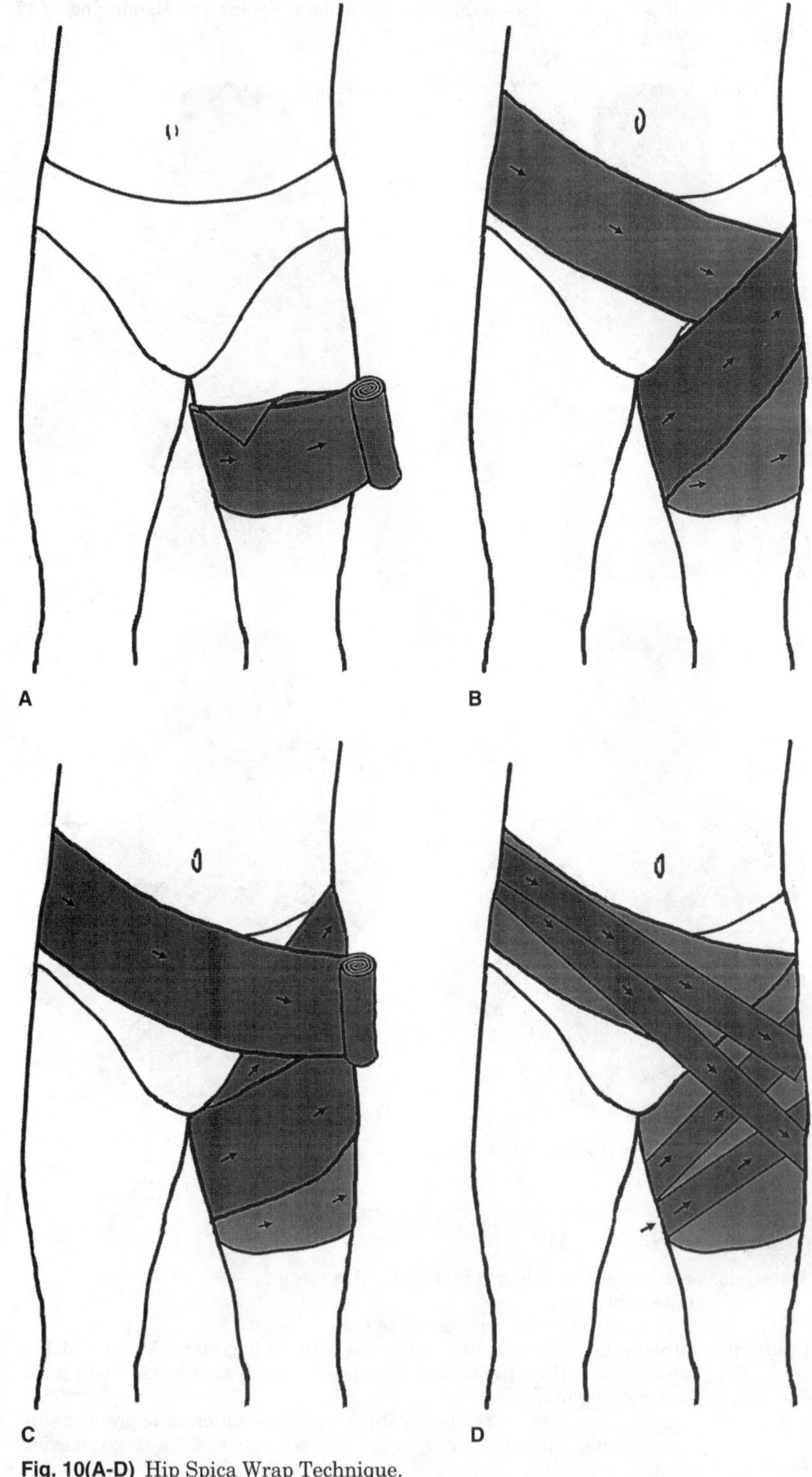

Fig. 10(A-D) Hip Spica Wrap Technique.

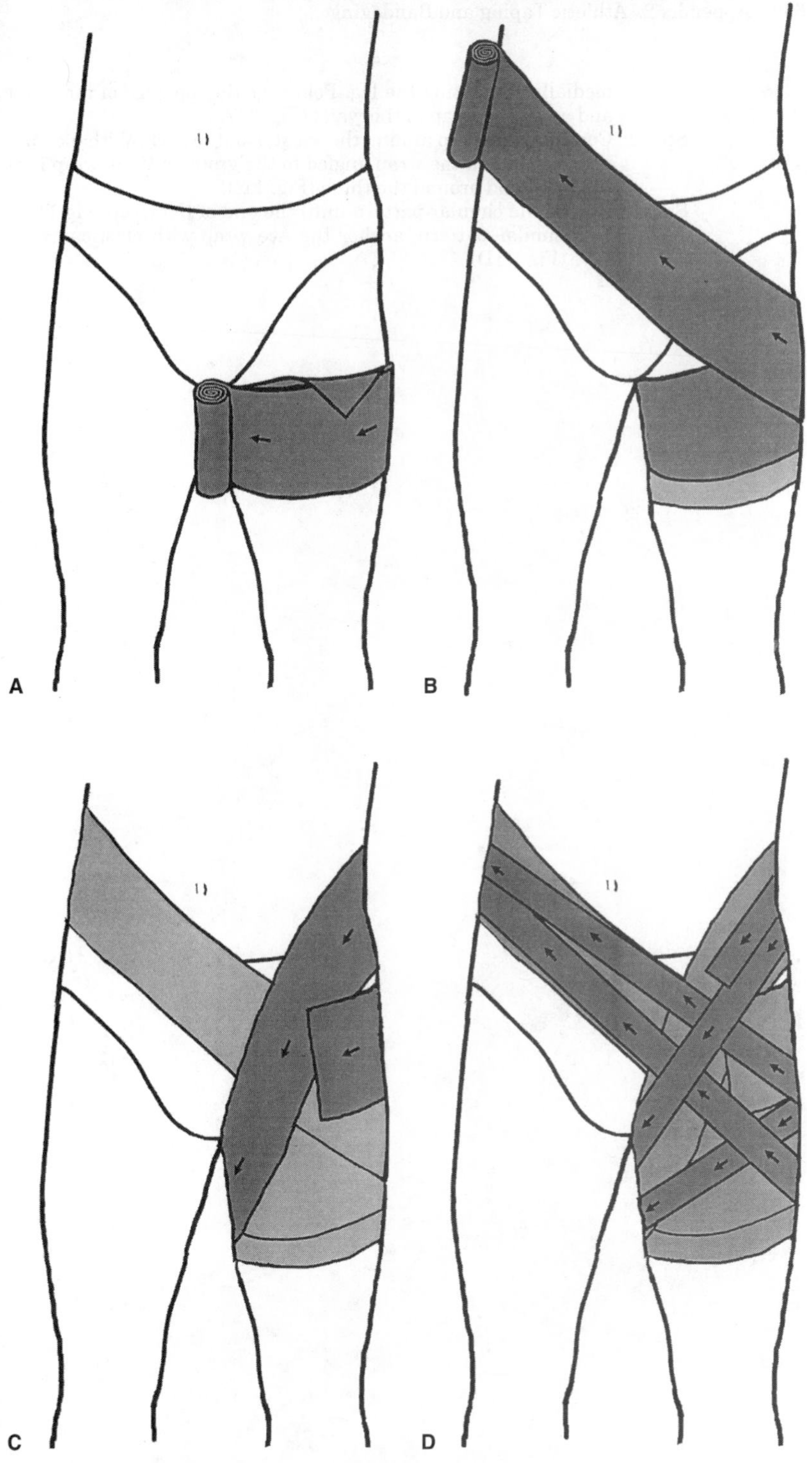

Fig. 11(A-D) Groin Spica Wrap Technique.

medially circulating the leg. Fold over the top edge of the wrap and angle the wrap to the waist (Fig. 11A).

Step 2: Continue the wrap around the waist, front to back. With increasing tension and the wrap angled to the groin, pull the wrap into the groin and around the thigh (Fig. 11B).

Step 3: Repeat the circular pattern until the end of the wrap (Fig 11C). In a similar pattern, anchor the Ace wrap with elastic stretch tape (Fig. 11D).

Appendix 3. **BANNED DRUGS**

Marc R. Safran

The following list contains classes of drugs that are not allowed in all or some sports by the National Collegiate Athletic Association (NCAA) and/or the U.S. Olympic Committee (USOC) guideline of 1996. Please refer to the specific agency for current guidelines and updates. Lists of specific drugs that are legal and banned are lengthy and differ with regard to which governing body is overseeing a given competition. These lists are obtainable by contacting the respective governing body.

* = Banned by USOC (1996)
+ = Banned by NCAA (1996–1997)
# = Banned by both USOC and NCAA

Stimulants (Generic names)

* Amfepramone
* Amfetaminil
* Amineptine
# Amiphenazole
# Amphetamine
# Bemegride
# Benzphetamine
# Caffeine (urine concentrations: USOC >12 mg/mL; NCAA >15 mg/mL)
* Cathine
# Chlorphentermine
* Clobenzorex
* Clorprenaline
# Cocaine
# Cropropamide
# Crothetamide
* Desoxyephedrine
# Diethylproprion HCl
# Dimethylamphetamine/Dimetamphetamine
+ Doxapram
* Ephedrine
* Etaphedrine
# Ethamivan
+ Ethylamphetamine
* Etilamfetamine
# Fencamfamine
* Fenetylline
* Fenproporex
* Furfenorex
* Isoetharine HCl
+ Isoprenaline
* Isoproterenol
* Ma huang (herbal ephedrine)
# Meclofenoxate
* Mefenorex
* Mesocarbe
* Metaproterenol
# Methamphetamine
* Methoxyphenamine
* Methylephedrine

Methylphenidate HCl
* Morazone
# Nikethamide
# Pemoline
# Pentetrazol/Pentylenetetrazol
# Phendimetrazine
# Phenmetrazine
# Phentermine HCl
* Phenylephedrine
* Phenylpropanolamine
# Picrotoxine
# Pipradol
* Prethcamide
# Prolintane
* Propylhexedrin
* Pseudoephedrine
* Pyrovalerone
* Selegiline
# Strychnine
And related compounds

Narcotic Analgesics (Generic Names)

* Alphaprodine
* Anileridine
* Buprenorphine
* Dextromoramide
* Dextropropoxyphen
* Diamorphine
* Dipipanone
* Ethoheptazine
* Ethylmorphine
* Fentanyl
* Hydrocodone
* Hydromorphone
* Levorphanol
* Meperidine
* Methadone HCl
* Morphine
* Nalbuphine
* Oxycodone
* Oxymorphone
* Pentazocine
* Phenazocine
* Propoxyphene
* Tincture Opium
And related compounds

Anabolic Steroids (Generic Names)

* Bolasterone
# Boldenone
# Clostebol
# Dehydrochlormethyltestosterone
* Dihydrotestosterone
+ Dromostanolone
# Fluoxymesterone
* Mestanolone
# Mesterolone
# Methandienone

Metenolone
* Methandrostenolone
# Methyltestosterone
# Nandrolone
# Norethandrolone
# Oxandrolone
# Oxymesterone
# Oxymetholone
# Stanozolol
# Testosterone
And other related compounds

Beta Blockers (Generic Names) (Specific Sports)

* Acebutolol
* Alprenolol
# Atenolol
* Betaxolol
* Bisoprolol
* Carteolol
* Carvedilol
* Esmolol
* Labetalol
# Metoprolol
# Nadolol
* Oxprenolol
* Penbutolol
# Pindolol
# Propanolol
* Sotalol
# Timolol
And related compounds

Diuretics (Generic Names)

Acetazolamide
* Amiloride
# Bendroflumethazide
# Benzthiazide
# Bumetanide
* Canernone
* Chlormerodrin
# Chlorthalidone
+ Chlorthiazide
* Diclofenamide
# Ethacrynic acid
+ Flumethazide
# Furosemide
* Glycerine
# Hydrochlorothiazide
+ Hydroflumethiazide
* Indapamide
* Mannitol
* Mersalyl
# Methylclothiazide
# Metolazone
+ Polythiazide
+ Quinethazone
# Spironolactone
* Torsemide

Triamterene
+ Trichlormethazide
* Urea
And related compounds and combinations

Beta$_2$ Agonists

* Bitoloterol
# Clenbuterol
* Fenoterol
* Metaproterenol
* Orciprenaline
* Pirbuterol
* Rimiterol
And related compounds

Miscellaneous

Heroin
Marijuana
THC (Tetrahydrocannabinol)
Alcohol
Erythropoietin
Growth Hormone,
Human Chorionic Gonadotropin
Corticotropin (ACTH)

Appendix 4. **CONTENTS OF THE MEDICAL BAG**

Marc R. Safran and George C. Fareed

The medical bag is important to help handle on the field injuries and routine medical problems during travel. The physician should be prepared for every foreseeable occurrence, regardless of severity. Therefore, it is important to maintain the constant presence of a well-stocked medical kit to allow the team physician to properly care for emergencies. The contents of the bag may vary depending on whether other sources of equipment are also available. Listed here are what are considered to be the minimum requirements for medical equipment and supplies. Each physician probably has his or her own preferences regarding some items, and the lists will need to be modified to reflect individual choices and practice methods. Requirements may also vary depending on whether the contest is "at home," "away," or "overseas," in warm climates, high altitude, etc. Special medications may be included for known medical conditions of athletes, coaches, or team officials. Some physicians feel that over-the-counter medications (such as aspirin, antacids, throat lozenges, etc.), nonemergent medications (such as nonsteroidal anti-inflammatories) and those that can be obtained with prescriptions (such as antibiotics) easily (depending on location) should not be carried routinely. After each event or trip, the supplies need to be restocked and updated and modified based on need. A consistent method of restocking with reference to a master list is advisable to prevent depletion.

Although most physicians do or should know how to perform cardiopulmonary resuscitation (CPR), as a practical reality, this skill is infrequently used by most physicians after leaving residency except by emergency/critical care specialists, trauma specialists, and cardiologists.

Physician's Bag

Ankle brace
Alcohol and Betadine (povidone-iodone) swabs
Bandages—elastic (Ace, Elasto-plast)
Bandages—plastic strips (Band-Aids)
Batteries
Bulbs
Benzoin
Blister pads/moleskin
Blood pressure cuff
Cotton-tip applicator swabs
Dental kit
  Hank's solution with container
Finger splints
  Formed Aluminum splints, different widths
  Foam rubber
Forceps
Gauze pads
Gelfoam
Gloves (sterile and nonsterile exam)
Hemostats
Hydrogen peroxide
Ice
Ice bags
Irrigation kit
Measuring tape
Nail clippers
Nasal packing (tampon)
Nonadhering sterile pads (Tefla)

Notepad/dictaphone
Otoscope/ophthalmoscope (with replacement batteries)
Pen / pencil
Penlight
Petroleum jelly
Prep razor
Prescription pad
Prewrap
Reflex hammer
Scalpel (#10, #11, #15)
Scissors
Scrub brushes
Slings
Splints
Sterile water
Steri-strips
Stethoscope
Superglue
Suture kit
  Absorbable suture
  Nonabsorbable suture (4–0, 5–0, 6–0)
Swiss Army Knife
Syringes (3 and 5 cc) and Needles (1 and 1.5 in., 20, 22, 25, and 27 gauge)
Tape (cloth, Micropore, Elastoplast)
Tape measure
Thermometer (oral and rectal)
Tongue depressors
Towel clamp
Vacutainer tubes, holder, and needles

Eye Kit
Eye chart
Eye patch
Fluorescein strips
Mirror
Ultraviolet penlight
Ophthalmic solutions (see below)

CPR Equipment
(In medical bag, see below for additional equipment)
Airway/endotracheal tube
Intravenous setups:
  Fluids: Liter bags of D_5W and D_5LR, ampules of D_{50}
  Intravenous tubing
  Intracath (Angiocath) needles (16 and 18 gauge)
Laryngoscope
Tracheostomy tube

Medications
Analgesics
  Aspirin
  Acetaminophen
  Codeine or synthetic analgesic tablets
  Ketorolac tromethamine (Toradol, oral and injectable—optional)
  Morphine sulfate or injectable meperidine HCL (Demerol)
Antibiotics
  Cephalosporin
  Erthyromycin
  Quinolone (optional)

- Tetracycline
- Penicillin
- Oxacillin
- Ampicillin/Amoxicillin

Antiinflammatory Agents

- Nonsteroidal antiinflammatory drugs (NSAIDs) (a few different ones, prescription strength and over-the-counter strength)
- Oral steroids (dexamethasone or Medrol Dose Pack)
- Topical antiinflammatories (over-the-counter and prescription nonsteroidal creams)
- Injectable corticosteroid

Cardiac Medications

- Atropine
- Beta blocker
- Digoxin
- Dopamine
- Epinephrine
- Furosemide
- Lidocaine
- Nifedipine
- Nitroglycerine
- Sodium bicarbonate
- Verapamil

Dermatologics

- Antibiotic ointment
- Antifungal cream
- Insect repellent
- Silver sulfadiazine cream
- Sunscreen
- Sunburn cream
- Zinc oxide powder

Eye-Ear-Nose-Throat Medications

- Acular drops
- Antibiotic ophthalmic drops
- Collyrium wash and eyedrops
- Corticosporin otitic
- Ear wax remover
- Prednisone ophthalmic solution
- Pseudoephedrine
- Scopolamine patch
- Tetracaine ophthalmic drops
- Vasoclear A (or Opcon A)
- Visine

Gastrointestinal Medications

- Antacids
- Antidiarrheals (Lomotil, Imodium)
- Antiemetic (Compazine/Tigan)
- Antiperistaltic (Loperamide)
- Antispasmodic (Donnatol)
- Bismuth subsalicylate (Pepto-Bismol)

Miscellaneous

- Albuterol Inhaler
- Aminophylline
- Ammonia capsules
- Anaphylaxis kit
- Antimalarial/antiparasitic medications
- Antihistamines (Benadryl/Claritin)
- Bupivacaine HCl (Marcaine)
- Clove oil

- Cough syrup
- Dental packing
- Diazepam, injectable
- Diphenhydramine
- Insulin, regular, human
- Ipecac
- Lidocaine (Xylocaine)
- Lip protector (Chapstick or Blistex)
- Muscle relaxants (Robaxin, Norflex, Parafon Forte, Valium)
- Naloxone
- Throat lozenges

Have available (not necessarily in the doctor's bag):

FIELD EQUIPMENT

Air splints
Blankets
Bolt cutters
Cervical collar (rigid)
Crutches
Sandbags
Screwdriver (helmet)
Spine board
Stretcher
Trainer's Angel (Football Helmet)

CPR EQUIPMENT

Airway/endotracheal tube
Bulb suction syringe
Cardiac monitor / defibrillator (not mandatory)
Crash cart with cardiac and anaphylactic medications
Esophageal obturator
Intravenous setups
- Fluids: liter bags of D_5W and D_5LR, ampules of D_{50}
- Intravenous tubing
- Intracath needles (16 and 18 gauge)

Laryngoscope
Oral and nasal oxygen with mask

Appendix 5. **REHABILITATION PROGRAMS**

W. Benjamin Kibler and Robert G. Watkins

Exercise Prescription for Rehabilitation of Acute Macrotrauma: Meniscal Injury

I. Acute Phase

A. *Goals*
1. Reduce effects of immobilization
2. Retard muscle atrophy of entire lower extremity
3. Neuromuscular control of the patella
4. Maintain components of fitness

B. *Effects of immobilization*
1. NSAID 48–96 hr if needed
2. Modalities 2–3 weeks
3. Patellar mobilization
4. Joint protection (brace/non-weight-bearing)
5. Range of motion

C. *Muscle atrophy / neuromuscular control*
1. Local
   a. Isometrics
   b. Straight-leg raises (avoid adduction and abduction for 2 weeks)
   c. Biofeedback—patellar control
2. Distant
   a. Open chain—nonpathologic areas (ankle, hip)
      i. Concentrics
      ii. Eccentrics

D. *Maintain components of fitness*
1. Aerobic endurance for upper body
   a. Ergometer
2. Strength for upper body and opposite leg
   a. Weights
   b. Machines

E. *Criteria for advancement*
1. Elimination of most swelling
2. Level II pain
3. Healing of injured tissue to allow mild tensile stress, range of motion (ROM), weight bearing
4. Straight-leg raise, 8 lb

II. Recovery Phase

A. *Goals*
1. Reestablish nonpainful active and passive ROM
2. Regain and improve lower extremity muscle strength
3. Improve lower extremity neuromuscular control
4. Normal arthrokinematics in single plane of motion

B. *Range of motion*
1. Dependent
   a. Patellar mobilization
   b. Manual capsular stretch and cross-friction massage
2. Independent
   a. Knee flexion and extension, active and passive
   b. Heel wall slides
   c. Bike and rowing machine
   d. Stretching—quadriceps, hamstring, iliotibial band, hip flexor, gastrocsoleus

- C. *Stretching*
  1. Dependent
     a. Proprioceptive Neuromuscular facilitation (PNF)
  2. Independent single planes (avoid aggressive hamstring work after posterior horn tear)
     a. Open chain
        i. Concentric and eccentric isotonics
        ii. Isokinetics
        iii. Tubing and free weights
     b. Closed chain
        i. Nautilus/Stairmaster
        ii. Lifeline/tubing
        iii. Free weights
- D. *Neuromuscular control*
  1. Balance board
  2. BAPS
  3. Fitter and slide board
  4. Minitrampoline
  5. Lifeline
- E. *Arthrokinematics*
  1. Joint mobilization
  2. Kinetic chain movement patterns, tennis-specific (for Tennis players)
     a. Flexion and extension
     b. Hip and leg rotation
     c. Acceleration and deceleration
- F. *Other activities*
  1. Practice service motion (for Tennis players)
  2. Hit ground strokes
  3. No intense play
- G. *Criteria for advancement*
  1. Nearly full active and passive nonpainful ROM equal to other side
  2. Quadriceps/ hamstring ratio 66% and strength 75% of noninvolved side
  3. Static balance on one leg times 1 min
  4. Normal smooth arthrokinematics with single-plane motion

III. Maintenance Phase

- A. *Goals*
  1. Increase power and endurance in lower extremity
  2. Increase normal multiple-plane neuromuscular control
  3. Sport-specific activities (for Tennis players)
- B. *Power and endurance* (avoid compressive and shear loads times 6–8 weeks)
  1. Multiple-plane motions
     a. Start and stop
     b. Side lunges
     c. Change of directions
  2. Plyometrics
  3. Anaerobic conditioning based on periodization
- C. *Neuromuscular control, multiple planes*
  1. Agility drills
  2. Footwork drills
- D. *Sport-specific training functional progression*
  1. Stage I
     a. Standing on one foot
     b. Jumping on two legs (forward, backward, sides)
     c. Jumping on a minitrampoline
     d. Jumping from stool, 40 cm (1 ft)
     e. Rope skipping on both feet
     f. Balance board with both feet (forward, side to side, 45-degree angle)
     g. Balance board with both feet (catch tennis ball)

2. Stage II
   a. Rope skipping on one foot
   b. Jumping from stool, 40 cm, land on one foot
   c. Jumping from stool, 80 cm, land on two feet
   d. Hopping one foot (forward, backward, sides)
   e. Jogging in place
   f. Jogging around court
   g. Jog figure eight (large and small)
   h. Jog figure eight backward
   i. Balance board with one foot (forward, side to side)
3. Stage III
   a. Running with direction changes
   b. Carioca running
   c. Running 1 to 1 1/2 miles
   d. Jumping: two-footed takeoff, land on one foot
4. Stage IV
   a. Anaerobic sprints with cutting on demand
   b. Split step
   c. Sport-specific training (tennis)
      i. Motions
         (a) Five-dot drill
         (b) Hexagon drills
         (c) Spider drills

IV. Criteria for Return to Play

A. Negative clinical exam
B. Normal ROM and flexibility equal to opposite side
C. Isokinetic strength 90% of normal side
D. Normal arthrokinematics in multiple plane
E. Pass functional exam—hop test, spider agility drill

Exercise Prescription for Rehabilitation of Chronic Microtrauma: Tendonosis

I. Acute Phase

A. *Goals*
   1. Reduce pain and inflammation
   2. Reestablish nonpainful active and passive ROM
   3. Reverse muscle atrophy
   4. Maintain components of fitness
B. *Pain and inflammation*
   1. NSAIDs for less than 2 weeks
   2. Modalities for 2–3 weeks
   3. Joint protection (braces and counterforce)
   4. Decrease activities
C. *Range of motion*
   1. Dependent
      a. Cross-friction massage (end of acute stage or with chronic)
   2. Independent
      a. Stretching of quadriceps, hamstrings, and iliotibial band
      b. Knee flexion and extension, active and passive
D. *Reverse muscle atrophy*
   1. Local
      a. Isometrics and gentle, pain-free straight leg raises
      b. Biofeedback patellar control
   2. Distant
      a. Open chain—nonpathologic areas (ankle, hip)
         i. Concentric
         ii. Eccentric
E. *Components of fitness*
   1. Eliminate most swelling
   2. Level II pain

3. Healing of injured tissue to allow mild tensile stress
4. Half squat without pain, body weight only

II. Recovery Phase

A. *Goals*
1. Regain and improve lower extremity muscle strength
2. Improve lower extremity neuromuscular control
3. Normal arthrokinematics in single plane of motion

B. *Strengthening*
1. Independent single planes
    a. Open chain
        i. Eccentric isotonics
        ii. Isokinetic
    b. Closed chain
        i. Nautilus/Stairmaster
        ii. Lifeline/tubing
        iii. Free weights

C. *Neuromuscular control*
1. Balance board
2. BAPS
3. Fitter and slide board
4. Minitrampoline
5. Lifeline

D. *Arthrokinematics*
1. Kinetic chain movement patterns (baseball activities)
    a. Flexion and extension
    b. Striding and follow through
2. Protective brace

E. *Other activities*
1. Short toss with stride—normal mechanics, no mound
2. Batting

F. *Criteria for advancement*
1. Full active and passive ROM to other side
2. Quadriceps/hamstring ratio 66% and strength 75% of noninvolved side
3. One-leg squat 10–15 reps without pain
4. Smooth arthrokinematics with single-plane motion

III. Maintenance Phase

A. *Goals*
1. Increase eccentric power and endurance in lower extremity
2. Increase normal multiple-plane neuromuscular control
3. Sport-specific activities (for baseball players)

B. *Power and endurance*
1. Eccentric work
    a. Quadriceps
    b. Hamstrings
    c. Gastrocnemius
    d. Hips
2. Plyometrics
3. Backward walking against tubing

C. *Neuromuscular control, multiple plane*
1. Agility drills
2. Footwork drills

D. *Sport-specific training functional progression*
1. Stage I
    a. Standing on one foot
    b. Jumping on two legs (forward, backward, sides)
    c. Jumping on a minitrampoline
    d. Jumping from stool, 40 cm (1 ft)
    e. Rope skipping on both feet
    f. Balance board with both feet (forward, side to side, 45-degree angle)
    g. Balance board with both feet (catch baseball)

2. Stage II
   a. Rope skipping on one foot
   b. Jumping from stool, 40 cm, land on one foot
   c. Jumping from stool, 80 cm, land on two feet
   d. Hopping on one foot (forward, backward, sides)
   e. Jogging in place
   f. Jogging around field
   g. Jog figure eight (large and small)
   h. Balance board with plant foot (forward, side to side)
3. Stage III
   a. Running with no direction changes
   b. Running 1 to 1 1/2 mi
4. Stage IV
   a. Spring start, slow stop
   b. Spring start, fast stop
   c. Jump on two feet, land on one foot
   d. Sport-specific training (for baseball)
      i. Crow hop to the mound
      ii. Crow hop from mound to half windup to full windup
      iii. Stride on mound
      iv. Full windup

IV. Criteria for Return to Play

A. Negative clinical exam
B. Normal ROM and flexibility equal to opposite side
C. Isokinetic test 90% of normal and 65% quadriceps/hamstring ratio
D. Normal arthrokinematics in multiple-plane motion
E. Pass functional exam—hop test, normal stride

Rehabilitation of Rotator Cuff Tendinitis

I. Acute Phase

A. *Goals*
   1. Reestablish nonpainful range of motion
   2. Retard muscle atrophy of entire upper extremity
   3. Neuromuscular control of scapula in neural glenohumeral position
   4. Reduce pain and inflammation

B. *Range of motion*
   1. Dependent
      a. Mobilization of glenohumeral, acromio-clavicular, and scapulothoracic joints
      b. Manual capsular stretching and cross-friction massage
      c. T-bar

C. *Muscle atrophy / neuromuscular control*
   1. Local
      a. Isometrics
      b. Scapular control
      c. Closed chain activities
   2. *Distant*
      a. Open chain—nonpathological areas (elbow, back)
         i. Concentrics
         ii. Eccentrics
   3. Aerobic/anaerobic activities

D. *Pain and inflammation*
   1. NSAIDs 48–96 hr
   2. Modalities 2–3 weeks
   3. Joint mobilization
   4. Joint protection

E. *Range of motion*
   1. Passive flexibility
   2. Active flexibility

F. *Criteria for advancement*
1. No swelling
2. Level II pain
3. Manual muscle testing strength 75% of strength in other muscles
4. Scapular control in neutral position

II. Recovery Phase

A. *Goals*
1. Regain and improve upper extremity muscle strength
2. Improve upper extremity neuromuscular control
3. Normalize shoulder arthrokinematics in single planes of motion
4. Improve active/ passive range of motion flexibility

B. *Strengthening*
1. Dependent
   a. Scapular proprioceptive neuromuscular facilitation
   b. Glenohumeral proprioceptive neuromuscular facilitation
2. Independent
   a. Concentric and eccentric isotonics
   b. Isotonics
   c. Tubing
   d. Rotator cuff isolation exercises (Jobe)

C. *Neuromuscular control*
1. Proprioceptive neuromuscular facilitation
2. Emphasis on force couples
   a. Scapular retractors/ protractors
   b. Glenohumeral elevators/depressors
   c. Glenohumeral internal/external rotators

D. *Arthrokinematics*
1. Joint mobilization
2. Kinetic chain movement patterns

E. *Criteria for advancement*
1. Full nonpainful scapulothoracic motion
2. Almost full nonpainful glenohumeral motion
3. Normal scapular stabilizer strength (lateral side asymmetry < 0.5 cm)
4. Rotator cuff strength 75% of normal
5. Normal throwing motion

III. Maintenance Phase

A. *Goals*
1. Increase power and endurance in upper extremity
2. Increase normal multiple-plane neuromuscular control (eliminate subclinical adaptations)
3. Sports-specific activity

B. *Power and endurance*
1. Multiple plane motions
2. Plyometrics
   a. Wall pushups
   b. Ball throws
   c. Tubing or other elastic resistance
   d. Medicine ball
3. Conditioning based on principles of periodization

C. *Sports-specific functional progression*
1. Long toss-short toss
2. Throwing
3. Pitching

IV. Criteria for Return to Play

A. Normal arthrokinematics in multiple planes

B. Isokinetic strength 90% of normal

C. Negative clinical examination

The Trunk Stabilization Program—Spine Rehabilitation

The trunk stabilization program followed at the Kerlan-Jobe Orthopaedic Clinic consists of a battery of eight types of exercises: "dead bug," partial sit-ups, bridging, prone exercises, quadriped, wall slides, ball exercises, and aerobics. Each category is further graduated through five levels requiring incrementally greater balance and strength. Within each level the intensity of performance is further graduated through such means as increasing the number of repetitions to be performed for a given exercise, varying the body positions held, and adding poundage when free weights are being used.

A primary objective of this program is to train the patient to make proper use of the abdominal and buttock muscles (as well as the chest muscles) when sitting, standing, walking, or running. Tightly controlled abdominal and buttock muscles are essential to building trunk stabilization.

The patient goes from an initially neutral, pain-free position for the spine to a safe, controlled position, then is gradually moved into increasingly advanced strengthening exercises. Eventually the patient learns to assume and control somewhat precarious positions that require greater balance and coordination.

Through this safe, progressive procedure, the therapist can determine the extent of rehabilitation attained and the type of daily living activities the patient may return to by ascertaining the patient's level of performance in each category. Very often, the patient will advance more quickly through one category than through another, such that he or she may be doing level 3 in dead bug exercises but only level 2 in prone exercises, for example. This is only natural, in that the therapist will have the patient advancing more quickly through exercises that the patient is better able to perform and has less pain doing.

Exercises used, in order, are as follows:

1. **Dead bug.** There is a minimal amount of back motion in this group of exercises. They are performed supine, with the knees flexed and feet on the floor. A trainer or therapist helps the patient push the lumbar spine back toward the mat without using exaggerated back flattening, or extreme force. Instead, the patient exerts a mild amount of painless force on the therapist's hand, which is placed under the patient's lumbar area. The patient is taught to maintain this neutral spine position by contracting abdominal and trunk muscles.
   - Level I: In the neutral position, with the patient's arms supported by the therapist, the arms are extended over the head and held for 2 min.
   - Level II: Without support from the therapist, the arms are extended over the head, and each leg is alternately extended for 3 min.
   - Level III: Weights are added to the legs, and the level II exercise is done for 7 min.
   - Level IV: Same as level III, done for 10 min.
   - Level V: Fifteen min of unsupported bilateral leg and arm extensions.
2. **Partial sit-ups.** The feet of the supine patient are placed firmly on the floor, arms beside the body, and the abdominal bracing is begun. The patient does partial sit-ups by placing the hands across the chest, bringing the head and shoulders off the floor, and holding that position. There should be a minimal amount of back motion in this exercise, so there's no need to fully sit up or have the legs extended.
   - Level I: One set of 10 repetitions.
   - Level II: Three sets of 10 repetitions.
   - Level III: Three sets of 10 repetitions. Then the arms are placed behind the head, and three sets of 10 repetitions are done in which the right elbow is touched to the bent left knee, then the left elbow to the right knee.
   - Level IV: Level III repetitions are increased to 20 and weights are placed on the chest.
   - Level V: Repetitions are increased to 30. Following these, while holding a weight, the patient pumps the arms over the body unsupported, then extends them backward over the head for a count of 10, brings then back up, and then to the chest.

3. **Bridging.** These exercises are done from the supine position, lifting the pelvis off the floor while maintaining the neutral, painfree position. Lifting is done with the legs, so that the back is not arched into a hyperextended position. Pain with this maneuver is produced only when there is too much hyperextension in the lumbar spine. This results when the patient is not properly using the gluteal muscles to stabilize the pelvis and back. Holding the bridged position helps to isolate trunk musculature in a different fashion than the dead bug exercises.

   All exercises using the green ball begin with the patient simply balancing on the ball, trying to get the feel and the appropriate proprioceptive input to maintain good balance. Then, to begin the exercises, the ball is positioned at about the midback. The patient's knees should be at 90 degrees, the chin tucked, head up, and both feet on the ground. Have the patient bridge by bringing the pelvis up, locked in the neutral position. Have the patient maintain that position, then relax.

   Level I: Raise the hips as far off the floor as possible without losing the painfree, neutral position, and hold for a count of 10. Do two sets of 10 repetitions.

   Level II: Do 20 repetitions with weights placed on the hips.

   Level III: While maintaining the neutral position, raise the hips from the floor, extend one leg, and hold for a count of 10. Do three sets of 20 repetitions with each leg. Follow by repeating the level II exercise. Then do 10 repetitions on the green ball.

   Level IV: Do four sets of 20 repetitions of the single-leg extensions. Do 10 repetitions on the green ball with weights placed on the hips.

   Level V: While bridging on the green ball with weights on the hips, alternately extend the legs for a count of 10. Do five sets of 20 repetitions.

4. **Prone exercises.** Begin the prone exercises with a cushion under the stomach for patients who suffer extreme pain with hyperextension. Again, the idea is to hold the back in a neutral position, not hyperextended. Alternating arm and leg extensions requires good trunk control to prevent hyperextension.

   Level I: The patient extends the arms and legs while rigidly holding the trunk musculature in a neutral, pain-free position. Hold for a count of 10. Then lift one arm off the ground and extend it while lifting the opposite leg off the ground and extending it. Hold for a count of 10. Relax, then repeat with the other arm and leg. Do one set of 10 repetitions.

   Level II: Do two sets of 20 repetitions.

   Level III: Repeat the level II exercise. Then do two sets of 10 repetitions of each of the following exercises with the abdomen resting on the green ball:

   1. *Swim:* Do an Australian crawl swimming motion with extended arms.
   2. *Superman:* Begin with the arms extended to the side, but with the elbows bent at 90 degrees. Simultaneously extend the elbows while extending the knees to roll forward. Hold the forward position, then roll back.

   Level IV: Do 10 sets of 20 repetitions of the Swim and Superman exercises, using arm weights with the Superman. Then do 10 sets of 20 repetitions of the following exercises:

   1. *Prayer:* Kneel on the floor with forearms on the ball. With the spine in the neutral muscle-control position, straighten the knees and rock forward, then rock back. Do not permit any lumbar motion.
   2. *Push-ups:* Starting from the level I position, extend the legs with the toes off the ground. Slowly lower the upper body, maintaining the neutral position, until the hands touch the floor. Return to the starting position.
   3. *Walkouts:* With feet apart, toes on the floor in the pushup position, and arms flexed at the shoulder and down to the floor, roll forward slowly. Extend the trunk out into mid-air while maintain tight trunk control. Hold for 10 sec before rolling back to the starting position.

Level V: Four sets of 20 repetitions of all the exercises in this group, all done with weights and with a body blade across the back. The patient must keep the blade from tipping or bending in any direction while maintaining good trunk control.

5. **Quadrupeds.** Down on all fours might appear to be an unusual position for learning how to stabilize the trunk, but this is really one of the best positions for relaxing the trunk muscles. Therefore, it is a good position for the patient to practice tightening the trunk musculature.

Level I: The patient, on all fours, tightens the trunk muscles and holds the spine in the neutral, painfree position for a count of 10 before relaxing. Once comfortable with this position, the patient should extend one arm and hold for 5 sec. Relax. Then the other arm and each leg in turn. Do one set of 10 repetitions.

Level II: As above, but extend one arm and one leg simultaneously and hold. Do two sets of 10 repetitions.

Level III: Same as level II, but using weights on legs and arms and doing three sets of 20 repetitions.

Level IV: Same as level II, but using weights and a body blade and holding the extended position for 10 sec instead of 5.

Level V: Same as level IV, but doing three sets of 20 repetitions while holding the extended position for 15 sec rather than 10 sec.

6. **Wall slides.** The patient rolls down a green exercise ball positioned between his or her back and the wall. An easy exercise that can be begun in the immediate postoperative period, it begins with a gentle flexion of the knees and with no real lower extremity or back strain. Quadriceps strength, once developed, indicates the patient's capacity to use his or her legs, rather than the back, for bending and lifting; patients with weak quads lock their knees and bend at the waist, which is exactly the opposite of what we want a back pain patient to do.

Level I: Begin with a slight knee flexion to go into a partial squat and hold for 10 sec. Gradually increase the distance traveled, working toward attaining a 90-degree bend in the legs and hips and a full squatting position.

Level II: Slide into a 90/90 position (90-degree of hip and knee flexion) and hold for 20 sec. Do 10 repetitions.

Level III: Same as level II, but hold for 30 sec. Follow with 10 lunges. These are done standing, striding forward with one foot from a neutral position, holding for three seconds, then returning to the neutral position. Do 10 repetitions with each leg.

Level IV: Hold the 90/90 wall slide position for 15 sec while holding weights. Follow with lunges using weights.

Level V: Same as level IV, but hold the weights at fully extended arm's length for the wall slides. When doing the lunges, again use the weights and hold the forward position for one minute.

7. **Ball exercises.** These exercises are all begun with the patient sitting on the ball, which has been placed in the small of the back. Chest and stomach are kept tight, and the feet stay on the floor. The patient should be able to balance on the ball before proceeding on through the various levels.

Level I: While balanced on the ball, keeping the chin tucked in to avoid straining the neck, roll back on the ball by straightening the legs. Then return.

Level II: Perform the level I exercise while alternately flexing the shoulders, lifting alternate arms over the head and holding them for a short count when fully extended. Then, with the ball under the patient's low back, arms folded across the chest, knees bent, and feet flat on the floor, do 20 sit-ups. Keep the pelvis stabilized and level using the abdominal and buttock muscles. Lift the shoulder blades and upper back while keeping the lower back in a neutral position and walking backward, pushing the ball. Bend at the waist to the maximum point that can be maintained while keeping the trunk rigid, hold for a count of 4 to 8, and return.

Level III: Do 20 sit-ups, as in the level II exercise. Then, with hands locked behind the neck, do 20 more sit-ups touching the left arm to the right knee and 20 more with the right arm touching the left knee.

Level IV: Adding weights, do three sets of 20 repetitions of the level III exercise.

Level V: Resistive exercises are done with the aid of a trainer or therapist holding one end of a baton or towel and pulling against the patient, who is seated on the ball and holding the other end. At maximum resistance, hold for a count of 10. Resistance can be provided alternately across the chest, to the side, or over the head with a baton, weighted stick, or with pulleys. At this time, the body blade may also be used.

8. **Aerobics.** Aerobic conditioning is a vital part of the program. The aerobically conditioned athlete is less likely to sustain injury than a deconditioned athlete, including injury to the trunk musculature supporting the axial skeleton. The problem with concentrating on just one type of aerobic exercise is that it can produce a tendinitis or strain due to constant activity in one particular body position. Good aerobic exercise, therefore, incorporates cross training.

   Level I: Walking in a swimming pool in chest- to neck-deep water is a conditioning method that provides the aerobic benefits of running without the jarring that is typical of dry land running. The water's buoyancy reduces the effects of gravity on the body, and the water provides gentle resistance to motion in any direction. We start patients walking in water as early as 3 weeks postoperatively. When the patient can comfortably walk on dry land, begin that activity too. Continue both of these activities at least through level II.

   Level II: Add 10 min on an exercycle to the activities of level I. The bent-forward position assumed on the exercycle can be very stabilizing. The seat should be set low enough that the feet are not reaching for the pedals at any point. When the patient has to reach for the pedals, it causes the pelvis to rock on the seat.

   Level III: If the patient knows how, start him or her swimming; if not, explain to the patient that swimming can be excellent exercise for someone willing to take lessons and do it properly. Be aware that a poor swimmer flailing about in the water is not engaging in productive exercise. Also, if the patient has the balance and coordination to handle a Nordic Trac, begin that activity, too.

   Level IV: The patient should spend 45 minutes on a climbing or stepping machine. Ensure that the patient is climbing with a very narrow step; this will provide the necessary aerobic conditioning without tilting the pelvis, as happens when the height of the step is too steep. Also have the patient skip rope. The shorter the rope, the better. This is an excellent technique for building trunk strength because the correct posture required for skipping rope—the back locked in a neutral position, leaning into a slightly bent-forward flexion position—can produce very tight trunk control while providing aerobic conditioning.

   Level V: Run for 1 hr. Good technique is as vital to running as to any other athletic exercise. If good posture is not maintained, it can lead to the development of contractures and weaknesses in isolated areas that are not being used.

Appendix 6. **PHYSICAL EXAMINATION–SPECIAL TESTS**

Marc R. Safran

The tests shown here are special tests for particular joints. The examinations shown here are not meant to supplant a complete history or physical examination. Joint motion and neurologic and muscle strength testing should still be performed and are well detailed in other texts (Magee, Hoppenfeld). When examining an injured athlete, examine the normal or unaffected limb, joint, or extremity first before proceeding with the injured side.

I. Wrist

A. **Shuck Test** (Fig. 1). Is a provocative maneuver that translates the lunate and triquetrum in opposite directions in the sagittal plane. The examiner faces the patient and grasps their wrist in slight flexion. The pisiform and triquetrum are grasped between the examiner's thumb and index finger with one hand and the lunate is grasped between the contralateral thumb and index finger. The examiner moves the different hands in opposite directions placing a shearing force at the lunotriquetral joint. Patients with lunotriquetral instability will have increased pain with this test.

B. **Watson's Maneuver** (Fig. 2). The patient is seated and their elbow rests on their lap. The forearm is pronated and the hand is brought into ulnar deviation. Pressure is applied to the distal pole of the scaphoid (Fig. 2A). The hand is then radially deviated while pressure is maintained on the distal pole of the scaphoid (Fig. 2B). This attempts to prevent the normal palmarflexion of the scaphoid with radial deviation. When the scaphoid is unstable, the proximal pole is subluxed dorsally with the maneuver, producing pain.

II. Elbow

A. **Elbow flexion test** (Fig. 3). The subject maximally flexes both elbows with the wrists in full extension. The subject holds this position for 3 min. This test is positive, indicating cubital tunnel syndrome, if symptoms of pain, numbness, and paresthesias occur in the distribution of the ulnar nerve (ulnar forearm, hand, and little and ring fingers).

B. **Valgus stress test** (Fig. 4). With the subject seated, the hand and wrist of the patient is held securely between the examiner's elbow, proximal forearm and body. The elbow must be flexed beyond 25 degrees. The examiner simultaneously palpates the ulnar collateral ligament (MCL) with the long finger of their free arm while varus and valgus stress are applied. Joint opening and end point laxity are assessed. (Reproduced with permission from Safran, et al. Chronic instability of the elbow. In: Peimer C, ed. *Surgery of the hand and upper extremity.* New York: McGraw Hill, 1996.)

C. **Milking maneuver** (Fig. 5). This test provides a valgus stress to the elbow to assess for valgus instability due to the ulnar collateral ligament. The patient may be seated or standing with the affected elbow flexed beyond 90 degrees. The patient's opposite hand is placed under the affected elbow to grasp the affected thumb, thereby exerting a valgus stress to the elbow. The ulnar collateral ligament and medial elbow joint space is palpated by the examiner for tenderness and joint line opening during this maneuver. (Reproduced with permission from Safran, et al. Chronic instability of the elbow. In: Peimer C, ed. *Surgery of the Hand and Upper Extremity.* New York: McGraw Hill, 1996.)

D. **Pivot shift test of the elbow** (Fig. 6). This test is utilized to assess for functional competence of the lateral ulnar collateral ligament (LUCL). Posterolateral rotatory instability of the elbow results from LUCL dysfunction. The patient lies supine on the examining table, the shoulder is flexed to 90 degrees and the examination is performed from the head of the table. The

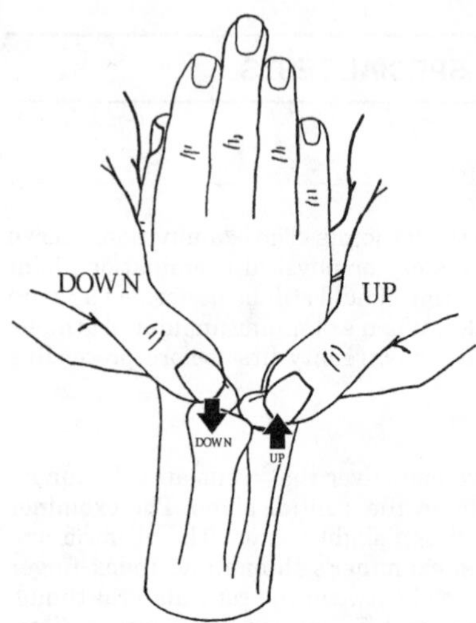

Fig. 1. Shuck Test

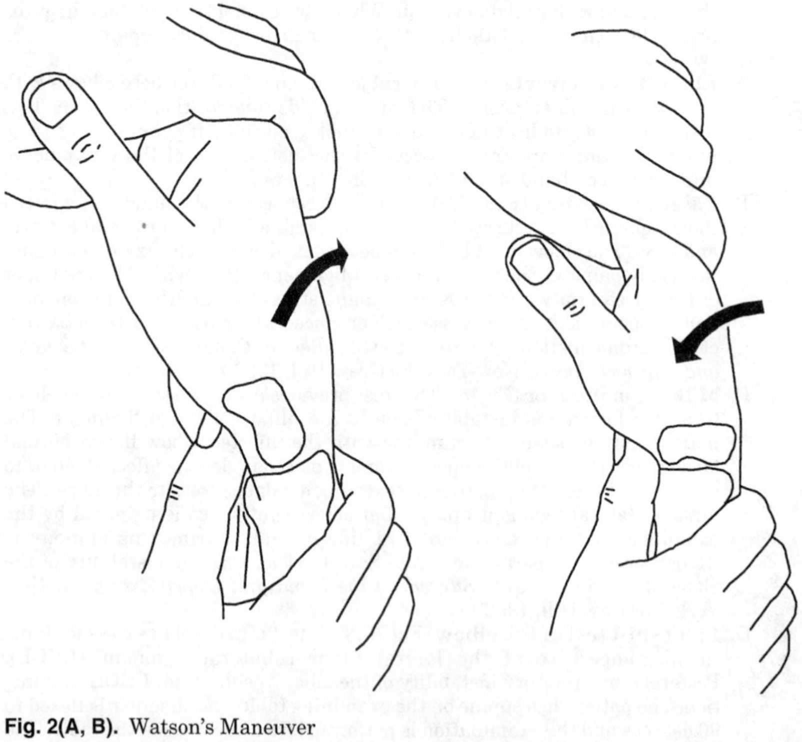

Fig. 2(A, B). Watson's Maneuver

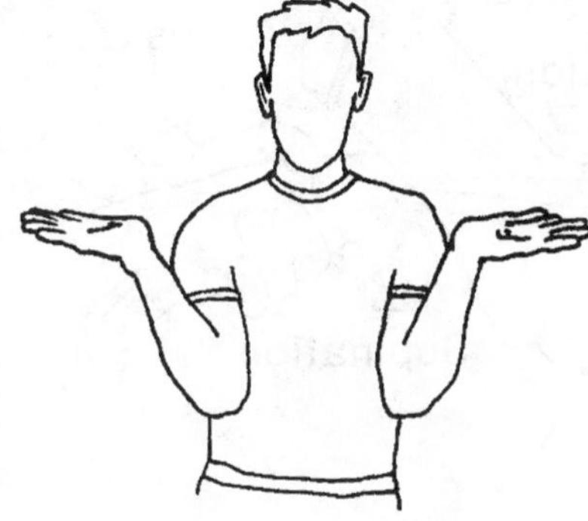

Fig. 3. Elbow Flexion Test.

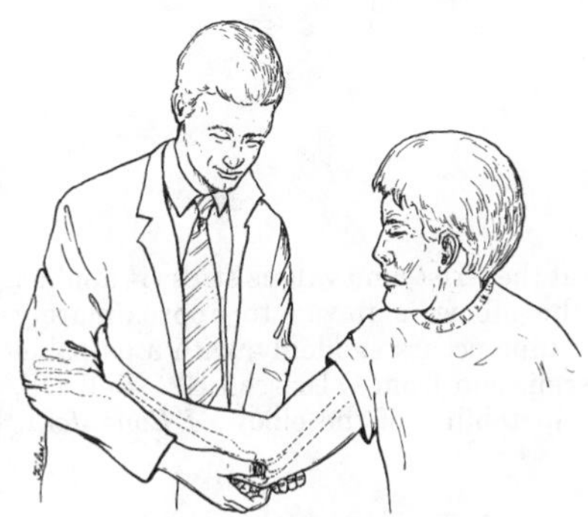

Fig. 4. Valgus Stress Test for the Elbow.

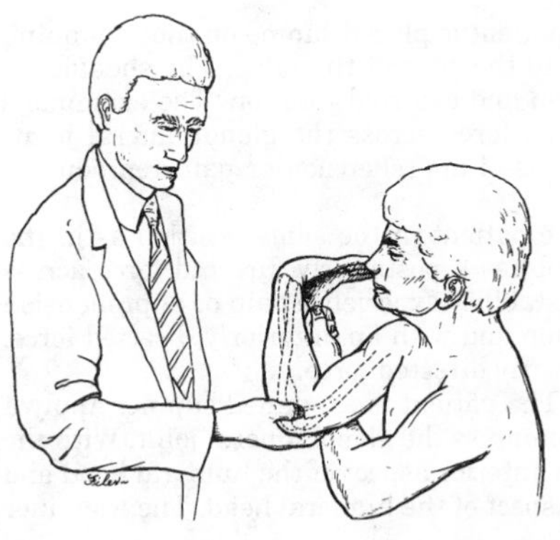

Fig. 5. Milking Maneuver.

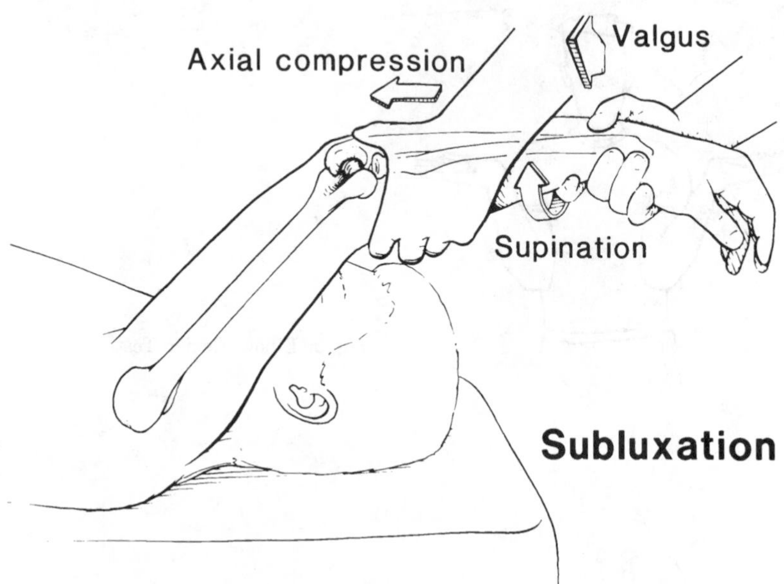

Fig. 6. Pivot Shift Test of the Elbow.

elbow is supinated with a mild force at the wrist, and valgus stress is applied to the elbow during flexion. As the elbow is flexed to approximately 40 degrees or more, reduction of the ulna occurs suddenly, with a palpable visible clunk. (Reproduced with permission from O'Driscoll SW, Bell DF, Morrey BF. Posterolateral rotatory instability of the elbow. *J Bone Joint Surg* 1991; 73A: 440–446.)

III. Shoulder

A. **Adduction load and shift test** (Fig. 7). The patient is seated and the examiner located just beside and behind the side to be examined. The examiner places the hand over the shoulder and scapula to stabilize the limb girdle and then, with the opposite hand, grasps the humeral head. The head is loaded (pushed lightly toward the glenoid) and then both an anterior and posterior stress is applied, noting the amount of translation. (Reproduced with permission from Rockwood CA Jr, Matsen FA III. *The shoulder.* Philadelphia: WB Saunders, 1990.)

B. **Apprehension test** (Fig. 8). The patient is placed supine on the examining table and the shoulder is brought to the edge of the table. The shoulder is then placed in 90 degrees abduction and external rotation. The examiner's hand creates an anteriorly directed force across the glenohumeral joint. During this maneuver, look for signs of apprehension or pain reproducing the patient's symptoms.

C. **Relocation test** (Fig. 9). With the patient in the same position as in the apprehension test, the examiner places a posteriorly directed force across the joint. Patients with anterior instability experience pain or apprehension with abduction and external rotation and with an anteriorly directed force. This pain disappears with a posteriorly directed force.

D. **Abduction load and shift test.** The patient is examined supine. Apply a force in line with the humerus to compress the glenohumeral joint. With the other hand place the thumb on the anterior aspect of the humeral head and the other fingers on the posterior aspect of the humeral head. The examiner

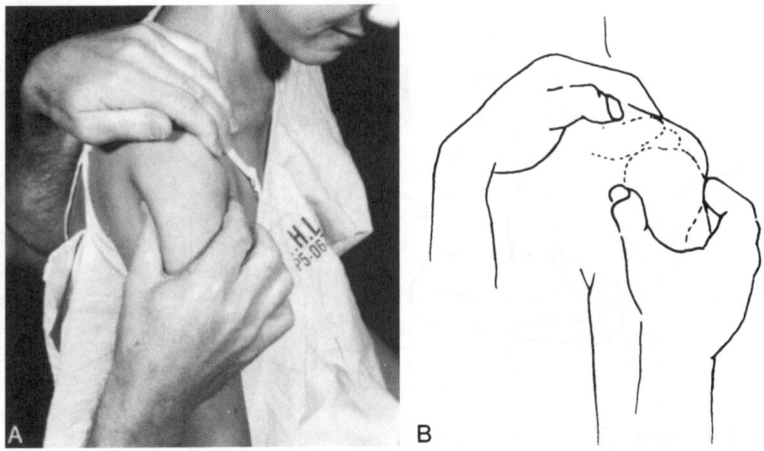

Fig. 7. Adduction Load and Shift Test of the Shoulder.

then feels the extent of anteroposterior motion in the glenohumeral joint by placing anterior and posteriorly direct forces alternately. A soft clunk may be sensed as the humeral head rides over the labrum and glenoid anteriorly or posteriorly. Gentleness when performing this maneuver will avoid pain and allow the patient to relax while performing this maneuver. This gives the examiner an idea of joint laxity, and side-to-side differences in glenohumeral laxity.

E. **Sulcus sign** (Fig. 10). The patient is seated with the arm to the side. The examiner grasps the elbow and applies inferior (downward) traction. The

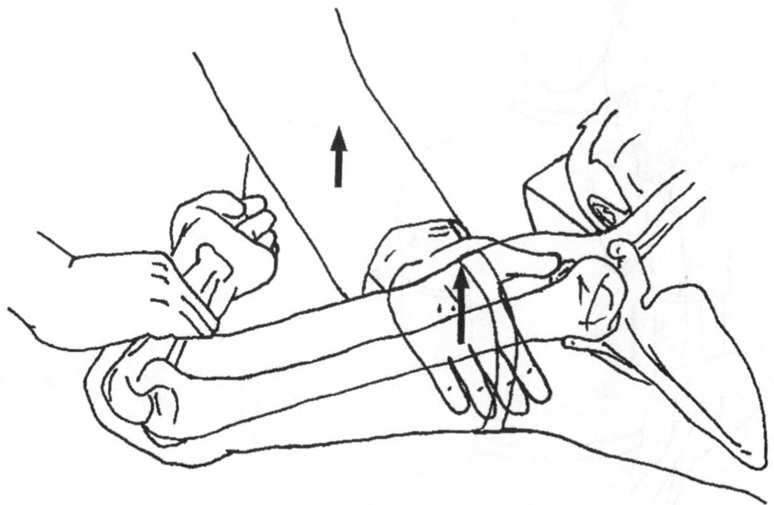

Fig. 8. Apprehension Test of the Shoulder.

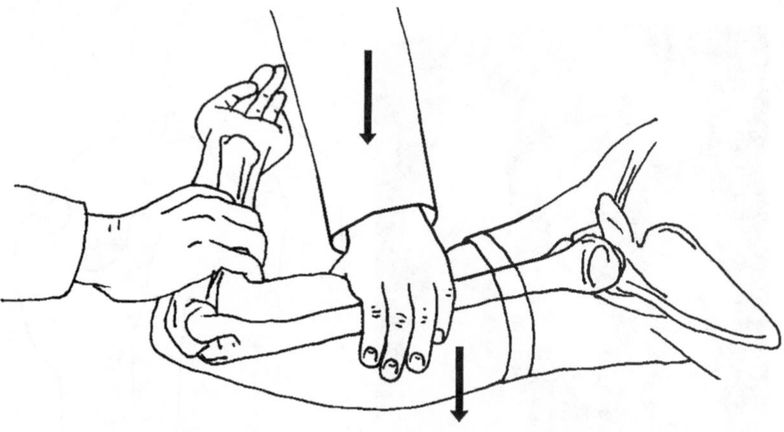

Fig. 9. Relocation Test of the Shoulder.

area adjacent to the acromion is observed and dimpling of the skin may indicate inferior laxity. The acromion and then the space underneath it is palpated to gain an impression of the amount of inferior humeral translation.

F. **Posterior stress test** (Fig. 11). This test is performed by stabilizing the medial border of the scapula with the hand as the patient is sitting up or having the patient lie down with the shoulder flexed 90 degrees with adduction and internal rotation. The examiner's other hand is then used to load

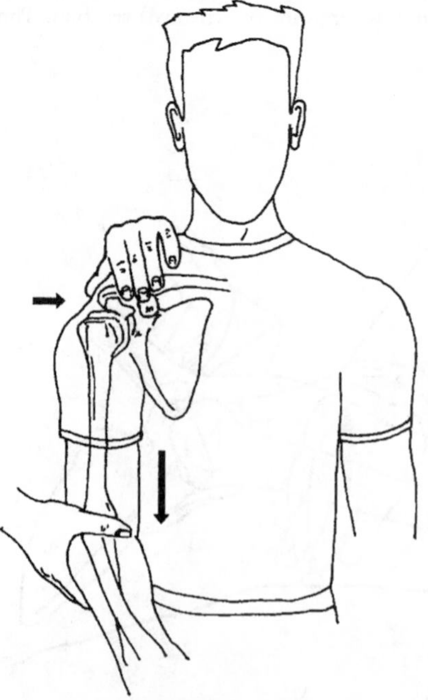

Fig. 10. Sulcus Sign.

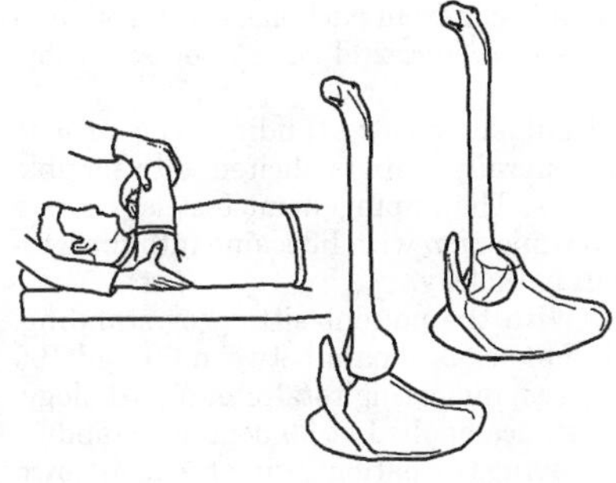

Fig. 11. Posterior Stress Test.

the humerus axially and posteriorly. A positive test, indicative of posterior shoulder instability, is confirmed if the patient has a palpable luxation of the humeral head over the posterior glenoid rim that reproduces his or her pain.

G. **Supraspinatus (empty the can) test** (Fig. 12). With the patient sitting or standing, the shoulder is abducted to 90 degrees and forward flexed 30 degrees with the athlete's thumbs pointing toward the floor (i.e., forearm internally rotated/ pronated). This position is maintained against manual resistance by the examiner. This test may be noted as positive for eliciting pain only or for pain and weakness. This test isolates the supraspinatus musculotendinous unit for testing. (Reproduced with permission from Nicholas JA, Hershman EB, eds. *The upper extremity in sports medicine,* 2nd ed. St Louis: Mosby, 1995.)

H. **Hawkin's sign** (Fig. 13). With the patient sitting or standing, the arm is passively brought into 90 degrees of forward elevation and then internally rotated. Pain is produced in this maneuver due to impingement of the supraspinatus tendon between the greater tuberosity and the coracoacromial ligament complex. It may also indicate coracoid impingement if the

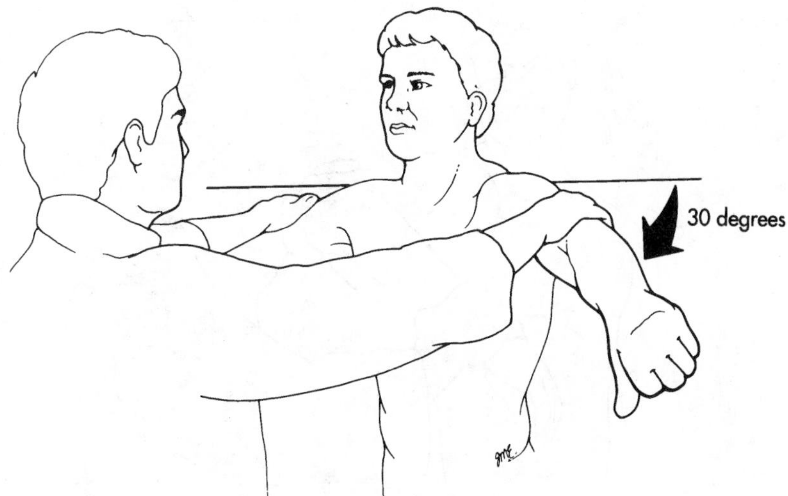

Fig. 12. Supraspinatus (empty the can) Test.

pain is anterior. (Reproduced with permission from Nicholas JA, Hershman EB, eds. *The upper extremity in sports medicine,* 2nd ed. St Louis: Mosby, 1995.)

I. **Impingement sign.** With the patient sitting or standing, the arm is brought into full forward elevation. Generally, pain is elicited with forcible forward elevation at 160 to 180 degrees. The impingement test is positive when this pain is then eliminated after injection with lidocaine into the subacromial space, indicating rotator cuff pathology.

J. **Painful arc (or abduction sign).** With the patient sitting or standing, abduction of the arm in the coronal plane causes pain between 60 and 100 degrees, usually maximally at 90 degrees, indicating rotator cuff pathology. This pain is often increased with resistance applied at 90 degrees of abduction. Another variation of this test is having the patient bring the arm down from full forward elevation. As the arm comes down in the 70- to 120-degree arc, the patient will note pain in the shoulder.

K. **Adduction sign.** With the athlete sitting or standing, the arm is brought into 90 degrees of forward elevation. The arm is then forcefully adducted across the body. Pain on the top of the shoulder [in the area of the acromioclavicular (AC) joint] is indicative of AC joint pathology, such as AC arthritis or distal clavicular osteolysis. Pain in the posterior shoulder may be indicative of posterior capsular tightness.

L. **Lift-off sign.** With the patient standing, the dorsum of the hand is brought to the L5-S1 area of the lower back. The patient is then asked to actively lift that the hand from the back with that same arm. Weakness or inability to lift the arm from the back in the face of full shoulder motion is indicative of subscapularis rupture or weakness.

M. **Speed's test.** With the patient standing or sitting, the patient brings the arm into 90 degrees of forward elevation, elbow fully extended and palm up. The patient resists a downward force by the examiner on the hand. Pain in the bicipital groove region of the anterior shoulder may indicate bicipital tendinitis or possibly SLAP (superior labrum, anterior and posterior) lesion.

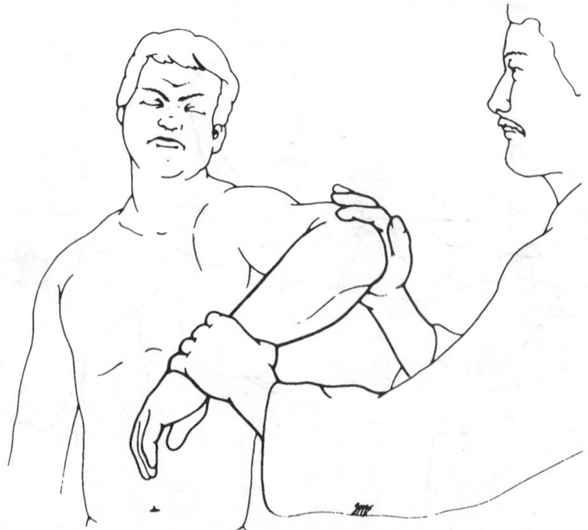

Fig. 13. Hawkin's Sign.

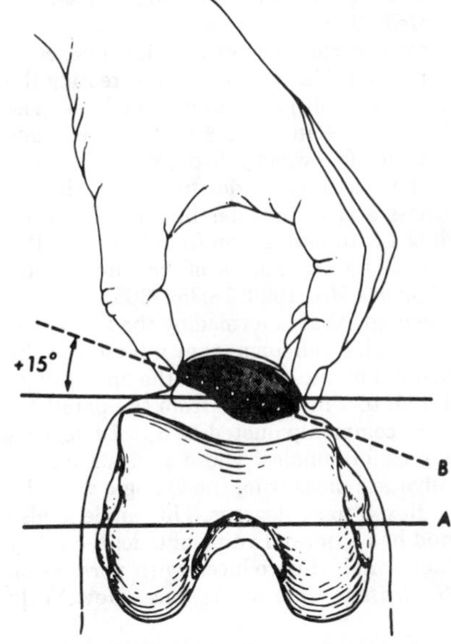

Fig. 14. Passive Patellar Tilt.

N. **Yergason's test.** The patient is standing or sitting facing the examiner with arm at the side (0° adduction) and elbow flexed. The patient tries to flex the elbow and supinate the wrist against the examiner's resistance. Pain in the anterior shoulder may indicate biceps tendinitis. Snapping in the anterior shoulder while performing this test with external rotation of the shoulder may indicate biceps instability.

IV. Knee

A. **Passive patellar tilt test** (Fig. 14). Is performed with the subject in the supine position, knee extended and quadriceps relaxed. Standing at the foot of the examination table, the examiner lifts the lateral edge of the patella from the lateral femoral condyle. The patella should remaining the trochlea and not be allowed to sublux laterally (this could affect the measurement). A tilt less than neutral (0 degrees) to the horizontal implies lateral retinacular tightness may exist. (Reproduced with permission from Kolowich PA, Paulos

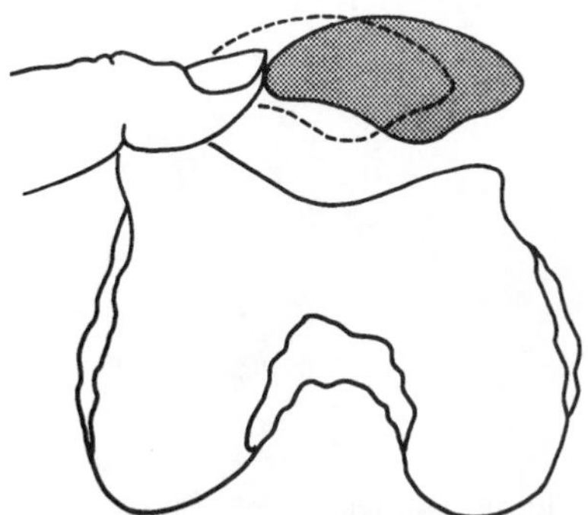

Fig. 15. Patellar Glide Test.

LE, Rosenberg TD, Farnsworth S: Lateral release of the patella: indications and contraindications. *Am J Sports Med* 1990; 18:359–365.)

B. **Patellar glide test** (Fig. 15). This test is performed with the knee flexed to 20 to 30 degrees and the quadriceps relaxed. This can be done by resting the knee over the examiner's thigh or with a small pillow under the knee. The patella is divided into longitudinal quadrants and then an attempt is made to displace the patella in a medial direction followed by displacement in a lateral direction under the guidance of the examiner's index finger and thumb. This determines parapatellar tightness and retinacular integrity laterally and medially, respectively. (Reproduced with permission from Kolowich PA, Paulos LE, Rosenberg TD, Farnsworth S. Lateral release of the patella: indications and contraindications. *Am J Sports Med* 1990; 18:359–365.)

C. **Q angle** (Fig. 16). The Q angle is the angle that is formed by the line of the pull of the quadriceps and that of the patellar tendon as they intersect at the patella. Clinically, this angle is measured by the angle from the anterosuperior iliac spine to the patella in relation to a line drawn from the patella to the tibial tubercle. Normal figures are commonly quoted as 8 to 10 degrees for males and approximately 15 degrees for females. These angles are measured in extension. Some authors advocate measuring the Q angle with the quadriceps contracted and the knee flexed to 90 degrees. This angle is also called the "tubercle sulcus angle" and has a normal value of 0 degrees. Any value greater than 10 degrees is abnormal. (Reproduced with permission from Tria AJ Jr, Klein KS. *An illustrated guide to the knee.* New York: Churchill-Livingstone, 1992.)

D. **Varus stress test** (Fig. 17). With the patient supine, the knee is placed in 20 to 30 degrees of flexion and neutral axial rotation. With one hand, the examiner stabilizes the femur and palpates the lateral joint line. With the other hand on the distal tibia, the examiner first exerts an axial load to place the joint surfaces in contact; this is the test starting position. The leg is then adducted while constraining axial rotation. The lateral joint space opening, as well as stiffness of the motion limit (end point) is estimated. If the test is

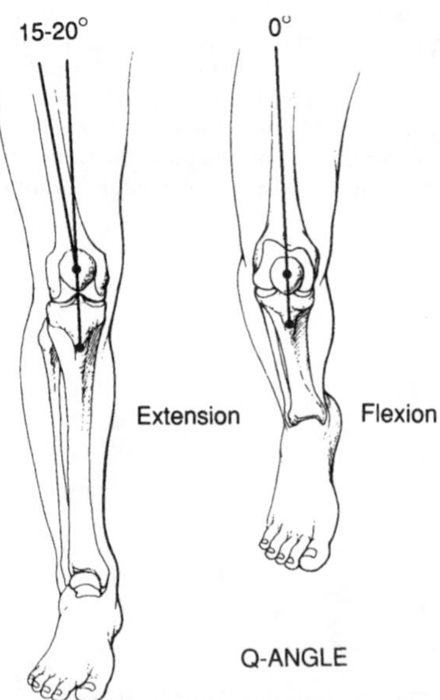

Fig. 16. Q-Angle

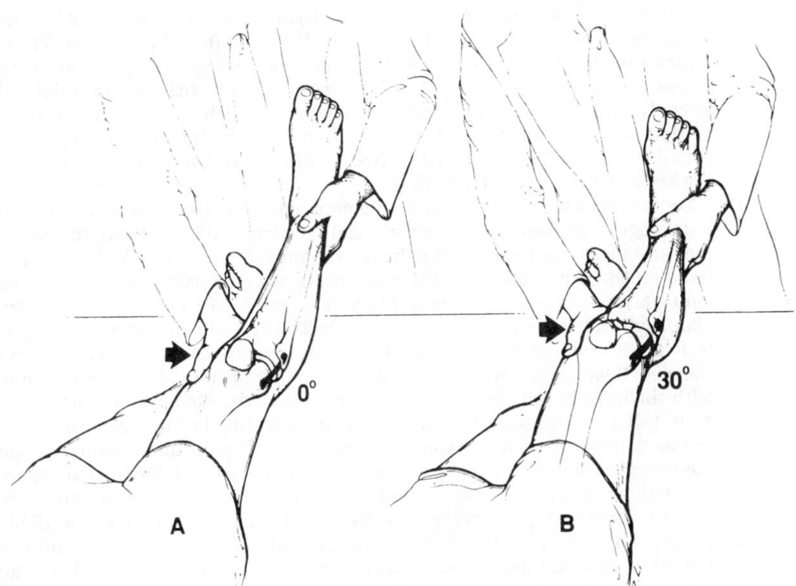

Fig. 17. Varus Stress Test of the Knee in Extension (A) and (B) 30° of Flexion.

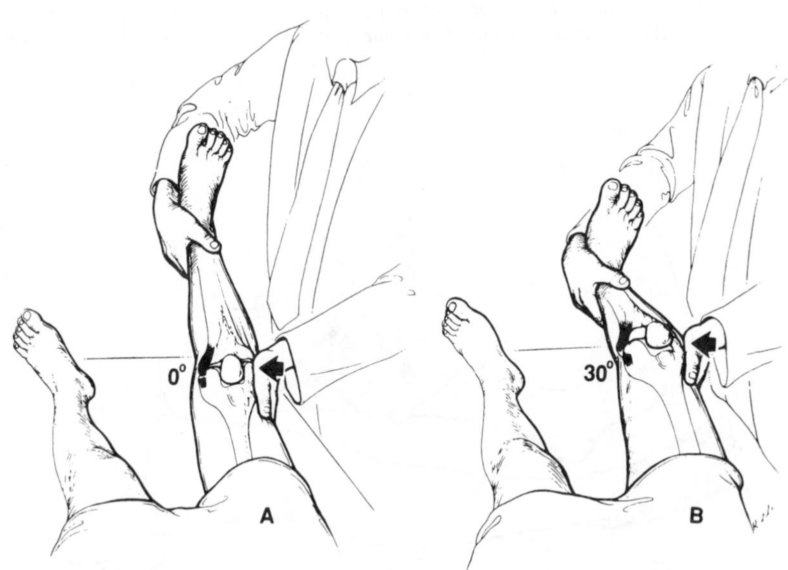

Fig. 18. Valgus Stress Test of the Knee in (A) Extension and (B) 30° of Flexion.

positive (increased opening of the lateral joint line as compared with the uninjured side), the test is repeated with the knee in full extension. These injuries to the Lateral Collateral Ligament (LC) are graded as I, pain with stress testing but no increased opening as compared with the contralateral knee; II, pain and opening of the lateral joint line with an end point to stress testing; and III, lateral joint opening with no endpoint. (Reproduced with permission from Tria AJ Jr, Klein KS. *An illustrated Guide to the knee.* New York: Churchill-Livingstone, 1992.)

E. **Valgus stress test** (Fig. 18). With the patient supine, the knee is placed in 20 to 30 degrees of flexion and neutral axial rotation. With one hand, the examiner stabilizes the femur and palpates the medial joint line. With the other hand on the distal tibia, the examiner first exerts an axial load to place the joint surfaces in contact; this is the test starting position. The leg is then abducted while constraining axial rotation. The medial joint space opening, as well as the endpoint is estimated. If the test is positive (increased opening of the medial joint line as compared with the uninjured side), the test is repeated with the knee in full extension. These injuries to the Medial Collateral Ligament (MCL) are graded as I, pain with stress testing but no increased opening as compared with the contralateral knee; II, pain and opening of the medial joint line with an end point to stress testing; and III, medial joint opening with no end point. (Reproduced with permission from Tria AJ Jr, Klein KS. *An illustrated guide to the knee.* New York: Churchill-Livingstone, 1992.)

F. **Lachman test** (Fig. 19). The patient is examined supine with the knee placed in 20 to 30 degrees of flexion. A small support under the thigh can provide this flexion angle. The clinician stabilizes the femur with one hand and applies an anterior displacement force to the proximal calf with enhancing or restraining axial rotation. The examiner senses the tibial displacement and the firmness of the displacement limit (end point). If both are normal, the Lachman test is negative. If either one is pathologic, then the Lachman test is positive suggesting injury of the Anterior Cruciate Ligament (ACL). (Reproduced with permission from Tria AJ Jr, Klein KS. *An illustrated guide to the knee.* New York: Churchill-Livingstone, 1992.)

G. **Pivot shift** (Fig. 20). This test has many variations described by many authors. The test produces anterior subluxation and internal axial rotation in early flexion as a result of anterior cruciate ligament (ACL) tear. The pos-

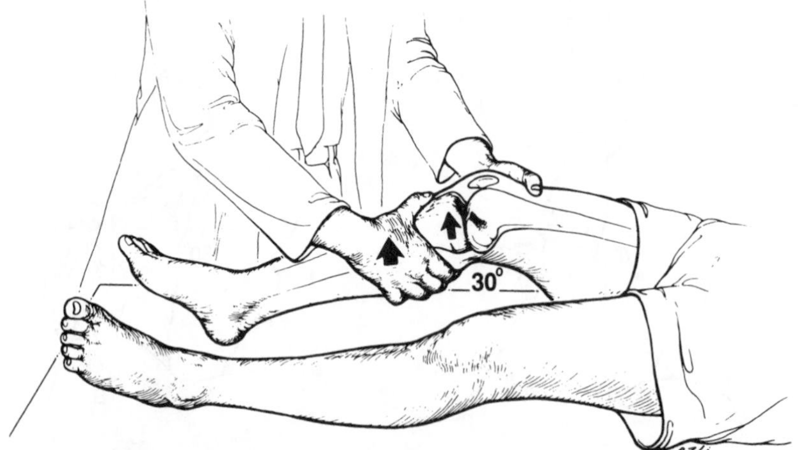

Fig. 19. Lachman Test.

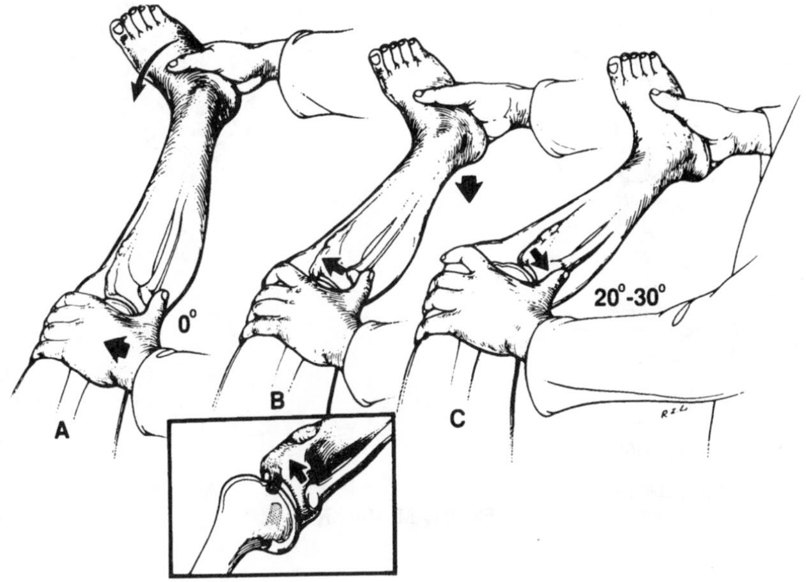

Fig. 20. Pivot Shift Test of the Knee.

terior pull of the iliotibial tract reduces the tibia at 20 to 40 degrees of flexion. With the patient supine, the knee is extended and the foot is held with internal rotation, allowing the femur to sag posteriorly. A valgus stress is applied to the lateral knee while flexing the knee. As flexion is commenced, the lateral tibia comes forward due to tightening of the iliotibial tract and then reduces with further flexion. It is the relocation event that is graded as 0 (absent), 1 + (slight slip), 2+ (moderate slip), or 3+ (momentary locking). (Reproduced with permission from Tria AJ Jr, Klein KS. *An illustrated guide to the knee.* New York: Churchill-Livingstone, 1992.)

H. **McMurray test** (Fig. 21). With the patient supine and the hip flexed to 90 degrees and the knee flexed fully, the examiner places one hand on the knee and the other on the patient's ipsilateral foot. By maneuvering the foot into abduction-adduction and external rotation-internal rotation, the examiner palpates the joint line for a click. Medially, this is demonstrated with external tibial rotation and varus stress as the knee is extended from a flexed position. Laterally, it is demonstrated with the tibia in internal rotation and valgus stress as the knee is extended. If positive, entrapment of the torn meniscus is demonstrated by a pop or click that is felt by the fingers, which are placed on the appropriate joint line. It has been shown that the posterior horn of the meniscus is torn when this maneuver yields these positive signs with the knee at full flexion or at approximately 90 degrees of flexion. The later in extension the click is identified, the more anterior the tear. (Reproduced with permission from Tria AJ Jr, Klein KS. *An illustrated guide to the knee.* New York: Churchill-Livingstone, 1992.)

I. **Posterior drawer** (Fig. 22). With the patient supine, the the knee is flexed 90 degrees and the hip flexed 45 degrees with the foot flat on the examining table or field and the extremity relaxed. The resting position of the femorotibial joint is noted. Usually, the anterior aspect of the medial tibial plateau is 10 mm anterior to the medial femoral condyle. If the tibia sags posteriorly (less than 10 mm in front of the femoral condyles), the tibia is

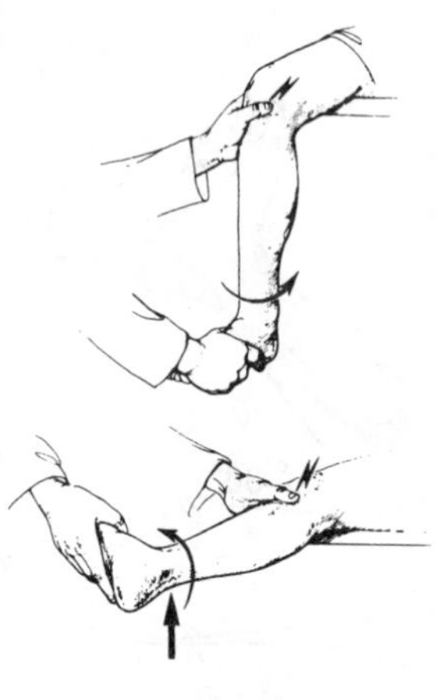
McMURRAY
A palpable click
is felt

Fig. 21. McMurray Test.

brought forward to its normal resting position. A posteriorly directed force is then applied to the proximal tibia and amount of posterior displacement is noted. The quality of the end point is also noted, but frequently a firm end point may be noted with significant posterior displacement. The amount of displacement is the important factor. In a grade I injury, the tibia is still anterior to the femoral condyles; grade II, the tibia is flush with the condyles; and grade III, the tibia plateau is posterior to the distal (anterior) aspect of the femoral condyles. (Reproduced with permission from Tria AJ Jr, Klein KS. *An illustrated guide to the knee.* New York: Churchill-Livingstone, 1992.)

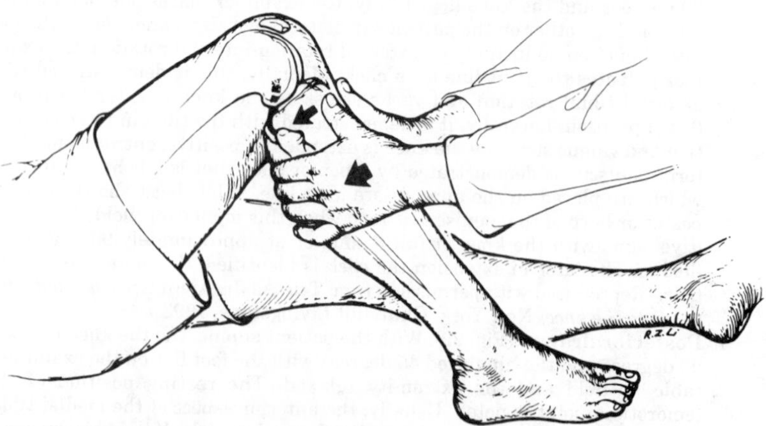

Fig. 22. Posterior Drawer Test of the Knee.

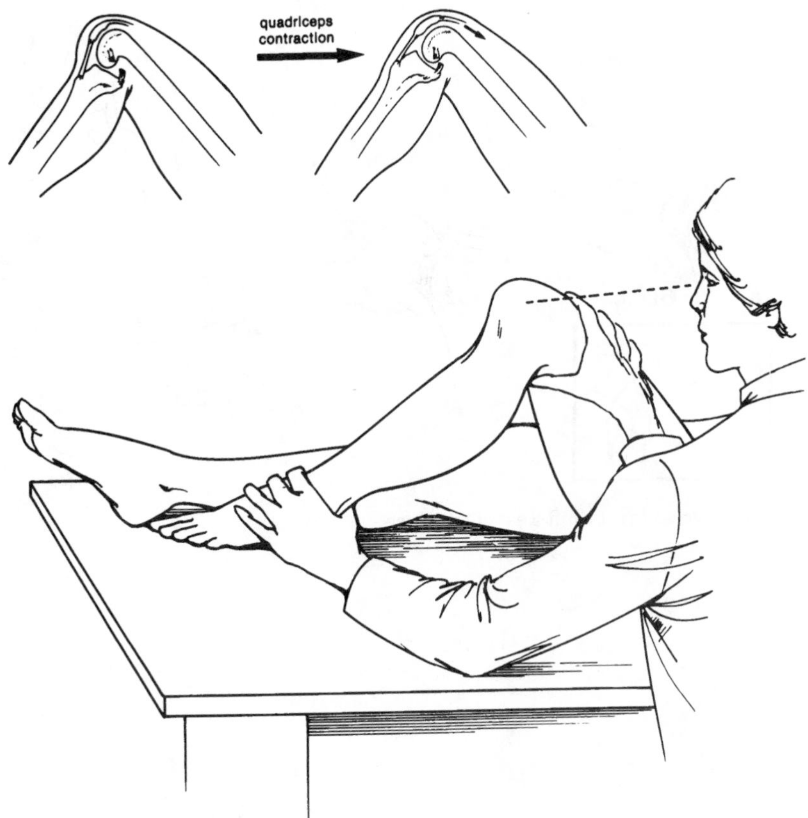

Fig. 23. Quadriceps Active Test.

J. **Quadriceps active test** (Fig. 23). With the patient laying supine and the knee flexed 90 degrees, the proximal tibia will sag posteriorly if the posterior cruciate ligament (PCL) is disrupted. The sag may be seen by looking at the knee in profile and palpated by feeling the femoral condylar-tibial step-off. This sag due to PCL disruption is confirmed by having the patient actively contract the quadriceps by trying to slide the foot down the table against some resistance. If a true sag exists, the proximal tibia will be pulled anteriorly, reducing the femoral condylar-tibial step-off. (Reproduced with permission from Daniel DM, Stone ML, Barnett P, Sachs R. Use of the quadriceps active test to diagnose posterior cruciate ligament disruption and measure posterior laxity of the knee. *J Bone Joint Surg* 1988; 70A:386–391.)

K. **Reverse pivot shift maneuver** (Fig. 24). The patient is supine and the limb is supported by the examiner's hand under the heel, thereby placing the knee in full extension and neutral axial rotation. With the examiner's other hand on the lateral aspect of the calf, a mild valgus stress is applied and the knee is flexed. In a positive test, indicative of injury to the posterolateral ligament complex, at about 20 to 30 degrees of flexion, the tibia will rotate externally; the lateral tibial plateau will displace posteriorly and will remain in this position during further flexion. When the knee is

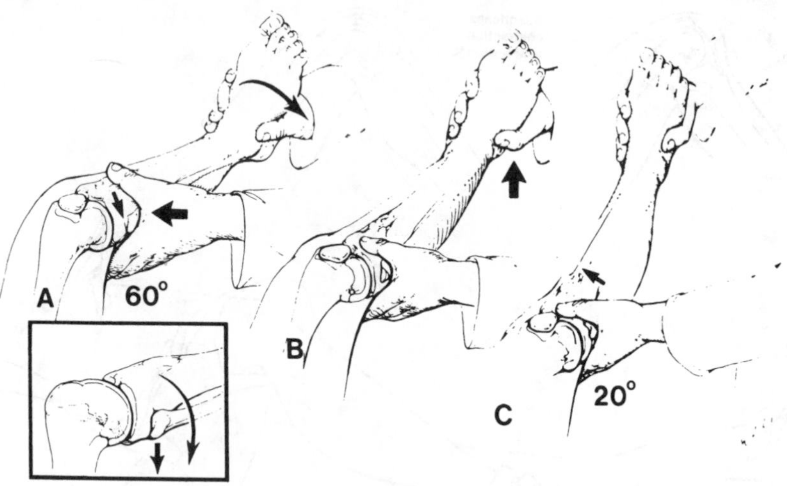

Fig. 24. Reverse Pivot Shift Test of the Knee.

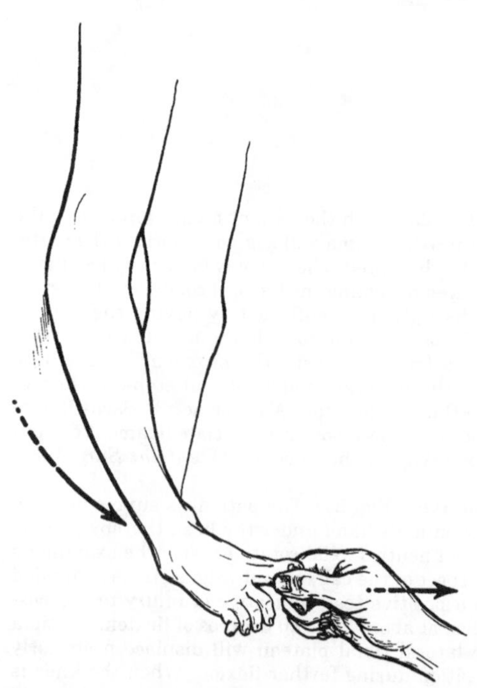

Fig. 25. External Rotation-Test Recurvatum

extended, the tibia will reduce. (thus, in the standard pivot shift, the tibia is anteriorly displaced in early flexion and then reduces between 20 and 40 degrees of flexion; while in the reverse pivot shift, the tibia is initially reduced and then the lateral tibial plateau displaces posteriorly at 20 to 30 degrees of flexion). (Reproduced with permission from Tria AJ Jr, Klein KS. *An illustrated guide to the knee.* New York: Churchill-Livingstone, 1992.)

L. **External rotation-recurvatum test** (Fig. 25). This test assesses for posterior capsular laxity by abnormal external rotation of the tibia on the femur associated with or in combination with excessive recurvatum. The test is performed with the patient supine. The knee is taken from 10 degrees of flexion to maximal extension. With increased external rotation and with an increase in recurvatum, a subtle varus deformity occurs. If the test finding is markedly positive, the PCL, lateral collateral ligament (LCL), and posterolateral corner must be torn. Hughston performs this test by simply lifting the leg of the patient by the great toe with the leg fully extended. In a positive finding, as the knee goes into hyperextension, the proximal tibia will shift into external rotation. (Reproduced with permission from Fu FH, Stone DA. *Sports injuries: mechanisms, prevention, treatment.* Philadelphia: Williams & Wilkins, 1994.)

M. **Dial test** (Fig. 26). This test can be performed supine, but the author prefers to perform this test with the patient prone. External rotation of the tibia on the femur at both 30 and 90 degrees of knee flexion is evaluated to test for injury to the posterolateral knee structures. The medial border of the foot in its neutral position is the reference point for external rotation. With the knee stabilized in the desired angle of knee flexion, the foot is externally rotated forcefully. The degree of external rotation of the medial border of the foot relative to the axis of the femur is measured and compared with the contralateral side. A difference of at least 10 degrees is significant. Increased external rotation at 30 degrees is indicative of injury to the posterolateral knee structures. Further increase in external rotation at 90 degrees is indicative of injury to the PCL and posterolateral corner. (Reproduced with permission from Veltri DM, Warren RF. Isolated and

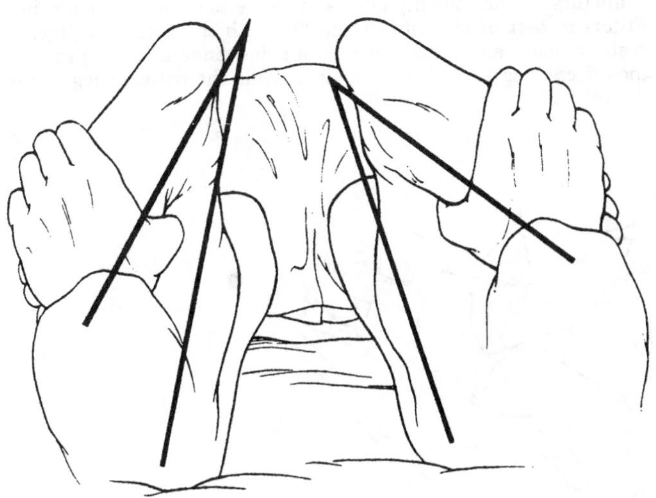

Fig. 26. Dial Test.

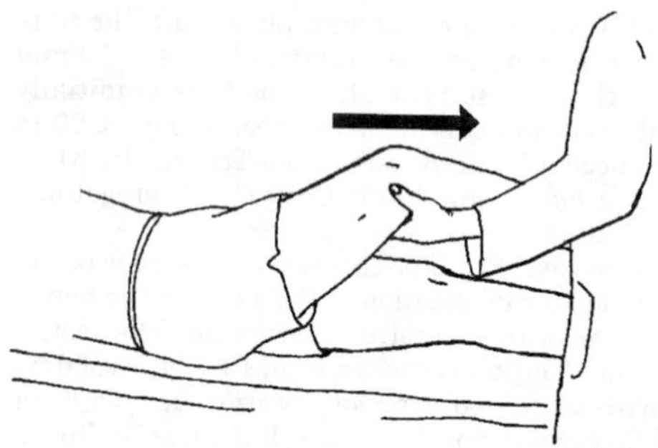

Fig. 27. Nobel Test.

combined posterior cruciate ligament injuries. *J Am Acad Orthop Surg* 1993; 1:67–75.)

N. **Nobel test** (Fig. 27). This test is for iliotibial band syndrome. With the patient supine, the thumb of the examiner is placed over the lateral femoral epicondyle and the patient actively flexes and extends the knee. Pain results and is usually maximal at 30 degrees of flexion at the level of the lateral femoral epicondyle.

O. **Garrick test.** With the patient supine, the knee is flexed 90 degrees, the leg is internally rotated, and the patient is asked to resist the examiner's attempt to externally rotate the tibia. This should elicit pain from the patient if the popliteus tendon is inflamed. Pain may also occur with passive stretching of the popliteus muscle by externally rotating the affected leg. This test assesses for popliteal tendinitis.

P. **Ober test** (Fig. 28). The patient lies on the side with the down hip and knee flexed; the examiner abducts the hip in neutral rotation and grabs the affected (up) knee and leg while extending the abducted hip and maintaining knee flexion and hip rotation. The examiner then allows the hip to adduct while maintaining hip extension and neutral rotation as well as knee flexion. If the knee does not drop below neutral (parallel to the ground), then the hip abductors are tight. Normal flexibility of the hip abductors is when the hip allows the knee to drop to or below neutral.

Q. **Fulcrum test of the tibia** (Fig. 29). With the patient supine, the leg is grabbed above and below the area of point tenderness. The examiner pulls the affected leg toward the examiner while the patient's leg is compressed

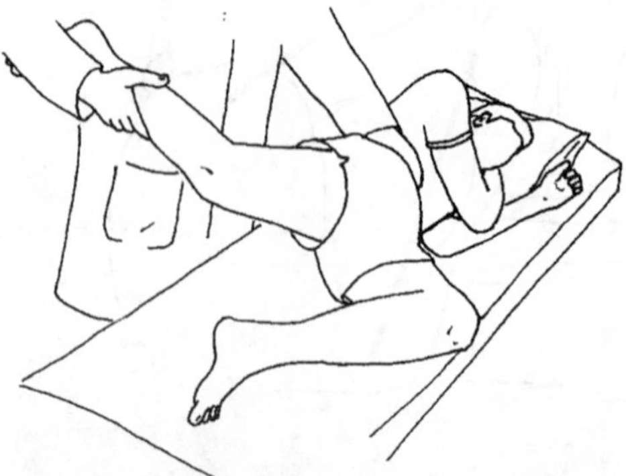

Fig. 28. Ober Test.

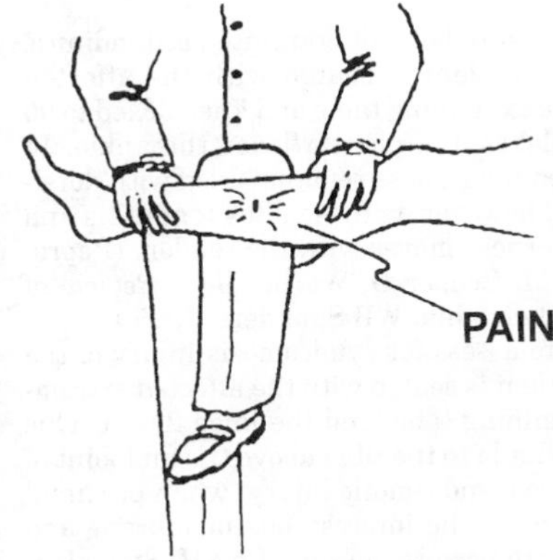

Fig. 29. Fulcrum Test of the Tibia.

against the examiner's knee / upper leg. The examiner's knee / leg is at the level of the patients point of maximal tenderness. This causes a fulcrum bending force at the level of maximal tenderness. Marked increase in pain with the fulcrum maneuver is considered a positive test and is indicative of tibial stress fracture. No increase in tenderness and nonfocal area of tenderness is more likely shin splints / tibial periostitis.

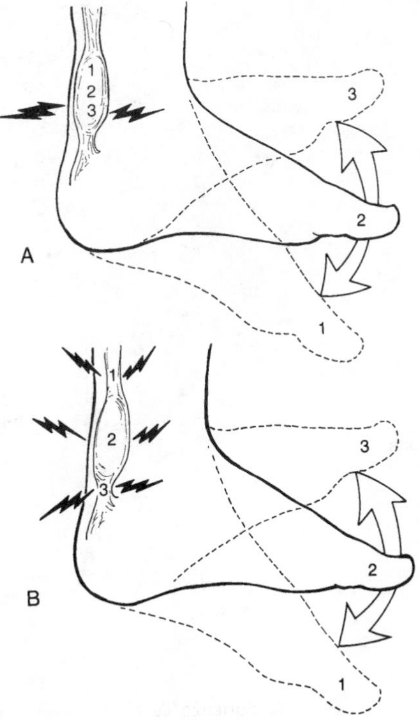

Fig. 30. Painful Arc Sign. (A) Peritendinitis, (B) Achilles Tendinitis.

V. Ankle

A. **Painful-arc sign** (Fig. 30). This is a test to help differentiate peritendinitis from actual Achilles tendinitis. The patient is seated with the affected extremity hanging over the edge of the examining table and knee flexed to 90 degrees. The patient actively dorsiflexes and plantarflexes the ankle. In peritendinitis (A), the area of localized tenderness remains fixed with dorsiflexion and plantarflexion of the foot; however, with Achilles tendinitis and partial rupture (B), the point of tenderness moves with the tendon. (Reproduced with permission from Miller M, Cooper D, Warner JJP. *Review of Sports medicine and arthroscopy*. Philadelphia: WB Saunders, 1995.)

B. **Squeeze test** (Fig. 31). This test is to assess for syndesmosis injury of the ankle (the high ankle sprain). The patient is seated with the affected extremity hanging over the edge of the examining table and the knee flexed. This test is performed by compressing the fibula to the tibia above the midpoint of the calf. The test is considered positive (syndesmotic injury) when proximal compression produces pain in the area of the interosseous membrane and syndesmotic ligament. (Reproduced with permission from Fu FH, Stone DA. *Sports injuries: mechanisms, prevention, treatment*. Philadelphia: Williams & Wilkins, 1994.)

C. **External rotation test** (Fig. 32). This is another test to assess for syndesmosis injury of the ankle (the high ankle sprain). The patient is seated with the affected extremity hanging over the edge of the examining table. This test is performed by applying external rotation stress to the foot and ankle with the knee held at 90 degrees of flexion and the ankle in neutral

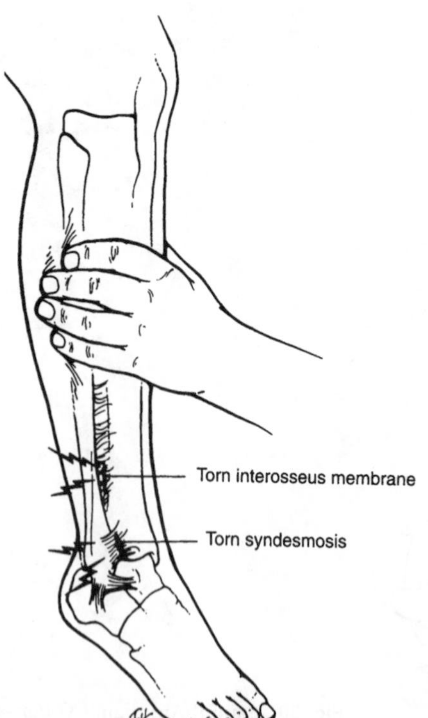

Fig. 31. Squeeze Test.

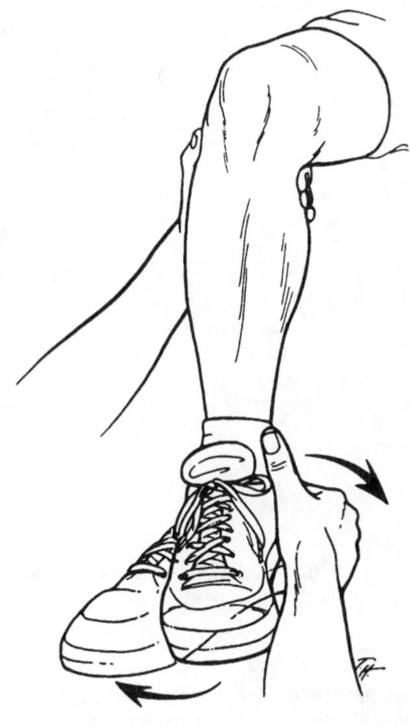

Fig. 32. External Rotation Test of the Ankle.

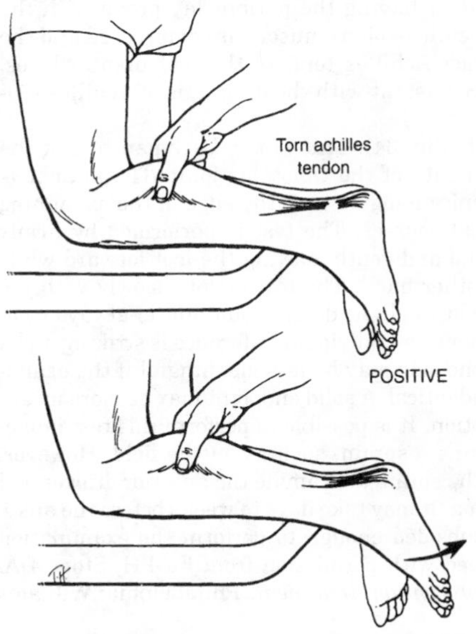

Fig. 33. Thompson's Test.

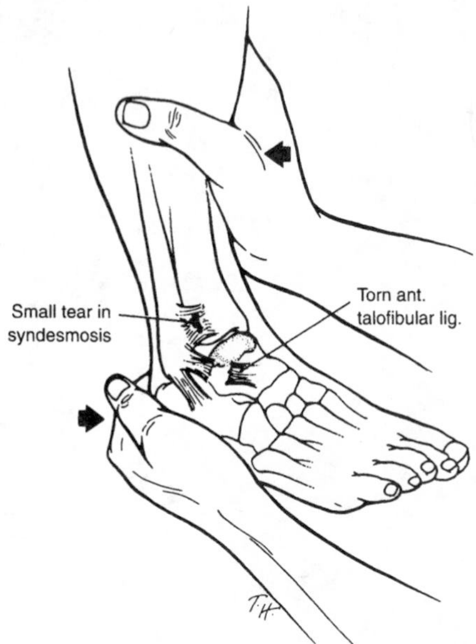

Fig. 34. Ankle Anterior Drawer Test.

position. A positive test produces pain over the anterior or posterior tibiofibular (syndesmotic) ligament(s) and over the interosseous membrane. (Reproduced with permission from Fu FH, Stone DA. *Sports injuries: mechanisms. prevention. treatment.* Philadelphia: Williams & Wilkins, 1994.)

D. **Thompson's test** (Fig. 33). This test is to assess disruption of the Achilles tendon. This test is performed by having the patient lay prone with the knee flexed. The calf (gastrocnemius-soleus muscle) is compressed and the foot is observed. With an intact Achilles tendon, the foot plantarflexes. Lack of foot plantarflexion is consistent with the diagnosis of Achilles tendon rupture.

E. **Ankle anterior drawer test** (Fig. 34). This is the Lachman test of the ankle to assess for excessive laxity of the tibiotalar joint. The patient is seated with the affected extremity hanging over the edge of the examining table and the knee is flexed 90 degrees. The test is performed by firmly grasping the heel with one hand and gently moving the foot forward while stabilizing the tibia with the other hand. The test is done slowly with the patient relaxed. The foot is held in slight dorsiflexion and is always compared to the other side. The amount of individual difference is striking and a "sloppy" feel of instability on one side may be less meaningful if the examination of the opposite ankle is identical. A solid endpoint may be more meaningful than the presence of motion. It is possible to perform this test immediately after the patient sustains a sprain, such as on the field. However, waiting just a few hours after the sprain to examine the anterior drawer will often be fruitless due to guarding. It may take days to weeks before the ankle swelling and guarding have subsided enough to perform the examination without anesthesia. (Reproduced with permission from Fu FH, Stone DA. *Sports injuries: mechanisms, prevention, treatment.* Philadelphia: Williams & Wilkins, 1994.)

VI. Spine

A. **Cram test (bowstring test)**. The patient is supine and the lower extremity is lifted with the knee extended, as in a straight-leg-raise test. Pressure is then placed on the sciatic nerve in the popliteal fossa with the extremity is elevated. The test is positive if it produces radiating pain above or below the popliteal fossa and there is more back pain than leg pain. The examiner should take care to press directly on the nerve only, whose location is directly medial to the lateral hamstring tendon.

SUBJECT INDEX

Subject Index

(Page numbers in *italic* refer to illustrations.)

A
Abdomen injuries
  assessment, 518–520
  boxing-related, 548
  limiting conditions, 28–29
  martial arts-related, 581
  pain, 268, 518
  preparticipation physical examination, 14–15
  prevention, 520
  return to play, 521–522
  sidelines management, 48
  treatment, 520–521
  types of, 518
Abrasions, 260
"Ace" bandages, 636
Achilles tendon
  dance-related injury, 553–554
  rupture, 463–464
  taping technique, 638
  tendinitis, 462–463
  ultrasonographic evaluation, 314
Acne, 264
Acquired immunodeficiency virus. *See* AIDS/HIV
Acromioclavicular joint injury, 362–365
Adductor muscle injury, 427–428
β-Adrenergic agonists, 246–247, 248
Advanced cardiac life support, 56–57
Aerobic capacity
  cerebral palsy athletes, 196
  developmental pattern, 163
  Down's syndrome athletes, 196
  for exercise, 69, 73–74
  gender differences, 171
  maximum oxygen uptake, 69, 73, 163
  wheelchair athletes, 191
  young athletes, 163
Aerobic conditioning
  cross-training, 75
  functional assessment, 69, 73–74
  guidelines, 74
  interval training, 74–75
  progression of training, 75–76
Aid stations, 59, 60
AIDS/HIV
  assessment and diagnosis, 206
  epidemiology, 206
  limiting conditions, 28
  pathophysiology, 206
  prevention, 206–207
  return-to-play considerations, 207
  sport-specific risk, 207
Alcohol
  effects on performance, 149–150
  patterns of use, 149
  physiology, 149
  testing, 150
  See also Drugs, recreational
Altitude illness. *See* High-altitude activity
Amenorrhea
  bone development and, 178, 179–180
  mechanism in athletes, 178–179
Amino acids, performance-enhancing, 143
Amphetamines, 144
Amputee athletes, 198
Anabolic agents, 142–144, 272
  prohibited substances, 652–653
  use in weight lifting/body building, 586
Anaphylaxis
  emergency protocols, 57
  exercise-induced, 27
  sidelines assessment/intervention, 46
Androgens, 142–143
Anemia
  clinical significance, 255
  foot-strike hemolysis, 257–258
  iron-deficiency, 256–257
  sports, 255–256
Ankle
  anatomy, 467
  anterior joint impingement, 472–473
  baseball-related injuries, 543
  basketball-related injuries, 545
  biomechanics, 467–468
  cricket-related injuries, 550
  dance-related injuries, 553–555
  diagnostic imaging, 307–308, 309
  fencing-related injuries, 564
  football injury patterns, 570
  gymnastics injury patterns, 574
  ice hockey injury, 576
  injection technique, 632–633
  injury patterns in endurance events, 558–559
  lacrosse injury patterns, 579
  martial arts injury patterns, 582

Ankle (*cont'd*)
  nerve entrapments, 473
  osteochondritis dissecans, 474
  peroneal tendon problems, 470–472
  physical examination, 688–690
  posterior impingement, 474
  posterior process fracture, 474
  posterior tibial tendon, 472
  preparticipation physical examination, *28*
  sinus tarsi syndrome, 475
  soccer-related injuries, 604–605
  sprains, 468–469
  subtalar instability, 473–474
  taping technique, 636–637
  tarsal coalition, 474–475
  tibiotalar instability, 469–470
  volleyball-related injury, 615
  wrestling-related injury, 621
Anorexia nervosa, 180
Anterior cruciate ligament injury, 173–175, 434–435
Anticholinergics, 247, 248, 252
Antihistamines, 248
Aortic valve stenosis, 24–25
Apophysitis, 170
Arrhythmias, 233–235, 579
Arthritis, 188
Arthrography, 313–314, 317
Assessment for limiting conditions
  abdomen, 28–29
  aerobic function, 69, 73–74
  AIDS/HIV, 206
  arrhythmias, 233–234
  asthma, 244–246
  athletic heart syndrome, 228
  body weight and composition, 135
  cardiomyopathies, 236
  cardiovascular, 21–25, 226–227
  chest pain, 229–230
  chlamydia, 204
  chronic obstructive pulmonary disease, 251
  congenital heart disease, 240
  dermatology, 27–28
  diabetes, 32, 217–218
  discoid meniscus, 442–443
  disordered eating, 180, 181
  Down's syndrome athletes, 195–196
  epilepsy, 299
  foot-strike hemolysis, 258
  gonorrhea, 203
  hepatitis, 207–208
  herpes simplex II, 205
  hydration status, 132
  hypertension, 232–233
  iron-deficiency anemia, 256–257
  liver dysfunction, 271
  menstrual dysfunction, 179
  mononucleosis, 201–202
  musculoskeletal, 29–31
  neurological, 25–26
  osteochondritis dissecans of knee, 445
  otitis externa, 209
  performance-enhancing drug use, 141
  pneumothorax, 249
  respiratory, 26–27
  sickle cell trait, 258–259
  sinusitis, 209–210
  sports anemia, 256
  station method, 11
  strep pharyngitis, 210
  syphilis, 204–205
  thyroid disorders, 222, 223
  upper respiratory infection, 211
  valvular heart disease, 238
  viral diseases, 27–28
  See also Physical examination, preparticipation
Assessment of injury
  abdomen, 48, 518–520
  Achilles tendon problems, 463
  acromioclavicular joint, 364
  acute cervical sprain, 282
  adductor muscles, 427
  ankle, physical examination, 688–690
  ankle impingement, 472–473, 474
  ankle nerve entrapments, 473
  ankle sprain, 468, 469
  axial load teardrop fracture, 284
  axillary nerve injury, 291
  biceps, 348, 349
  bunions, 483
  capitellar osteochondrosis, 378–379
  cardiac concussion, 515
  carpal instabilities, 382
  carpal tunnel syndrome, 390
  clavicle fractures, 361
  coracoid impingement, 346
  corns, 486
  cuff contusion, 346–347
  deltoid disruption, 359
  dental, 49–50, 500–502
  dislocations, 50–51
  effort thrombosis, shoulder, 358
  elbow, physical examination, 669–672
  elbow dislocations, 370
  elbow fractures, 368, 369
  elbow tendons, 373, 374, 375
  epicondylitis, 371
  exercise-induced collapse, 55–56, 96–97
  exertional leg pain, 461–462
  eye, 48–49, 498–499
  facet joint syndrome, 405
  femoral shaft fractures, 429
  on field, 33–34, 44, 45
  foot neuropathies, 485, 486
  fractures, 50, 316–317, 319–320
  genitourinary system, 523–526
  hallux rigidus, 483
  hamstring, 427
  hand/finger, 393
  hand/finger fractures, 393–394

hand/finger ligament injuries, 395–396, 397, 398
hand/finger tendon injuries, 399, 400, 401
hand/wrist fractures, 383–384
hand/wrist tendinitis, 389–390
head, 46–48, 275–277, 278
heat illnesses, 51–52, 95–102
heel compression syndrome, 482
heel pain syndrome, 480–481
herniated disc, 404–405
hip, 418, 419, 420
hip neuropathies, 423
hip soft tissue injury, 421, 422, 423
interosseous nerve syndrome, 376
knee, physical examination, 677–687
knee dislocation, 438–439
knee ligament, 432, 433, 434–435, 436–437
knee pain, 448
laryngeal, 46
lateral knee pain, 451–452, 453
Lisfranc fracture-dislocation, 479
Little Leaguer's elbow, 378
low back pain, 402–403, 560
maxillofacial, 489
medial knee pain, 449–450
median nerve compression, 376–377
meniscal cysts, 444
meniscal tears, 440–441
metatarsal fractures, 478, 479
multidirectional shoulder instability, 356–357
muscle, 425
myocardial contusion, 514
myocardial infarction, 52–53
olecranon bursitis, 370
olecranon osteochondrosis, 379
osteochondral fractures, 446–447
osteolysis of distal clavicle, 365
patellofemoral disorders, 455–456
pectoralis major, 349
pelvic/groin region, 412–413
pelvis, 48
peripheral nervous system, 287–288, 289
peroneal nerve entrapment, 465
peroneal tendon problems, 470, 471–472
physician responsibilities, 33
plantar nerve entrapment, 481
pneumothorax, 516–517
portable diagnostic kit, 43
posterolateral rotary instability, 373
pulmonary contusion, 516
quadriceps strain, 426
rib fracture, 511, 512
scapular fracture, 513
shoulder, physical examination, 672–677
shoulder impingement, 343–344, 345
shoulder instability, 352–353, 355
shoulder stress fracture, 359–360
on sidelines, 35
sidelines physician, 44, 45–53
sinus tarsi syndrome, 475
snapping scapula, 357–358
soft tissue, 338–339
spear tackler's spine, 284
spine, 48, 281, 691
spondylilisthesis, 407–408
spondylosis, 409–410
sternoclavicular separation, 366
sternum fracture, 512–513
stress fractures, 173
subscapularis rupture, 347
subtalar joint instability, 473
suprascapular nerve injury, 291
syncope, 229
talus fracture, 474
tarsal coalition, 474
tarsal fractures, 475, 476, 478
tennis leg, 464
thoracic nerve palsy, 290–291
thoracic outlet syndrome, 290
toenail problems, 484
tooth fracture classification, 500–502
tooth luxation, 502
in training room, 35–36
transient quadriplegia, 282–283
triangular fibrocartilage tears, 388
turf toe, 484
to ulnar collateral ligament, 372
ulnar neuropathy, 375
valgus extension overload syndrome, 377
wrist, physical examination, 669
wrist ligament, 381
Asthma
diagnosis, 244–246
management, 246–248
pathophysiology, 244
prevalence, 244
prevention, 248–249
sidelines assessment/intervention, 46
Athletic heart syndrome, 228
Athletic trainer
on-field injury assessment, 34
responsibilities, 4
Axillary nerve injury, 291
Axonotmesis, 288

B

Back flexion, *20*
Back pain
in golfers, 571
running-related, 560
swimming-related problems, 610
in tennis players, 612
Back strain, 402
Bacterial infection, dermatological, 262–263
Badminton, 612
Barotrauma, 114–115
pulmonary, 115
Baseball/softball
injury patterns, 541–543
protective equipment, 124
Basketball
injury patterns, 544–545

Bee stings, 264
Bennet's fracture-dislocation, 394
Beta agonists, prohibited, 653
Beta blocking agents, 187
  prohibited, 653
Biceps injury, 347–349
  distal tendon, 374
Bladder dysfunction, in wheelchair athletes, 194
Bladder injury, 523–524
Bleeding, 53
Blisters, 260
Blood disorders, 255–259
  gastrointestinal bleeding, 269–270
Blood doping, 146
Blood flow
  in energy production, 92–93
  warmup exercises, 166
Blood testing, enzyme-based lactate analysis, 73–74
Body building, 586–588
Body temperature
  dehydration effects, 132
  heat injury, 95–96
  variation in, 91
Bone
  arthrographic assessment, 313–314
  computed tomography, 312–313
  diagnostic imaging, 305–308
  disorders among cerebral palsy athletes, 196–197
  magnetic resonance imaging, 308–310
  menstrual dysfunction and, 177–180
  radionuclide bone scan, 310–312
  See also Fractures; Musculoskeletal assessment;
    Musculoskeletal disorder;
      Musculoskeletal injury;
    specific bone
    sidelines injury management, 50–51
Boutonniere deformity, 400
Boxer's knuckle, 401
Boxing
  amateur vs. professional, 546
  dental injuries, 548
  ear injuries, 547
  eye injuries, 546–547
  facial injuries, 546
  jaw injuries, 548
  musculoskeletal injuries, 548
  neurologic injuries, 546
Braces, protective, 121
Brachialis tendon strain, 373–374
Breast injury, 511
Bronchitis, 253, 254
Bronchodilators, 246–247
Bronchospasm, exercise-induced, 26–27, 610
Bulimia, 180
Bunions, 483–484, 555
Burners/burner syndrome, 26, 289–290, 569
Bursitis
  hip, 421–422
  olecranon, 370
  pelvic region, 416
  pes anserinus syndrome, 449–450
  tibial collateral ligament, 450

C

Caffeine, 144–145
Calcaneus fractures, 478, 558
Calcium requirements of female athlete, 182
Canadian Academy of Sports Medicine emergency kit, 38–43
Cancer
  androgen-associated risk, 142
  smokeless tobacco-associated, 153
Canoeing/kayaking/rafting, 592–594
Capitellar osteochondrosis, 378–379
Carbohydrates
  in fluid replacement, 133
  requirements, 129–130
Cardiac arrest, 56–57
  sidelines assessment/intervention, 46
Cardiomyopathy
  dilated, 236
  hypertrophic, 21, 236
    clinical features, 236
  nonspecific, 236–237
  right ventricular, 236
Cardiovascular system
  adaptations to exercise, 227–228
  androgen effects, 142
  aortic diseases, 242
  arrhythmias, 233–235, 579
  assessment, 226–227
  athletic heart syndrome, 228
  cardiac concussion, 514–515
  cardiac murmers, 227
  cardiac rupture, 514–515
  chest pain evaluation, 229–230
  cocaine effects, 151
  congenital heart disease, 238–242
  contraindications to exercise, 226
  coronary artery disease, 237–238
  exercise testing, 228–229
  hypertension, 231–233
  infective carditis, 22–23
  limiting conditions for sports participation, 21–25
  maintenance of fitness in rehabilitation, 530
  myocardial contusion, 514
  pericardial tamponade, 515
  preparticipation physical examination, 14
  sudden death, 230–231, 544
  syncope evaluation, 229
  thoracic injury, 514–515
  valvular heart disease, 238
  vessel rupture, 515
  weight lifting/body building effects, 586
  wheelchair athletes, 191
  See also Cardiomyopathy
Carditis, infective, 22–23

Carpal instabilities, 382
Carpal navicular fracture, 312–313
Carpal tunnel syndrome, 193, 390
Carpi radialis, flexor, 389–390
Carpi ulnaris, extensor/flexor, 389
  instability, 391–392
Cartilage synovium, 337–338
Cerebral edema, high-altitude, 112
Cerebral palsy, 196–197
Chain exercises, 534
Chest
  anatomy, 509, *510*
  breast injury, 511
  cardiovascular injury, 514–515
  contusion, 509–511
  costochondral fracture, 513
  lacrosse injury patterns, 579
  martial arts injury patterns, 581
  muscle strain, 511
  pain, 229–230
  pulmonary injury, 516–517
  rib fractures, 511–512
  scapular fracture, 513
  sternum fracture, 512–153
  wrestling-related injury, 621
Chewing tobacco, 151–153
Chillblains, 107
Chlamydia, 204
Chronic obstructive pulmonary disease, 188, 250–252
Clavicle
  acromioclavicular joint injury, 362–365
  distal, osteolysis, 365
  fractures, 361–362
  lacrosse injury patterns, 578
  sternoclavicular separation, 366–367
Cocaine
  adverse effects, 151
  effects on performance, 151
  patterns of use, 150
  physiology, 150–151
  testing, 151
Coccyx fracture, 415
Cold injury
  pernio, 261
  physiologic response, 106
  predisposing conditions, 109
  risks for wheelchair athletes, 194
  types of, 106–109. *See also specific type*
Computed tomography, 312–313
  abdomen, 520
  patellofemoral problems, 456
Concentric muscle action, 79
Concussion, 276
  assessment, 25
  boxing-related, 546
  cardiac, 514–515
  football-related, 568
  ice hockey injury, 575
  recommendations for athletic participation, 25–26
  sidelines assement/intervention, 47
Condylar fractures, 395
Constipation, 271
Consultants, 4–5
Contagious disorders, 27
Contusion
  abdominal wall, 520
  cerebral, 47
  chest, 509–511
  hip pointer, 569–570
  muscle, 332
  myocardial, 514
  osteochondral, 338
  pelvic region, 416
  pulmonary, 516
  quadriceps, 428
  rotator cuff, 346–347
Coracoid impingement, 346
Cornea, 49
Corns, 260, 486, 555
Coronary artery, congenital anomalies, 24
Coronary artery disease, 237–238
  exercise-related sudden death, 231
  risk in older athletes, 187–188
  screening, 24
Coronoid process fracture, 368
Cortisone, 625
Costochondral fracture, 513
CPR equipment, 656, 658
Cram test, 691
Creatinine, 143
Cricket, 549–550
Cricothytoidotomy, 46
Cross-country skiing, 601
Cross-training, 75
Cruciate ligament injury
  anterior, 173–175, 434–435
  football injury patterns, 570
  posterior, 436–438
  skiing-related, 600
Cryotherapy, 532
Cubital tunnel syndrome, 375–376
Cutting weight, 135–136
Cycling-related injuries
  in endurance events, 560–561
  palsy, 390–391
  patterns, 551–552
  predicted incidence, 54
  protective equipment, 124
  risks for disabled athletes, 197
Cystic fibrosis, 250
Cysts, meniscal, 443–444

D

Dance-related injuries
  acute, 553–554
  chronic/overuse injuries, 554–555
  dancer's fracture, 479
  instructor-physician interaction, 555
  rehabilitation, 554

Deaf athletes, 197
Decathlon, 614
Decompression sickness
  pathophysiology, 115–116
  treatment, 116–117
Defibrillators, 46
Dehydration
  adverse effects, 132
  for rapid weight loss, 135–136
  risk among older athletes, 186
Dental problems
  anatomy, 500
  boxing-related injury, 548
  fracture classification, 500–502
  headache etiology, 294
  lip laceration, 502
  prevention, 504
  sidelines management, 49–50
  smokeless tobacco use and, 153
  tooth avulsion, 49–50, 503–504
  tooth extrusion, 503
  tooth intrusion, 503
  tooth luxation, 502
DeQuervain's tenosynovitis, 389
Dermatological conditions, 264–266
  abrasions, 260
  acne, 264
  bites/stings, 264
  blisters, 260
  corns, 260
  dermatitis, 265, 577
  infectious, 261–263
  infestations, 264
  limiting conditions, 27–28
  pernio, 261
  psoriasis, 265
  purpura, 260
  sunburn, 261
  surfing-related, 606–607
  urticaria, 265
  wilderness exposure, 592
  wrestling-related, 621
  See also Skin
Destot's sign, 414
Diabetes
  as limiting condition, 32
Diabetes mellitus
  exercise in, 217, 219–221
  management, 219–222
  pathophysiology, 216–217
  presentation, 217–218
Diaphragm trauma, 268
Diarrhea, 268–269
Diet and nutrition
  body fat loss, 134–135
  carbohydrate requirements, 129–130
  diabetes management, 219–220
  electrolyte requirements, 133
  energy requirements, 129
  fat, 130
  in female athlete, 182
  fluids, 130–133
  for gymnasts, 573
  iron-deficiency anemia, 256
  potassium sources, 133
  protein requirements, 130
  rapid weight loss, 135–136
  for weight lifting/body building, 586
  for weight/strength gain, 136–137
Digitorum communis tendon, 400
Disabled persons
  amputees, 198
  benefits of exercise, 190
  cerebral palsy athletes, 196–197
  cycling risks, 197
  definition, 190
  Down's syndrome athletes, 195–196
  hearing impaired, 197
  multiple sclerosis athletes, 198
  preparticipation physical examination, 190
  sports participation trends, 190
  visual impairment, 197
  wheelchair athletes, 191–194
Discus, 614
Disordered eating
  assessment, 181, 573
  contributory factors, 181
  definition, 180
  female athlete triad, 175–177
  health consequences, 181
  prevalence, 180–181
  treatment, 182
Diuretics, prohibited, 653–654
Diving-related illnesses
  arterial gas embolism, 115, 116–117
  barotrauma, 114–115
  decompression sickness, 115–116
  drug use and, 118
  inert gas narcosis, 117
  pathophysiology, 114
  predisposing conditions, 118
  pulmonary barotrauma, 115
  See also Swimming and platform/springboard diving
Documentation, 65
Down's syndrome, 195–196
Drug testing
  alcohol, 150
  analysis, 159
  cocaine, 151
  costs, 160
  emerging technologies, 159–160
  evasion techniques, 159
  informed consent for, 156, 157
  marijuana, 154
  notification for, 157–158
  off-season, 157
  penalties, 160
  procedure, 158–159

selection for, 157
types of, 156–157
U.S. programs, 156
Drugs, performance enhancing
adverse effects, 141
assessment, 141
definition, 141
drug testing program, 156–160
efficacy, 141
ethical/legal issues, 142
pattern of use, 141
program and policy issues, 146–147
prohibited substances, 651–654
types of, 141. *See also specific type*
Drugs, recreational
health costs, 148
patterns of use, 148–149
risk factors for abuse, 148
See also Alcohol; *specific drug*
Dynamic constant external resistance, 79

E

Earle's sign, 414
Ear(s)
auricular hematomas, 491–492
barotrauma, 114, 493, 494
boxing-related injuries, 547
diving-related injury, 557
external injury, 491
external otitis, 492–493
frostbite, 493
headache etiology, 294
inner injuries, 494
ossicular chain injury, 493–494
preparticipation physical examination, 14
surfing-related injury, 606–607
tympanic perforation, 493
Eccentric muscle action, 79
Elbow
boxing-related injury, 548
capitellar osteochondrosis, 378–379
coronoid process fracture, 368
diagnostic imaging, 306
dislocations, 51, 369–370
distal humerus, fracture of, 368–369
diving-related injury, 557
epicondylitis, 371–372
football injury patterns, 569
golf injury patterns, 572
gymnastics injury patterns, 573
ice hockey injury, 576
injection technique, 628–629
injury patterns in rafting-type activities, 593
intercondylar fracture, 369
lacrosse injury patterns, 578
Little Leaguer's, 377–378
medial epicondylar osteochondrosis, 377–378
nerve injuries, 375–377
olecranon fracture, 368
olecranon osteochondrosis, 379
overuse injuries, 370–371
physical examination, 669–672
posterolateral rotary instability, 373
preparticipation physical examination, *22*
radial head fracture, 369
range of motion, *22*
tendon injuries, 373–375
ulnar collateral ligament injury, 372–373
valgus extension overload syndrome, 377
Velpeau bandage, 644–646
wrestling-related injury, 621
Electrical stimulation, 532
Electrolytes, 133
Embolism, diving-related, 115, 116–117
Emergency intervention
cardiac arrest, 46
epileptic seizure, 301–302
exercise-related headache, 298
eye injury assessment, 498–499
eye injury emergency kit, 499, 656
for fractures, 318
head injury, 275–277
preparation. *See* Preparation for emergencies
spine injury, 280–281
Endocrine function
anatomy and physiology, 216
in diabetes mellitus, 216–217
in muscle metabolism, 216
thyroid disorders, 222–224
Endurance events
diabetes management in, 221
gender differences in performance, 171
injury patterns, 54–55, 558–561
role of medical staff, 558
thermal injury risk, 57–58
Endurance training
aerobic, 74
aerobic capacity of young adults, 163
interval, 75
protein intake, 130
sports anemia in, 255–256
Energy metabolism
efficiency, 92
heat gain, 92–93
heat loss, 92
intersport variation, 129
nutritional requirements, 129
Environmental conditions
cold injury prevention, 108–109
cycling-related injury, 552
golf injuries, 572
heat injury prevention, 103–104
heat injury risk, 57–58
performance in cold environments, 109
risk for mountain climbers, 584
in thermoregulation, 91

Ephedrine, 145
Epicondylitis
  baseball-related injuries, 542
  elbow, 371–372
Epilepsy
  classification, 299
  definition, 299
  long-term management, 300–301
  mortality, 300
  sports participation and, 299, 300, 302
  team physician's role, 301–302
  treatment, 299
Epiphysitis, 391
Epistaxis, 495, 547
Epstein-Barr virus, 201–202
  limiting conditions, 28
Equestrian sports. *See* Horseback riding
Erythrasma, 263
Erythropoietin, 145
Ethical decision-making, 7–8
Ethical issues
  assessment of injury, 33
  performance-enhancing drug use, 142
Exercise
  cardiovascular adaptations, 227–228
  cardiovascular assessment, 226–227
  in diabetes mellitus, 217, 219–221
  by disabled persons, 190
  HIV infection and, 207
  hypertension and, 232
  infection and, 201
  by older persons, 184–186, 187
  spine rehabilitation program, 665–668
  warmup, 166
Exercise-associated collapse, 96–97
Exercise capacity
  aerobic function assessment, 69, 73–74
  high-altitude, 112
Exercise-induced conditions
  anaphylaxis, 27
  asthma, 244–249
  breast pain, 511
  bronchospasm, 26–27
  bronchospasms, 610
  emergency protocols, 55–56
  hypothermic, 56
  leg pain, 461–462
  sudden death, 230–231
  See also Headaches, exercise-related; Heat injury
Exercise testing, 228–229
  asthma assessment, 245–246
Exostosis, 592–593, 606
Eye(s)
  basketball-related injuries, 544
  blood in, 49
  boxing-related injuries, 546–547
  common injuries, 498
  danger signs, 498
  emergency care, 48–49, 499
  headache etiology, 294
  ice hockey injury, 575
  incidence of injury, 497
  injury assessment, 498–499
  mechanisms of injury, 497–498
  medical kit, 656
  one-eyed athletes, 31, 498
  orbital blow out fractures, 49
  prognosis, 499
  protectors, 499
  retinal detachment, 49
  retinal hemorrhage, 49
  wrestling-related injury, 620

F
Fabella syndrome, 452
Face. *See* Maxillofacial injuries; *specific structures*
Facet joint syndrome, 406–407
Fat
  body fat loss, 134–135
  dietary, 130
Female athlete, 171
  anemia risk, 256
  field hockey injury patterns, 567
  genitourinary injuries, 524, 525–526
  gymnasts, 573–574
  musculoskeletal considerations, 172–175
  nutritional concerns, 182
  physiology, 171
  preventive interventions, 183
  sport-specific risks, 172
  stress urinary incontinence, 182–183
  triad, 175–177
Femur
  neck fractures, 420, 560
  shaft stress fractures, 429–430
Fencing, injury patterns, 564–565
Field hockey, 566–567
  protective equipment, 123
Fingers. *See* Hand and fingers
Flexibility exercises, 532–533
Fluid replacement, 104–105
  determinants of, 132–133
  diabetes management, 219
  electrolytes in, 133
  methods, 133
  monitoring hydration status, 132
  in older athletes, 186
  for rapid weight loss, 135–136
  requirements, 130–131
  thermoregulation, 132
Foot
  diagnostic imaging, 307–308, 309
  fungal infection, 261–262
Foot injuries
  baseball-related, 542–543
  bunions, 483–484
  corns, 486
  cricket-related, 550
  dance-related, 553–554, 555

fencing-related, 564
foot-strike hemolysis, 257–258
football-related, 570
great toe problems, 482–483
heel compression syndrome, 481–482
heel pain, 481–489
ice hockey-related, 576
injection technique, 633–634
lacrosse-related, 579
Lisfranc fracture-dislocation, 479–480
martial arts-related, 582
metatarsal fractures, 478–479
neuropathies, 485–486
patterns in endurance events, 558
plantar nerve entrapment, 481
soccer-related, 605
taping and bandaging techniques, 636–641
tarsal fractures, 476–478
toenail problems, 484–485
turf toe, 484, 570
wrestling-related, 621
See also Ankle
Football
injury patterns, 568–570
protective equipment, 121–122
spine injury prevention, 280
Footballer's ankle, 472–473
Fractures
ankle, posterior process, 474
assessment, 316–317, 319–320
axial load teardrop, 284
baseball-related injuries, 541, 542–543
carpal navicular, 312–313
clavicle, 361–362
computed tomography, 312–313
costochondral, 513
cycling-related, 551
definition, 316
diagnostic imaging, 309–310, 311
elbow, 368–369
etiology, 316
femoral shaft, 429–430
hallux sesamoid, 312
hand and wrist, 382–385, 393–395
hip, 419–421
horseback riding-associated, 562
ice hockey-related, 575
injury patterns in endurance events, 558, 560
laryngeal, 46, 496
leg, stress, 461
limits to sports participation, 30
martial arts injury patterns, 581
maxillofacial, 490
medial epicondylar, 377–378
metatarsal, 478–479
natural history, 317
nose, 494–495
orbital blow out, 49
osteochondral, 446–447, 477
overuse injuries in young athletes, 168–170
pelvic/groin region, 414–415, 560
physeal injuries in young athletes, 168, *169*
prevention, 317, 320
proximal femur, *311*
rib, 511–512
risk among female athletes, 172–173
rugby injury patterns, 596
Salter-Harris classification, 168
scapular, 513
shoulder, 359–360
sidelines management, 50
spine, 30
sternum, 512–513
stress type, 319–321
tarsal, 476–478
terminology, 316
tooth, 500–502
treatment, 317–319, 320–321
Frostbite, 107
ear, 493
Frostnip, 106–107
Fungal infections, 261–262
Furunculosis, 27
Fusion, spine, 30, 31, 286
Futsal, 602–603

G
Garrick test, 686
Gastrocnemius strain, 554
Gastrocnemius tear, 464
Gastroesophageal reflux, 267–268
Gastrointestinal disorders, 272
abdominal pain, 268
bleeding, 269–270
constipation, 271
diarrhea, 268–269
gastroesophageal reflux, 267–268
inflammatory bowel disease, 270
irritable bowel, 270
nausea, 267
peptic ulcer, 270
prevalence among athletes, 267
trauma, 268
Gender differences, 171
Genitalia
boxing-related injury, 548
female injuries, 525–526
male injuries, 524–525
preparticipation physical examination, 15
Glasgow coma scale, 276
Glenohumeral joint, 342
instability, 351, 352
Glucocorticoids, 247
Glucose metabolism, 216
Golf-related injuries, 571–572
Gonorrhea, 202–203
Great toe, 482–483

Groin and thigh
adductor injuries, 427–428
anatomy, 424
femoral shaft fractures, 429–430
hamstring injuries, 426–427
hernia, 428–429
ice hockey injury, 576
injury patterns in endurance events, 559, 560
martial arts injury patterns, 581
muscle injury, 424–426
quadriceps contusion, 428
quadriceps strain, 426
rugby injury patterns, 595–596
spica wrap, 646–650
See also Pelvic/groin region
Guyon's tunnel syndrome, 390–391
Gymnastics, 573–574

H

Hallux rigidus, 482–483
Hammer throw, 614
Hamstring syndrome, 416, 423
groin injuries, 426–427
Hand and fingers
assessment, 393
condylar fractures, 395
dislocation of finger, 51
ice hockey injuries, 576
ligamentous injuries, 395–398
metacarpal fracture, 393–394
mountain climbing injuries, 584–585
phalangeal fractures, 394–395
preparticipation physical examination, *21*
range of motion, *21*
rugby injury patterns, 595
skiing-related injuries, 600
soccer-related injuries, 605
taping techniques, 643–644
tendon injuries, 398–401
volleyball-related injury, 615
Hand and wrist injuries
acute ligamentous, 381
baseball-related, 542
boxing-related, 548
cricket-related, 550
diagnostic imaging, 307, 309, 314, 381
diving-related, 557
epiphysitis, 391
extensor hood injury, 314
football-related, 569
fractures, 382–385
golf-related, 572
Guyon's tunnel syndrome, 390–391
gymnastics-related, 573
ice hockey-related, 576
injection technique, 629–630
instabilities, 391–392
Kienböck's disease, 385–386
lacrosse-related, 578–579
martial arts-related, 581
neuropathies, 390–391
physical examination, 669
radioulnar dislocation, 312
in rafting-type activities, 593
risk, 381
splinting, 386
taping techniques, 641–643
tendinitis, 389–390
tennis-related, 611
triangular fibrocartilage tears, 388–389
ulnocarpal abutment, 385
Hawkin's sign, 675–676
Head injury
assessment, 275–277, 278
baseball risk, 124
boxing-related, 546–547
in canoeing-type activities, 592
cerebral concussion/contusion, 47
cycling-related, 551
diving-related, 557
emergency protocols, 57
football risk, 121, 568
hematomas, 47–48
in ice hockey, 575
in lacrosse, 578
martial arts risk, 581
mechanism, 275
recognition of, 275
recovery, 278–279
second-impact syndrome, 275–277
sidelines assessment/intervention, 46–48
soccer-related, 605
treatment, 277
wrestling-related, 620
Headaches, exercise-related
epidemiology, 293
etiologies, 293–295
treatment, 295–298
Heart disease
congenital, 238–242
valvular, 238
See also Cardiomyopathy; Cardiovascular system
Heat cramps, 51–52
Heat exhaustion, 95
pathophysiology, 97–99
sidelines management, 52
Heat injury
exercise-associated collapse, 96–97
medical preparation, 105
physiologic mechanism, 91
prevention, 52, 102–105
rectal temperature, 95–96
risk, 57–58
risk for young athletes, 163–164
risks for wheelchair athletes, 194
sidelines management, 51–52
sunburn, 261
types of, 95. *See also specific type*
wet bulb globe temperature calculation, 57–58, 103

Heat stroke, 95
  pathophysiology, 99–101
  sidelines management, 52
Heat syncope, 95
  pathophysiology, 97
Heel compression syndrome, 481–482
Heel pain, 481–489
Helmets
  baseball, 124
  football, 121–122
  hockey, 122
  in-line skating, 124
  lacrosse, 123
Hematoma
  abdominal wall, 521
  auricular, 491–492, 620
  epidural, 47
  iliacus syndrome, 423
  intracerebral, 47
  intracranial, 277
  septal, 547
  subdural, 47–48
  subungual, 485
  testicular, 577
Hemolysis, foot-strike, 257–258
Hemorrhoids, 272
Hepatitis, 271–272
  assessment and diagnosis, 207–208
  epidemiology, 207
  limiting conditions, 28, 29
  natural history, 208
  prevention, 208
  return-to-play considerations, 208
  treatment, 208
Hepatomegaly, 29
Heptathlon, 614
Hernia
  groin and thigh region, 428–429
  inguinal, 29
  pelvic region, 416
Herpes gladiatorum, 263
Herpes simplex, 27, 205–206, 263
High-altitude activity
  acute mountain sickness, 110–111, 583
  adaptation, 110
  maladaptation, 110
  mountaineering, 583–585
  training, 112–113
High jump, 614
Hip
  anatomy, 418
  assessment, 418
  avulsion fractures, 419
  bursitis, 421–422
  diagnostic imaging, 307
  dislocations, 50, 420
  epiphyseal injury, 419–420
  football injury patterns, 569–570
  hamstring syndrome, 423
  injury patterns in endurance events, 559–560
  neuropathies, 423
  piriformis syndrome, 422–423
  snapping-hip syndrome, 422
  Spica wrap, 646
  stress fractures, 420–421
  types of injury, 418
Hip pointer, 569–570
Hives, 265
Hockey. *See* Ice hockey; Field hockey
Hoffa's disease, 448
Hook of hamate fracture, 385
Hormones
  peptic ulcer pathogenesis, 270
  See also Endocrine function
Horseback riding
  injury patterns, 562–563
  mortality, 563
  professional jockeys, 563
  rodeo, 589–591
Human chorionic gonadotropin, 143
Human growth hormone, 143
Human immunodeficiency virus. *See* AIDS/HIV
Humerus, distal fracture, 368–369
Hurdlers, 613
Hydraulic resistance exercise, 79
Hyperglycemia
  acute, treatment, 221
  in diabetes mellitus, 221
Hyperreflexia, autonomic, 194
Hypertension, 21–22
  athletic eligibility, 232
  diagnosis and evaluation, 232–233
  epidemiology, 231–232
  management, 233
Hyperthermia risks for wheelchair athletes, 194
Hyperthyroidism, 223–224
Hypertrophy, idiopathic concentric left ventricular, 24
Hyphema, 49
Hypoglycemia
  acute, treatment, 221
  after exercise, 217
  emergency protocols, 57
  See also Diabetes mellitus
Hypotension medication, 187
Hypothermia
  classification, 108
  pathophysiology, 107–108
  prevention, 108–109
  risk for mountain climbers, 583
  risks for wheelchair athletes, 194
Hypothermic exercise-associated collapse, 56
Hypothyroidism, 222–223

I

Ice hockey
  injury patterns, 575–577
  protective equipment, 122–123

Iliacus hematoma syndrome, 423
Iliopectineal bursitis, 416
Iliotibial band syndrome, 422, 451–452
  physical examination for, 686
Immersion foot, 107
Immunizations, 212
Impaired competitors, 58
Impetigo, 27, 262–263, 622
In-line skating. *See* Skating, in-line
Infectious disorders
  dermatological, 261–263
  exercise and, 201
  horse bites, 562–563
  immunization, 212
  liver dysfunction, 271–272
  return-to-play criteria, 211–212
  risk for mountain climbers, 583
  sexually transmitted, 202–208
  upper respiratory, 210–211, 252–254
  viral diseases, limiting conditions, 28
  wilderness exposure, 592
  wrestling-related, 621–622
  See also specific disorder; specific pathogen
Inflammation management, 529
Inflammatory bowel disease, 270
Influenza, 212, 253–254
Informed consent, for drug testing, 156, 157
Injections, intraarticular
  ankle, 632–633
  contraindications, 625
  cortisone, 625
  elbow, 628–629
  goals, 625
  knee, 630–632
  metatarsal phalangeal, 634
  plantar fascia, 633
  shoulder, 626–628
  supplies, 625
  technique, generally, 625–626
  wrist, 629–630
Insulin deficiency, 216–217
Insulin growth factor, 143
Insulin shock, 57
Interosseous nerve syndrome, 376
Interval training, 74–75
Iron
  deficiency anemia, 256–257
  in female athlete, 182
Irritable bowel syndrome, 270
Ischial bursitis, 416
Isokinetics, 79
Isometric training, 77
  for young athletes, 166
Isotonic training, 79

J
Javelin, 613
Jaw injuries, 548
Jersey finger, 399–400
Jock itch, 262
Jogger's foot, 485–486
Joint function
  ankle, 467–468
  isometric training, 77
  limiting conditions, 31
Joint injections. *See* Injections, intraarticular
Jones fracture, 478–479
Jumper's knee, 614

K
Kayaking, 592–594
Keratolysis, 263
Khellin derivatives, 247–248
Kidneys
  ice hockey injury, 577
  injury, 523
  single-organ athletes, 31
  trauma, 521
Kienböck's disease, 385–386
Knee injury
  anterior pain, 448
  baseball-related, 543
  cycling-related, 551
  diagnostic imaging, 307, 309
  dislocation, 50, 438–439
  in endurance events, 559
  football-related, 570
  gymnastics-related, 574
  ice hockey-related, 576
  injection technique, 630–632
  lacrosse-related, 579
  martial arts-related, 582
  medial pain, 449–450
  meniscus. *See* Meniscus
  osteochondral fractures, 446–447
  osteochondritis dissecans, 444–446
  pain in young athlete, 165–166
  physical examination, 677–687
  preparticipation physical examination, *27*
  rugby-related, 596
  skiing-related, 600–601
  soccer-related, 604
  swimming-related, 610
  tarsal coalition, 312
  uncommon sources of pain, 448
  volleyball-related, 615
Knee ligament
  anatomy, 431
  lateral collateral injury, 433–434
  medial collateral injury, 431–432
  multiple injuries, 438–439
  sprain classification, 431
  See also Cruciate ligament

L
Lachman test, 680
Lacrosse
  injury patterns, 578–579
  protective equipment, 123

Larva migrans, 264
Laryngeal injury, 496, 575
  cricothytoidotomy, 46
  sidelines assessment/intervention, 46
Leg injury
  Achilles tendon problems, 462–464
  anatomy, 460
  assessment, 460–461
  basketball-related, 545
  compartment syndromes, 461–462
  cramp, 56
  exertional pain, 461–462
  medial head gastrocnemius tear, 464
  medial periostalgia, 462
  patterns in endurance events, 559
  peroneal nerve entrapment, 465
  stress fracture, 461
Legal issues, 7
  performance-enhancing drug use, 142
  preparticipation physical examination, 20
Lice, 264
Lifestyle factors, 18–20
Ligament injury, 337
  ankle anatomy, 467
  ankle sprains, 468–470
  baseball-related, 541–542
  basketball-related, 544–545
  cricket-related, 550
  endurance event risks, 559
  hand/finger, 395–398
  knee, 432–439
  tibial collateral bursitis, 450
  ulnar collateral, 372–373
  wrist, 381
Light-intensity training, 6
Limiting conditions
  abdominal disorders, 28–29
  cardiovascular, 21–25
  dermatological, 27–28
  diabetes, 32
  musculoskeletal disorders, 29–31
  neurological, 25–26
  respiratory, 26–27
  sickle cell trait, 32
  single-organ athletes, 31–32
  viral diseases, 28
  See also Assessment for limiting conditions
Lip laceration, 502
Lisfranc fracture-dislocation, 479–480
Little Leaguer's elbow, 377
Liver
  disease, 271–272
  limiting conditions, 29
Long QT syndrome, 25

M

Magnetic resonance imaging, 308–309
  patellofemoral problems, 456
Mallet finger, 398–399
Marathon running
  cardiac arrest, 56
  fluid replacement, 55
  incidence of injury, 54
  See also Endurance events; Endurance training
Marfan's syndrome, 24, 242
Marijuana, 153–154
Martial arts, 580–582
Mass-participation event planning, 54–65
Maxillofacial injuries
  anatomical considerations, 489
  assessment, 489
  boxing-related, 546
  in canoeing-type activities, 593
  fractures, 490
  in ice hockey, 575
  incidence, 489
  rugby injury patterns, 595
  soccer-related, 605
  soft tissue repair, 489–490
  wound care, 489
  wrestling-related, 620
  See also specific structures
Maximum oxygen uptake, 69, 73
  in young athletes, 163
McMurray test, 681
Measles, 212
Median nerve compression, 376–377
Medical kits
  CPR equipment, 656
  eye injury, 656
  portable emergency, 38–43
  sidelines physician, 44
  standard medical bag, 655–658
Medical team
  for care of female athletes, 183
  mass-participation events, 60
  responsibilities, 4–5
Meniscus
  anatomy, 440
  cysts, 443–444
  discoid, 442–443
  macrotrauma rehabilitation program, 659–661
  tears, 307, *310*, 440–442
Menstrual function
  assessment, 179
  athletic performance and, 171
  bone concerns in disorders of, 177–180
  female athlete triad, 175–177
  in gonorrhea, 202–203
  interventions for dysfunction, 179–180
  irregularity, 135
  luteal phase dysfunction, 178, 180
Meralgia paresthetica, 423
Metacarpal fracture, 393–394
Metatarsal fractures, 478–479, 558
Methylprednisolone, 281
Methylxanthines, 247
METs, 69
  normative values, 73
Miserable misalignment syndrome, 173, *175*

Mitral valve prolapse
  diagnosis, 23–24
  recommendations for athletic participation, 24
Molluscum contagiosum, 27, 263
Mononucleosis, 201–202
  splenomegaly and, 29
Morton's neuroma, 485
Motivation of older athletes, 186
Mountaineering and climbing, 583–585
Multiple sclerosis, 198
Muscle
  anatomy and function, 424
  baseball-related injuries, 541–542
  basketball-related injuries, 544
  chest strain, 511
  classification of injury, 425
  cramps. *See* Muscle cramps
  cricket-related injury, 550
  delayed onset soreness, 334, 425
  glucose metabolism, 216
  mechanism of injury, 424–425
  metabolism, 424
  neurologic control, 533–534
  skeletal, 424
  tennis-related injuries, 611–612
  See also Musculoskeletal assessment; Musculoskeletal disorders/injuries; *specific muscle or region*
Muscle cramps, 95
  pathophysiology, 101–102
  sodium depletion, 133
Musculoskeletal assessment
  androgen effects, 142
  arthrographic, 313–314, 317
  chest pain, 229–230
  computed tomography, 312–313
  female athlete, 172–173
  imaging of injury, 305. *See also specific imaging modality*
  magnetic resonance imaging, 309–310
  preparticipation physical examination, 15–18
  radiography, 305–308
  radionuclide bone scan, 310–312
  ultrasonography, 314
Musculoskeletal disorder/injury
  among wheelchair athletes, 191–194
  boxing-related injury, 548
  cardiovascular system, 242
  cerebral palsy athletes, 196–197
  diagnostic imaging, 305
  diving-related, 556–557
  in Down's syndrome athletes, 195–196
  fencing-related, 564–565
  field hockey risk, 566–567
  in figure skating, 598–599
  football risk, 568–570
  headache etiology, 294
  horseback riding risk, 562–563
  in in-line skating, 598
  in indoor soccer, 602
  lacrosse patterns, 578–579
  limiting conditions, 29–31
  in martial arts, 580–582
  in outdoor soccer, 604–605
  rugby patterns, 595–596
  in speed skating, 597–598
  surfing-related, 607
  in waterskiing, 618–619
  in weight lifting/body building, 588
  sidelines management, 50–51
Musculoskeletal injury
  See also Fractures; Musculoskeletal assessment; Soft tissue injury; *specific anatomical site*
Myocardial contusion, 514
Myocardial infarction
  cocaine-related, 151
  sidelines management, 52–53
Myocarditis, 237
Myositis ossificans traumatica, 334, 428
Myotatic reflex, 84–85
Myxedema, 222–223

N

Narcosis, nitrogen, 117
Narcotics, prohibited, 652–653
National Collegiate Athletic Association
  drug testing policy, 156–160
  prohibited drugs, 651–654
  spine injury prevention rules, 280
National Operating Committee on Standards for Athletic Equipment, 121
Nausea, 267
NCAA. *See* National Collegiate Athletic Association
Neck injury
  cycling-related, 552
  football-related, 568
  lacrosse-related, 578
  laryngeal fracture, 46, 496
  martial arts risk, 581
  soccer-related, 605
  vessel injury, 496
  wrestling-related, 620
Neck range of motion, *24*
Necrosis, 324
Nerve entrapments, 193–194
  ankle, 473
  foot, 485–486
  peroneal, 465
  plantar, 481
Neural injury
  baseball-related, 541
  boxing-related, 67
  cycling-related, 552
  elbow, 375–377
  in endurance events, 558, 560–561
  foot, 485–486

in football, 569
headache etiology, 294
hip, 423
limiting conditions, 25–26
peripheral, 287–292
preparticipation physical examination, 18
rehabilitative muscle strengthening, 533–534
risks for wheelchair athletes, 193–194
in wrestling, 620
Neurapraxia, 288
Nicotine, 145
effects on performance, 153
physiology, 152–153
See also Tobacco
Nipple rash, 511, 606
Nobel test, 686
Nonsteroidal antiinflammatory drugs, 269
Nose
boxing-related injuries, 547
epistaxis, 495
fractures, 494–495
headache etiology, 294
preparticpation physical examination, 14

O
Ober test, 686
Odontoid agenesis, 30
Odontoid hypoplasia, 30
Older persons, 189
arthritis, 188
benefits of exercise, 184
chronic lung disease, 188
coronary artery disease, 187–188
cost of access to physical activities, 186
exercise goals, 184–186, 187
exercise-related sudden death, 231
hazards of exercise, 184
master's athletes, 189
medication use, 187
safety of exercise, 186
Olecranon
bursitis, 370
fracture, 368
osteochondrosis, 379
Oligomenorrhea, 177–180
Onychomycosis, 261
Osteitis pubis, 415
Osteoarthritis, 188, 560
Osteochondral contusion, 338
Osteochondral fractures, 446–447, 477
Osteochondritis dissecans, 170, 310, *312*, 338
ankle, 474
capitellum, 542
elbow, 378–379
shoulder, 444–446
Osteoporosis
definition, 178
female athlete triad, 175–177
menstrual dysfunction and, 177–180
Otitis externa, 208–209
Overload injuries, 325
Overuse injuries
among young athletes, 168–170
assessment, 36
cycling-related, 551
dance-related, 554–555
definition, 325
elbow, 370–371
iliotibial band syndrome, 451–452
nature of, 168
preventive stretching, 87

P
Pads, protective, 121
Pancreas, trauma, 521
Panner's disease, 738
Patellofemoral disorders, 173, *174*
anatomic considerations, 454
arthroscopy, 457–458
cerebral palsy athletes, 196
dance-related, 554
definitions, 454
diving-related, 557
injury patterns in endurance events, 559
pain evaluation, 455
prognosis, 459
radiography, 456
treatment, 456–457
types of, 454–455
Patent foramen ovale, diving and, 118
Pectoralis major injury, 349–350
Pediculosis, 264
Pelvic inflammatory disease, 202–203
Pelvis/groin
anatomy, 412
assessment, 412–413
bursitis, 416
contusion injuries, 416
diagnostic imaging, 307
fractures, 414–415, 560
hamstring syndrome, 416
hernia, 416
inflammatory conditions, 202–203, 415
injury patterns in endurance events, 560
muscle tendon injuries, 415–416
risk of injury, 412
sidelines assessment/intervention, 48
treatment for injury, 413–414
tumors, 416–417
See also Groin and thigh
Penile injury, 524
Peptic ulcer, 270
Periodization of training, 82–83
Peripheral nerve injury, 287–292
Pernio, 261

Peroneal nerve entrapment, 465
Peroneal tendon problems, 470–472
Pes anserinus syndrome, 449–450
Phalangeal fractures, 394–395
Phalangeal joint injuries, 395–396
Pharmacotherapy
  asthma management, 246–248
  asthma prevention, 248
  chronic obstructive pulmonary disease, 251–252
  diving and, 118
  emergency treatment of spine injury, 281
  epilepsy management, 299
  exercise-related headaches, 295–297
  gastroesophageal reflux, 268
  hypertension management, 233
  older athletes, 187
  in rehabilitation, 531
  soft tissue injury, 339
  standard medical kit, 656–658
Pharyngitis, 210
Physeal/epiphyseal injuries, 168, *169*
  hip anatomy and assessment, 418
  hip injuries, 419–420
Physical examination, preparticipation
  abdomen, 14–15
  ankle, *28*
  athletes with disabilities, 190
  back flexion, *20*
  body symmetry, *25*
  cardiovascular system, 14
  clearance, 18
  concerns of female athletes, 183
  disordered eating evaluation, 181
  Down's syndrome athletes, 195
  elbow range of motion, *22*
  evaluation form, *12–13*
  genitalia, 15
  goals, 20
  hand and finger range of motion, *21*
  head, eyes, ears, nose and throat, 14
  height and weight, 14
  history-taking, 11–14
  implementation, 10
  knee, *27*
  legal considerations, 20
  lifestyle factors, 18–20
  lower extremities, *18–19*, 173–175
  musculoskeletal system, 15–18
  neck range of motion, *24*
  neurological, 18
  pulmonary system, 14
  rotator cuff function, *26*
  setting, 11
  shoulder range of motion, *23*
  skin, 15
  strength training program, 166
Physician responsibilities, 6–7, 8–9
  athlete with epilepsy, 301–302
  during competition, 5–6
  generally, 4
  injury assessment, 33, 34
  postcompetition, 6
  precompetition, 5
Piriformis syndrome, 422–423
Plantar fasciitis, 558
  taping/bandaging, 638–641
Plantar nerve entrapment, 481
Pneumatic resistance exercise, 79
Pneumonia, 253, 254
Pneumothorax, 249–250, 516–517
  sidelines assessment/intervention, 46
Poison ivy, 28
Pole vault, 614
Pollicis brevis, abductor/extensor, 389
Pollicis longus, extensor, 390
Polycythemia, 145
Popliteus tendinitis, 450–451
Postcompetition, 6
Postinjury period, 5–6
  See also Assessment of injury
Postseason, 5
Potassium, 133
Power lifting, 586–588
Precompetition, 5
Preparation for emergencies
  Alpine skiing events, 600
  cardiac arrest, 46
  clinical protocols, 38
  communication, 38, 65
  documentation, 65
  educational efforts, 58
  environmental conditions, 58–59
  equipment, 37, 60
  eye care, 499
  heat injury, 105
  identifying hazardous conditions, 57–59
  impaired competitor policy, 58
  mass participation events, 54
  medical bag, 655–658
  mountain climbers, 584
  personnel, 37–38, 60
  physician training, 38
  portable emergency kit, 38–43
  protocols, 55–57
  risk assessment, 54–55
  risk of severe injury, 37
  at rodeos, 589–590
  tertiary care, 38
  transportation, 38, 57
Preseason practice
  body fat loss in, 135
  physical examination, 10
  See also Aerobic conditioning
Prevention
  abdomen injury, 520
  Achilles tendon rupture, 463
  acute mountain sickness, 110
  anterior shoulder instability, 353
  cardiac concussion, 515
  chlamydial infection, 204

competitor education, 58
dental injury, 504
environmental considerations, 57–59
eye injury, 497
with female athletes, 183
football injuries, 568
fractures, 317, 320
golf injury, 571
gymnastics injuries, 574
heat illness, 102–105
heat injury, 52, 102–105
hepatitis, 208
herpes simplex II, 205
high-altitude pulmonary edema, 111–112
HIV, 206–207
Hoffa's disease, 448
hypothermia, 108–109
impaired competitor policy, 58
of injury among young athletes, 170
inner ear injury, 494
iron-deficiency anemia, 257
knee ligament injury, 432, 433, 435, 437, 439
menstrual dysfunction, 179–180
middle-ear barotrauma, 494
mononucleosis, 202
muscle cramps, 102
muscle injury, 426
otitis externa, 209
pelvic/groin injury, 413
pes anserinus syndrome, 450
recurrent epistaxis, 495
respiratory infection, 252
of rodeo injuries, 591
soccer-related injuries, 605
spine injury, 280
stretching, 87
sudden death, 231
surfing-related injuries, 608
syphilis, 205
tennis leg, 464
See also Protective equipment
Pronator syndrome, 376–377
Proprioceptive neuromuscular facilitation, 85–86
Prostheses/orthoses, 198
Protective equipment, 124
for eyes, 499
function, 121
hand/wrist splints, 386
importance of fit, 121
regulation, 121
in rugby, 596
for single-organ athletes, 31–32
technical development, 121
types of, 121
See also specific sport
Protein
requirements, 130
strength training, 137
Protocols, emergency intervention, 38, 55–57
Pseudoephedrine, 145
Pseudonephritis, 526
Psoas tendon syndrome, 422
Psoriasis, 265
Psychological functioning
androgen effects, 142
headache etiology, 295
marijuana effects, 154
in rehabilitation, 530
Pulmonary edema, high-altitude, 111–112
Pulmonary function test, 245
Pulmonary system
airway injury, 516
contraindications to diving, 118
contusions, 516
pneumothorax, 516–517
preparticipation physical examination, 14
sidelines assessment/intervention, 45–46
thoracic injury, 516–517
wheelchair athletes, 191
See also specific disorders of
Purpura, 260

Q
Quadriceps
contusion, 428
strain, 426

R
Racketball, 612
Radial collateral ligament, 397
Radionuclide bone scan, 310–312
Radioulnar dislocations, 312
Radius fracture, distal, 382–383
Rafting, 592–594
Range of motion
elbow, *22*
flexibility conditioning program, 85–86
flexibility defined, 84
hand and finger, *21*
neck, *24*
neurophysiologic basis, 84
rehabilitation, 535, 536
return-to-play considerations, 29
shoulder, *23*
stretch reflex, 84–85
therapeutic stretching, 86–88
Rating of perceived exertion, 74
Raynaud's phenomenon, 109
Rehabilitation
acute macrotrauma meniscal injury, 659–661
acute phase, 535
for chronic microtrauma tendonosis, 661–663

Rehabilitation (*cont'd.*)
cryotherapy, 532
dance-related injuries, 554
electrical stimulation, 532
establishment of diagnosis, 529
eye injury, 499
flexibility exercises, 532–533
functional phase, 536–537
goals, 529
herniated disc, 406
initial injury management, 531
maintenance of general fitness, 530
management for proper healing, 530
minimization of local effects, 529–530
muscle strengthening, 533–534
pharmacotherapy, 531
postcompetition, 6
recovery phase, 535–536
rest, 531
return to play, 531
for rotator cuff tendinitis, 663–665
spondylilisthesis, 409
spondylosis, 411
stretching, 6
surgery, 531–532
therapeutic program, 534, 537
trunk stabilization program, 665–668
ultrasound therapy, 532
Relaxants, 146
Resistance training
objectives, 77
for older athletes, 186
periodization, 82–83
protein intake, 130
types of, 77–79. *See also specific type*
workout design, 79–81
for young athletes, 166, 167
Respiratory system
infections, 252–254
limiting conditions, 26–27
oxygenation-enhancing agents, 145–146
sidelines assessment/intervention, 45–46
upper respiratory infection, 210–211
Retina
detachment, 49
hemorrhage, 49
Return-to-play
after abdomen injury, 521–522
after Achilles tendon injury, 464
after acute cervical sprain, 282
after ankle sprain, 469
after anterior cruciate ligament injury, 435
after axial load teardrop fracture, 284
after axillary nerve injury, 291
after chlamydial infection, 204
after clavicle fracture, 362
after costochondral fracture, 513
after deltoid disruption, 359
after effort thrombosis, 359
after elbow dislocation, 369
after elbow fracture, 369
after elbow surgery for instability, 373
after elbow tendon injury, 374
after epicondylitis of elbow, 371
after eye injury, 499
after fabella syndrome, 452
after gonorrhea infection, 203
after head injury, 278–279
after hepatitis infection, 208
after herpes simplex II infection, 206
after infectious disorder, 211–212
after lateral collateral knee ligament injury, 434
after medial collateral knee ligament injury, 432
after medial epicondylar osteochondrosis, 378
after meniscal cysts, 444
after meniscal injury, 442, 661
after microtrauma tendonosis, 663
after mononucleosis infection, 202
after muscle injury, 425–426
after myocardial contusion, 514
after olecranon bursitis, 370
after olecranon osteochondrosis, 379
after osteochondral fractures, 447
after osteochondritis dissecans of knee, 446
after osteolysis of distal clavicle, 365
after otitis externa, 209
after Panner's disease, 379
after patellofemoral problems, 459
after pectoralis major injury, 350
after pelvic/groin injury, 413–414
after peripheral nerve injury, 289–290
after peroneal nerve entrapment, 465
after pneumothorax, 517
after popliteus tendinitis, 451
after posterior cruciate ligament injury, 437–438
after proximal biceps injury, 348, 349
after pulmonary contusion, 516
after rehabilitation, 531
after rib fracture, 512
after rotator cuff tendinitis, 663
after scapular fracture, 513
after semimembranosus tendinitis, 449
after shoulder instability, 354, 356
after shoulder stress fracture, 360
after sickle cell trait diagnosis, 259
after sinusitis, 210
after snapping scapula treatment, 358
after spine fusion, 286
after spine injury, 284–286
after sternoclavicular separation, 366–367
after sternum fracture, 513
after strep pharyngitis, 210
after syphilis infection, 205
after tarsal fractures, 477
after tennis leg, 464
after tibial collateral bursitis, 450

after tibiofibular joint instability, 453
after tooth avulsion, 504
after tooth extrusion, 503
after tooth fracture, 500, 501, 502
after tooth intrusion, 503
after tooth luxation, 502
after ulnar collateral ligament injury, 372
after ulnar neuropathy, 375–376
after valgus extension overload, 377
diabetes management, 219, 222
with hand/wrist splints, 386
with HIV infection, 207
with Hoffa's disease, 448
injury assessment, 34, 35
musculoskeletal assessment, 29–31
sidelines decision making, 44
with spear tackler's spine, 284
with thyroid disorders, 224
with transient quadriplegia, 283
Rhabdomyolysis, exertional, 95
Rib fractures, 511–512
Ringworm, 262
Rodeo, 589–591
Rotator cuff function
anatomy, 342
baseball-related injuries, 541
contusions, 346–347
ice hockey injury, 576
impingement syndrome, 343–346, 541
preparticipation physical examination, *26*
risks for wheelchair athletes, 193
tendinitis rehabilitation, 663–665
ultrasonographic evaluation, 314
Roux's sign, 414
Rugby, 595–596
Running
aid/fluid stations, 59, 60
course considerations, 59
endurance events, 558–561
gastrointestinal problems, 267, 268–270
injury patterns, 613
medial knee pain, 449–450
predicted incidence of injury, 54
sprinters, 613
thermal injury risk, 57–58

S
Sacroiliitis, 415
Salter-Harris classification of fractures, 168
Scabies, 27, 264
Scaphoid fracture, 383–384
Scapular fracture, 513
Scrotum trauma, 521, 525
Seizure disorder, 25
diving and, 118
See also Epilepsy
Semimembranosus tendinitis, 449
Sexually transmitted diseases, 202–208
Shepherd's fracture, 474
Shin splints, 462
Shot-put, 613
Shoulder
dislocations, 50–51
range of motion assessment, *23*
Shoulder injury
anatomy, 342
anterior instability, 351–354
baseball-related, 541
biceps tendon, 347–348
boxing-related, 548
coracoid impingement, 346
cricket-related, 549–550
cuff contusion, 346–347
cycling-related, 552
deltoid disruption, 359
diagnostic imaging, 305–306, *306*, 309, 313–314
diving-related, 556–557
effort thrombosis, 358–359
football-related, 569
golf-related, 572
gymnastics-related, 574
ice hockey-related, 575–576
impingement syndrome, 343–346
injection technique, 626–628
instability, generally, 351
lacrosse-related, 578
multidirectional instability, 356–357
muscle tendon, 342
pectoralis major, 349–350
physical examination, 672–677
posterior instability, 354–356
proximal biceps, 348–349
in rafting-type activities, 593
snapping scapula, 357–358
stress fracture, 359–360
subscapularis rupture, 347
swimming-related, 609
tennis-related, 611
Velpeau bandage, 644–646
volleyball-related, 615
Shuck test, 669
Sickle cell trait, 258–259
as limiting condition, 32
Sidelines physician
abdomen injury management, 48
airway management, 45–46
cardiac arrest intervention, 46
dental injury management, 49–50
eye injury management, 48–49
head injury management, 46–48
heat injury management, 51–52
medical equipment, 44
myocardial infarction management, 52–53
orthopedic injury management, 50–51
pelvis injury management, 48
return-to-play decisions, 44
sidelines management, 48
spine injury management, 48

Single-organ athletes, 31–32
Sinusitis, 209–210
Skating, figure, 598–599
Skating, in-line
  injury patterns, 598
  protective equipment, 124
Skating, speed, 597–598
Skiing
  injury patterns, 600–601
  predicted incidence of injury, 54
  water, 618–619
Skin
  chest contusions, 509–511
  injury patterns in endurance events, 560
  injury risks for wheelchair athletes, 192
  mountain climbing injuries, 584–585
  preparticipation physical examination, 15
  See also Dermatological conditions
SLAP lesion, 347–348
Smokeless tobacco, 151–153
Snapping-hip syndrome, 422
Snapping scapula, 357–358
Snowboarding, 601
Snuff, 151–153
Soccer
  ball-to-head injury, 605
  indoor, 602–603
  injury patterns, 604–605
  protective equipment, 123
Sodium, 133
Soft tissue injury
  aging and, 324, 340
  assessment, 338–339
  chest, 509–511
  chronic microtraumatic, 329–330
  degeneration, 324
  delayed onset muscle soreness, 334, 425
  hand/wrist, 388–392
  healing, 324, 339–340
  hip, 421–423
  horseback riding-associated, 563
  inflammation, 323–324
  ligament, 337
  load and use concepts, 325
  maxillofacial repair, 489–490
  mechanisms, 326–327
  muscle, 332–334
  myositis ossificans traumatica, 334, 428
  necrosis, 324
  pathophysiology, 327–330
  principle of transition, 327
  profile, 330–331
  risks for wheelchair athletes, 192–193
  sources of pain, 331–332
  spectrum, 322–324
  synovial, 338
  tendon, 334–337
Spear tackling, 280, 283–284, 568
Speed's test, 676
Spine, congenital anomalies of
  fusion, 30, 31, 286
  limits to sports participation, 30–31
Spine injuries
  limits to sports participation, 30, 31
Spine injury
  acute cervical sprain, 281–282
  axial load teardrop fracture, 284
  in baseball, 542
  bowstring test, 691
  degenerative disc disease, 560
  diagnostic imaging, 308, 309
  diving-related, 556
  emergency management, 280–281
  epidemiology, 280
  facet joint syndrome, 406–407
  in football, 569
  in gymnastics, 574
  herniated disc, 289, 403–406
  in horseback riding, 563
  in ice hockey, 575
  intervertebral disc tear, 402–403
  low back strain, 402
  lumbosacral assessment, 413
  peripheral nerve injury, 289–290
  prevention, 280
  return-to-play guidelines, 284–286
  spear tackling, 280, 283–284
  spondylilisthesis, 407–409
  spondylosis, 409–411
  surfing-related, 607
  transient quadriplegia, 282–283
  transportation of patient, 281
  trunk stabilization program for
    rehabilitation, 665–668
  in wrestling, 621
Spleen
  ice hockey injury, 577
  limiting conditions, 28–29
  rupture, 520, 521
Splenomegaly, 28–29
Splints
  hand/wrist, 386
  protective, 121
Spondylolisthesis, 407–409
Spondylolysis, 311–312, 313
Spondylosis, 409–411
Sports injury, 322. *See also* Soft tissue injury
Sports medicine
  ethical decision-making, 7–8
  medical team, 4–5
  physician responsibilities, 5–7, 8–9
  unique features, 3–4
Sprinting, 613
Squash, 612
Staph infection, 262–263
Steeplechase, 613
Sternoclavicular injury
  ice hockey risk, 576
  separation, 366–367